SPINAL CORD INJURIES
COMPREHENSIVE MANAGEMENT
AND RESEARCH

Spinal Cord Injuries

COMPREHENSIVE MANAGEMENT
AND RESEARCH

BY

PROFESSOR SIR LUDWIG GUTTMANN

CBE, FRS, MD, FRCP, FRCS, HonD Sc(Liverpool),
HonD Chir(Durham), HonLLD(Dublin), HonFRCP(C)
Founder and Former Director of the National Spinal
Injuries Centre, Stoke Mandeville Hospital, Aylesbury, Bucks
Director of the Stoke Mandeville Sports Stadium for
the Paralysed and other Disabled

SECOND EDITION

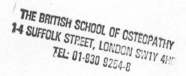
Blackwell Scientific Publications
OXFORD LONDON EDINBURGH
MELBOURNE

© 1973, 1976 Blackwell Scientific Publications
Osney Mead, Oxford
8 John Street, London WC1
9 Forrest Road Edinburgh
P.O. Box 9, North Balwyn, Victoria, Australia

British Library Cataloguing in Publication data
Guttmann, Sir Ludwig
Spinal cord injuries : comprehensive management
and research. – 2nd ed.
Bibl. – Index
ISBN 0–632–00079–1
1. Title
617′.1 KD 594. 3
Spinal cord – Wounds and injuries

First published 1973
Second edition 1976

Distributed in the U.S.A. by
J. B. Lippincott Company, Philadelphia,
and in Canada by
J. B. Lippincott Company of Canada Ltd.,
Toronto

Printed in Great Britain by
Adlard & Son Ltd
Dorking, Surrey
and bound by
Mansell (Bookbinders) Ltd.,
Witham, Essex

THIS BOOK IS DEDICATED TO

THE MEMORY OF

Dr George Riddoch (1888-1947)

Neurologist, The London Hospital and the
National Hospital for Nervous Diseases.
Pioneer Advocate of Specialized Units
for the Treatment of Sufferers from
Spinal Cord Lesions

'. . . and the breath came into them, and they lived, and stood upon their feet, an exceeding great army.'

Ezekiel 37, 10

'You are the living demonstration of the marvels of the virtue of energy. . . . You have given a great example, which We would like to emphasize, because it can give a lead to all: You have shown what an energetic soul can achieve, in spite of apparently insurmountable obstacles imposed by the body.'

H.H. Pope John XXIII on the
occasion of the 1960 International
Stoke Mandeville Games in Rome

CONTENTS

D. GUNSHOT INJURIES AND STAB WOUNDS

E. COMPLICATIONS

F. NEUROPHYSIOLOGICAL AND CLINICAL ASPECTS OF SPINAL CORD INJURIES

PREFACE TO SECOND EDITION

A second edition of this book has been called for, following its wide circulation in many countries, thanks to the generous reception given it by the medical, para-medical and legal professions. In view of the steadily increasing interest in the many medical and social problems of this multi-disciplinary subject of spinal paraplegia and tetra-plegia, the author decided to amplify the first edition by taking into account results of recent experimental and clinical research as well as new developments in the clinical management of spinal cord sufferers. This applies in particular to the chapters on spinal shock and animal and clinical experiments on ischaemia following compression and contusion. The mechanism and classification of spinal injuries are discussed in greater detail and it has been also necessary to re-write or expand the chapters on deep vein thrombosis, para-articular ossification, respiratory, bladder and renal complications, as well as settlement and legal aspects. The opportunity has also been taken to correct a few errors and enlarge references and index.

Dr Dennis Guttmann's help in amending the chapter on renal deficiency is very much appreciated.

PREFACE

In 1950, I wrote a monograph on my experience on 570 spinal paraplegics and tetra-plegics, of whom 458 were traumatic lesions, mainly war casualties, treated at the National Spinal Injuries Centre, Stoke Mandeville Hospital in Aylesbury, since its inception on 1 February 1944. This monograph, published in 1953 in Volume Surgery of the British Medical History of the Second World War, laid down the principles of a synthesis between all clinical procedures and measures of social and professional rehabili-tation in a subject which, throughout all ages, had been considered as one of the most depressing and neglected in medicine: Spinal Paraplegia.

The idea of giving spinal cord sufferers a comprehensive treatment and care from the start and throughout all stages is now more and more universally recognized, as against the customary approach of fragmentation of the initial and early treatment of these patients from their social rehabilitation, erroneously called 'Third Phase' of management. In this respect, the congregation of paraplegics and tetraplegics in Spinal Centres under the care of a specialized staff has proved beyond all doubt to be the best basis for such comprehensive management of these most severely disabled victims of accidents and disease, and consequently the idea of setting up of Spinal Injuries Centres, originated during World War II in Great Britain, is now spreading all over the world.

New and significant disclosures have been made in our research throughout the many years since that monograph was published, which were applied in the practical management of the spinal man, and the consequence was a steady stream of publications by myself and my co-workers on numerous aspects of that complex multidisciplinary speciality of medicine, surgery and social science.

One can point to progress in many directions, but some of the more outstanding may be mentioned here: the participation of the isolated cord through co-ordinated reflexes in the restoration and maintenance of the upright position of the paralysed, reorientation of postural and vasomotor control by special methods, prevention and treatment of pressure sores and infection of the urinary tract in the immediate and later stages, restoration of the respiratory function in tetraplegics and a new approach to the sexual problems. Our findings of the highly significant role played by autonomic mechanisms, especially the cardio-vascular system, in the function of the organism below and above the transection of the spinal cord have opened new vistas into future research. Ways have been revealed in which the dysfunction of internal organs in the paralysed part of the body excite abnormal discharge of the various components of the autonomic system and also how the autonomic hyperreflexia can be controlled and avoided. In the psychological readjustment of the paralysed the introduction of sport and vocational training of the paralysed have proved invaluable for their social re-integration into community life.

This book is the product of about 30 years' personal experience of more than 4,000 paraplegics and tetraplegics treated at Stoke Mandeville. In this work, my previous research on neurophysiological and clinical problems since 1923 in Breslau and from 1939–43 in Oxford has helped me immensely towards the understanding of the many aspects of the physiology and pathology in spinal man.

It was not the purpose of this book to describe in detail all the various surgical and other procedures employed as these can easily be obtained from existing specialized text books, but rather to evaluate the most debatable procedures carried out on traumatic paraplegics and tetraplegics. Therefore, only certain specific procedures introduced at Stoke Mandeville have been described in detail.

In planning this book, special attention had to be paid to the details of the multifarious and diverse physical and psychological effects which spinal injuries exert on the organism. Therefore, all these aspects had to be organized and moulded into an homogeneous and meaningful pattern.

While this book gives an account of my own concept of comprehensive management of paraplegics and tetraplegics, the experiences and publications of other workers in this field are widely mentioned and discussed in relation to our own experiences.

I recognize that no book on paraplegia can be complete or perfect, but I trust that this book will be of interest and guidance to everyone concerned with the treatment and social readjustment of spinal paraplegics and tetraplegics.

I have been most fortunate in having a team of enthusiastic, loyal and hard working medical and para-medical co-workers and many volunteers with me throughout the years. Various research projects have been carried out co-operatively with some of my medical colleagues, mentioned individually in the text of this book, and my gratitude to them is deeply felt. I am equally grateful to those colleagues of this and other hospitals as well as to members of the Department of Physiology in Oxford, who co-operated in carrying out special techniques in which they were experts.

The development of the Stoke Mandeville Spinal Centre to its national status would not have been possible without the co-operation of the various administrative authorities concerned and I would like to place my sincere appreciation to them on record.

To Else, my wife, I am deeply grateful for her enduring patience, encouragement and active help in my work.

I had the good fortune to have Joan Scruton as lay administrator of the National Spinal Injuries Centre at my side from the beginning of my work, who, with her calm efficiency and loyalty, shared a great deal of the administrative burden with me. She and Kate Lambrechts have been of indispensable help in preparing the manuscript in its various stages, and I owe much to their devotion and accurate work.

I am also very appreciative of the excellent work of our photographers, Arthur Riddle and, in particular, Derek Standen, who have been responsible for most of the illustrations in this book.

Last, but by no means least, my warmest thanks are due to the publishers of this book, Blackwell Scientific Publications, for their understanding and great trouble they have taken to comply with my wishes.

Ludwig Guttmann

A · Introduction

CHAPTER 1
HISTORICAL BACKGROUND

Of the many forms of disability which can beset mankind, a severe injury or disease of the spinal cord undoubtedly constitutes one of the most devastating calamities in human life. This is readily understood if one realizes the paramount physiological importance of the spinal cord not only as the main transmitter of all impulses and messages from the brain to all parts of the body and vice versa but also as a nerve centre in its own right, controlling vital functions such as voluntary movements, posture, bladder, bowel, and sexual functions, as well as respiration, heat regulation, and blood circulation. Therefore, a severance or severe injury of the spinal cord, whether caused by trauma or disease, always results in a disablement of great magnitude from the site of the lesion downwards.

It is obvious that such an affliction has always aroused medical interest, and references to spinal cord injuries have already been found in records from very early periods of civilization. The Edwin Smith Surgical Papyrus, written about 5,000 years ago by an Egyptian physician (translated by the famous Egyptologist, Dr Breasted), contains a clear description of the cardinal symptoms of a complete lesion of the cervical cord, following dislocation or fracture of the spine: paralysis of all four extremities, complete sensory loss, loss of bladder control, priapism, and involuntary seminal ejaculations. Reference is even made to conjunctival congestion—today recognized as the result of vasodilatation due to paralysis of the vasomotor control in these high lesions. In discussing the prognosis and therapy of such patients (cases 31 and 33 of the Papyrus), the comment of the unknown author is as brief as it is significant: 'an ailment not to be treated'. It is not known whether this ancient author has generalized his defeatist attitude to spinal cord lesions at any level, but it cannot be denied that the sentiments thus expressed have prevailed throughout thousands of years amongst most members of the medical profession in all countries, towards sufferers from severe lesions of the spinal cord.

Medical history is very sketchy between the Egyptian and Greek periods. Homer made reference in the tenth chapter of the *Odyssey* to Elpenor, the youngest of Odysseus's companions, who, having got drunk and longing for fresh air, slept on the roof of Circe's house. Roused in the morning by the bustle of his companions' departure, he leapt up suddenly and, forgetting the right way down, toppled headlong from the roof, breaking his neck, 'and his soul went down to Hades'.

Hippocrates, about 400 BC, in the chapter περὶ τῶν ἐντοσ παθῶν describing chronic paraplegia, mentions constipation and dysuria, as well as oedema of the lower limbs and bedsores, as complications of paraplegia. It is interesting to note that he already advocates a large intake of fluid and a special diet for these patients, consisting of four to nine pints of milk, preferably from an ass, combined with honey, and he also recommends a special mild white wine from Mendes in Egypt. Hippocrates also introduced various methods of reduction of deformities of the spine by traction, and his famous extension bench—better known, through the work of Aulus Cornelius Celsus, as scamnum—was employed in various modifications by physicians throughout the centuries to reduce fractures as well as other deformities of the spine by forceful and brisk procedures. They

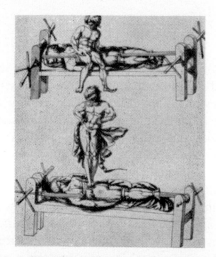

FIG. 1. Vidus Vidius manuscript, Bibliotheque Nationale, Paris.

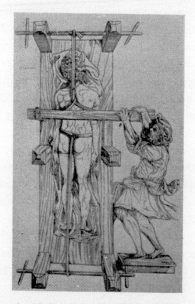

FIG. 2. De Machinamentis (Oribasius). In: Vidus Vidius: Chirurgia, è Graeco in Latinum connersa, Paris 1544.

were described by Oribasius (324–400) and Paulus of Aegina (625–690), and Figs. 1 and 2 are illustrations of the technique employed, as published in *Chirurgia, è Graeco in Latinum connersa* (Paris 1544), by Vidus Vidius. The victim, lying on a bench in prone position, was pulled extended from the shoulder upwards and distally from the hips, while the medical attendant either stood or sat on the gibbus, or a cross-bar was pressed onto the gibbus until it disappeared. Avicenna (980–1037), while following Paulus of Aegina's treatment for dislocation of the thoraco-lumbar spine, reduced the cervical spine by extension in supine position followed by fixation of the neck through splints. It was Roland of Parma, professor at Salerno, who, in his *Chirurgia* (1210), discarded the use of Hippocrates' bench and used manual extension only. For dislocation of the thoraco-

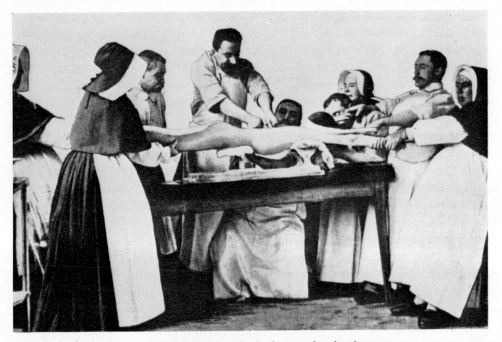

FIG. 3. Calot's method of manual reduction

lumbar spine, the patient was placed in supine position and the medical attendant pulled on his legs, while an assistant held the upper part of the body. For the reduction of the cervical spine, the patient was placed in sitting position, the physician braced his feet on the patient's shoulders and pulled his head briskly with a folded cloth passed underneath his chin. However, the famous French surgeon, Ambroise Paré, in his *Dix-Livres de Chirurgie* (1564), reverted to Hippocrates' extension method in prone position but used it with greater caution by reducing the fracture of dislocation by manual pressure and immobilizing the vertebral column after reduction by splints or specially designed lead plates. The patient was then turned on his back and kept in that position for a long time. This extension technique in prone position with manual reduction of the vertebral fracture or dislocation was still used in the nineteenth century by Jean Francis Calot, manipulating the spinal deformity with his fists (Fig. 3). I myself witnessed this method even in 1917, when, before taking up medicine, I worked as an orderly in the Accident Hospital for Coalminers (Knappschaftslazarett) in my home town of Königshütte in Upper Silesia, Germany, now Chorzow, Poland. It was executed by the surgeon in charge, Dr Hartmann, in a case of fracture-dislocation of the thoraco-lumbar junction of the spine. The only difference between his and Paré-Calot's technique was that the patient was held in the air in supine position by two assistants extending the patient under the armpits and two extending the pelvis and legs, while the surgeon reduced the dislocation by forceful manipulation with his fists from below. After this procedure, the patient was put in a plaster cast. He died four weeks later from sepsis and cachexy as a result of urinary infection and multiple pressure sores.

Surgical intervention in spinal injuries and operations on the spinal cord have been discussed and described long before the modern principles of asepsis were discovered. Amongst authors of ancient times, Galen, 131, may be mentioned, who reported about experiments on the effect of longitudinal and transverse incisions of the spinal cord. He found that, whilst a longitudinal incision in the cord had no demonstrable effect on function, transverse incision resulted in paralysis of the body below the level of the lesion. Paulus of Aegina, who modified Hippocrates' method of traction for vertebral dislocations by external fixation of the reduced spine by a thin sheet of wood fixed along the spine extending above and below the site of injury, can also be considered as the originator of decompressive laminectomy and he also advocated removal of a fractured spinous process causing pain. Antrine Louis (1762) successfully removed a bullet lodged in the spine.

An important contribution at the end of the eighteenth century to the subject of traumatic paraplegia, as a result of a fracture-dislocation of the 12th thoracic vertebra, is the treatise of the German surgeon, J.Sömmering (1793): *Bemerkungen über Verrenkung und Bruch des Rückgraths*. In 1814, Henry Cline, a London surgeon, carried out a laminectomy, but the patient died nine days later. It was in this first quarter of the nineteenth century that arguments on indication and value of this operation were widely discussed amongst leading members of the medical profession, and the management of spinal injuries became a topic of real interest in England and other countries.

Throughout the nineteenth century, the general tendency in the treatment of spinal cord injuries was to be conservative, and leading neurologists and surgeons threw the weight of their authority against surgical treatment. There were a few prominent supporters of operative treatment, such as Astley Cooper (1827), but, on the whole, Charles Bell's view (1824)—'laying a patient upon his belly and by incisions laying bare the bones of the spine, breaking up these bones and exposing the spinal marrow itself, exceeds all belief'—was widely accepted. One of the famous personalities in British history of that time, Lord Nelson, was one of the victims of a spinal cord injury, as a result of a gunshot wound during the battle of Trafalgar, when the bullet, after penetrating the chest, lodged in the thoracic spine, producing a paraplegia below the breast. The final scene in Nelson's life was recorded by Beatty, the ship's surgeon, and has been described in detail in Oliver Warner's book *Trafalgar*, from which the following is quoted: 'Mr Beatty was called by Dr Scott to Nelson, who said—"Ah, Mr Beatty! I have sent for you to say what I forgot to tell you before, that all power of motion and feeling below my chest are gone: and you very well know I can live but a short time .... You know I am gone". The surgeon's reply was: "My Lord, unhappily for our Country, nothing can be done for you." ' Nelson died within a few hours. It is also of historical interest that, on 2 July 1881, the 20th President of the United States of America, James A.Garfield, became a victim of a spinal injury as a result of a gunshot injury resulting in an incomplete conus-cauda lesion, and died 79 days later. The Museum of the Armed Forces Institute of Pathology in Washington has preserved the specimen of President Garfield's shattered vertebrae. There is another vertebral specimen on show in the same Museum —namely, the upper cervical vertebrae of John Wilkes Booth, who made history as the murderer of President Abraham Lincoln and who received a bullet wound through the cervical cord. Recently (1972) Governor George Wallace of Alabama became a victim of a spinal cord injury, following a gunshot wound during his election campaign. He survived but is still chairbound.

The great developments in surgery in the Listerian period, Pasteur's work on bacteriology, the introduction of ether anaesthesia, and later the discovery of X-ray by Röentgen have, no doubt, modified the extreme conservative view, and the field of spinal cord surgery has steadily been extended. However, the prognostic outlook of sufferers from severe lesion of the spinal cord has remained extremely poor, and the mortality rate in both peace and war has been very high. The hopeless frame of mind, held even by experts, has been appropriately summarized by Wagner & Stolper (1898) on page 576 of their book: *Die Verletzungen der Wirbelsäule und des Rückenmarks* (the injuries of the spine and spinal cord), a book which up to the First World War was considered as a standard work on the subject of spinal injuries. Their views are expressed as follows: In complete lesions it is the physician's forlorn task, even while knowing that the patient is approaching an early death, to keep him alive for weeks and months on end, only to see him wretchedly fade away, despite all skill and efforts.

In the Balkan wars, the mortality rate after spinal cord injury was over 95 per cent, and recollections of casualties with spinal cord injuries from the First World War and the after-war period have also left depressing memories of hopelessness and helplessness. The literature of that time in every country, though containing many excellent publications on problems of pathology and physiology, reveals a profound defeatist attitude of the medical profession towards these unfortunate sufferers, when dealing with the problem of prognosis and rehabilitation.

Harvey Cushing, the world famous neuro-surgeon and Consultant in Neurosurgery to the American Army during the First World War, gave in 1927 a vivid description of the pitiful fate of battle casualties with spinal cord injuries, 80 per cent of whom died in the first two weeks. 'The conditions were such', he wrote 'owing to pressure of work, as to make it almost impossible to give these unfortunate men the care their conditions required. No water beds were available, and each case demands undivided attention of a nurse trained in the care of paraplegics. Only those cases survived in which the spinal lesion was a partial one.'

The mortality rate of traumatic paraplegics in the British Army was similar. The early mortality (death within the first few weeks or months) varied from 47 to 65 per cent (Vellacott & Webb-Joynson, 1919), and the overall mortality after three years was estimated at 80 per cent (Thompson-Walker, 1937). Most of those men who managed to survive dragged out their lives as useless and hopeless cripples, unemployable and unwanted. They were doomed to spend the rest of their lives as pensioners at home or in institutions, dependent on other people's assistance and, as a rule, with no incentive or encouragement to return to a useful life. On the contrary, the existing legislation and regulations regarding war pensions or workmen's compensation made it quite impossible for these 100 per cent disabled men to return to remunerative employment, for fear of losing their pensions and compensation. Indeed, until the Disabled Persons' Act (1944) was passed in this country, society still adhered to the ancient Greek conception, as recorded in Lysias' oration περὶ τοῦ ἀδυνάτου (about 400 BC), that 100 per cent disablement excluded a cripple from remunerative work.

In the inter-war period and even during the Second World War, the defeatist attitude of most members of the medical profession in this and other countries was still prevalent, and the general attitude of despondency is revealed in the report of the Medical Research Council of 1924: 'the paraplegic patient may live for a few years in a state of more or less ill-health'. Martin (1947) aptly summed up the unsatisfactory situation as follows: 'The record attained in World War I is not a very enviable one and it is quite apparent that the methods of treatment of traumatic paraplegia were not improved by the rich experience of that War.' Gowland (1934, 1941) gave the following account of the conditions of traumatic paraplegics from the First World War treated at the Star and Garter Home, founded after the First World War in Richmond, Surrey, for disabled ex-servicemen—'Two or three times a week, the patient is bathed: this means he must be lifted from his bed to his ward chair and wheeled into the bathroom, where his pyjamas and nightclothes are removed, and he is placed in a very warm bath and washed by an orderly.' In discussing the problem of painful, reflex spasms and contractures, he points out: 'The position is often terrible. I suppose there is more morphia, atropine and hyoscine used in this Home, which I look after, than in any other place of the same size in the country'. To quote further statements of this author: 'When the vertebral lesion had consolidated—say some eight to twelve months after injury—it is well to encourage the paraplegic to sit up and get about in a wheelchair or hand-propelled or motor tricycle.' Such views which reflect very well the conception held generally, in these years, that nothing or very little could be done for these unfortunate people, was hardly designed to encourage the paramedical professions—nurses, physiotherapists, occupational therapists and society at large, in particular the Ministry of Labour and employers—to help these men to return to a useful life and employment. These victims of war, road and industrial accidents did not establish a social problem as, in the vast majority of cases, their life expectancy was very short, as a rule 2–3 years to the utmost, as a result of sepsis from infection of bladder and kidneys on the one hand and pressure sores on the other —complications which were considered inevitable. Therefore, any attempt to restore such a person to his former social activities seemed to be out of the question and the view generally held was the sooner he died the better for all concerned. It is, therefore, not surprising that, in all discussions on rehabilitation during the years 1939–42, the subject of rehabilitation of victims of spinal paraplegia was hardly mentioned in spite of the fact that the modern principles of rehabilitation had been successfully applied for a number of years to other forms of disablement such as blind, amputees and other crippling diseases. In this connection the first 'Discussion on Rehabilitation of Injuries to the Central Nervous System' held in 1941 in the Royal Society of Medicine may be mentioned. Four speakers discussed brain injuries and one (myself) peripheral nerve injuries, while the subject of spinal cord injuries was not even mentioned.

A NEW APPROACH

A fundamental step forwards in a new approach to the problem of management of spinal cord sufferers was taken during the Second World War by the Peripheral Nerve Committee of the Medical Research Council, under the leadership of Dr George Riddoch, Neurological Consultant to the British Army and the Ministries of Health and Pensions, who decided to congregate spinal cord casualties in special Spinal Injuries Units within various E.M.S. and Ministry of Pensions Hospitals in Great Britain, for it was anticipated that the number of war casualties with spinal cord injuries would be considerably increased by air raid casualties amongst civilians. There were several reasons for this decision: first of all, it was generally agreed that conditions for a systematic study of the many aspects concerned with the treatment and rehabilitation of spinal paraplegics were infinitely more favourable in a spinal unit than when these cases lay scattered in general medical or surgical wards, from which, as a rule, they were transferred to chronic wards or homes for incurables. Even if they were admitted to neurological, neurosurgical, orthopaedic or urological units, the facilities available were limited to the study of specialized problems and short-term treatment only. Above all, these departments were so busy with their many other afflictions in their own specialities that, as a rule, it was quite impossible for both the medical and nursing staff to give spinal paraplegics let alone tetraplegics, that meticulous care and attention which these patients need day and night, especially during the acute stages.

During the course of the war, twelve spinal units were gradually set up in various parts of this country, where most of the 700 odd casualties with spinal cord lesions were collected (Winwick, Warrington; Barnsley Hall, Basingstoke; Warncliffe, Sheffield; Chapel Allerton, Leeds; Ronkswood, Worcester; Dunstan Hill, Newcastle; Rookwood, Cardiff; Llandrindod Wells; Stanmore, London; Leatherhead, Surrey; and Edinburgh).

However, in those days, it was not generally recognized by both the medical and administrative authorities that, in order to prevent these spinal units becoming merely an accumulation of doomed cripples, the provision of certain arrangements was indispensable.

1 Most important of all, supervision of such a unit by an experienced physician or surgeon, who was prepared to give up part of his own speciality in order to devote his full time to the work which demanded meticulous attention to detail, to plan and organize the many details of treatment and lastly but by no means least to correlate the sometimes conflicting interests of the visiting medical and surgical specialists concerned with the immediate and long term management of paraplegics and tetraplegics. The organization should be such that the paralysed patient is never in doubt which is the doctor who is looking after him.

2   Nursing and other paramedical staff such as physiotherapists and occupational therapists sufficient in number to cope with the many details involved in the work, in particular, avoidance of the usual practice of changing the nursing staff from one department to another at short intervals.

3   Adequate technical facilities such as workshops for the social rehabilitation of these long-term patients, in particular pre-vocational training.

4   Arrangements for domestic and industrial resettlement of paraplegics.

5   After-care by regular check-ups of patients discharged from hospital.

It is, therefore, not surprising that these early units did not prove satisfactory, indeed no great encouragement was given to those medical men who were charged with the task to run them. D.Allen (1964) recalled his appointment to the job as Medical Officer in charge of the Spinal Unit at the E.M.S. Hospital at Leatherhead as follows: 'In the spring of 1944, I was called to group headquarters for interview with the group officer, a surgeon of formidable character. "Allen", he said to me, "I am sorry to have to inflict this on you, but we have been ordered to open a spinal unit at Leatherhead Hospital, and I want you to take charge of it. Of course, as you know, they are hopeless cases—most of them die, but you must do your best for them." With these words of encouragement I returned home sadly.'

T.B.Dick (1949, 1969) has given an excellent account of the unsatisfactory conditions prevailing in the early years of the war, in one of the first spinal units to be set up, where some 40 cases were treated. Although a neurosurgical team was in charge of the spinal unit, he states—'no one member of that team devoted more than a part of his time to the care of spinal injury cases'. Dick, describing two examples of inadequate treatment which he has chosen at random, continues, 'It was not uncommon at this period on a ward round to find virtually every case of paraplegia with persistent pyrexia. There did not appear as yet to be any definite plan or end in view of the rehabilitation of even the more fit patients'. From my own observations which I made during visits to other spinal units at the request of the Ministry of Pensions, it can be stated that conditions were very similar in that period of war. It was little consolation that, at that time, the results in other countries such as Australia, Canada and U.S.A. were no better. Even as late as 1944, American authors (Everts & Woodhall) were still able to write: 'Certainly it cannot be said that any striking advance has been made in the late care of spinal cord injuries.'

CHAPTER 2

THE STOKE MANDEVILLE NATIONAL
SPINAL INJURIES CENTRE

INTRODUCTION OF A COMPREHENSIVE TREATMENT AND
REHABILITATION SERVICE

In 1943 I was given the task by the British Government authorities to set up a new Spinal
Unit at the Ministry of Pensions Hospital, Stoke Mandeville in Aylesbury, as one of the
medical preparations for the Second Front planned for the Spring Offensive in 1944,
when an increased number of spinal cord casualties was anticipated.

With the opening of this unit on 1 February 1944 with one patient and 26 beds, a
concept of comprehensive treatment and rehabilitation was introduced for spinal cord
sufferers. The basic principle of the new concept was the aim to provide for spinal
paraplegics as well as tetraplegics a comprehensive service from the start of their injury
or disease and throughout all stages involving *all* aspects of this multi-disciplinary subject
of medicine—to rescue these men and women from the human scrap-heap and to return
most of them, in spite of their profound disability, to the community as useful and
respected citizens. The chief object was not just to preserve the lives of paraplegics and
tetraplegics, but to give them a purpose in life. To achieve this object it was a fundamental task to establish a synthesis between all clinical procedures and all measures
to be taken for the social resettlement of these patients, which were not considered as
separate entities but, *a priori*, and throughout all stages to be planned and carried out
as one common operation.

Naturally, the practical application of this philosophy was no simple task, considering
the thousands of years' old prejudice towards spinal cord sufferers. Moreover, although
Stoke Mandeville Hospital, built on ground level without steps or stairs, and with a wide
open space around the hospital, appeared to be most suitable for a Spinal Injuries Centre,
the facilities available for a comprehensive management of these patients were hopelessly
inadequate, and the paramedical staff delegated to the unit quite unprepared and
untrained. My first nursing staff consisted of a young registered sister, commanded by the
Matron to take on the job as sister-in-charge of the ward, a female auxiliary nurse and
eight medical orderlies seconded from the Army. When I enquired of the first orderly
about his experience as a medical orderly in the Army, his answer was 'Shovelling coal,
Sir,'! The attitude of physiotherapists in those days towards spinal paraplegics was as
defeatist as that of most members of the nursing profession, and an illuminating account
has been published in 1949 by one of my former physiotherapist-pupils in *Cord*, the
journal of paraplegics founded in 1947 at Stoke Mandeville by Captain P.F.Stewart and
five other patients of the unit 'to promote the best interests of all those suffering from
spinal troubles and to employ the influence and machinery of the British Legion in all
Pension matters and such problems as Housing and Employment; to spread abroad

9

all information of particular interest to paraplegics; and to foster in civilian life that spirit of comradeship that has grown up in the services and in hospital'. It was this staff, joined soon by Miss Joan Scruton as Secretary and later Administrator of the Unit—the only volunteer at that time who wanted to work in a Spinal Unit—who were trained in the details of meticulous care and various aspects of treatment and who developed into an enthusiastic and devoted team, inspiring the patients to active and full co-operation. Naturally, the defeatist attitude of the many visitors had to be changed (see chapter on Psychological Aspects). Indeed, in the first two years of our work the question that was put to me with almost monotonous regularity by visitors from the medical and paramedical professions as well as administrators was 'Is it really worth while?'

Radical changes in the medical and psychological approach to the whole problem were introduced, as has always been done in other pioneer work in medicine, to overcome dogmas and prejudice. It was quite unorthodox in those days to reject the conventional methods of recumbency and immobilization of traumatic paraplegics in plaster casts and plaster beds as well as to abstain from hasty, indiscriminate operative procedures, such as laminectomy and open reduction, as initial treatment of the broken spine and to replace them by new methods aimed at the mobilization of the natural forces of repair and readjustment so inherent in the human organism. It was, at that time, a new approach for both medical and nursing staff to teach that bedsores resulting in osteomyelitis and sepsis or ascending infection of the upper urinary tract and renal deficiency were by no means inevitable consequences of spinal paraplegia, as commonly accepted, but that these complications, as well as others such as contractures and intractable spasticity could, by introducing new methods of management, not only be controlled but altogether prevented. The continuous drainage of the paralysed bladder by immediate suprapubic cystotomy, which in the Second World War was considered by most surgeons as the method of choice for the initial treatment of the paralysed bladder, was rejected from a point of principle as unphysiological. This method was replaced by the non-touch technique of intermittent catheterization carried out in the acute stages by the medical attendant himself and not, as was the custom, by nurses or orderlies. Above all, it was quite revolutionary to teach and impress on the authorities of medical and social services, in particular the Ministry of Labour and Housing Authorities, that the mere fact that a person was a paraplegic did not justify care in one of the institutions for incurables, but that in spite of permanent and severe physical handicap, rehabilitation to a useful life and employment was possible. With this object in view, regular work and sport were introduced from the beginning as essential parts of the clinical treatment of these patients which, in due course, proved so very successful for their physical, psychological and social rehabilitation.

Actually, the first industrial experiment to prove that paraplegics in their wheelchairs could work in a factory side by side and in competition with able-bodied workers was carried out with our first six rehabilitated paraplegic ex-servicemen at the end of 1944. Naturally, this achievement had a remarkable, psychological effect on the rest of the patients and gave them encouragement and hope for their future. It was the team-spirit on the part of my initial staff and the early patients which enabled us to prove within a short period of $1\frac{1}{2}$ years that the new philosophy in the approach to the management of these patients could be put into practice (Guttmann 1945).

POST WAR DEVELOPMENT OF THE UNIT INTO A NATIONAL CENTRE

Already at the end of the War the number of beds in the Unit was gradually increased to 100 as several of the original units in this country were closed and their patients transferred to Stoke Mandeville. Moreover, after the War the number of civilian paraplegic men, women and children steadily increased. By 1951, when Stoke Mandeville Hospital was taken over by the National Health Service, the Unit had a complement of 160 beds which in due course was increased to 195 beds. The Unit was then designated as a National Spinal Injuries Centre admitting patients from all parts of the United Kingdom and many other countries, the latter according to Ministry of Health's regulations as private patients.

With the growth of the Centre, the facilities of auxiliary services were also gradually increased. This applied to physiotherapy, occupational therapy, vocational training, as well as school education for the children. The patients are accommodated in 6 male and 2 female wards and a special children's annexe has been added, thanks to a grant of £35,000 from the Sir William Coxon Trust. The Children's Annexe built in 1965 has been a great improvement for the accommodation and management of paraplegic children,

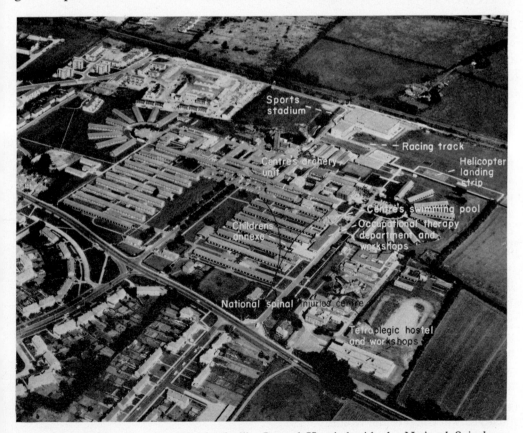

FIG. 4. Aerial view of Stoke Mandeville General Hospital with the National Spinal Injuries Centre and Sports Stadium for the Paralysed and Other Disabled.

including those suffering from spina bifida. Moreover, facilities for sport and recreation were greatly improved by the building of a recreation hall, where training in indoor archery and table tennis could be carried out. Moreover, the building of a large indoor swimming pool, as well as the allocation of a large field of 11 acres for sports competitions, proved very important additions to the facilities for the work of the Centre. Recently, an intensive care unit for acute injuries, especially tetraplegics, has been constructed as part of the Centre.

The medical staff of the Centre consists of a clinical director (after my retirement in 1966, Dr J.J.Walsh was appointed), 3 consultants, a clinical assistant, a senior registrar and 4 junior grades, dealing with all aspects of spinal paraplegia and tetraplegia. The Centre has its own secretarial staff, records department and 2 welfare officers. Fig. 4 shows the lay-out of Stoke Mandeville Hospital with its National Spinal Injuries Centre which represents the largest department of this General Hospital. Alas—shortage of nursing staff has forced the Unit to close wards during recent years and the number of beds is at present about 155. So far, 5935 patients have been treated in this Centre.

AUXILIARY UNITS

In addition to the 195 patients who receive their comprehensive clinical treatment and social re-adjustment at the Centre, a Hostel in the proximity of the Centre was built in 1965 and opened in 1966 for those tetraplegics and other severely handicapped spinal cord sufferers who for one reason or another could not be accommodated in their own homes and for those who lived at home but whose families were no longer able to continue to care for them. This Hostel had a complement of 30 beds and was divided into single, 2 bedded and 4 bedded rooms and represented a pilot scheme for the whole country (Fig. 5a and b). It was hoped that more of these hostels would be built in the vicinity of spinal units in other parts of the United Kingdom where such cases could be accommodated. A workshop was connected with the Hostel which enabled the residents to carry out some remunerative work under sheltered conditions. Moreover, the residents also take part in the sports activities of the Centre. This Hostel, called Sir Ludwig Guttmann Hostel, has been rebuilt and enlarged to 40 beds and is now part of the new Stoke Mandeville District Hospital. It is still the only one of its kind in Great Britain.

In addition to the 195 paraplegics and tetraplegics at the Centre and its Hostel, there are several auxiliary units affiliated to and medically guided by the N.S.I.C.:

1   Spinal Unit at the Star and Garter Home for Ex-servicemen, Richmond, Surrey, set up in 1946 with 24 beds. This unit is, of course, run on the modern management of paraplegics and tetraplegics which is vastly different from that described by Gowland in 1934–41. Drugs such as morphia and hyoscine mentioned by Gowland have been completely discarded and the Unit is run on Stoke Mandeville principles.

2   Chaseley Home, Eastbourne, also for paralysed ex-servicemen, started in 1946 with 40 beds. Some of the residents are employed outside the hostel, others are working in the sheltered workshop of the Home.

3   Duchess of Gloucester House, Isleworth, Middlesex. This is a Hostel with 78 beds (72 male and 6 female) which was specifically built for paraplegics and opened in 1949

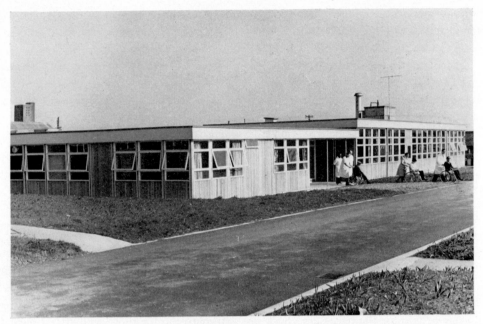

FIG. 5a. Former Sir Ludwig Guttmann Hostel at Stoke Mandeville Hospital (recently rebuilt)

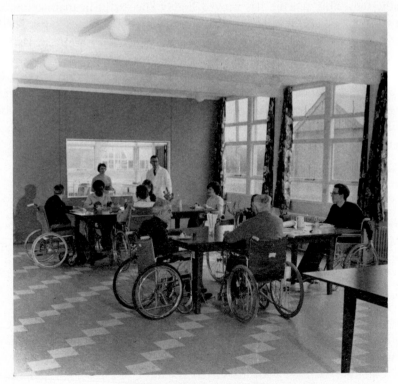

FIG. 5b. Sir Ludwig Guttmann Hostel, interior.

by the former Ministry of Pensions. It is under the administration of the Ministry of Labour and Social Security and only those paraplegics are admitted who are able and willing to take up full time employment outside the Hostel in open industry.

4 Settlement for paraplegic ex-servicemen Lyme Green, Macclesfield in Cheshire, opened in 1946 by the Joint Committee of the Red Cross Society and the Order of St John of Jerusalem, where paraplegics live with their families in bungalows and work in sheltered workshops within the Settlement.

5 Settlement for paraplegic ex-servicemen at Garston Manor, Watford. The residents live in bungalows and all are employed outside the Settlement in open industry.

AFTER CARE SERVICE

A systematic out-patient service was organized in 1951 to deal with routine clinical check-ups for the increasing number of patients discharged to their homes, paraplegic settlements and other institutions, in particular for those who had found employment and were anxious to have as little time off work as possible (see Chapter on Statistics). When distance prevents out-patient check-ups, the paraplegic or tetraplegic is readmitted for a day or two for the necessary check up. Alternatively, for those who are employed, X-ray, blood and urine check-ups are carried out in their nearest hospital and results are sent to the Centre for review to decide whether or not readmission for in-patient treatment is indicated. This scheme has proved highly successful in maintaining so many former patients in good health and employment for many years. For ex-service pensioners, the Ministry of Pensions and Social Security has for many years arranged visits by their regional doctors and welfare officers to the paraplegic's home and they will get in touch with this Centre if any special social or medical problems arise. This after-care service has also proved important in advising local authorities in the adjustment of the paraplegic's or tetraplegic's home, by providing garages, widening doors, adjusting toilets and bathrooms, building ramps, etc. A close relationship between the Centre and the patient's family-doctor is established once the patient is discharged from hospital.

TYPE OF CLINICAL MATERIAL—TIME OF ADMISSION

Patients are admitted to the Spinal Centre at varying intervals after injury or onset of disease and in many cases their condition is extremely serious. The patients admitted can conveniently be divided into the following groups.

1 *Patients admitted immediately or at an early date after injury*

During the war they were admitted from first aid posts of the Normandy front or bombed cities, arriving often with gaping wounds caused by bullets or shell fragments with or without discharging cerebro-spinal fluid, or with associated injuries to other organs, or, especially in air-raid victims, with associated fractures of ribs, skull and extremities. Since the war, when the great majority of traumatic cord injuries have been due to closed fractures or fracture-dislocations, patients have been admitted in ever increasing numbers either immediately or within the first few days after injury from casualty departments of general hospitals, or from accident, neurosurgical or orthopaedic hospitals. This has been more and more recognized by surgeons as the most satisfactory procedure to avoid early infection of the paralysed bladder and the development of other complications, especially pressure sores. In 1963, at a symposium on spinal cord injuries at the Royal College of Surgeons in Edinburgh, I reported that of 396 traumatic paraplegics and tetraplegics admitted during the first 15 days between 1957–63, out of a total admission of 744 cases, 85 were admitted on the day injury, and 234 within 48 hours, 109 of them on the day after injury. The largest group of immediate admissions were the tetraplegics (87), the second largest the thoracic lesions between T6-T12 (78). It may be noted that many of these cases were also suffering from associated injuries of various kinds. The beneficial effect of an immediate or very early admission of these casualties will be discussed in the chapters on pressure sores and urological aspects. In traumatic patients, who for one reason or another are not immediately transportable, the medical or surgical officer in charge of the case often contacts the director of the Spinal Centre to discuss the case and seek advice about aspects of early management, especially the paralysed bladder, or the director or one of his senior colleagues is called in for immediate consultation. Early admission of non-traumatic patients include those following operative procedures for the removal of tumours or prolapsed intervertebral discs, acute vascular lesions, transverse myelitis and epidural abscesses.

2   Patients admitted at later dates

(a) These are cases admitted with signs of septic absorption resulting from infection of the urinary tract producing calculosis or hydroureter, hydro- and pyonephrosis or patients suffering from pressure sores of various size and depth, often producing osteomyelitis with or without destruction of joints. Many of this group show signs of nutritional deficiency and, especially during the early years of our work, showed extreme degrees of malnutrition comparable with those found in inmates of concentration camps. (Belsen type of paraplegics). Fig. 6 demonstrates a woman who was stabbed by her husband and sustained a severe incomplete thoracic cord injury. She was admitted in a pitiful state of malnutrition from a general hospital 4 months after injury suffering from sepsis as a result of pressure sores and infection of the urinary tract. The following pictures show various stages of rehabilitation. Nothing can explain more strikingly the difference between inadequate treatment and proper comprehensive management in traumatic paraplegia than the facial expression of one of our early patients—an ex-serviceman—at the time of admission to the Spinal Centre and time of discharge. (Fig. 7).

(b) Another group of late arrivals are patients where pain and intractable spasticity overlaid by contractures are found in the foreground of the clinical symptomatology. Fig. 8 shows a young soldier admitted from a General Hospital after 4 months, following traumatic tetraplegia below C6/7 with profound flexion contractures of the forearms due to faulty positioning. The agony of suffering from pain is shown in the patient's face when

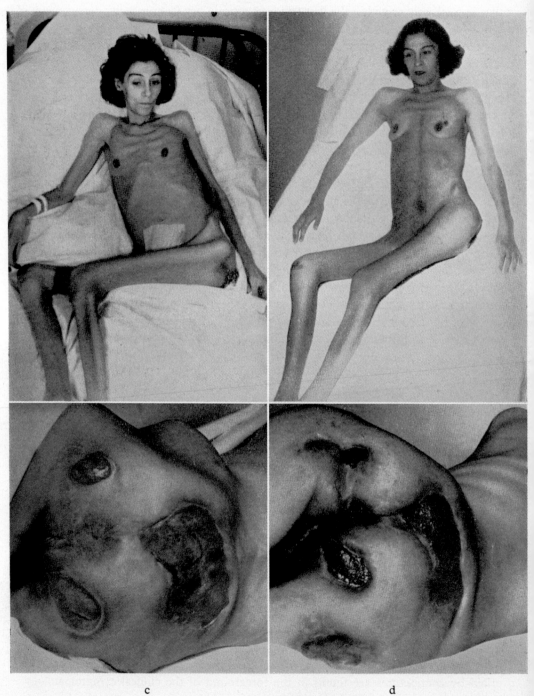

FIG. 6.

a, 9th March, 1949.   b, 23rd April, 1949.   c, 9th March, 1949.   d, 23rd April, 1949.

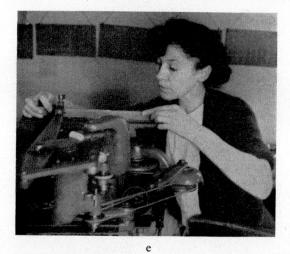

e

FIG. 6. Profound nutritional deficiency in a case of incomplete traumatic transverse spinal syndrome below T_1, due to the septic absorption and loss of protein from multiple sores, and stages of rehabilitation following complete healing of sores.

the sister tried to extend the forearm. However, by appropriate measures (see Chapter on Physiotherapy) the severe contractures could be overcome, as shown in the photographs made during the later stages of management. This group also includes patients with flaccid paralysis who, through inadequate treatment or neglect, have developed deformities of spine and limbs.

(c) A further group of late arrivals are those with more or less satisfactory physical condition but who are demoralized as a result of prolonged and enforced inactivity in hospitals, institutions or at home. This group includes paraplegics who have been treated in so-called general Rehabilitation-Departments, where they form a minority and where the medical and paramedical staff is so busy dealing with other afflictions that they have not the time to give paraplegics and tetraplegics the attention necessary to prevent them from becoming disgruntled and retiring into their disability.

(d) Ex-patients of the Spinal Centre either discharged to their own homes, institutions or settlements are re-admitted for routine check-ups or inpatient treatment for flare ups of their urinary infection or other afflictions such as renal deficiency, hypertension, gastro- or duodenal ulcers, lung complications, cancer, etc. Some have to be readmitted for treatment of recurrent pressure sores as a result of inadequate care at home or institutions or due to personal indifference and neglect, in spite of all the instructions they have received during their initial inpatient treatment at the Centre. Some of our former patients living at home were admitted to their local hospitals for treatment of acute complications such as pneumonia or fractures of long bones as a result of an accident but have had to be readmitted to the Spinal Centre because they developed pressure sores in the local hospital, where they could not receive that specialized care needed day and night during their acute illness.

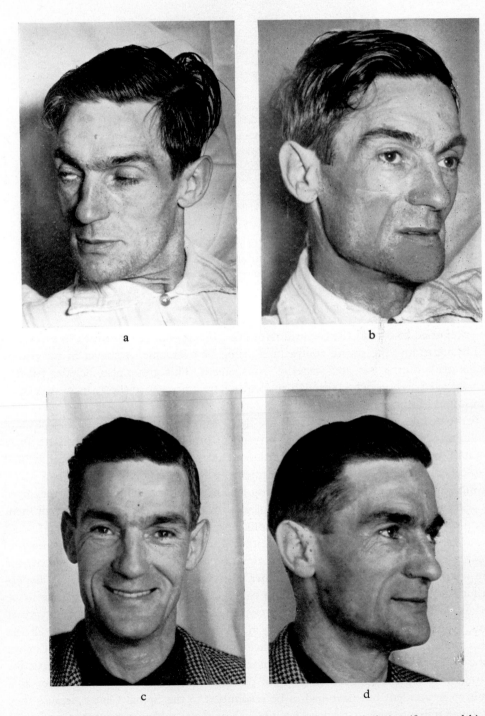

FIG 7. Traumatic paraplegic with severe septic absorption on admission (figs. a and b) at the time of discharge, recovered and fully rehabilitated for employment (c and d).

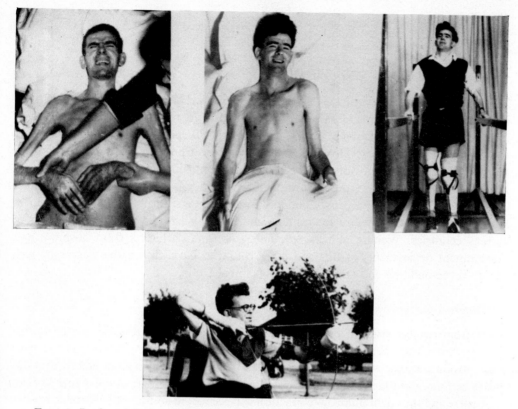

FIG. 8. Profound flexion contracture of the elbow in a patient with complete lesion below C6/7, due to faulty positioning when admitted to Stoke Mandeville from a general hospital 4 months after injury. The following photographs show the improvement of the contractures and the various stages of rehabilitation.

THE IMPORTANCE OF TEAM WORK

All this reveals the great multitude of problems the medical and paramedical staff of a Spinal Centre have to cope with in this multi-disciplinary speciality of medicine and surgery. The whole rehabilitation of the spinal man represents a composite of acute treatments and long-term management, which makes this subject on the one hand so complicated but on the other so fascinating. This can only be solved satisfactorily by team work, in which the director of the unit is the co-ordinator with the final responsibility. The secret of teamwork is that every member of the team must consider his or her job as the most important but at the same time must respect the work of the other members of the team, be they the medical officer in charge of the case or an orderly.

TEACHING

For many years, this Centre has been engaged in teaching undergraduates and postgraduates of the medical profession as well as of the nursing, physiotherapy and occupational therapy professions and welfare officers, and this activity has increased in recent years.

1 Medical staff, welfare officers and administrators

The great majority are physicians, surgeons and medical students from many hospitals in this country and abroad. The Centre takes part in regular postgraduate courses arranged by the Health Service, British Council for Orthopaedic Surgeons organized by the Stanmore Orthopaedic Hospital, as well as those from the National Hospital for Nervous Diseases, Queen Square, London, and the medical services of the Army and Air Force. In recent years, the Centre has been included in the postgraduate courses of the Royal College of Surgeons, London. Physicians and surgeons from other countries have been sent to this Centre for training and have, as a result, set up spinal units in various countries. Welfare officers, administrators and architects from hospitals and Government departments of this and other countries have visited the Centre to seek advice in the building and administration of Spinal Units.

2 Postgraduate courses for nurses

Apart from regular visits of groups of nurses who are sent to this Centre for formal lectures through the Royal College of Nursing, four-monthly postgraduate courses have been introduced since 1953 which are attended by nurses from hospitals and institutions in this country and indeed from all over the world. They take part in the actual work of the Centre and thus gain immediate practical experience; in addition they receive regular lectures by senior members of the medical staff. Some of the postgraduate nurses have continued working in the Centre after the course to gain more detailed experience. The Centre is, of course, included in the training programme of student and pupil nurses of the Aylesbury Nursing School, mainly in their second and third years.

3 Physiotherapy and occupational therapy staff

In addition to full day visits of individuals and groups of physiotherapists and occupational therapists from teaching schools and hospitals, annual postgraduate courses for physiotherapists have been held for a number of years which have become very popular and are greatly supported by the British Chartered Society of Physiotherapy.

4 Teaching outside the Centre

Throughout the years, members of the medical staff as well as the former Lay Administrator, Miss Scruton, and Welfare Officer of the Centre have delivered a great number of lectures to teaching hospitals, training schools and many organizations such as Red Cross, St John's Ambulance Brigade, W.V.S., British Legion, Rotary and Round Table Clubs, Government departments, etc. Members of the medical staff have been invited to lecture at international congresses and visit other countries to lecture on the problems of paraplegia. Meetings of medical and scientific organizations, such as the Neurological and Orthopaedic sections of the Royal Society of Medicine, the British Biochemical

Society and sections of international congresses such as the International Congress of Physical Medicine and International Society for the Rehabilitation of the Disabled (recently called Rehabilitation International), have been held at this Centre throughout the years. Moreover, regular international Scientific Meetings on Paraplegia have been organized since 1953 on the occasion of the annual International Stoke Mandeville Games for the Paralysed. Having regard to the ever increasing interest of members of the medical profession in this problem as a result of these meetings, the International Medical Society of Paraplegia was founded in 1961 at Stoke Mandeville, which holds its annual meetings at Stoke Mandeville and in the Olympic year in the country of the Olympic Games. This Society has now over 700 members representing many countries and has its own international journal, *Paraplegia*, which is published by Livingstones of Edinburgh, and Longman, London, and which appears quarterly. So far 14 volumes of *Paraplegia* have been published.

RESEARCH

From the beginning of our work, research went hand in hand with the clinical work, and many aspects of paraplegia have been the subject of intensive clinical and experimental research. Since 1954, the Centre has had its own research department, consisting of a biochemical and physiological laboratory with a biochemist, technician and senior research assistant carrying out research work in co-operation with the clinical staff and visiting research workers from other departments of this country and abroad. Moreover, for several years an electro-mechanical laboratory was included in the research department which was concerned with the development of electronic controls for tetraplegics. As a result, the patient operated selector mechanism—called POSSUM—was developed by Mr R.G.Maling and D.C.Clarkson and their co-workers, which enables tetraplegics with high lesions and with complete paralysis of all muscles of the upper limbs to control through a tube by sucking and blowing with the mouth various types of apparatus to make them relatively independent and restore contact with the outside world. They are thus able to open and close the door of the house, switch on and switch off lights, radio and television, control an electric typewriter and, by a special adjustment of the telephone, are able to communicate with the outside world. The Post Office authorities have been very helpful in supplying special telephones. The most important aid is the electric typewriter which puts a tetraplegic into the category of a disabled person who is capable of competing in the labour market. The disadvantage of this apparatus is that it is rather expensive.

Throughout the years, a great number of publications have been produced on many aspects of paraplegia, and members of the medical staff have regularly read papers at the annual scientific meetings of the International Medical Society of Paraplegia since its inception. Further details about the results of the research of the Centre are given in the individual chapters of this book.

CHAPTER 3

DEVELOPMENT OF OTHER SPINAL
INJURIES CENTRES
1. THE UNITED KINGDOM

There are seven other Spinal Injuries Units of smaller size which were set up after the Second World War in various parts of the United Kingdom which, like Stoke Mandeville, are built on ground level.

LODGE MOOR, SHEFFIELD

The Unit at Lodge Moor Hospital in Sheffield has a complement of 60 beds and Dr A.Hardy, F.R.C.S., is the Consultant-in-charge. The Unit was first opened in 1945 at the Warncliff Hospital, a mental hospital, and was transferred to Lodge Moor in 1951. Since its inception over 1,500 cases were treated until 1969, over 90 per cent being new traumatic cases. In the first 10 years, over 200 miners were admitted, since Sheffield is situated near the Yorkshire coal-mining area. However, the numbers of coal miners with spinal injuries has declined during the last 10 years.

The Unit takes part in postgraduate teaching but undergraduates from the Orthopaedic Department of Sheffield University also come periodically to Lodge Moor to be instructed in the problem of paraplegia. Dr Hardy sees virtually all new spinal injuries which are admitted first to orthopaedic and accident departments. Although the Unit has no personnel or facilities for research, Dr Hardy and his deputy Dr Watson have published most valuable papers on various clinical and social aspects of paraplegia. Lodge Moor very soon included sport in the rehabilitation of paraplegics and takes part regularly in the annual Stoke Mandeville Games. The unit is provided with a swimming pool.

MIDLAND SPINAL INJURIES UNIT

This Unit is part of the famous Robert Jones and Agnes Hunt Orthopaedic Hospital at Oswestry, Shropshire, and was set up in 1965 with a complement of 60 beds (20 for females). Mr T.McSweeney, M.CH., F.R.C.S., is the director of the Unit and Dr B.F.Jones, M.R.C.P., his deputy. Before 1965, cases of spinal injuries were treated in various wards of the hospital under the care of various 'firms', which did not prove satisfactory. Oswestry had, however, been orientated towards the problems of paraplegia since the foundation of the hospital in 1920, for this hospital became a Centre for the treatment of tuberculosis of the spine and has done pioneer work on Pott's paraplegia. From 1960–69, 380 paraplegics and tetraplegics were treated, of these 295 were traumatic cases (140 tetraplegics).

The catchment areas of the unit are the Birmingham region and part of the Manchester and Welsh regions. Oswestry being a 500 bed specialized orthopaedic hospital has its own physiotherapy school, and students carry out much of the day to day physiotherapy under the direction of a supervisor who is attached to the Spinal Unit. There is a heated swimming pool in which regular classes are held for paraplegics. There is also a well-equipped occupational therapy department for wood-working and metal-working tools as well as lighter crafts, and electric typewriters are available and put into much use by tetraplegics. A senior Occupational Therapist devotes all her time to the Spinal Unit and directs the activities of students who are seconded to Oswestry from the O.T. School, Dorset House, Oxford. Art therapy is also available which has proved most valuable for the paralysed. The establishment of an Industrial Rehabilitation Unit adjoining the hospital has been planned but not yet materialized. Sport is also included in the rehabilitation treatment of the paralysed and the Unit participates in the annual Stoke Mandeville Games.

The Unit has the full time services of a Medical Social Worker who at an early stage secures co-operation of the local authorities, medical and welfare departments to facilitate the domestic and industrial resettlement of the patients.

SPINAL UNIT AT PINDERFIELD HOSPITAL, WAKEFIELD

This, the second Spinal Injuries Unit for Yorkshire started in 1954 and has a complement of 30 beds. The unit is attached to the Department of Neurology and Dr J.B.Cook, M.D., F.R.C.P., who also holds the post of Clinical Lecturer in Neurology at Leeds University and Postgraduate Clinical Tutor, is the Consultant Neurologist in charge of the unit. There is both undergraduate and postgraduate teaching on the unit, and the unit is also involved in the training scheme for Senior Registrars, Orthopaedic and Urological Surgeons. The unit also has a Research Assistant concerned with the investigation of bladder function. Specialized equipment for renal function such as isotope scanning and renal flow estimation are available.

Most traumatic paraplegics are admitted within 48 hours and are sent directly to the Spinal Unit. From 1960–69 altogether 527 patients were admitted (145 new cases), amongst them 62 coal miners (Wakefield is also situated in a coal-mining area).

SOUTHPORT SPINAL UNIT AT PROMENADE HOSPITAL

This is the Liverpool Regional Paraplegic Centre, a unit of 34 beds (30 male and 4 female) which was opened in 1947. Until 1965 Dr Damanski, an urological surgeon, was in charge of the unit with Mr Osborne, F.R.C.S., orthopaedic surgeon, Mr Sutcliffe Kerr, F.R.C.S., neurosurgeon, Mr Maisels, F.R.C.S., plastic surgeon, Mr Cosbie Ross, F.R.C.S., and Mr Gibbon, F.R.C.S., urological surgeons, all acting as visiting consultants. After Dr Damanski's retirement, Dr J.Silver, M.R.C.P.E., former registrar and senior research assistant at Stoke Mandeville, took over but returned to Stoke Mandeville in 1970 as a Consultant in Paraplegia and was replaced by Dr Krishnan, F.R.C.S., neurosurgeon and a former trainee at Stoke Mandeville.

Since its inception there have been 2,207 admissions, amongst them 768 new patients. The traumatic lesions were admitted within 48 hours of injury. The teaching activities of the unit have expanded during recent years for both undergraduate and postgraduate teaching. In addition, the unit also deals with the training and postgraduate teaching of nurses. The unit has been particularly engaged for many years in research of urological problems of spinal cord injuries, carried out by Mr Cosbie Ross, Mr Gibbon and Dr Damanski, and Dr Silver did research on problems of spasticity and continued research on chest movements in paraplegia which he started with me at Stoke Mandeville. The Southport Unit has also been represented for many years at the annual Stoke Mandeville Games. There have been discussions to transfer the unit to Liverpool with a great increase of the number of beds, but so far nothing has materialized.

EDENHALL SPINAL UNIT, MUSSELBURGH, SCOTLAND

This small unit of 22 male and 6 female beds was opened in 1959, but before the setting up of the unit a number of ex-service paraplegics were treated at Edenhall when the hospital was under the administration of the former Ministry of Pensions and also an increasing number of civilian cases when this hospital was taken over in 1956 by the Ministry of Health. Mr W.Kerr, F.R.C.S.E., who was also a consultant to the Appliance Department, was in charge of the unit and his statistic of a period from 12 July 1959 to 31 October 1969 show 268 new patients admitted, not immediately after injury but some time, even several months, later. During the same period, 271 former patients were readmitted for treatment, largely as a result of pressure sores and urological complications. Owing to the very small size of the unit, it soon became impossible to admit patients for routine review unless they came from a very long distance and 545 reviews were carried out on outpatients.

The problem of immediate access to new traumatic cases is still complicated by the small size of the unit and because of differences between the neurosurgical and orthopaedic departments in Edinburgh. Therefore, the unit has still to rely on orthopaedic and neurosurgical consultants to carry out the initial treatment and such care as they can give during the first period of treatment. Although the standard of care has improved during the last 20 years, this fragmentation between the initial treatment and the long term rehabilitation and care is still not satisfactory. It is only very recently that the consultant in charge of the spinal unit has had access to the acute cases admitted to the Royal Infirmary of Edinburgh University. However, the Regional Hospital Board hopes to replace the present unit with a larger, up-to-date unit in the future building plan.

Very little research activities are carried out but a great deal of teaching is done and every undergraduate student of Edinburgh University had a lecture on paraplegia from Mr Kerr in a half-day visit to the unit, the students reporting in groups of 12 every month. Moreover, postgraduate students working for the Fellowship of the Royal College of Surgeons have a postgraduate day of lectures and demonstrations once a year. Furthermore, all nurses from two of the Edinburgh Schools of Nursing have a half-day of lectures and demonstrations and postgraduate neurological nurses attend in groups of 2 or 3 for one week six times a year. All pupil physiotherapists, occupational therapists and medical social workers attend for a half-day of lectures and demonstrations, while each physiotherapy pupil is attached for one week and a few of the occupational therapists are attached for 2–3 months at a time. After Kerr's death Dr Elizabeth McClemont has taken charge of the unit.

SPINAL UNIT AT PHILIPSHILL HOSPITAL, NEAR GLASGOW, SCOTLAND

This new unit of 25 beds under the Directorship of Mr MacDougall, F.R.C.S., has been opened very recently and I had the honour to perform the official opening. This unit, which is part of the Orthopaedic Department of Glasgow University, is well equipped and has a particularly good occupational therapy and art therapy department, which is under the administration of the Department of Education. This unit works in close co-operation with the Department of Neurology of Glasgow University.

SPINAL UNIT ROOKWOOD HOSPITAL, CARDIFF, WALES

This unit of 35 beds, which was started by me in 1952 with Dr R. Thomas in charge, admitted, during the time when I was its consultant, traumatic paraplegics and tetraplegics immediately after injury. When Dr Thomas left after my retirement from the Health Service it came under the charge of Dr Lewis as the unit was taken over by the Orthopaedic Department of the Prince of Wales Hospital, where the acute cases are first admitted. However, Dr Lewis also left and the fragmentation of treatment unfortunately still continues.

NEED FOR INCREASED FACILITIES

In view of the greatly increased life-expectancy of both paraplegics and tetraplegics and the steadily increasing number of these patients from year to year, there is a great need for enlarging some of the existing Spinal Centres in the United Kingdom and creating new units in certain parts of the country. Representations to the Department of Health have been made in this connection by the leaders of the existing Centres since the late sixties. Although the need was recognized by the authorities concerned, no concrete measures have been taken so far to remedy the unsatisfactory situation. The same applies to the setting up of hostels, and that at Stoke Mandeville is still the only one in existence. It may be noted that the recently published Tunbridge Report on Rehabilitation, recognizing the need for increasing the facilities for the specialized treatment and rehabilitation of spinal paraplegics and tetraplegics, has recommended the setting up of two more Spinal Injuries Centres for England and Wales.

CHAPTER 4

DEVELOPMENT OF OTHER SPINAL
INJURIES CENTRES

2. OTHER COUNTRIES

ARGENTINA

There is one large Rehabilitation Centre in Buenos Aires under the leadership of Dr José Cibeira. This is run by a voluntary institution called Asociación Cooperadora del Instituto nacional de Rehabilitacion del lisiados (A.C.I.R.) which is supported by the Government. This is a general rehabilitation centre but with a large complement of locomotor lesions such as polio, spina bifida, and also includes traumatic paraplegics and tetraplegics. The latter group has gradually increased in recent years and Dr Cibeira is building a Spinal Injuries Unit. This Rehabilitation Centre is equipped with good research facilities and a number of publications have been produced by Dr Cibeira and his colleagues, who take part regularly at the annual meeting of the International Medical Society of Paraplegia. Argentine is the first country in South America which has from an early stage included sport in its rehabilitation programme, which has proved most valuable, and the Argentine paraplegic team has for many years taken part in the International Stoke Mandeville Games and distinguished themselves by their excellent skill.

AUSTRALIA

Since 1954, Spinal Injuries Centres have been established in Perth, Western Australia, Melbourne, Victoria, Adelaide, South Australia, Sydney, New South Wales, and Brisbane, Queensland. All these units are attached to teaching hospitals. The most highly developed Centre is that under Dr G.Bedbrook and Dr E.R.Griffiths at Shenton Park, Perth, which has excellent facilities for micro-biological and pathological research which have been conducted by Drs Pearman and Kakulas respectively. Dr Bedbrook has been repeatedly called to countries in the Far East to advise in the setting up of Spinal Injury Centres.

At Austin Hospital in Melbourne, the Spinal Centre has been completely reorganized since my visit in 1957, undertaken at the request of the Nuffield Foundation. In 1960 this Unit came under the leadership of Dr D.Cheshire, who developed it to a high standard. After his resignation in 1972 (he is now Director of Research at the Spinal Injuries Centre in Phoenix, U.S.A. of which Dr John Young is the Director), Dr David Burke became his successor, and in 1974, Dr Gerald Ungar, former Senior Registrar at Stoke Mandeville, was appointed as his deputy.

In recent years, the Spinal Injuries Centre at North Shore Hospital, Sydney, which for many years has laboured under unsatisfactory accommodation, has been rebuilt, and Dr J.Yeo, a neurologist, is in charge of the Unit and the neurosurgeon is Dr John Grant. Dr Yeo is engaged in animal experimental research on spinal cord injuries and regeneration of the spinal cord.

All the Spinal Centres in Australia admit spinal injuries immediately after accident and are in a position to give their patients a comprehensive management from the start. In view of the great distances in Australia, many patients are transferred immediately to the Spinal Centres by air transport.

AUSTRIA

In Austria it was the late Dr G.Neubauer, a surgeon, who after the Second World War, following his visit to Stoke Mandeville, pioneered the modern management of traumatic paraplegia and tetraplegia in his Rehabilitationcenter Tobelbad, near Graz, which was set up by the Austrian Insurance Organization. This well built Institute, equipped with all facilities for the medical and social rehabilitation of spinal cord sufferers and which works in close association with the orthopaedic department of Graz University, was the first of its kind to be established in a German speaking country. The present director is Dr Zrubecky, a surgeon, who himself is a paraplegic. Sport plays an essential part in the work of this Centre and Austria was one of the first countries to take part in the International Stoke Mandeville Games for the Paralysed. In 1972 another rehabilitation centre was set up in Häring under the leadership of Dr Stipicic who has organized a Spinal Injuries Unit of 40 beds, which is functioning well.

BELGIUM

Professor P.Houssa and his associate Dr A.Tricot have for many years specialized in the treatment and rehabilitation of traumatic paraplegics and tetraplegics on Stoke Mandeville principles. Professor Houssa is the founder of the Centre de Traumatologie et de Réadaptation at the Hôpital Universitaire Brugman in Brussels where he has pioneered in problems of traumatic paraplegia. He and Dr Tricot have been the promotors of sport for the paralysed and other severely disabled people in Belgium and since 1953 Belgium has taken part regularly in the Stoke Mandeville Games. This Centre has developed excellently and is now associated with the University Hospital of Brussels.

Professor Houssa has now retired after 25 years of pioneer work and Professor Tricot is now in charge of the Centre.

CANADA

The outstanding Spinal Injuries Centre in Canada is Lyndhurst Lodge in Toronto founded by the Canadian Paraplegic Association in 1945 and working under the direction of Dr A.Jousse who reported on 958 traumatic patients under his care (1967). This is an autonomous Centre but has been associated in later years with Toronto University. Lyndhurst Lodge has been rebuilt and is equipped with much better clinical and research facilities. Dr A.Jousse, who has given outstanding service to this Centre, has recently retired and his place has been taken by Dr W.O.Geisler, who, for many years, was Dr Jousse's associate. In recent years, a small Unit of 14 beds was set up in Manitoba. Dr B.Grogono who was in charge of this unit gave in 1968 a thorough statistical survey of spinal cord lesions in Canada. According to this author, the total incidence of spinal cord injuries in Canada is about 12 per cent per million population, as compared with 15 per cent per million in the U.S.A. He came to the conclusion that in Canada a fully co-ordinated system of treatment and care of paraplegics and tetraplegics has yet to be established, especially for early care, accommodation and research. Recently, 1975, Professor E.H.Botterell who, for many years was the neuro-surgical consultant at Lyndhurst Lodge, has, with his colleagues at Lyndhurst Lodge, surveyed the situation regarding care of acute spinal injuries in the Province of Ontario and has stressed that the total management is still fragmented, which has proved un-satisfactory, and a high percentage of pressure sores and infection of the urinary tract is still prevailing. They highly recommend the setting up of Regional Spinal Injuries Centres which should be affiliated to a university. Acute cord injury patients should, as a rule, be transferred by road or air transport to these Regional Centres and should *not* be transported routinely to the hospital nearest to the accident. They also emphasize that one specialist in paraplegia (paraplegist) must be responsible for the over-all care and management of the spinal cord injured patient, whether paraplegic or tetraplegic, and other consultants and specialists 'should revolve around the patient and the para-plegist'. Such a spinal centre called 'acute cord injury centre' should give these patients a comprehensive management from the start and throughout all stages of their re-habilitation.

One can only hope that this system, which has proved so successful in England and other countries, will be adopted not only in Ontario but in all other parts of Canada.

Canada and U.S.A. were the first countries to follow Great Britain's example in later stages of the Second World War to congregate spinal cord war casualties in special Units. Canada is a founder nation of the American Wheelchair Games, the first of which took place in Winnipeg in 1966, and Dr R.W.Jackson was the chairman of the Canadian Paraplegic Sports Association.

CZECHOSLOVAKIA

In recent years a Spinal Injuries Centre has been set up under the leadership of Dr V. Knapek at Ostrava in the coal-mining and industrial district of Czechoslovakia, which is run on Stoke Mandeville lines. Dr Knapek has also included sport as part of the rehabili-tation of these patients and in recent years paraplegic teams from Czechoslovakia have taken part in the Stoke Mandeville Games.

FRANCE

After the Second World War, it was the neurologist Professor A.Grossiord who, in co-operation with Dr J.Bénassy, an orthopaedic surgeon, specialized in the treatment and rehabilitation of spinal cord afflictions including traumatic lesions at Raymond Poincaré Hospital, Garches, near Paris. Other specialized units are the Centre de Reeduca-tion Motrice in Fontainebleau, Paris, under Dr M.Maury, who spent some time for specialized training at Stoke Mandeville. Grossiord, Maury and Bénassy are founder members of the International Medical Society of Paraplegia and have made important contributions in various aspects of paraplegia and tetraplegia. Another unit is that of the Invalides, Paris, for ex-servicemen. A Spinal Injuries Unit of 40 beds with an operating theatre and intensive care unit has been built within the very modern General Rehabilitation Centre in Mulhouse under the leadership of Dr Paul Dollfus, a graduate of Stoke Mandeville. Dr Dollfus is also Consultant to the Traumatological and Orthopaedic Unit at Colmar where he works with Dr Molé and sees all acute spinal injuries immediately after admission, and recently he has been elected as an Honorary Consultant to the Spinal Injuries Centre at Basle, Switzerland.

GERMANY

During the last 20 years, as a result of the initiative taken by some leading members of the medical profession, the V.D.K. (Verband Deutscher Kriegsopfer) and the Industrial Insurance Organisations (Berufsgenossenschaften), active steps were taken in Germany for the establishing of a comprehensive management of traumatic paraplegics and tetraplegics. Medical, nursing and physiotherapy personnel were sent to Stoke Mandeville for training from hospitals for ex-servicemen (Versorgungskrankenhäuser), such as Pyrmont and Bayreuth and other hospitals. The Berufsgenossenschaften were the first to organize Spinal Injuries Units such as in Koblenz, Bochum, Duisburg, Frankfurt, Murnau, Tübingen and Ludwigshafen. Instructions were given to all administrative regional divisions of their organization to ensure that their insured workers who sustained spinal cord injuries were admitted immediately or as soon as possible to their own Spinal Units. Cases admitted to other hospitals should be checked to ensure that they are receiving adequate treatment. An investigation through the medical adviser of their organization is requested to clarify the circumstances in instances where, through deliberate retention in a hospital, avoidable complications are reported. In due course, these measures have proved very beneficial in congregating traumatic paraplegics and tetraplegics in these spinal units. In view of the steadily increasing number of traumatic spinal cord lesions in Germany as a whole, the administration of the Berufsgenossenschaften have increased the number of beds in their Spinal Units since 1964 from 263 to 324 to make some beds available for non-insured victims of road accidents and industry. Dr Meinecke (1968), who was in charge of the Spinal Injuries Centre, Bochum, has given a comprehensive report about 615 patients with spinal cord lesions treated since the end of the war at the Accident Hospital Bergmannsheil in Bochum. Five hundred and ninety-five were traumatic lesions and 57·1 per cent of these had associated injuries.

In February 1967, the Spinal Injuries Centre in Heidelberg, Schlierbach, was opened. This Centre, which was created by the late Professor K.Lindemann, represents the first Spinal Injuries Centre in a German University and is part of the Orthopaedic University Clinic. It consists of two magnificent buildings, the clinical department (Ludwig Guttmann-Haus) with 60 beds and a department of 60 beds for vocational and social rehabilitation with a boarding-school and training workshops (Kurt Lindemann-Haus). This is indeed the ideal model of a modern Spinal Injuries Centre, equipped with all facilities to provide a comprehensive service for traumatic and non-traumatic spinal cord sufferers (Fig. 9). Unhappily, Kurt Lindemann did not live to see the realization of his creation. The Centre is directed by Professor V.Paeslack, a general physician, who, with members of his nursing and physiotherapy staff, received specialized training at Stoke Mandeville. Recently, Professor Paeslack added a ward for spina bifida children as part of the Centre.

The most recent, specially built Spinal Centre of the Berufsgenossenschaften is that in Murnau, Bavaria, opened in January 1969. It is part of an Accident Hospital and was founded by its former director, Professor A.Lob. At present, it has a complement of 60 beds but will be enlarged to 100 beds. This Centre has its own operation theatres and all facilities for a comprehensive paraplegia service and like the Heidelberg Centre can serve as a model for other centres.

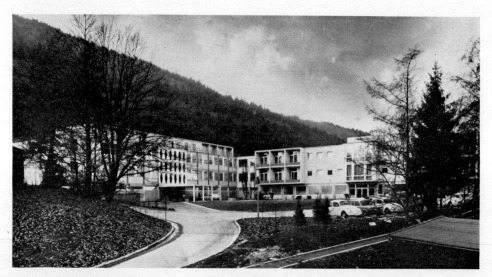

FIG. 9. The Spinal Injuries Centre in Heidelberg–Schlierbach.

In Cologne, Professor Scheid founded in 1967 a Rehabilitation Centre as part of the Neurological University Clinic for neurological disabilities, amongst them spinal cord afflictions, and in recent years acute traumatic paraplegics and tetraplegics were admitted to give these patients a comprehensive treatment from the start. This centre is under the direction of Professor K.Jochheim and until 1970 Dr H.Wahle. Another Spinal Unit is part of the Neurological Department of the Versorgungskrankenhaus in Bayreuth, as part of the Veterans Hospital, where Dr L.Lemberg, a former trainee of Stoke Mandeville, is in charge. This unit has been enlarged in 1975 to 100 beds for ex-service paraplegics and tetraplegics. Other developments in Germany in recent years for the rehabilitation of paraplegics have been the Industrial Rehabilitation Units, the Johannes Straubinger Haus in Wildbad under Mr W.Weiss, built by the Charitas Organization, and that of Mr Peters in Krayburg, Bavaria. Furthermore, a very modern industrial training centre including domestic settlement, called Berufsförderungswerk, has been established near Heidelberg by Mr W.Boll for disabled people, where paraplegics can live with their families. This spacious and excellent industrial Rehabilitation

Centre in Heidelberg has been the venue of the XXI International Stoke Mandeville Games where 1,000 paraplegic athletes and 400 escorts representing 45 countries were accommodated.

In East Germany a Spinal Injuries Centre was set up in Berlin–Buch in the early sixties which is run on Stoke Mandeville principles.

HOLLAND

At the end of the Second World War, following a study visit of medical and administrative officers from the Dutch Army to Stoke Mandeville, a Rehabilitation Centre with a unit for paraplegics was set up for disabled ex-servicemen at Aardenburg, near Doorn under Dr van Gogh. He and his successor Dr Kayser brought in 1952 the first paraplegic sports team to England to compete in the Stoke Mandeville Games for the paralysed, which was the beginning of these Games as the annual International Sports Festival for the Paralysed, the Olympics for the Paralysed. In due course, the Dutch military authorities set up a settlement for paraplegics and other severely disabled ex-servicemen. Holland also has established a large Rehabilitation Centre mainly for polios and paraplegics at The Hogstraat, for some years under the direction of Dr Miedema. There is also a small Spinal Injuries Unit in Amsterdam under Dr Hofmann as part of a hospital of chronic diseases, and one can only hope that Dr Hofmann, a very devoted surgeon in this speciality, will be given better facilities.

Recently interest in setting up one or two other Spinal Units in Holland is increasing.

IRELAND

In 1961, a Sanatorium for Tuberculosis outside Dublin, run by an order of nuns, the Sisters of Mercy, was converted into the National Medical Rehabilitation Centre under the direction of Dr T.Gregg. The Centre has 120 beds, 45 of which are designated for a comprehensive management of spinal injuries from the start and throughout all stages. Moreover, recently a specialized service of 18 beds for spina bifida children has been added. Specialized teams were trained at Stoke Mandeville, and Dr C.Wilmot, who is in charge of the Dublin Spinal Unit, was a member of my staff for about two years. Dr J.J. Walsh, my successor as Director of the Stoke Mandeville Centre, was appointed as Hon. Consultant and pays regular visits to the Dublin Centre to deal with special surgical problems. The Centre is closely associated with the National Organization for Rehabilitation (N.O.R.). A hostel of 20 beds will be opened in the near future for paraplegics whose home conditions are unsatisfactory but who can be employed in the Dublin area. From 1961–67, 146 new traumatic cases were admitted, the majority 109 (28 complete and 81 incomplete) were cervicals (Gregg, 1967). Dr Gregg and his team have made an important contribution to the immediate transfer of traumatic paraplegics and tetraplegics to the Centre by organizing a 'flying squad' consisting of a doctor, a nurse and an orderly who, on request, will immediately bring in the paralysed, either by ambulance or helicopter, from the place of accident or any hospital in the country. This immediate admission has proved both a life saving measure and the best prevention of early urinary infection and pressure sores caused by inadequate initial management in hospitals neither acquainted with nor equipped for the specialized treatment of these patients. Sport is included in the rehabilitation, and the Irish team has taken part regularly in the Olympics for the Paralysed.

ISRAEL

Until recently there has been fragmentation of the management of traumatic paraplegics and tetraplegics in Israel and acute cases were treated in orthopaedic units such as Tel Hashomer or in neurosurgical or general surgical units, while the long-term rehabilitation was carried out in physical medicine departments such as Hadassah Hospital, Jerusalem, or in a general rehabilitation hospital such as Assaf Harofe, Zrifin, where Dr Ralph Spira, a former medical officer at Stoke Mandeville Centre is engaged in the rehabilitation of polios and paraplegics in later stages. He has done detailed and most valuable research on sport in these patients. At the Loewenstein Hospital Rehabilitation Centre, Raanana, under Dr T.Nejemson (120 beds) 20 beds have been set aside for the treatment of paraplegics. The late Professor Adler, Chief of the Department of Physical Medicine at the Hadassah, gave in 1968 a survey of his paraplegic patients who were transferred to him for rehabilitation either with infected urinary tract or pressure sores (Adler, 1968). The authorities concerned have been increasingly dissatisfied with the fragmentation of management of traumatic paraplegic patients and having regard to the increased number of war casualties and road accidents, the Ministry of Defence in co-operation with the Ministry of Health have taken the initiative at the instigation of Mr A.Fink, the Director of Rehabilitation, to build a Spinal Injuries Centre at Tel Hashomer—now named Sheba Hospital—for the comprehensive treatment and rehabilitation of spinal paraplegics and tetraplegics. I had the honour of laying the foundation stone of the Centre at a ceremony on 26 October 1972. This Centre will bear my name. Medical, nursing and physiotherapy staff have been trained at Stoke Mandeville and Dr Rozin is the Director of the unit. He and his staff have given an excellent service to spinal injured during the Yom Kippur War. Sport for the disabled is highly developed in Israel and since 1954 a team of paralysed athletes has taken part in the International Stoke Mandeville Games. Moreover, the XX Games in 1968 took place in Israel with 750 competitors and 300 escorts.

ITALY

It was the Italian National Institute for Labour Accident Insurance (I.N.A.I.L.) which in 1957 set up for their injured workers an autonomous Spinal Injuries Centre of 110 beds at Ostia-Lido di Roma under the direction of Professor A.Maglio, which is run on Stoke Mandeville principles. This Centre has pioneered in Italy the modern concept of treating spinal paraplegics and tetraplegics and, up to 1967, 1,700 patients have been treated there. More than 300 new cases due to industrial accident are added to the 5,000 stabilized cases in Italy (Maglio, 1963). The Centre is organized as a completely autonomous hospital and equipped with all clinical social and educational facilities. It has its own workshops for manufacturing calipers and repair of wheelchairs. Special emphasis has been laid on the development of sport. Actually, the first International Stoke Mandeville Games ever held in the Olympic year in connection with the Olympic Games took place in Rome in 1960, when 400 paralysed sportsmen and women representing 23 countries were accommodated in the Olympic Stadium. However, the industrial resettlement of paraplegics in Italy is handicapped through the still existing laws in that country which do not allow severely disabled people in receipt of full pensions to take up employment. The Spinal Centre at Ostia has since been taken over by the Health Service of Italy and Professor Masserelli a former assistant of Professor Maglio is now in charge of the Centre. Work in the Ostia Centre has become more and more difficult as the building has greatly deteriorated. There is also a small Spinal Unit for ex-servicemen in Rome under Dr Palcinelli set up by the Italian Government (Opera Nazinale Pergli Invalidi Di Guerra, O.N.I.G.) and another in Milan under Dr Bruno and Professor Ascoli, an urologist.

Moreover, the Clinica 'Santa Lucia' in Rome, under the leadership of Dr Enzo Zucchi is also very much concerned with the treatment and rehabilitation of spinal cord injuries. It has good facilities for physiotherapy and vocational training and a large sportsfield has recently been added. Two years ago, the Italian Medical Association of Paraplegia was founded which holds regular annual meetings.

JAMAICA

Paraplegics and tetraplegics are first treated at the Orthopaedic department of the University under Professor Golding. However, in the early '60's a Rehabilitation Centre (The Mona Rehabilitation Centre) mainly for paralysed people and especially polios was built in Kingston, thanks to the great efforts of Mr Sammy Henriques, which has good facilities for rehabilitation, in particular, sport. There the Second Paraplegic Commonwealth Games were held in 1966 under the leadership of Professor Golding, which were opened by H.R.H. the Duke of Edinburgh, accompanied by Prince Charles and Princess Anne. This event was a great success and aroused great interest in the community of that country and other parts of the West Indies. Ever since, teams from Jamaica have taken part in the Stoke Mandeville Games and the Pan American Games.

JAPAN

The whole approach of the medical profession and the public towards spinal paraplegics fundamentally changed in Japan after the return of Dr Nakamura and Professor Tamai, both orthopaedic surgeons, from Stoke Mandeville, where they gained extensive experience during many months training. It was Dr Nakamura from Beppu who in 1962 brought the very first small team of Japanese paraplegics to England to take part in the International Games, which on the team's return, aroused increasing interest in the rehabilitation of traumatic paraplegics in Japan. In the Olympic year of 1964, the Stoke Mandeville Games were held immediately after the Olympic Games in the magnificent Olympic Stadium of Tokyo, under the leadership of Mr Kasai and his committee, when more than 100,000 people watched the excellent sportive performances of the 350 paraplegic athletes representing 23 countries. The athletic performances, endurance and standard of these paralysed athletes were also an extraordinary inspiration to the Japanese Government, private organizations and employers to help their paraplegic fellow men in their social and industrial resettlement. Within 6 months after the Games, the first factory, specially built for the paralysed, called Nagano Plant, 70 miles west of Tokyo was opened for 56 paraplegics in an area of many factories producing cameras and communication machinery. In 1967, Professor Amako reported that two more of such factories had been established, one in Beppu where Dr Nakamura is in charge and the other at the Fuji factory of Musashino Electric Co-operation, not very far from the National Spinal Injuries Centre, Hakone, set up under the direction of the late Dr Tomita. According to the late Dr Tomita's statistical survey (1968), the number of paraplegics in Japan had reached the 10,000 mark.

There are now 4 of these factories for paraplegics and other severely disabled which are called Sun Industries.

Recently, the Far East and South Pacific Games for the Paralysed and other Disabled (FESPIC) have been founded and the first sports event was held in Oita in June, 1975, in which representatives of Japan, Korea, India, Pakistan, Sri Lanka, Phillipines, Bangladesh, Burma, Thailand, Fiji, New Guinea (Papua), Australia, and New Zealand took part: indeed, an important demonstration of the development of sport of the paralysed and other severely disabled in the Far East. The city of Osaka has built a magnificent sports stadium for the paralysed and other disabled on the lines of the Stoke Mandeville Sports Stadium for the Paralysed and other Disabled, which was opened in June, 1974.

NEW ZEALAND

For many years, leading surgeons of various specialities have made great efforts to induce the authorities concerned to set up Spinal Injuries Centres for a comprehensive management and rehabilitation of these patients. However, no progress was made mainly owing to financial difficulties and statutory restrictions in the social field. For instance, according to the regulations of the New Zealand State Health Service, paraplegics can receive their wheelchairs only on loan for 9 months after which time they have to buy the wheelchair. This regulation is in striking contrast to the provisions made for appliances and aids for other disabilities, such as contact lenses, and help for the blind, artificial limbs for amputees and artificial hip joints, which are given free under the existing regulations. Moreover, the only small unit of 10–12 beds segregated for the treatment of spinal cord injuries at the Christchurch General Hospital is at present hopelessly inadequate. During my recent visit (1971) to that beautiful country, undertaken at the request of the New Zealand Paraplegic Federation, I was given every opportunity to study this whole medical and social problem of paraplegia and tetraplegia. As a result of many discussions with the hospital, municipal and governmental authorities, including the Minister of Health, the Government has now given financial help to set up two Spinal Injuries Centres, one at Auckland and the other at Birwood Hospital, Christchurch.

POLAND

In 1949, a Centre for Rehabilitation of Paraplegics was established within the Institute for Rehabilitation at Konstancin, near Warsaw, under Dr Marian Weiss. This unit was at first concerned mainly with paraplegics transferred from other hospitals suffering from serious complications. In due course, with the growing problem of paraplegia and with increasing facilities for the management of paraplegics and tetraplegics, a unit for paraplegic children and another for acute traumatic lesions were added. In 1964, by a decree of the Ministry of Health and the general management of hospitals in Warsaw no surgical hospital is allowed to admit paraplegics, all of whom have now to be congregated at Konstancin, which has greatly improved the standard of the initial treatment of traumatic paraplegics and tetraplegics. Beds are still reserved for the admission of cases with complications, but, as a rule, the medical officer in charge of such a case is requested to stay at Konstancin for at least six weeks to receive training for proper management of his own case. Acute traumatic paraplegics and tetraplegics are transferred to Konstancin by helicopters of the Sanitary Ambulance Service or, if this is not possible, by a military 'plane. The Konstancin Centre has good facilities for clinical and social rehabilitation, including excellent sport facilities, with easy access for paraplegics from the Spinal Centre. Moreover, with the help of the Co-operative Society for Invalids and Sheltered Workshop, paraplegics with distal lesions can be trained in special professional schools as medical laboratory assistants, radio and television technicians and in precision engineering. Dr Weiss, who is now professor at the School of Medicine of Warsaw University, and his staff are engaged in research and teaching and recently other Spinal Units have been set up in Poznan and Upper Silesia. Poland was the first country behind the 'Iron Curtain' which for some years has taken part in the Stoke Mandeville Games.

PORTUGAL

There is a General Rehabilitation Centre at Estoril (Centro de Medicina de Reabilitacao) started by Dr Victor M.Santana Carlos. Paraplegics and tetraplegics were treated amongst other patients in that Centre as they were in Orthopaedic and Neurosurgical departments of general hospitals in Lisbon. However, in view of the increased number of paraplegics and tetraplegics as the result of the combat in Angola, the Ministry of Defence is very anxious to start a proper spinal injuries centre, and Dr Carlos has segregated a ward for these casualties and other traumatic injuries of the spinal cord. There is also a well built hostel in Lisbon for the institutional care of Portuguese ex-servicemen.

SCANDINAVIAN COUNTRIES

There are no proper Spinal Injury units in any of the Scandinavian countries which can give paraplegics and tetraplegics a comprehensive treatment and rehabilitation from the start. In these countries there still exists the fragmentation of treatment and the initial and early treatment is carried out in neurosurgical or orthopaedic departments and patients are then transferred to General Rehabilitation Centres. Dr Bodil Eskesen of

Orthopaedisk Hospital, Copenhagen, Denmark, has taken particular interest in the long
term management of paraplegics and tetraplegics and has been particularly interested in
the development of sport of these patients who, in recent years, come regularly to the
International Stoke Mandeville Games, as do paraplegics from Finland, Norway and
Sweden.

SOUTH AFRICA

There are now several Spinal Injuries Centres in this large country to cope with the
steadily increasing problem of spinal cord affliction. When I visited South Africa in
1957 there was only one Spinal Injuries Unit established for comprehensive management,
that set up in 1955 under Dr R.Lipschitz, neurosurgeon, at the Baragwanath Hospital
outside Johannesburg, for coloured people only. At that time, the great majority of
spinal cord injuries were caused by stab wounds. In 1967, Lipschitz reported at the
annual meeting of the International Medical Society of Paraplegia on 252 stab wounds
of the spinal cord collected during a period of 12 years. During my recent visit in March
1969, the number of stab wound injuries in that unit had greatly diminished, and this
was the result of improved socio-economic conditions amongst the Africans living in and
around Johannesburg. The other large Spinal Injuries Centre was opened in 1963 by
the urologist Dr T.Retief and Dr A.Key at the Conradie Hospital, Cape Town, which
copes with all traumatic paraplegics and tetraplegics from the whole Cape Province,
which extends about 800 miles north and 1,000 miles east of Cape Town. Conradie is
a general hospital of single-storeyed bungalow type with a complement of 660 beds, very
suitable for the 120 wheelchair patients of the Spinal Centre. From its inception, this
Spinal Centre insisted on the immediate admission of patients and this has been achieved
by the ready co-operation of the Hospital Administration of the Cape Province. Dr Key,
who is now in charge of the Centre, has given an excellent survey of the first 300 new
cases of a total of 487 admissions between 1963 and 1967. The majority of new injuries
were admitted within 48 hours and 52 within a week. One hundred and five patients
from hospitals outside Cape Town were transferred by air. The ratio male to female was
9 : 1. Amongst the causes of spinal cord lesions, 70 (23) were due to stab wounds.
According to Dr Key's latest statistic (1971) this number has increased to 200 (see chapter
on Stab Wounds). The majority (135) were cervical injuries. The mortality rate by 1967
was 13 per cent. Two hundred and fifty-four were discharged, of these 219 to their
own homes and 29 to hostels. The Cape Town Spinal Centre has also organized a follow-
up service of its patients. Only those too far afield are supervised by the nearest provin-
cial hospital, general practitioner or district surgeon. There have been smaller Spinal
Injuries Units set up in South Africa in recent years: one at the Orthopaedic University
Clinic in Pretoria and one at the Hospital of the Gold Mines for African workers, most
of whom are re-employed as surface workers under sheltered conditions after completion
of their rehabilitation. Sport plays an important part in the rehabilitation and teams
have taken part in the Stoke Mandeville Games.

In 1975, the South African Government agreed to send a mixed racial team to the
1975 Olympics of the Paralysed. This was indeed the first breakthrough in sport in

the apartheid problem. During my recent visit to Capetown, I witnessed several basketball matches between mixed racial teams.

SPAIN

The first Spinal Injuries Centre in Spain (Instituto Guttmann) was founded in 1965 in Barcelona by Señor Gonzales, a former tetraplegic patient of Stoke Mandeville. This Centre has been set up in a dilapidated hospital for venereal diseases which was given rent free to Mr Gonzales by the Government and which had to be completely reconstructed for the purpose of an autonomous Spinal Injuries Centre. The medical director is Dr M.Sarrias Domingo, an orthopaedic surgeon and former trainee of Stoke Mandeville. The Centre is legally connected with the National Association of Civilian Invalids. The Centre has its own operating theatre, X-ray equipment, laboratory and all facilities for the immediate and long-term management, including educational and recreational facilities and sport. The Unit was started with 25 beds but has been gradually increased to 70 beds. The excellent work this Unit has been doing since its inception has no doubt stimulated other organizations in Spain to organize better facilities for the treatment of spinal cord afflictions. Small units have since been set up in Madrid and Toledo, another in the General Hospital at Barcelona and one recently in Valencia within a general Rehabilitation Centre. The Valencia unit, at present with 40 beds, is under the leadership of Dr V.Forner, one of my former co-workers. At the invitation of a committee set up by the Spanish Government, I advised in the setting up of a National Spinal Injury Hospital of 200 beds in Toledo, which was opened on the 7 October 1974 by Prince Carlos and Princess Sophia of Spain. This is a magnificent three-storey hospital of 200 beds with several lifts and no architectural barriers whatsoever. It has all facilities for a comprehensive management for the immediate and long term management of spinal paraplegics and tetraplegics, including vocational training and industrial resettlement and excellent indoor and outdoor sports facilities.

The Centre is connected with the City of Toledo by a specially constructed wide bridge over the river Tago. Dr Manuel Santz is the Administrator and Dr Vincente Forner, a former graduate of Stoke Mandeville, is in complete charge as the Director of the whole clinical treatment as well as social rehabilitation. His deputy is Dr Jose Mendoza.

SWITZERLAND

In 1957 I was asked by a Swiss Committee consisting of civilian as well as Army authorities, including members of the medical profession, to advise in the establishment of a Spinal Injuries Centre for a comprehensive management of paraplegics and tetraplegics, as it was realized how much such an institution was needed. Finally, it was decided to build this Centre in Basle, a German-speaking canton within the grounds of an institution for chronic invalids, called *Milchsuppe* (milk soup), as there already existed workshops and facilities for vocational training as well as for sheltered work. However, mainly due to financial difficulties, progress in the realization of the project was slow and it was not until June 1967 that this Centre was opened. However, the original idea that this Centre should admit traumatic paraplegics and tetraplegics immediately or in the early days after injury for comprehensive treatment and resettlement was not implemented, due to financial restrictions made by the Insurances concerned regarding immediate admission of the patients. Moreover, this Centre had a difficult start due also to friction between members of the medical staff and the lay administrator, which resulted in the resignation of two senior medical members, one of them the medical director of the Unit. Following investigations made by the governing authorities of Basle, Dr G.Zäch was appointed three years ago as the Medical Director and Dr W.Seiler as his Associate. Moreover, a new Administrator was appointed and they and their entire staff are doing excellent work.

The Spinal Centre in Basle, which is a National Centre is now doing excellent work in the immediate and long term management of spinal cord injuries. While the cost of maintenance has been mainly the responsibility of the Council of Basle, it is now certain that the 22 Cantons of Switzerland will contribute as the Basle Centre admits patients from all over Switzerland. Therefore the future of this Centre seems to be secure.

While the Spinal Unit at Basle was being planned and its construction started, the University Hospital 'Beau Sejour' in Geneva took the initiative in 1963 to set up its own Spinal Injuries Centre within the reorganized Department of Physical Medicine (Director Professor Fallet), which was opened in 1965 under the leadership of Dr A.Rossier, himself a traumatic paraplegic, to serve the French-speaking regions. Dr Rossier had part of his training at Stoke Mandeville. This unit started with 20 beds but has been enlarged to 40 beds to cope with the demand of other French-speaking cantons. Rossier (1967) has given details about his Unit. The Unit admits male and female patients at and over the age of 15 years and has all the facilities of the University Hospital at its disposal. Acute traumatic cord lesions are admitted to the Emergency Department of the hospital where they are seen immediately by the Director of the Spinal Unit in consultation with the neurosurgeon and where the necessary X-rays are taken. Provided that there are no specialized surgical or other procedures indicated, the patient is immediately admitted to the Spinal Unit, alternatively the patient is visited in any other specialized department by Dr Rossier at least twice daily and thus a continued observation of the patient from the start by the head of the Spinal Unit is guaranteed. Dr Rossier has carried out intensive research and published valuable papers on various problems concerned with paraplegia and has been made lecturer (Dozent) at the Medical Faculty of the University. Recently he has received a professorship in Spinal Cord Injuries and Social Medicine at Harvard University, Boston, U.S.A., and has been elected Director of the Spinal Unit at the V.A. Hospital, West Roxburg, as successor of Dr Talbot. His successor in Geneva is Dr H.Hachen who is also very active in research and has repeatedly reported results of his studies at the annual Scientific Meetings of the International Medical Society of Paraplegia. In recent years a closer relationship has developed between the Belgian, French, German and Swiss Spinal Units by holding meetings where mutual interests are discussed.

U.S.A.

Before the entry of the U.S.A. into the Second World War after Pearl Harbour, Donald Munro, former neurosurgeon at the City Hospital, Boston, Mass., made important and original contributions to the problem of spinal paraplegia. Although tidal drainage was originally introduced by Lover in 1917, at Guy's Hospital in England, it was Dr Munro who pioneered and developed this method for the initial treatment of the paralysed bladder, which became widely used, especially during the Second World War. Moreover, his method of anterior rhizotomy has been accepted by many neurosurgeons for the treatment of intractable spasticity. Munro always believed in the social rehabilitation of paraplegic patients and became a strong advocate of their social and industrial resettlement. In those years it was also Dr Deaver of the Institute for Cripples in New York who specialized in the physical rehabilitation of patients with spinal cord afflictions, especially polio victims.

In the U.S.A., it was the Veterans Administration of the Government which set up Spinal Units in 8 of their Veterans Hospitals. Bors (1967) has given an excellent survey of the development of his Centre at Long Beach, California, which had its origin in 1944–45 at the Hammon General Hospital at Modesto, Calif., and later at the Birmingham General Hospital in Van Nuys, Calif. Up to 1967, altogether 2,232 patients had passed through Bors' Unit, 2,073 of them with traumatic lesions of the spinal cord. Bors' views as an urologist towards the complex problem of spinal paralysis, based on such long experience, are absolutely identical with my own as a neurological surgeon. 'It is logical', he writes, 'that anyone, irrespective of his speciality, who wishes to serve these patients afflicted with a neurological disorder, should familiarize himself with the basic principles of neuroanatomy, neurophysiology and neurologic examination. . . . It also goes without saying that such a man will have to forgo some of his work connected with his original speciality, whether this was surgery, medicine or their respective sub-specialities, physical medicine, psychiatry, neurological surgery or neurology, because that physician will have to devote his attention to all aspects of a patient whose requirements are multi-disciplinary.' Following Dr Bors' retirement his associate for many years, Dr E.Commar became director of the Long Beach Centre and after his retirement Dr Metha is in charge of the Centre. The other two larger V.A. Spinal Injuries Centres are that at Hines V.A. Hospital, Chicago, and, especially, that at West Roxbury, Mass., until recently under the leadership of Dr H.Talbot, a urological surgeon who, like Bors and Commar, has been a pioneer in the urological aspects of paraplegia. He was elected Professor at Harvard University.

The Spinal Injuries Centres of the Veterans Administration in U.S.A. are still confronted with serious disadvantages. They are restricted to spinal cord injured patients who are or have been members of the Armed Forces. Moreover, the vast majority, if not all of these patients are not admitted immediately after onset of paraplegia or tetraplegia to receive a comprehensive treatment from the start but are transferred at later stages from hospitals concerned with their initial treatments, consisting of immediate or early laminectomy or fusions as methods of choice, while the all-important initial management of the paralysed bladder or the prevention of pressure sores are not fully understood or are even neglected. The patients are transferred after weeks or months to the Spinal Injuries Centres of the V.A., often with serious complications, especially of the urinary tract, for 'rehabilitation'. Only recently, a detailed account of this unsatisfactory state of affairs resulting from such dichotomy of management has been given by Jacobson & Bors (1970) concerning war casualties of spinal cord lesions from the Vietnamese Combat. Civilian patients with spinal cord afflictions, including traumatic lesions, are treated in private hospitals mainly by neurosurgeons or orthopaedic surgeons and later in general Rehabilitation Centres, and there is indeed a great shortage of proper Spinal Injuries Centres for civilians in the U.S.A. This has been realized by leading members of the medical profession and the House of Representatives of the U.S.A., and it is significant that an outstanding surgical society such as the Cushing Society of the American Neurosurgeons, at their Congress in Chicago, 1967, passed a resolution urging the Government and Congress to establish Spinal Injuries Centres for civilians. Efforts are recently being made by the authorities concerned to set up regional Spinal Centres for civilians, and the first of this kind has been set up at Phoenix under Dr J.Young and Dr D.Cheshire has joined him recently as director of research. Dr Young who formerly was director of the Craig Rehabilitation Centre in Denver (Ohio), is very determined to develop a comprehensive management of paraplegics and tetraplegics from the start and throughout all stages in his Centre. Other Regional Spinal Injuries Centres are being set up.

Sport amongst paraplegics in U.S.A. has been practised since 1947, first almost exclusively in basketball, and the U.S.A. teams have excelled themselves by their skill in this sport at the Stoke Mandeville Games for many years. Gradually they also have included many other events in their sports and Mr Ben Lipton of the Bulova Industrial Training Centre for watch-making, New York, has played a leading part in the development of sport for paraplegics.

YUGOSLAVIA

In 1971 I attended a Congress on Sport for the Disabled in Belgrad where one of the main topics was spinal paraplegia. Ever since, the interest in a comprehensive management of spinal cord injuries has increased in this country and, in particular, Professor Grobelnik and Dr R.Turk are engaged in their Rehabilitation Centre particularly with spinal cord injuries. Teams of Yugoslav paraplegics have taken part in the International Stoke Mandeville Games in recent years.

CHAPTER 5

DEVELOPMENT OF OTHER SPINAL
INJURIES CENTRES
3. PROBLEMS IN DEVELOPING COUNTRIES

AFRICA

In contrast to the United Kingdom, the European Continent, America, Australia and South Africa where trauma plays a very essential part causing spinal cord lesions, in tropical Africa and also Asia infectious conditions such as tuberculosis of the spine, polio and transverse myelitis represented until recently the major causes. Most surgeons took still a very defeatest attitude toward the traumatic paraplegics, let alone tetraplegics. It was significant that at the first Symposium on Rehabilitation in Africa at Kampala (Uganda) in March 1964 A.Roper, from Bulawayo, Rhodesia, made the following statement: 'The surgeon, faced with the request from another hospital to accept two patients of the same age, one with Pott's paraplegia, the other with traumatic paraplegia, must accept the former.' At the same meeting, J.Golding, from Kingston, Jamaica, pointed out: 'In my view, a complete cervical lesion, showing no signs of improvement by three weeks, is best sent home.' Both surgeons considered a special centre for the rehabilitation of these patients unnecessary, Roper even as 'luxury'. However, with the increase of traumatic spinal cord lesions in African countries, as a result of increase of industrialization and motorized vehicles, the attitude of members of the medical and para-medical professions is changing, and the discussions at the second (Addis Ababa, 1966) and third African conferences on rehabilitation (Lusaka, 1968) sponsored, like the first, by the British National Fund for Research into Crippling Diseases under the leadership of Mr Duncan Guthrie showed that the establishment of Spinal Units where patients suffering from traumatic and non-traumatic lesion could be congregated for comprehensive treatment and social resettlement, far from being a luxury was an increasing necessity. D.Wilson (1966) reported in Addis Ababa about his experience at the Institute Medical Evangelique, Kimpisa in Congo Central Province, on 47 spinal cord lesions, 23 of whom were due to accidents, amongst them 4 cervicals. Five were caused by road accidents, while in the majority (13) falls from palm trees were the cause. Two of the non-traumatic and 3 of the traumatic lesions (2 tetraplegics) died. To meet the needs of these patients who could not return to their own villages the building of a 'Paraplegic Village' in the vicinity of the hospital was planned. At the third African Conference, held in 1968 in Lusaka (Zambia), the subject of spinal cord injuries was one of the main topics of the discussions, which revealed the growing interest in this problem.

KENYA

A small Spinal Unit was set up at Nairobi due to the efforts of Mr John Britton, himself a paraplegic and former member of the English Paraplegic Sports Association. This

Unit is supported by the Kenyan Government. Following Mr Britton's departure to U.S.A., Mrs Dorothy Hughes is in charge of the Unit and small teams of paraplegics have taken part in the International Stoke Mandeville Games in recent years.

UGANDA

There is no Spinal Injuries Unit in this country, but the Orthopaedic Surgeon, Professor Huckstep, has done great pioneer work in the treatment of polio victims, and has con-gregated in an annexe of his department, polios with the most grotesque deformities one can imagine, who were sent to him following neglect and inefficient treatment. Following my visit to his hospital of Makerere University at Kampala, he sent nursing personnel to Stoke Mandeville for training and care of traumatic paraplegia and tetra-plegia. A small paraplegic team took part in 1971 and 1972 International Stoke Mandeville Games. Unfortunately, Professor Huckstep left Uganda to become Professor of Ortho-paedic Surgery in Sydney, Australia. It remains to be seen whether his work for spinal cord victims, both medical and traumatic lesions, will be continued.

In Ethiopia, Kenya and Zambia, leading members of the medical profession and administrative authorities have become more and more aware of the need to establish specialized units for a comprehensive treatment and social resettlement of both trau-matic and non-traumatic spinal cord lesions at present scattered in orthopaedic or general surgical departments. However, judging from personal observations and in view of the political unrest and financial and economic difficulties in some of these countries, it will take a very long time for a satisfactory solution of this problem. However, Kenya has made a beginning through the activity of Mr John Britton, a paraplegic himself and one of the outstanding paraplegic sportsmen in England. Following his visit to Kenya and negotiations with the Kenyan Government and the Cheshire Home, a spinal unit of 40 beds is being set up by the Kenyan Government for a comprehensive management of paraplegics and tetraplegics. This unit will also be provided with a hostel for those patients who, for one reason or another, cannot return to their homes. Kenya was represented at the 1972 International Stoke Mandeville Games in Heidelberg.

HONG KONG

A small Spinal Unit has been set up in 1965 at the Grantham Hospital, which originally was designated for patients suffering from tuberculosis of bones and joints. Since 1965, 28 paraplegics and tetraplegics due to other causes as well as 30 victims of tuberculosis of the spine were treated there. At any one time, the unit was occupied by 20–24 patients. This unit suffers from the fact that owing to the shortage of doctors in Hong Kong there is no leader to organize and supervise a comprehensive management of these patients (Miss Sheila Iu, 1968). Recently, a closer relationship has been established for the training of medical and para-medical personnel between Grantham Hospital and the units of Dr Bedbrook in Perth and Dr Cheshire in Melbourne, Australia. During my last visit to Hong Kong in 1971 I was pleased to learn that the setting up of two spinal units is contemplated. In the meantime, sport for paraplegics has been organized and

Hong Kong has been represented in increasing numbers at the International Stoke Mandeville Games. Recently, a Spinal Injury Unit has been set up in Kowloon and the Medical Officer in charge was sent to Lodge Moor Spinal Unit, Sheffield and Stoke Mandeville to be trained in our methods.

INDIA

In recent years, progress in dealing constructively with the ever increasing problem of spinal paraplegia has been made in various parts of this huge sub-continent, where many other medical and social problems for the disabled and able-bodied alike are so pressing. At the Military Hospital in Poona, a Spinal Centre of 40 beds has been set up under the leadership of Lt.Col. Chahal. This Unit has done excellent work during the war with Pakistan. Lt.Col. Chahal had some specialized training at Perth Spinal Centre, Western Australia. He reported about the work of his Unit at the 1974 Annual Scientific Meeting of the International Medical Society of Paraplegia. Recently, a hostel has been set up for those paralysed people who cannot go home.

A small Spinal Unit has been set up at the Department of Traumatic and Orthopaedic Surgery in the J.J. Hospital, Bombay under Dr K.S.Masalawala, which I opened in 1969. Dr Masalawala reported about the first 60 cases at the 1974 Scientific Meeting of the Society.

Another Spinal Centre has been set up at the Orthopaedic Hospital of the Medical College in Lucknow. There, Dr S.Varma, a former Registrar of Stoke Mandeville, has been in charge for several years and is doing an excellent work under primitive conditions. However, it is hoped that better accommodation will be built for the Unit.

Sport amongst paraplegics in India has no doubt promoted public interest in these severely disabled, as it has done in other countries, and India has already been three times represented in the Olympics for the Paralysed.

MALAYSIA

At the request of the Foreign and Commonwealth Office and the invitation of the Malaysian Government in 1973, I spent several weeks in Malaysia to advise the Malaysian Government in the setting up of a National Spinal Injuries Centre. I visited Kuala Lumpur, Ipoh, Penang and Kota Bharu to study conditions regarding spinal cord injuries in that huge country. Following discussions with the authorities of the Ministry of Health, it was decided to build a National Spinal Injuries Centre of 100 beds with all clinical, surgical and training facilities as part of a new hospital to be set up in the South of Kuala Lumpur.

INDONESIA

At the 4th Pan Pacific Rehabilitation Conference at Hong Kong in 1958, the late Dr R.Soeharso gave a report about paraplegic care in Indonesia. Although his Rehabilitation Centre was already set up in 1951, it was not, as he pointed out, until 1963 that the interest in paraplegia led to the opening of a special ward for paraplegics. However, there were still great limitations in the services that could be offered. Only selected cases of paraplegia could be accepted, namely those who still had bladder control and were free from sores. From Dr Soeharso's report, it is difficult to assess the present standard of that unit, and it would appear that the management of complete paraplegics, let alone tetraplegics, is still far from satisfactory. This may apply to the prevention and treatment of infection of the urinary tract, the problem of pressure sores and the prevention and treatment of contractures. It is significant of this unsatisfactory situation that Soeharso did not 'hesitate to advise bilateral above-knee amputation in cases of fixed deformities of joints and bad health (decubitus etc.)'. At least a special home for paraplegics has been established, which offers sheltered work and living quarters for those patients who otherwise would not survive in their village homes.

Dr G.Bedbrook has recently been asked by the Indonesian Government to advise, in the setting up of a Spinal Injuries Centre in Jakarta and the first ward of eight patients has been formed at Fatmawati Hospital. The medical and nursing staff was trained at Perth Spinal Centre.

PAKISTAN

When I visited this country in 1953, at the request of the Pakistani Government and the World Veterans Federation, to investigate the facilities for rehabilitation in the Military Cantonments, paraplegic ex-servicemen were congregated in a hostel of the Red Cross in Sialkot. Their conditions were most unsatisfactory and they lived in a ward without any incentive for an active life, although there were already good facilities for the social re-integration of amputees. The condition of the few civilian paraplegics I saw at Jinnah Hospital in Karachi was quite hopeless. At that time, the country had still to cope with the resettlement of several millions of refugees from India. Conditions have considerably changed since, and Jinnah Hospital, which I visited in 1968, is well equipped for a Spinal Injuries Unit, which has been established as part of the Orthopaedic Department. Professor Kazi and Dr Kermani are very anxious to increase the unit under its own director, as the number of paraplegics is increasing from year to year due to increasing industrialization and road accidents. The problem of spinal cord injuries will no doubt have considerably increased during the latest conflict with India.

SOUTH KOREA

There is little known of the treatment and care of civilian paraplegics in Korea. However, the Veteran Administration in Seoul has made considerable progress in the rehabilitation of ex-servicemen. They are well trained in sport and a Korean team has taken part in the International Stoke Mandeville Games in increasing numbers during the last few years.

CHAPTER 6
CONCLUSIONS

During the last 21 years, I visited 46 countries, some of them several times, at the invitation of governments, universities and various organizations to study the problem of paraplegia in the respective countries and advise in the management of these patients. From all my observations, some of which are now recorded in this book, the following conclusions may be made:

1 There is no doubt that today spinal paraplegia and tetraplegia are a world-wide problem. It is no longer a medical problem alone but has developed also into a social problem, increasing in size from year to year in all countries of the world, including the so-called developing countries. One can already foresee that in 15–20 years at the latest spinal paraplegia will be one of the major social problems of disablement.

2 The advances made in the medical and social rehabilitation of spinal cord sufferers from injuries and diseases during the last 25 years is mainly due to the congregation of these patients in Spinal Injuries Units under a specialist staff. By far the most favourable results have been achieved in those Centres with their own director in charge, prepared to forgo some of his original speciality for the multi-disciplinary speciality of spinal paraplegia, which should have an equal status to that of any other sub-speciality of medicine and surgery, such as chest, opthalmology, E.N.T., dermatology, etc.

3 The fragmentation of the management of the spinal paraplegic and tetraplegic into immediate, intermediate treatment and the long-term physical, psychological and social readjustment including domestic and professional or industrial resettlement, called rehabilitation, has, as a rule, proved unsatisfactory, and from all that I have seen in many countries often disastrous. For, those who advocated such fragmentation were—and, alas, still are—concerned only with the treatment of some special procedures in which they are skilled but on the other hand overlook and even neglect other vital aspects in the immediate and early treatment of these patients, in particular the proper care of the paralysed bladder. Only in those hospitals where the spinal specialist himself has no surgical facilities but has access to and control of the whole management of these patients from the start, have satisfactory results been achieved. In this respect, the Spinal Centres at Heidelberg in Germany and Geneva in Switzerland can be quoted as excellent examples.

4 It is of lesser importance whether a Spinal Injuries Centre is established as part of a General Hospital, Accident Hospital or other specialized departments such as Ortho-paedic, Neurological, Neurosurgical, Urological Units or General Rehabilitation Centre, or built as an autonomous centre such as those in Ostia-Rome, Barcelona and Toledo, Spain. The vital point is that a Spinal Injuries Centre must have its own director who is familiar with all aspects of this complex problem of spinal paraplegia and can co-ordinate the work of his whole team, as is done in any other speciality.

5 Amongst the various facilities necessary for a comprehensive management from the start and throughout all stages, the provision of an operating theatre, facilities especially

for urological diagnoses and treatment, X-ray facilities, adequate provisions for physio-therapy, work-therapy and sport are the most important necessities.

6 The size of a Spinal Injuries Centre has been under discussion for some time. In particular, it was feared that a Spinal Centre of larger size in a general hospital might be a hindrance to the development of other specialities. The Stoke Mandeville Centre has proved, beyond any shadow of doubt, that a centre, even of its large size which, as a national institution, served the whole country for many years, has been no detriment to the development of other medical or surgical specialities. On the contrary, for those specialities serving the local or regional population, such as medical, surgical, rheumatic, paediatric, plastic surgery, geriatric units, etc., the existence of the Spinal Centre, far from being a hindrance, has afforded facilities which these units have been able to utilize most advantageously for their own purposes. On the other hand, the spinal centre, as any other unit, has been using the facilities of the general hospital, such as X-ray department, operating theatre, pathology laboratory, etc., and has enjoyed throughout the years a close co-operation with the consultants of other units who have been readily available when the need arose. Therefore, from all our experience, it can be concluded that the setting-up of a spinal centre in a general hospital, as a speciality of its own, represents at least one satisfactory solution.

From all my experience gained during my visits to so many countries in all parts of the world, I have come to the conclusion that for industrialized countries the most economical size of a Spinal Injuries Centre, equipped with all facilities for a comprehensive manage-ment of paraplegics and tetraplegics through their acute and later stages, should be at least 50 beds, divided for men, women and children. This figure should not be taken dogmatically and, whatever the initial number of beds for the start may be, provision should be made immediately for a final complement of 100 beds.

7 A Spinal Centre should be attached to, or at least work in close co-operation with, a Teaching Hospital of a University and should take part in the training of undergraduate and post-graduate medical and para-medical personnel. This is the best guarantee to disseminate understanding and knowledge of the whole complex problem amongst the medical and paramedical professions.

8 The establishment of a hostel in the neighbourhood of the centre, equipped with a sheltered workshop, is essential for the accommodation of tetraplegics and paraplegics, who for one reason or another are unable to return to their own homes. This is of parti-cular importance for the developing countries, where the return of spinal paraplegics, let alone tetraplegics, to their villages in the bush following successful rehabilitation in hospital usually means immediate deterioration and early death, thus wasting all the public money which was spent for the rehabilitation of the paralysed, quite apart from the humanitarian aspect. The establishment of a 'Flying Doctor' service which has proved to be very successful in Australia and Ireland for transferring to the Centre acute traumatic paraplegics and tetraplegics from the place of accident or hospitals which are not equipped for their treatment, is indeed highly recommendable, as this will obviate early complications such as infection of the paralysed bladder and the development of pressure sores which occur so very often in hospitals lacking in knowledge and facilities for a comprehensive treatment of these complicated patients.

9 There is still a great need for research on many aspects of paraplegia and tetraplegia. Therefore, a Spinal Injuries Centre should be provided with proper facilities in this respect.

10 Every Spinal Centre should be provided with adequate facilities for an outpatient- and after-care service. In the latter domiciliary visits to former in-patients of the Centre by a medical member and welfare officer of the staff of the Centre to study the home conditions should be included, as these can be of immense value for assessment and proper records as well as of help to the patients.

11 A Spinal Injuries Centre should be attached wherever possible to a University and should take part in the teaching of medical students and post graduates. The Director of the Unit should be entitled to receive a Professorship in the same way as leaders of other specialities. In this respect the Universities of Harvard, at Boston, Heidelberg and Brussels are shining examples.

12 The recognition by Governmental Health Authorities of spinal paraplegia and tetraplegia as a specialty in its own right is really overdue having regard to the important part it plays today in the field of medicine. This would be not only a great help to those presently engaged in this complex problem of medicine, surgery and social medicine, but an incentive to younger members of the medical profession to take up this specialty as their career.

B · Anatomy, Neuropathology and Regeneration

CHAPTER 7

ANATOMICAL DATA ON VERTEBRAL COLUMN AND SPINAL CORD

Most textbooks on anatomy and histology deal adequately with the structures of the vertebral column as well as with the basic structures of the spinal cord, and textbooks on anatomy such as Gray's, Sobotta–Becher, Braus and Rauber–Kopsch's are easily accessible. Readers who wish to study more details of the vertebral structures are referred to the textbooks of Fick (1911), Hovelaque (1937), Lob (1954), Brocher (1955), Schlüter (1964) and Schmorl & Junghanns (1968). Those who are interested in detailed neuro-anatomical and histological research on the spinal cord are referred to the comprehensive review of Pollack (1935), and the work of Romanes (1951, 1965) and Balthasar (1952).

Neuro-histology developed as a special branch of anatomy since Clarke (1851) and Stilling (1857) gave detailed description of the nucleus in the medial portion of the posterior horn, named ever since the Clarke–Stilling column. During the nineteenth and twentieth centuries a great deal of information on neuro-histology has accumulated and the reader is particularly referred to the pioneer work of men such as Golgi (1886), His (1893), Cajal (1895–1935), Nissl (1903), Hortega (1920, 1932) and Spielmeier (1922). Moreover, in recent years electron-microscopy has greatly advanced our knowledge of the highly organized and detailed morphological structures of synapses and intracellular structures of ganglion cells of the spinal cord. The time has passed when the spinal cord was called in anatomical textbooks 'the simplest and most primitive part of the nervous system'.

The present account is confined to anatomical data related especially to the clinical and anatomical pathology of the spinal cord.

VERTEBRAL COLUMN

The vertebral column represents an elastic and flexible bony structure consisting of 24 independent vertebrae—7 cervical, 12 thoracic and 5 lumbar—which although firmly connected by articulations and ligaments allow a limited amount of movement on one another. The elastic quality of the vertebral column is secured by the cartilaginous intervertebral discs interposed between two neighbouring vertebrae. There are no inter-vertebral discs between atlas and axis, the first being between 2nd and 3rd cervical

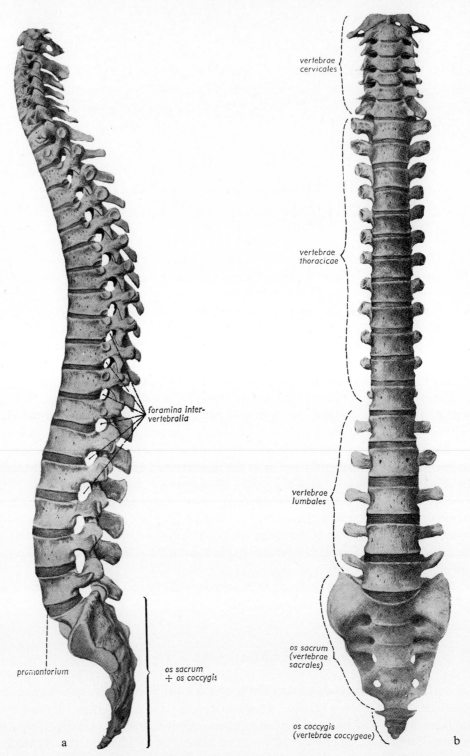

vertebrae
cervicales

vertebrae
thoracicae

foramina inter-
vertebralia

vertebrae
lumbales

os sacrum
(vertebrae
sacrales)

promontorium

os sacrum
+ os coccygis

os coccygis
(vertebrae coccygeae)

a   b

FIG. 10. Vertebral column (lateral and ventral) from *Atlas der Anatomy* (Sobotta–Becher)
Part I, 16th Edition, Munich–Berlin–Wien 1967.

vertebrae and the last between 5th lumbar vertebra and sacrum. Altogether there are 23 intervertebral discs. The vertebral column showing ventral convex curves in the cervical and lumbar regions and a concave curve in the thorax region is connected cephalad through the atlas with the skull and caudal through the 5th lumbar vertebra with the os sacrum which is provided with 5 vertebrae and which in turn is connected with the 4 vertebrae of the os coccyx (Figs. 10a and b). Fig. 10a shows the foramina interverte-bralia, the most proximal between the 2nd and 3rd cervical vertebrae, the most distal between the 5th lumbar vertebra and sacrum. There is one intervertebral foramen on each side between two neighbouring vertebrae providing the communication of the spinal nerves and vessels with the spinal cord and its meninges.

The individual vertebrae consist of the anterior part, the vertebral body, and the posterior part, the vertebral arch consisting of a pair of pedicles and a pair of laminae and is provided with seven processes—four articular, two transverse and one spinous process. The vertebral bodies and arches form the vertebral canal which contains and protects the spinal cord. In the thoracic region each rib of the thoracic cage also forms an essential part of each vertebral arch.

There are two superior and two inferior articular processes which arise from the junction of the laminae and pedicles and are in contact with the corresponding processes of the adjacent vertebrae. Their function is to control and restrict the range of vertebral movement.

The transverse processes spring laterally from the junctions of the pedicles and laminae. They provide the attachment of ligaments and muscles and while, in the thoracic region they limit the movements of the ribs, they act as a fulcrum for lateral and rotatory movements of the vertebrae in the other regions.

The spinous processes originating from the junction of the laminae and projecting in backward and downward directions also serve the attachments of ligaments and muscles.

There are great variations in size, shape and direction of the individual vertebrae in accordance with their functions as levers of extension, flexion and rotatory movements in the various regions of the vertebral column. Figs. 11–16 demonstrate the main varieties of vertebrae at various levels of the spine.

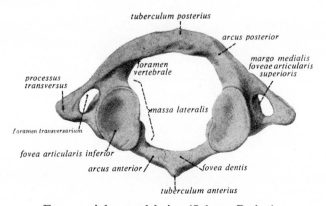

FIG. 11. Atlas, caudal view (Sobotta–Becher).

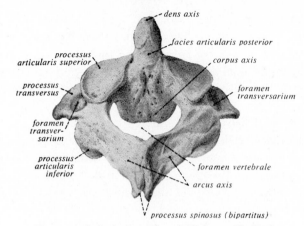

FIG. 12. Axis (epistropheus) (Sobotta–Becher).

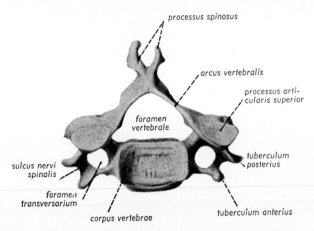

FIG. 13. 7th cervical vertebra (cranial view) (Sobotta–Becher).

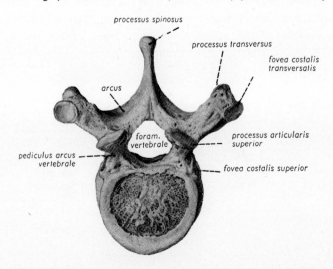

FIG. 14. 6th phoracic vertebra (cranial view) (Sobotta–Becher).

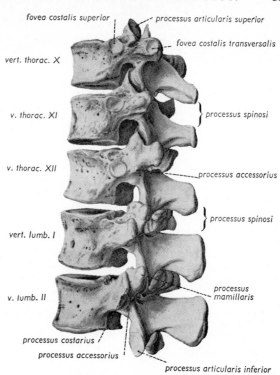

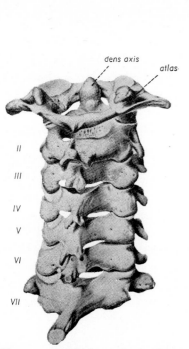

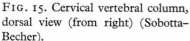

FIG. 15. Cervical vertebral column, dorsal view (from right) (Sobotta–Becher).

FIG. 16. The three caudal thoracic and two upper lumbar vertebrae (lateral view) (Sobotta–Becher).

It is beyond the scope of this book to describe in detail the congenital abnormalities of the vertebral column but some of them, relevant to the effects of spinal injuries may be mentioned here (see also later). The number of vertebrae may vary, and it is not uncommon to find six lumbar vertebrae and, on the other hand, a sacralization of the 5th lumbar vertebra which may be bilateral or unilateral. Assimilation of the atlas with the base of the skull is relatively rare. There are also anomalies of the ribs, and the most well known are the 13th rib connected with the 1st lumbar vertebra and the super-numery rib of the 7th cervical vertebra or an enlargement of the tuberculum anterius of that vertebra. Another common anomaly is the spina bifida of the 5th lumbar and 1st sacral vertebrae which may appear as spina bifida occulta, as a congenital defect without herniation of neural tissue or meninges, or another form of vertebral defect, spina bifida cystica, associated with external swelling containing spinal cord tissue and meninges. Butterfly forms of congenital vertebral anomalies have been reported by Frets (1911) and Junghanns (1968).

INTERVERTEBRAL DISCS

The intervertebral discs, closely coherent to the anterior and posterior longitudinal ligaments, form the chief connection of the vertebrae. They consist of a central nodular fluid matrix containing collagen fibrils, the nucleus pulposus. At birth, it is soft and gelatinous and consists of mucoid material, but by the end of the first decade a gradual replacement of the mucoid material takes place by fibrocartilage originating from the annulus fibrosis and from the covering cartilagenous plates of the upper and lower surfaces of the vertebrae (Walmsley, 1950; Tondury, 1958). Its differentiation from the annulus fibrosis is then less distinct and in due course it becomes amorphous and loses its elasticity (Püschel, 1930). Although the anatomy of the intervertebral discs was known for many centuries it is only during the last 40 years or so that their importance in the pathology of the spine in relation to the pathology of the spinal cord and spinal roots has been appreciated (Schmorl, 1927–32; Galland, 1930; Mixter & Barr, 1934; Bradford & Spurling, 1945; Armstrong, 1957; and Frykholm, 1970).

The shape of the intervertebral discs is adapted to that of the vertebral bodies but its thickness varies. While their thickness is fairly uniform in the thoracic region it is increased in the cervical and lumbar regions, more anteriorly and posteriorly so that the nucleus pulposus lies eccentrically and more close to the posterior longitudinal ligament. Therefore, it is exposed to stresses such as distortion and tearing caused by fractures and dislocations of vertebral bodies but also by occupational stress, lifting and carrying of heavy weights, sportive activities, etc.

The discs are avascular apart from the supply of their peripheral parts from adjacent blood vessels and they receive their nutrition from the spongy bone of the upper and lower surface of the vertebrae.

LIGAMENTS

Figs. 17 and 18 demonstrate the ligamentous connections of the vertebrae. The most important ligaments are the anterior and posterior longitudinal ligaments and the

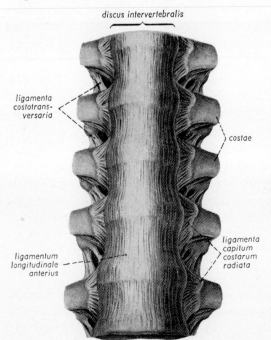

discus intervertebralis

ligamenta costotrans-versaria

costae

ligamentum longitudinale anterius

ligamenta capitum costarum radiata

FIG. 17. Ligaments of the caudal part of the thoracic column with ribs, ventral view (ligamentum longitudinalis anterius) (Sobotta-Becher).

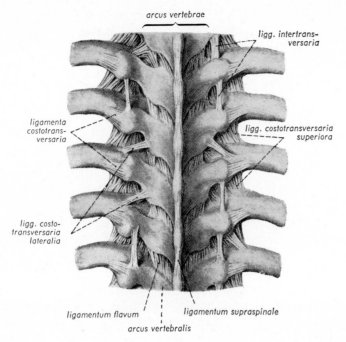

FIG. 18. Ligaments of the middle and caudal thoracic vertebrae and ribs (dorsal view) (Sobotta–Becher).

ligamenta flava. The anterior longitudinal ligament, beginning at the tuberculum anterius of the atlas and consisting of longitudinal fibres, is firmly fixed to the anterior surface of the vertebral bodies and intervertebral discs and ends at the sacrum. Its attachment to the vertebrae is more firm on the upper and lower anterior surfaces of the vertebrae than on the middle part (Fig. 17).

The posterior longitudinal ligament is fixed on the posterior surfaces of the vertebral bodies within the spinal canal and its attachments reach cranially the axis and caudally the sacrum and, as mentioned before, they also connect with the intervertebral discs.

The ligamenta flava, consisting of yellow elastic fibres, connect the laminae of adjacent vertebrae, being attached to the lower margin of the anterior surface of the superior lamina and to the posterior surface of the upper margin of the inferior lamina of the vertebrae. Through their attachments they control the movements of the vertebrae and prevent excessive flexion.

Other components of the ligamentous complex of the spine are the ligamentum nuchae which extends from the external protuberance of the skull to the 7th cervical vertebra, furthermore, the supraspinous and interspinous ligaments, which are connected with the spinous processes, while the intertransverse ligaments interposed between the transverse processes are connected with the deep back muscles and the ligamenta costotransversaria (Fig. 19).

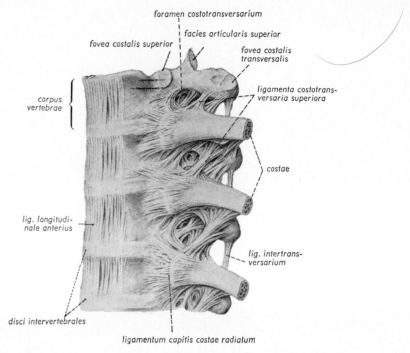

foramen costotransversarium

facies articularis superior

fovea costalis superior

fovea costalis transversalis

corpus vertebrae

ligamenta costotransversaria superiora

costae

lig. longitudinale anterius

lig. intertransversarium

disci intervertebrales

ligamentum capitis costae radiatum

FIG. 19. Ligaments of the middle and caudal thoracic vertebrae and ribs (lateral view) (Sobotta–Becher).

MUSCULAR ATTACHMENT TO THE SPINE

The muscles of the trunk are not only essential to restore the upright position and for the readjustment of postural sensibility in the paraplegic (see chapter on Sensibility), but their attachments on the vertebral column is vital in securing the normal configuration of the spine and in preventing deformities such as scoliosis and kyphosis. Therefore, it is essential to keep these muscle groups of the trunk attached to the spine in the best possible condition, following traumatic lesions of the spinal cord resulting from fractures and fracture-dislocations of the spine. Their additional damage must be avoided which may result from local pressure from plaster casts and plaster beds, or hasty and indiscriminate operative procedures; for the impact of the original violence to the vertebral column at the time of injury always results also in damage of these muscles at the site of bone injury.

The trunk muscles, which are attached to the vertebral column either directly or through their fasciae, can be divided into superficial and deep groups. The superficial group includes splenius capitis, rhomboidei, trapezius, latissimus dorsi and serratus posterior, while the deep or intrinsic muscles of the back include the erector spinae (sacrospinalis) with its upward continuation to the thoracic and cervical regions, furthermore, semispinalis, interspinalis, transverse-spinalis, multifidus, intertransversaria

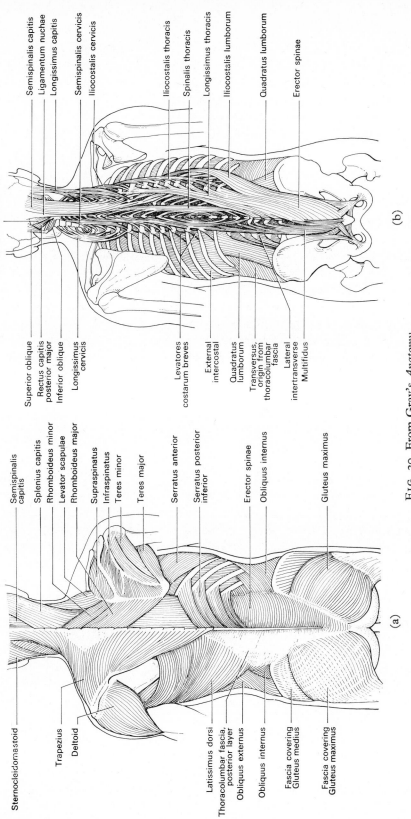

Sternocleidomastoid

Semispinalis capitis
Splenius capitis
Rhomboideus minor
Levator scapulae
Rhomboideus major

Supraspinatus
Infraspinatus
Teres minor

Teres major

Serratus anterior

Serratus posterior inferior

Erector spinae

Obliquus internus

Gluteus maximus

Trapezius

Deltoid

Latissimus dorsi

Thoracolumbar fascia, posterior layer
Obliquus externus

Obliquus internus

Fascia covering Gluteus medius

Fascia covering Gluteus maximus

(a)

Rectus capitis posterior minor

Semispinalis capitis
Ligamentum nuchae
Longissimus capitis

Semispinalis cervicis
Iliocostalis cervicis

Iliocostalis thoracis

Spinalis thoracis

Longissimus thoracis

Iliocostalis lumborum

Quadratus lumborum

Erector spinae

Superior oblique
Rectus capitis posterior major
Inferior oblique
Longissimus cervicis

Levatores costarum breves

External intercostal

Quadratus lumborum

Transversus, origin from thoracolumbar fascia

Lateral intertransverse

Multifidus

(b)

FIG. 20. From Gray's *Anatomy*.

rotatores and quadratus lumborum. The position of all these muscles and their relationship to the spine is comparable to struts on the mast of a ship or inserted in framework to bear weight, pressure and other stresses, in the direction of its length. Their relationship and attachment to the spine is best demonstrated in two excellent preparations, published in Gray's *Anatomy*, and may serve as a constant reminder to all concerned with the initial treatment and physical readjustment of paraplegics and tetraplegics (Fig. 20a and b).

SPINAL CORD

External structure

The spinal cord, medulla spinalis, is the caudal continuation of the oblongata and extends distally from the level between occiput and upper border of the atlas to the lower border of the first or upper border of the second lumbar vertebra. In length it is about 45 cm in the male and 42 cm in the female and is divided into cervical, thoracic and lumbar regions. The cord contains two enlargements:
1 the cervical enlargement (intumescentia cervicalis) extending from C3 to T2, the largest circumference being at the level of C5/6;
2 the lumbar enlargement (intumescentia lumbalis) which extends from T10 to T12 tapering down into the conus terminalis from which the filum terminale descends to the periost of the 2nd segment of the coccyx.

Spinal nerve roots

Thirty-one pairs of spinal roots spring from the spinal cord, divided into anterior and posterior roots: 8 cervical, 12 thoracic, 5 lumbar, 5 sacral and 1 coccygeal nerve. While the upper cervical roots run almost horizontally to enter their respective intervertebral foramina, the roots of the other regions take a more oblique downwards course, and in the lumbar region they run almost vertically forming the cauda equina around the filum terminale. Thus C1 and C2 segments lie beneath spinous process C1, and C3 segment beneath C2 spinous process. As a result of the longer course the successive spinal roots take caudalwards to enter their respective intervertebral foramina Th1 segment is in alignment with spinous process C6, L1 segment with spinous process Th12 and S1 segment with Th12 process. The knowledge of these anatomical facts is essential for the clinical diagnosis and surgical treatment of pathological processes, in particular tumours. Each anterior root joins the corresponding posterior root distally from the spinal ganglion of the latter, forming the spinal nerve. Fig. 21 shows the topographic relationship of the spinal cord segments, spinal roots to the individual spinous processes and vertebral bodies.

The anterior roots conduct all efferent fibres for the innervation of the skeletal muscles and through the pre-ganglionic sympathetic fibres for the autonomic system, while the posterior roots consist of afferent fibres. With regard to the problem of efferent fibres running in the posterior roots see section of Vasomotor Control.

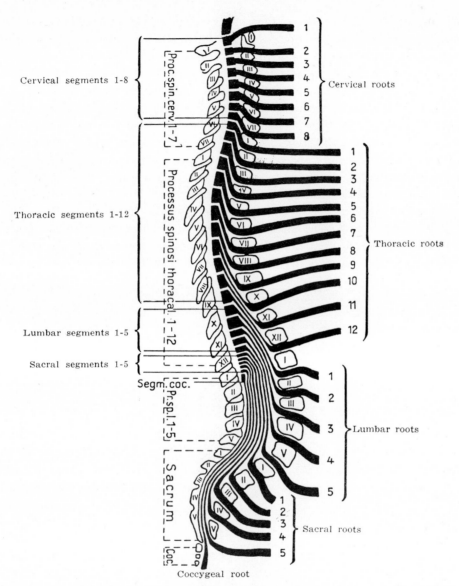

FIG. 21. Topographical correlation between spinal cord segments and vertebral bodies, spinous processes, and intervertebral foramina. From Bing–Haymaker's *Local Diagnosis* in *Neurological Diseases*.

Meninges

The spinal cord is protected by three layers of covers: Dura mater, Arachnoidea and Pia.

The spinal dura mater is the continuation of the inner layer of the cerebral dura, the outer layer of which ceases at the foramen magnum and is replaced by the periosteum lining the vertebral canal. It is separated from the spinal dura mater by the extradural space containing fat and a venous network. The dura also envelopes the spinal roots, spinal ganglia and the spinal nerves themselves as they pass through the foramina inter-vertebralia. The dura consists of dense fibrous tissue, and in contrast to the cerebral dura has little vascular supply. The dura ends in a sack at the level of the 2nd or 3rd sacral vertebrae forming the filum durae matris spinalis.

The arachnoidea which is a continuation of the cerebral arachnoid is a delicate, cobweb-like membrane consisting of fine elastic fibrous tissue and containing vessels of varying size which can be large enough to be damaged by lumbar or cysternal punctures resulting in more or less extensive haemorrhage. The interspace between the surface of the spinal cord and the dura mater (cavum subdurale) is filled with the cerebro-spinal fluid circulating within the space formed by arachnoid and pia. With regard to the mechanics and dynamics of the cerebro-spinal fluid the reader is referred to the writer's monograph, published in Vol. VII (2) pages 1–114 of the *Handbuch der Neurologie* of Bumke & Foerster (1936). On opening the dura the arachnoid can be easily detached from the innerside of the dura, but it is firmly fixed to the pia and partly penetrates into the anterior median fissure, posterior median sulcus and posterior intermediate sulcus.

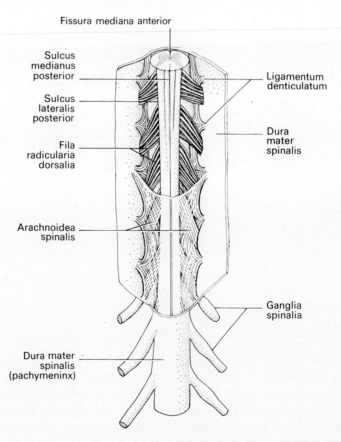

FIG. 22. Part of the spinal cord with its meninges (dorsal view) (Sobotta–Becher).

Ligamentum denticulatum

In the cervical and thoracic regions the arachnoid thickens between the anterior and posterior roots and on each side forming the ligamentum denticulatum through a tooth-like process which is fixed to the innerside of the dura. There are 20 denticulate ligaments in the cervical and thoracic regions, the last being at the level of the 12th thoracic and first lumbar spinal roots.

The pia mater covers the whole spinal cord and is firmly adherent to it and also lines the wall of the anterior median fissure. Below the conus medullaris the pia is continued as filum terminale. Fig. 22 demonstrates the relationship of the spinal cord to its meninges.

Inner structure

The spinal cord is divided into the grey and white matter, the latter surrounding the grey substance.

The grey matter

The grey matter, substantia grisea, runs throughout the whole length of the spinal cord and forms a column which on cross section has the shape of a butterfly and consists of anterior, lateral and posterior horns. The two symmetrical columns of the grey matter are connected by a bridge of the intermediate central substance, containing in the middle the central canal which is surrounded by the substantia gelatinosa centralis. The central canal containing cerebro-spinal fluid runs through the cord caudally to the conus terminalis and partly the filum terminale and continues cephalad through the distal part of the oblongata into the 4th ventricle. Transverse sections through the spinal cord at various levels show considerable differences in shape and extent of the grey matter, and in the cervical and lumbar enlargement and also sacral cord it takes a large space as compared with the upper cervical and thoracic regions (Fig. 23).

HISTOLOGICAL STRUCTURES

One has to distinguish between neuronal and supporting tissues. The neurones have their cell bodies in the grey matter sending out long axons. There are receptor, effector and connector (internuncial) neurones. Neurones and their dendrites are linked with other neurones by synapses, a Greek term—συναπτω: to clasp—introduced by Sherrington (1897)—to explain the transverse membranes which separate two neurones at close contiguity. In the grey of the anterior column the ganglion cells which are multipolar and their axons representing the 'final common motor path', innervate the striated muscles, some of them, specifically, the neuromuscular bundles, through the intrafusal fibres. The number of synapses connected with the effector cells of the anterior grey column is particularly large.

Receptor neurones consist of bipolar or pseudo-unipolar nerve cells, while the internuncial neurones are, like the effector neurones, multipolar.

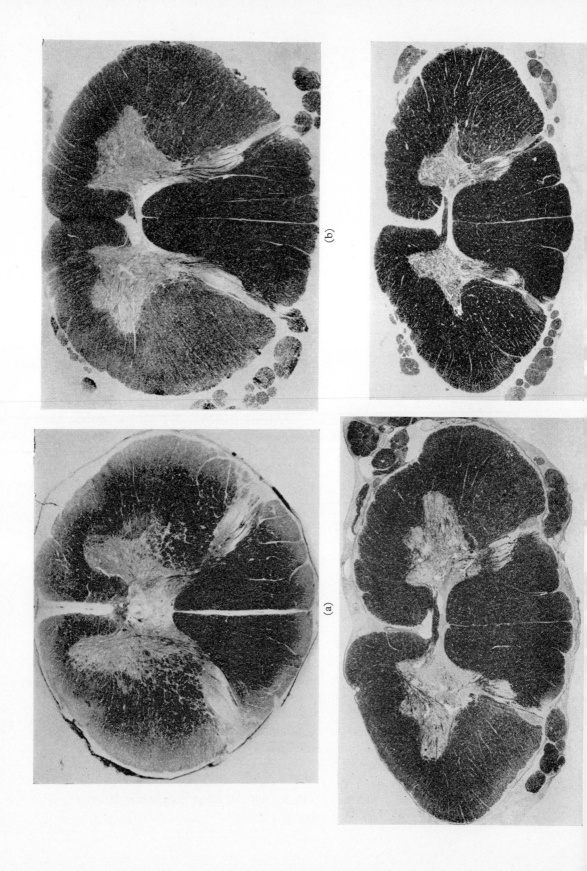

(a)

(b)

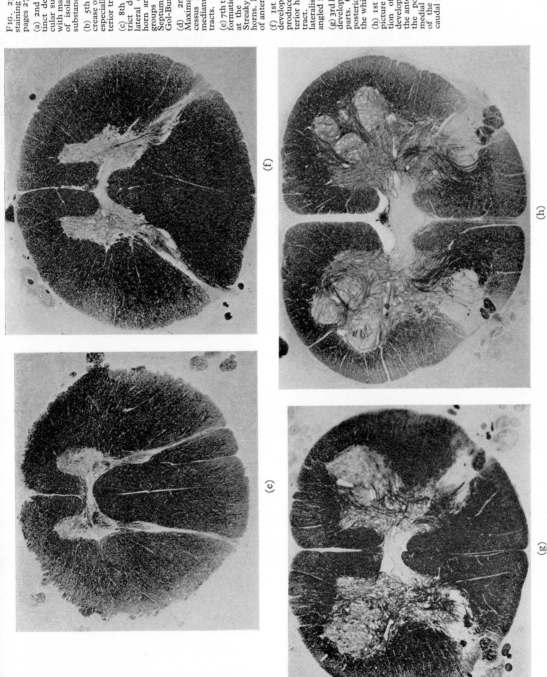

FIG. 23. Kulschitzky myelin staining (from Pollack (1935), pages 276-280).

(a) 2nd cervical segment. Distinct development of the reticular substance in lateral tracts with marbled appearance. Onset of isolation of the gelatinous substance of posterior horns.

(b) 5th cervical segment. Increase of fronto-dorsal diameter especially marked in the posterior tracts.

(c) 8th cervical segment. District development of dorso-lateral cell groups of anterior horn and lateral horn. Medial groups are still not developed. Septum para medianus between Gol-Burdach in posterior tracts.

(d) 2nd thoracic segment. Maximal development of processus lateralis. Septum para medianum in the posterior tracts.

(e) 7th thoracic segment. Typical formation of Clarke's column at the base of posterior horn. Streaky appearance of posterior horns. Right-angled basic form of anterior horns.

(f) 1st lumbar segment. The development of Clarke's column produces swelling of the posterior horn against the posterior tract. Distinct processus lateralis and typical right-angled form of anterior horns.

(g) 3rd lumbar segment. Distinct development of the medial parts. Change of form of the posterior horns and increase of the white matter.

(h) 1st sacral segment. Typical picture of intumescence formation of caudal part. Marked development of lateral groups of the anterior horns in contrast to the poor appearance of the medial parts. Typical widening of the posterior horns of the caudal part of the spinal cord.

The posterior roots conduct all afferent impulses to the spinal cord. These are transmitted directly to the brain via the white posterior tracts or the afferent fibres, forming
connections with intercalated neurones of the posterior grey column cells, either synaptic-
ally with efferent cells of the anterior grey column (monosynaptic reflex arcs) or inter-
segmentally with intercalated neurones in segments above and below. Commissural
axons are those which cross to the opposite side of the cord. Fibres of the intersegmental
neurones may either remain in the grey matter or may travel in the white matter adjacent
to the grey and intermingle (reticular formation of the cord).

The cells of the lateral grey column form the intermediolateral group of cells and
their axons travel in the anterior roots as pre-ganglionic sympathetic fibres and through
the white rami communicanes into the ganglia of the sympathetic chain. In the sacral
section this cell group sends its axons to the anterior roots through the anterior rami of the
corresponding sacral nerves and thus represent a contribution to the para-sympathetic
system.

Electron-microscopy and the work of Eccles and his school has clarified to a great
deal the hitherto obscure physiology of the synapses (Eccles, 1963) and also helped in
solving the old controversy between the exponents of the neurone theory (His, 1886;
Forel, 1887; Cajal, 1888–1934) and those of the reticular theory (Gerlach, 1871; Golgi,
1885; Held, 1905, 1929) in favour of the neurone theory.

The supporting tissue of the spinal cord consists of the three types of glia, macro,
micro and oligodendron glia. In addition there are the ependymal cells, forming the
central canal, furthermore, connective tissue in the form of collagen fibres and fibroblasts
accompanying the vascular endothelial cells of the blood vessels. The variety of all these
cells has its bearing on their reactions to injury of the cord.

The white matter

The anatomical arrangement of the white substance of the spinal cord consists of three
columns (funiculi): anterior, lateral and posterior. Within each of these funiculi there are
ascending and descending tracts conducting afferent and efferent impulses of great variety.

ANTERIOR FUNICULUS

(a) *Ascending tract*

Anterior spino-thalamic tract. The anterior spino-thalamic tract is an additional pathway
for some touch and pressure sensibility. The afferent fibres after entering the cord ascend
two or three segments in the posterior funiculus before synapsing with cells of the posterior
grey column of the same side which sends their axons to the white commissure from
where they cross to the contralateral anterior funiculus and enter the anterior spino-
thalamic tract to ascend to the brain.

(b) *Descending tracts*

(*1*) *Anterior cortico-spinal tract.* This tract is situated alongside the anterior median fissure and is much smaller than the lateral cortico-spinal tract, moreover, its size diminishes as it descends to the middle of the thoracic region.

(*2*) *Vestibulo-spinal tract.* This tract has its origin in the lateral vestibular nucleus and descends uncrossed alongside the periphery of the anterior funiculus. Its fibres are connected with the cells of the anterior grey column serving postural control.

(*3*) *Tecto-spinal tract.* This tract arises in the superior colliculus side and after crossing in the oblongata runs on the opposite side in the spinal cord adjacent to the anterior median fissure forming synapses with cells of the anterior grey column, particularly in the cervical region. It is an efferent pathway for spino-visual reflexes, the afferent pathway of which is the spino-tectal tract.

(*4*) *Reticulo-spinal tracts.* These are fibres scattered mainly through the medial part of the anterior fasciculus arising from the brain stem and ending on motor cells of the anterior grey.

LATERAL FUNICULUS

(a) *Ascending tracts*

(*1*) *Posterior spino-cerebellar tract* (Flechsig). This tract commences at the level of the upper lumbar nerves and ascends in the periphery of the posterior part of the lateral funiculus to the cerebellum through the inferior cerebellar peduncle. It conveys proprioceptive impulses for the co-ordinated control of locomotion and is mainly concerned with conveying impulses from the lower limbs and trunk.

(*2*) *Anterior spino-cerebellar tract* (Gowers). This tract begins in the upper lumbar region and ascends in the lateral funiculus in front of the posterior spino-cerebellar tract to the upper part of the pons, from there it descends into the superior cerebellar peduncle to terminate in the cerebellum. Like the posterior spino-cerebellar tract it also serves conducting proprioceptive impulses for the co-ordinated control of locomotion.

(*3*) *Lateral spino-thalamic tract.* This tract conveys pain and other nociceptive and emotional sensations (see section on Sensibility) as well as temperature sensibility from the side of the body opposite to the side of the spinal ganglia. The first neurones of this pathway are in the spinal ganglia, from there their axons enter the spinal cord via posterior roots. They enter the substantia gelatinosa after having ascended a short distance in the posterior-lateral tract. The great majority of fibres synapse with cells of the posterior grey column. From there the axons progress forwards, traverse the white commissure to the lateral funiculus of the opposite side of the cord and ascend to the brain, terminating eventually in the ventral nucleus of the thalamus. There is clinical evidence that some of the fibres originate in the posterior grey of the same side.

(*4*) *Spino-tectal tract.* This tract is topographically closely related to anterior spino-cerebellar and lateral spino-thalamic tracts. Its fibres arise in the posterior grey column and soon cross to reach the opposite lateral funiculus. Afferent impulses ascending in the spino-tectal tract are concerned with head and eye movements.

(5) *Posterior-lateral tract.* It is formed by fibres of the posterior roots which are divided into ascending and descending branches. The fibres ascend one or two segments in the posterior tract and give up collaterals which terminate around cells of the posterior grey column, from where the new axons travel to the opposite lateral spino-thalamic tract and convey nociceptive and thermal sensibility.

(b) *Descending tracts*

(*I*) *Lateral cortico-spinal tract.* This is the most important upper motor neuron tract originating from the giant pyramidal cells in the motor cortex, descending through the capsula interna and traversing the pedunculus cerebri and pons into the oblongata. In the lower part of the oblongata two-thirds of the fibres decussate and descend in the lateral funiculus of the spinal cord, while the rest of the fibres descend into the same side of the cord forming the anterior cortico-spinal tract. The majority of the cortico-spinal fibres terminate in the cord opposite to the side of the cortex from which they spring and synapse either directly with motor ganglion cells of the anterior grey column or they synapse on internuncial neurones in the neighbouring part of the base of the anterior grey column. From these neurones they are brought into contact with the motor cells of the anterior grey column.

(*2*) *Rubro-spinal tract.* This tract originates from cells of the red nucleus of the tegmentum and descends on the opposite side of the cord anteriorly to the lateral cortico-spinal tract, forming synapses in the anterior grey column. Thus this tract brings the cells of anterior grey column into contact with the corpus striatum.

(*3*) *Olivo-spinal tract.* The fibres of this tract, which originate in the olivary nucleus of the oblongata, synapse with ganglion cells of the anterior grey column in the cervical region only.

(*4*) *Descending autonomic tracts.* These are crossed and uncrossed fibres originating from the hypothalamic and other stations of the brain stem regulating functions of the autonomic system. They descend to the spinal cord mainly in an area between the posterior border of the spino-thalamic tract and the anterior border of the pyramidal tract and synapse to the lateral funiculus.

(*5*) *Lateral retro-spinal tract.* This is another important descending upper motor neuron tract which originates from the reticular formation of the brain stem and descends mainly in the contralateral side of the spinal cord and synapses with the internuncial and motor cells of the anterior grey column. Its significance in connection with the reflex behaviour in spinal cord lesions will be discussed in the section on Neurophysiology.

Posterior funiculus

Ascending tracts (fasciculus gracilis and fasciculus cuneatus). These two tracts occupy practically the whole funiculus posterior and transmit cephalad the proprioceptive sensibility including sense of position and movement, vibration, two-point discrimination, appreciation of figure-writing, deep pressure and also touch sensation. The fasciculus gracilis (Goll) receives fibres from the posterior roots of the distal parts of the body (thoracic, lumbar, sacral and coccygeal regions). The fibres coming from the sacral part are displaced medially by fibres which enter at higher levels. In the upper regions of the cord the fasciculus gracilis lies in the medial part of the posterior funiculus while the funiculus cuneatus (Burdach) subserving these modalities of sensibility in the upper part of the body occupies the lateral part. The fibres of the two fasciculi ascend uncrossed to the oblongata and after taking part in the decussation of the lemnisci ascend on each side to the ventral nucleus of the thalamus and from there they are conveyed to areas 1–3 of the postcentral gyrus of the cortex.

Descending tracts. There are some descending fibres in the cervical, upper thoracic and lower thoracic regions in the posterior funiculus which are mainly intersegmental and represent collectively the septomarginal tract.

Intersegmental tracts. There are intersegmental fibres in the anterior, lateral and posterior funiculi which mingle with ascending and descending tracts; some of them cross to the opposite side.

SOMATOTOPIC ARRANGEMENTS WITHIN THE SPINAL CORD

There exists a somatotopic division of lamellated type representing the various parts of the body within ascending and descending tracts which is particularly conspicuous in the cervical region. This has important bearing on the clinical symptomatology following injuries and other afflictions of the spinal cord (see chapter on Clinical Symptomatology). There exists also a somatotopic grouping of motoneurones associated anatomically as well as functionally with particular types of muscles (Gehuchten & de Neef, 1900; Bikeles & Franke, 1905; Romanes, 1951; Balthaser, 1952) and Fig. 24 shows Glee's adaptation (1961) from Sharrard's publication (1956).

Vascular supply of the spinal cord

Since Adamkiewicz (1882) described details of the arterial supply of the spinal cord this problem has been studied by numerous workers in this field (de Kadyi, 1889; Tanon, 1908; Adachi, 1928; Tureen, 1938; Bolton, 1939; Su & Alexander, 1939; Mettler, 1948; Zülch, 1951; Lazorthes *et al.*, 1957–58; Tönnis, 1963; Romanes, 1965; Tellinger, 1966; Piscol, 1972; Dommisse, 1975, and others). Although there is some disaccord about certain details amongst authors, there is general agreement that the spinal cord receives its arterial supply from various sources.

The anterior spinal artery originates on either side from the intracranial end of the vertebral arteries at the distal part of the oblongata. After forming a solitary trunk this

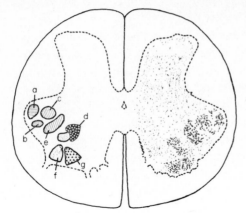

FIG. 24. A representation of the lower limb muscles in the motor cell columns at the level of lumbar 5. (*a*) long toe extensors; (*b*) peroneal muscles; (*c*) calf muscles; (*d*) hamstring muscles; (*e*) posterior tibial muscle; (*f*) hip adductors; (*g*) tensor fasciae lateae (from Gleer, *Experimental Neurology*, adapted from Sharrard, *British Surgical Progress*, p. 83, 1956).

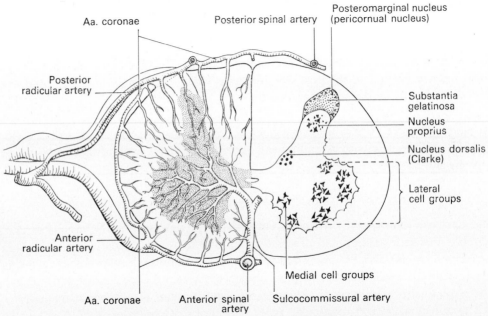

FIG. 25. The arterial beds and cell aggregates of the spinal cord as seen in cross section (from Bing's *Local Diagnosis*, 14th Edition).

artery descends along the anterior median fissure of the cord to the upper thoracic region. It receives radicular reinforcements from branches of the cervical part of the vertebral arteries, and the most constant branch enters at the level of the 5th and 6th cervical segments. Another constant branch is the arteria radicularis magna of Adamkiewicz which enters the cord between the level of the 9th thoracic and 1st lumbar segments. Lazorthes *et al.* divided the arterial supply of the cord into three zones:

1 the superior zone supplying the cervical segments including the first three upper thoracic segments. This vascularization is rich and depends on three to four arteries;

2 the inferior zone at the level of the thoraco-lumbar enlargement including the two distal thoracic segments. This vascular supply is also rich;

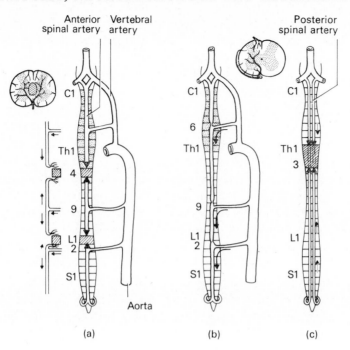

FIG. 26. The arterial supply of the spinal cord. *A* (after Zülch, 1954) is based on clinical and pathological studies. The chief sources of blood are through the radicular arteries of segments C6, Th10, and L2. The postulated direction of blood flow in the arteriae coronae is indicated. Regions of apposition of arterial beds, namely, segments Th4 and L1 (diagonal-hatch), are said to be weak points in the circulation on the basis (diagram to extreme left) that arterial pressure is lowest in the terminal vessels of a system. For the same reason, the central grey matter and the ventral part of the posterior column also represent weak points (diagonal-hatch) in the circulation (inset).

B and *C* (after Bolton, 1939) are based on anatomical studies. The sources of arterial supply of the cord are the same as in *A*. The postulated direction of blood flow is indicated. The region of poorest circulation (diagonal-hatch) is said to be at upper thoracic levels. The arterial beds of the anterior and posterior spinal arteries as seen in cross section are indicated (inset). The stippled areas in the upper part of the cord in *A* and *B* represent the two views as to the segments supplied from the cervical branches of the vertebral artery (from Bing's *Local Diagnosis*, 14th Edition).

3   the intermediate zone involving the mid-thoracic segments which is relatively poorly vascularized, especially at the level of the 4th thoracic segment. This area has been considered particularly vulnerable to vascular conclusion and ischaemia as found by Bolton (1939) in his injection studies and later by Zülch (1954). Fig. 25 taken from Bing's *Local Diagnosis in Neurological Diseases* (14th edition) as revised and enlarged by Webb Haymaker (1956) demonstrates the arterial beds and cell aggregates of the spinal cord as seen in cross section and Fig. 26 shows the blood supply of the spinal cord according to Bolton (1939) and Zülch (1954) respectively. Romanes (1965) reported about 22 spinal cords in which he studied the feeding vessels to the anterior spinal arteries. He found that while the chance of feeding vessels on the right and left side was about equal in

the cervical and lumbar regions, there was a marked preponderance on the left in the thoracic region where the majority of the vessels entered, the sites of entry of the great spinal arteries being between T8 and T11 on the left.

From the central anterior spinal artery sulcocommissural branches spring which pass into the anterior median fissure and one passes alternatively to the right and left to vascularize the anterior, lateral and also the anterior part of the posterior horn of the grey matter but also part of the lateral and anterior white tracts (Mair & Druckman, 1953). The capillary network is much more dense in the grey than in the white matter which explains its greater vulnerability following fractures and dislocations of the spine.

The posterior arteries also arise from the intercranial part of the vertebral arteries but do not join into one single trunk but descend as a pair along the medial edge of the posterior roots. According to Romanes these long vessels are reinforced by a greater number of feeding vessels than the anterior spinal artery. In the region of the conus medullaris there may be communications between the posterior and anterior arteries as shown in Fig. 27a of one of Romanes' cases. Large communications between the posterior spinal arteries were found in both enlargements of the cord, especially in the lumbar-sacral region as shown in Fig. 27b of another case studied by Romanes. The posterior spinal arteries supply the posterior horns and together with the arteriae coronae most of the white matter.

Recently, Piscol (1972) published results of his studies on the blood supply of the spinal cord based on 50 preparations in adults. The methods employed consisted in morphological description, contrast filling and measuring of the calibres of the vessels. He found that the upper cervical cord receives its arterial supply from the vertebral arteries while the distal cervical region is mainly supplied by ascending cervical and upper

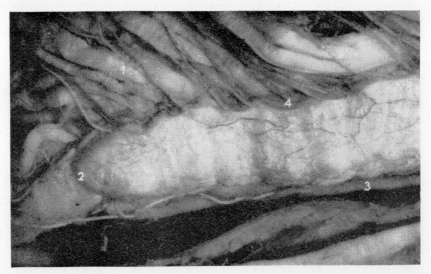

FIG. 27a. Lateral view of the sacrococcygeal region of the spinal cord. (1) Dorsal rootlet. Note the number of small feeding vessels to the posterior spinal artery on the dorsal rootlets. (2) Large communication between anterior (3) and posterior (4) spinal arteries (from Romanes (1965), *Paraplegia*, **2**, 199).

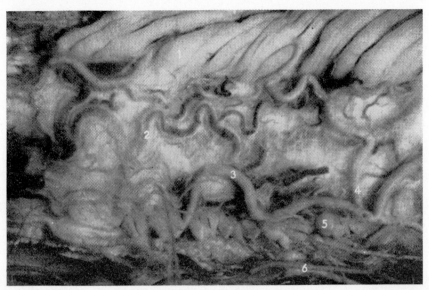

FIG. 27b. Dorsal view of the sacral region of the spinal cord. (1) Dorsal rootlet. (2) Posterior spinal vein. (3) Posterior spinal artery; particularly large on this side because of a large feeding vessel entering cranial to this photograph. Note large communications (4) with smaller left posterior spinal artery. (5) Cut dorsal rootlet. (6) Two small feeding vessels to the posterior spinal artery dissected off the cut dorsal rootlets (from Romanes (1965), *Paraplegia*, **2**, 199).

thoracic arteries. In certain cases, however, the whole cervical cord down to C7 segment receives its supply from the vertebral arteries only. Figs. 28a and b show variations in the descending branches of the vertebral arteries. While in Fig. 28a the descending branch is well developed on the right side, the left branch is only rudimentary. Fig. 28b shows both descending branches well developed and united at the level of C1 into one single branch. On the other hand the anterior spinal arteries may descend separately over several segments of the cervical cord as shown in Fig. 28c.

With regard to the anterior radicular arteries, 296 were accounted for, of these, 138 in the cervical, 118 in the thoracic, 31 in the lumbar and 9 in the sacral region, and a distinction is made between large, medium, small and minute sizes. Fig. 28d shows a synoptic segmental representation of these 4 arterial categories in the various regions of the cord. In the cervical region there is a prevalence of a great number of vessels of all 4 categories between C4 and C8 segments in particular of medium, small and minute sizes, while the thoraco-lumbar region, T9–L1 is supplied mainly by large vessels.

In accordance with previous workers Piscol found the contrast filling of posterior radicular arteries more difficult because of their smaller calibre. In 39 preparations he found 431 posterior radicular arteries, of these, 94 in the cervical and 229 in the thoraco-lumbar region. The largest supply of medium and small size vessels were found in the cervical areas between C4 and C7 corresponding to the cervical intumescence, while the supply with the largest size vessels was found between T10 and L2, in particular, in T12 and L1.

The venous return from the spinal cord takes place through veins accompanying the anterior and posterior roots which drain into the spino-vertebral venous plexus, which at thoracic and lumbar level empties into the azygos vein and has, therefore, connections with the venous system of lungs and the abdominal and pelvic cavities.

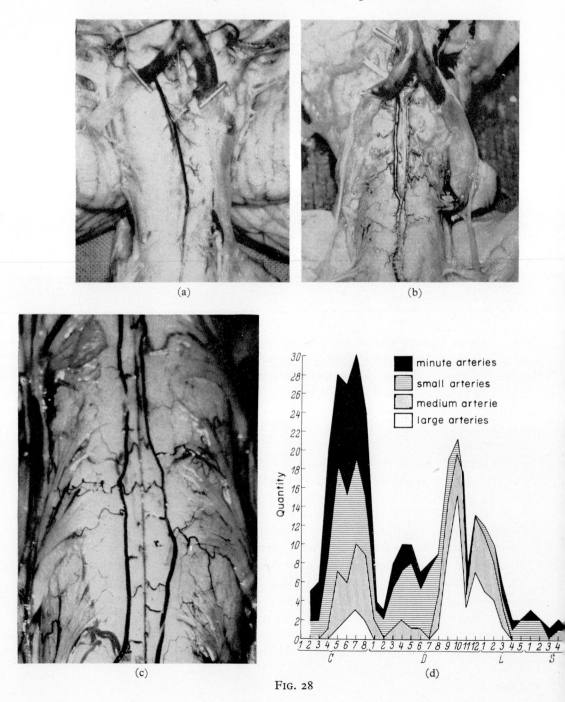

(a)

(b)

(c)

(d)

Fig. 28

A most meticulous and comprehensive study on the vascular supply of the spinal cord has recently been published by G.E.Dommisse (1975) in his book *The Arteries and Veins of the Human Spinal Cord from Birth*. Five techniques were employed, the principal one of which consists of a detailed micro-dissection on 42 cadavers, amongst them thirty neonates, one infant, four adolescent and seven adult cadavers. The results obtained are recorded in many photographs, amongst them a considerable number of coloured ones, in graphs, diagrams and tables demonstrating the intricacy of the vascular supply of the spinal cord at various levels. His findings on the complex venous system reveal the relationship of veins of the spinal cord and vertebral column to the neighbouring structures. Moreover, the findings on the collateral arterial circulation and its compensatory function help one to understand the varying degrees of neurological deficit following occlusion of spinal cord arteries.

CHAPTER 8

NEUROPATHOLOGY OF THE SPINAL CORD
AND SPINAL ROOTS

The pathological changes in the neural elements and blood supply of the spinal cord resulting from closed injuries differ from those following gunshot and stab wounds in that in the two latter conditions the dura in most cases is opened and C.S.F. leakage and infection such as meningitis, epidural and subdural abscess formation, may not uncommonly occur. An extensive literature exists on this subject in many countries, especially those involved in the two world wars, and the reader is referred to the publications and comprehensive reviews of Jacob (1919), Roussy & L'Hermitte (1920), Guillain & Barré (1917), Hassin (1923), Foerster (1929), Marburg (1936), Davison (1945), Scarff & Pool (1946), Greenfield (1958) and in more recent years Zülch (1954, 1967), D.Tönnis (1963), Jellinger (1966), Wolman (1964), Hughes (1965), Klaue (1969) and Mayer & Peters (1971).

In the following, an account is given of the pathological changes in the spinal cord and its vascular supply, as found in our own clinical material following concussion, contusion, laceration and transection of the cord resulting from closed injuries of the vertebral column. In addition details of pathological changes in the cord produced by angiomatous malformation will also be presented.

CONCUSSION (COMMOTIO MEDULLAE SPINALIS)

Since Obersteiner (1878) advanced the theory of the 'molecular disturbances of neurones' as the underlying cause of concussion, this condition has been differently defined by various authors. L'Hermitte (1932), for instance, postulated for the diagnosis of concussion the integrity of the spine—a view which cannot be accepted. Most authors share Hartmann's view (1900), that spinal cord concussion is a totally reversible functional disorder of the spinal cord. However, as Marburg (1936) rightly emphasized, the proviso is the speedy recovery of the initial transverse cord syndrome within 24–48 hours—a view which is also held by the present writer. True concussion is very rare following vertebral injuries, and Marburg has seen only four cases in his large material of the First World War who fulfilled this condition. I have seen only one case during the Second World War, a man, who, while sitting in his room, was thrown to the ground by the blast of an exploding bomb nearby. On admission to the Spinal Unit he showed an incomplete transverse syndrome at mid-thoracic level. X-ray was normal but the lumbar puncture showed a high C.S.F. pressure of 250 mm. However, the fluid was not xantochromic nor was there increase of protein or cells. He recovered completely within 24 hours from his symptoms, including pyramidal signs. Foerster's (1929) two patients, who recovered only after 10 and 11 days respectively, cannot be considered as concussion in the strict sense. It is probable that in these cases some petechial haemorrhages, followed by oedema, may have been the cause of the delay in functional recovery. It must be admitted that the underlying mechanism of spinal cord concussion is still obscure. However, in the light of the modern advances made on the interneurone function of synapses and their afferent and efferent connections and the chemical transmission between neurones, one cannot help feeling that Obersteiner's concept of the 'molecular disturbance of neurones' may be after all an acceptable explanation of the mechanism involved in spinal cord concussion.

CONTUSION, LACERATION, TRANSECTION

Contusion, the most frequent type of injury of the spinal cord, produces a great variety of detectable organic alterations in the axons, parenchyma, vascular supply and meninges which may be combined or independent of each other. The damage to the spinal cord is caused by the impact of the violence, leading to acute compression of the cord and resulting in destruction of the nervous elements and their blood supply at the site of the main impact of the violence but also producing pressure, squeezing and stretch effects on several segments above and below the main injury. The alterations in the tissues consist of petechial haemorrhages due to rhexis or diapedesim, haematomyelia, thrombosis, resulting in softening of the parenchyma with demyelination and necrosis, cyst formation and fibrotic and glial scarring. At some stage, there is proliferation of vessels and glial cell proliferation. Several authors (Kienbëck, 1902; Klaue, 1969; Mayer & Peters, 1971) have drawn special attention to vacuolization in the white matter of the cord, forming distinct fields of vacuoles (Lückenfelder). They represent the breaking down of the myelin tubes surrounding the axons, which themselves undergo chromatolysis, and the disappearance of the Nissl bodies from the centre of the cell.

Three stages in the pathological changes of the cord as a result of contusion can be distinguished, although the transition from one to another is rather fluent.

Acute stage

The macroscopic appearance of the cord following contusion is shown in Fig. 29. The cord at the site of the impact of the violence is swollen, of bluish-red discoloration, and

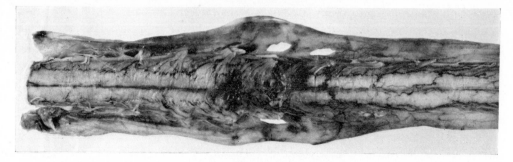

FIG. 29.

the pia-arachnoidea haemorrhagic and there are also patches of haemorrhages on the inside of the dura. The line of the long spinal artery is interrupted.

Microscopically, the first stage is characterized by haemorrhages involving very extensively the highly vascularized and spongious and therefore most vulnerable grey substance, especially in the centre but also spreading to varying degrees into the white matter.

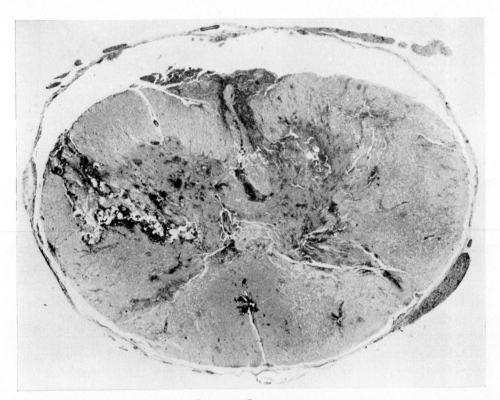

FIG. 30. C5 segment.

Figs. 30 and 31 demonstrate sections of the cervical cord of a young man of 21 who was admitted on 18 February 1961, three days after a motor cycle accident, in which he sustained a severe head injury with fracture of the left parietal bone and severe cerebral concussion, multiple fractures of long bones and a fracture-dislocation of C4/5 resulting in complete tetraplegia with areflexia. He died one day later (4 days after injury) as a result of his severe brain lesion.

The main damage to the spinal cord is situated in the segments of C6 and C5, demonstrating a mass of haemorrhages scattered mainly over the whole grey matter but also spreading into the white substance. In fact, there is a large infarction in the postero-lateral tract with multiple vacuoles, especially marked in C5 segment (Fig. 30). The normal architectural distinction between grey and white matter has practically disappeared in C6 segment (Fig. 31) and the butterfly-like shape of the grey matter is only indicated. The main haemorrhage, partially thrombosed, occurred in the anterior spinalis

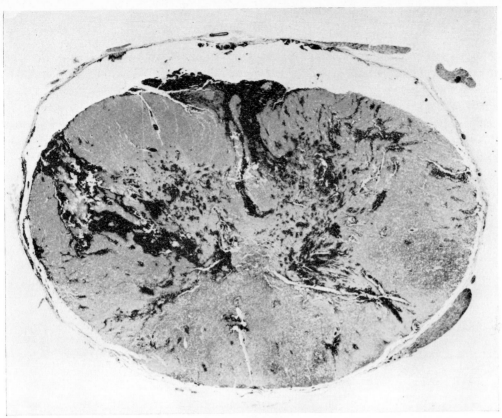

FIG. 31. C6 segment.

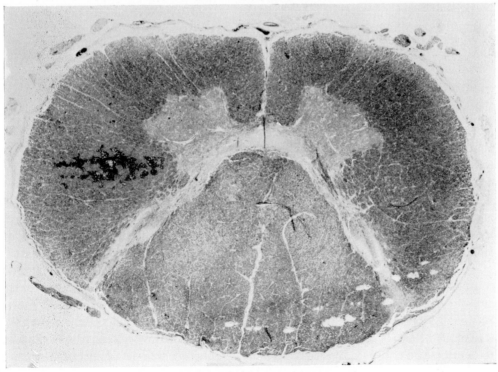

FIG. 32. C4 segment.

artery as seen in C6 and C5 segments. The upwards spread of the cord damage is shown in C4 segment by haemorrhages in the left lateral tract (Fig. 32). There is also a 'core' to be seen in the upper ventral part of the left posterior column, which is also present though small in C5 and C6 segments. The downwards spread of the damage is seen in C7 segment by a round haemorrhagic 'core' in the ventral part of the left posterior column. The left posterior horn appears swollen as compared with the right, containing haemorrhages and vacuoles. The ventral parts of the posterior columns show definite paler colour than the dorsal parts, as expression of early demyelination, and show a field of multiple vacuoles (Fig. 33). The early demyelination is particularly striking over the whole left

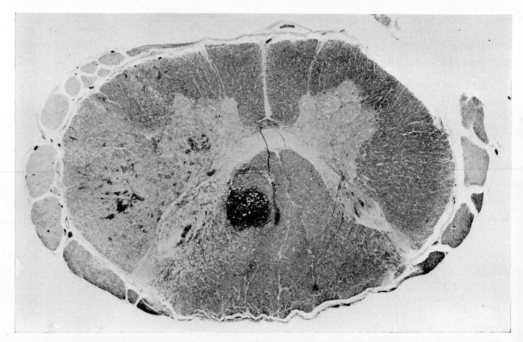

FIG. 33. C7 segment.

postero-lateral column, dotted with some small scattered haemorrhages and a large field of small vacuoles fairly corresponding to the infarction seen in C5 and C6 segments and demonstrating early breakdown of the myelin tubes surrounding the axons.

The ganglion cells in this early stage show chromatolysis and disappearance of the Nissl substance with eccentricity of the nucleus, and the whole shape of the ganglion cells is altered. The axis cylinders are fragmented, beaded (Hughes, 1965) and tortuous. In the subsequent phase of the acute stage, there is a massive invasion of polymorphs.

Another type of spinal cord damage as the result of fracture dislocation of the spine is shown in Figs. 34a–f of a man, aged 46, who sustained a very severe fracture dislocation of C6/7 with a fracture of the spinal process of C7 in a car accident on 12 March 1963, and was admitted to Stoke Mandeville on the same day. He showed a complete tetraplegia below C5 on the left and C6 on the right. Before his accident he was suffering from asthma and chronic bronchitis. A lumbar puncture showed xantochromic fluid, a

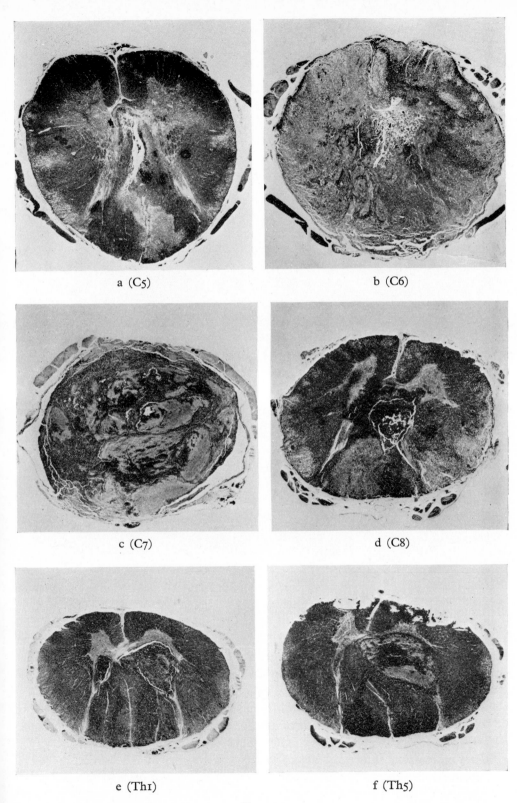

a (C5)

b (C6)

c (C7)

d (C8)

e (Th1)

f (Th5)

Fig. 34.

pressure of 145 mm and complete block. He was put on respirator and head traction. He died 3 days later from a total collapse of the right lung due to mucuous plugging. The findings in this case are shown in Figs. 34a–f. The segments C6 and C7 show complete disintegration of the normal architecture of the cord and disappearance of the distinction between the grey and white substances. The whole shape of the segments is distorted and the neural tissues are replaced by necrotic tissue intermingled with haemorrhages. There was a profound extension of the cord damage cephalad to C2 and caudal to T5/6. Figs. 34a–f illustrate the effect of the concussion in caudal direction from C8 to T5

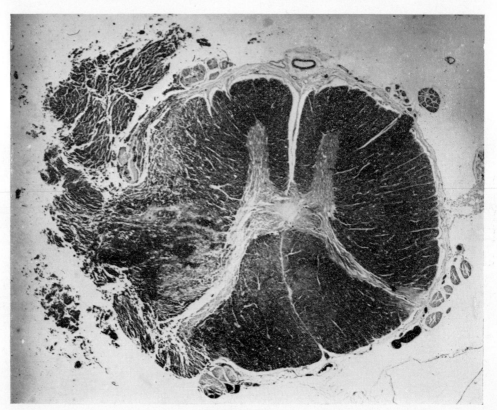

FIG. 35.

segments. C8 segment shows a large central necrosis containing debris and involving the greater part of the grey substance surrounded by several haemorrhagic patches. This picture shows strikingly in the haemotoxilin–eosin staining the early demyelination in the posterior, lateral and anterior white columns with vacuolization. T1, T3 and T5 segments illustrate the central necrosis which is particularly haemorrhagic in T1. In T5, the two solitary necroses have been united into one single large one, showing haemorrhage in its central part, and surrounded by a pigmented wall.

While the violence at its main impact usually produces a complete transection of the cord, segments above or below may sustain only unilateral laceration, as shown in Fig. 35 of T8 segment in a case with complete crushing of the whole cord at T10/11.

Intermediate and late stages

These stages of absorption and reparative organization, which may take many weeks and months after the acute stage has elapsed, are described together as they are inter-mingled, especially in the more progressed stage of reparative organization. The early intermediate stage is characterized by invasion of lymphocytes and there is also macroglial proliferation—the latter provided the parenchyma has not been completely destroyed initially—and by large macrophages. According to Greenfield *et al.* (1958) and Hughes (1965), the most striking cell everywhere is the lipid phagocyte or compound granular corpuscle. Their function is the absorption of necrotic tissue. The replacement of the perished parenchyma is carried out by fibroblasts. Therefore, according to the time which has elapsed after the acute stage, one will find various phases of reparative organiza-tion in those cases of severe contusion with extension to segments cephalad and caudal from the main destruction of the cord.

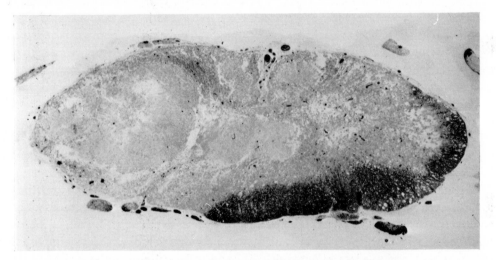

FIG. 36. C7 segment, final stages of post-traumatic changes.

The final stage is characterized by the formation of fibrous and glial scars, and macro-scopically the spinal cord at the site of the main lesion may be shrunken. Fig. 36 shows the final scar of the 7th cervical segment of a case with complete traumatic tetraplegia. The original segmental architecture is abolished, the parenchyma destroyed and replaced by fibrous and glial scar tissue leaving only a narrow myelinated margin of the anterior and lateral columns dotted with multiple vacuoles of different size. Klaue (1971) has recently drawn attention to the marked swelling of the axis cylinders within the network of vacuoles.

Late myelopathy (remote post-traumatic cord lesions)

The formation of cysts of smaller or larger size may also occur in later stages of cord damage. These may develop even months and years after the original trauma in remote areas of the spinal cord above the original spinal cord lesion.

Marburg (1936) described as 'vasopathia traumatica' post-traumatic alterations of the vascular supply leading to thrombosis and softening of the tissues. Zülch (1954) described pencil-like softening of the thoracic cord following cervical injury as a result of defective blood circulation. However, there are discrepancies of opinion amongst workers in this field regarding details of the vasogenic origin of the remote post-traumatic cord lesions (Becker & Hess, 1954; Becker, 1958; Schneider, 1955; Tönnis, 1963). Jousse (1971) reported about 13 out of 729 patients who developed late myelopathy.

One of the latest cases of late development and progression of the spinal symptomatology I have seen is a woman, aged 51, who sustained a complete paraplegia below T4/5 on 2 August 1969 following fracture of the spine. She was treated originally at the Spinal Injuries Centre, Oswestry. In February 1970 (7 months after injury) she experienced unpleasant tingling sensation around the right elbow which gradually spread over the right arm and neck and also over forearm and fingers of the right hand. Moreover, she noticed clumsiness in her right hand and fingers, especially when knitting. On examination she had, in addition to a complete transverse lesion below T4 of spastic type in extension, a thermo-analgesia below C2 on the right side. There was also impairment of postural sensibility in the fingers of the right hand, especially the 4th and 5th and there was slight ataxy in the right arm on finger–nose test. The deltoid, triceps and supinator reflexes were absent on the right side but present on the left. Of special interest was the cutaneous vasomotor response to a stroke or needle prick over the whole area of analgesia, as compared with the corresponding normal areas of the left side. Every stroke and needle prick produced marked and long lasting weal eruption, while on the corresponding areas of the left side the same stimuli produced the normal short-lasting local vasodilatation surrounded by a small line of vasoconstriction.

Motor function in all muscles of the right upper limb, including finger and thumb muscles, were intact. In this case, the late development of post-traumatic vascular pathology, most probably of thrombotic nature, has affected the distribution of the right posterior spinal artery, resulting in gradual ascending deterioration of the right posterior horns up to C2 and to a lesser degree also of the posterior column on the same side. That this has resulted in softening of the affected tissue forming a tapering pencil-like cavitation can only be assumed at the present juncture.

Another case of this type is a former naval lieutenant (I.S.) aged 26, who on 30 July 1969 was involved in a car accident while a front seat passenger. He sustained a complete paraplegia below the chest as a result of a fracture dislocation of the 5th/6th dorsal vertebra. He was up in a wheelchair 6 weeks after the injury and took part in all the activities of the Lodge Moor Spinal Injuries Centre where he was treated.

During his stay in hospital he noticed one day that he could not feel cold in his left hand and arm. This impairment of sensation to temperature and also to painful stimuli increased in due course until it reached the left side of the neck.

When I saw this man first in 1970 he had a complete motor paralysis below T5 with loss of control of bladder and bowels, but the sensibility below that level was not completely lost. However, he had a dissociated sensory loss over the whole left arm, neck, including the 2nd and 3rd cervical segment.

On re-examination on 7 July 1972 the neurological condition below T5 was unchanged and so was the loss of pain and temperature sensibility on the left side up to C2. In contrast to the previous case there were no disturbances of posterior column sensibility.

Fig. 37 demonstrates a cyst of larger size containing fluid and debris involving the posterior horn on the left side. These cysts, developing in particular in the central and ventro-posterior part of the grey matter and involving several segments, have been wrongly termed traumatic syringomyelia. They may increase in size, in due course, and give rise to increased neurological symptoms. Kautzky described increase of clinical symptoms in a case of traumatic lesion of the cervical cord following grenade injury. At operation a cyst containing clear fluid was found. The clinical symptoms improved after operation.

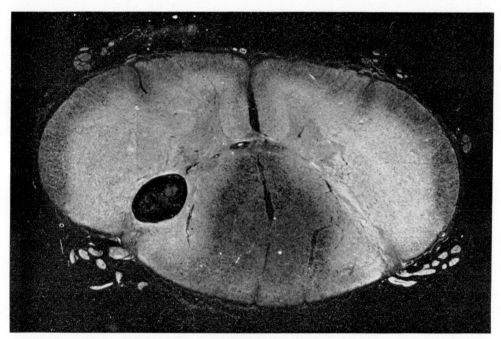

FIG. 37.

CONUS–CAUDA EQUINA LESIONS

These are very frequent sequelae of closed injuries of the 12th thoracic and the three upper lumbar vertebrae. In lesions of the 12th thoracic and the two first lumbar vertebrae, the conus and epiconus is often destroyed. Some of the anterior and posterior roots may have escaped injury while others are crushed or transected. Transection of spinal roots are common in gunshot injuries. The late changes following gunshot injury of the epiconus and conus are shown in a man who was wounded in Normandy in 1944 and admitted to Stoke Mandeville in 1947 with a complete flaccid paraplegia below T12, with ascending infection of the urinary tract following suprapubic cystotomy, which was then closed. He died in 1957 from a cancer of the bladder. The cord in the lower thoracic and lumbar region was firmly adhered to the meninges. The whole lumbar and sacral cord showed microscopically complete destruction and was replaced by glial and fibrous scar. Many spinal roots were embedded in dense fibrous adhesions and showed demyelination. The vessels showed various degrees of thrombosis. These changes are shown in Fig. 38, and Fig. 39 demonstrates the extensive ascending demyelination in the fasciculus gracilis of the posterior column and also lateral demyelination in the marginal anterior and posterior spino-thalamic tracts of the 7th thoracic segment.

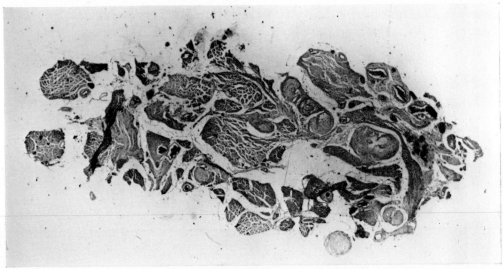

FIG. 38.

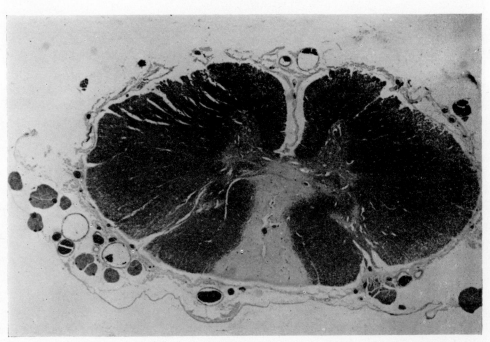

FIG. 39.

HAEMANGIOMA OF THE SPINAL CORD

Of the non-traumatic afflictions of the spinal cord, the writer has chosen this case of angiomatous malformation as the patient combines discrete vascular abnormalities of the cord, including thrombosis, with the effects of gradual compression of the cord.

This man, aged 30, was admitted on 18 November 1955 with an incomplete transverse spinal syndrome below T7, which was complete below T10. The motor paralysis was of flaccid type with areflexia. The arm reflexes were exaggerated in both upper limbs but there was no muscular impairment or disturbance of sensibility. In November 1943 he had started with weakness in both lower limbs, more in the left than the right, which had gradually increased, and in September 1944 he developed difficulty in starting micturition and in controlling his bowel function. By February 1945 he had a practically complete paraplegia below T10 and at operation at that time carried out by the neurosurgeon Mr Harvey Jackson, an angioma was found starting at the level of the distal cervical segment and involving the whole spinal cord in the thoracic area. He had deep X-ray treatment afterwards in 1945–46. In the following years he had repeated hospital treatments elsewhere for infection of the urinary tract and pressure sores.

On admission to Stoke Mandeville he was suffering from marked renal deficiency and hypertension 185/110, with a blood urea of 208 mg per cent, and protein excretion of 13·1 g daily in the urine. Urine was infected with proteus. Hb 64 per cent, serum albumin 3·55, serum globulin 2·4. He had a residual urine of 60 oz, bilateral hydronephrosis and ureteric reflux. Blood transfusions combined with Bull's diet and antibiotics resulted in improvement of blood urea to 146 mg per cent and anaemia (79–85 per cent Hg). The paraplegia remained unchanged. After his first discharge on 5 May 1956 he was repeatedly readmitted because of deterioration in his renal and heart insufficiency and he died from uraemia on 24 September 1956.

The necropsy revealed a large haemangioma of the whole spinal cord with the main vascular anomalies in the mid-thoracic and lumbosacral regions where the dilatation of the tortuous vessels was most striking. The radicular veins of the cauda equina were also dilated.

Microscopically, sections below T7, including lumbar and sacral segments showed a complete disappearance of the normal architecture of the cord and almost no distinction between grey and white structures, while in the upper thoracic and cervical segments this distinction was maintained. All segments were surrounded by greatly dilated vessels many of which showed various stages of thrombosis. In T7/8 an enormously dilated and thrombosed vessel had invaded and compressed the spinal cord substance. There was also a 'core' of small vessels lying proximal to the thrombosed vessel (Fig. 40a). The profound vascular proliferation within the tissues of the cord was most conspicuous in T10 and T11 segments, as shown in section of T9 (Fig. 40b). The compression of the cord tissue as a result of the invasion of a large external vessel was particularly conspicuous in L1 segment, which also showed in addition to diffusely scattered vessels of various sizes, a circumscribed 'core' of small vessels on the left half of the cord (Fig. 40c). The whole L1 segment was greatly demyelinated, especially on the side of the compression. Further indentations and compression of the cord through large vessels were also seen in the

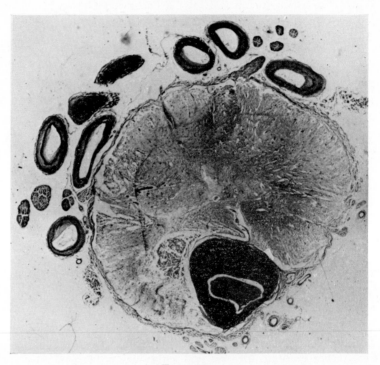

Fig. 40a.

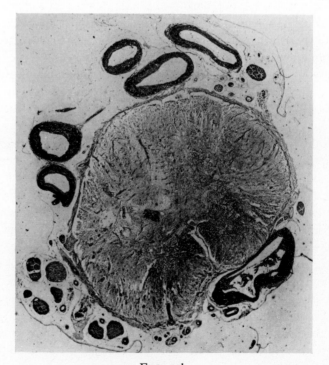

Fig. 40b.

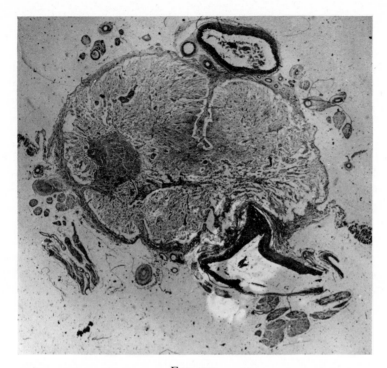

Fig. 40c.

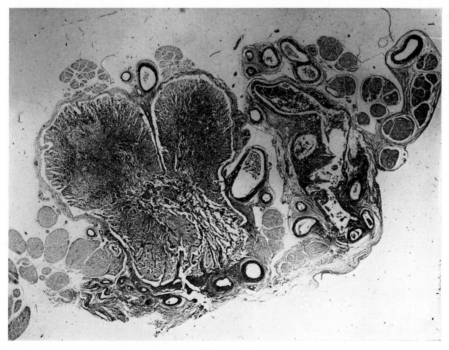

Fig. 40d.

lower lumbar and sacral segments as shown in Fig. 40d of S1 segment. This figure also shows numerous demyelinated spinal roots with completely or partly thrombosed vessels. The ascending demyelination of the posterior, lateral and anterior tracts is demonstrated in C7 segment which showed the normal architecture of the cord divided into grey and white substances and also the ascending degeneration in the nucleus gracilis as well as demyelination in the marginal zones of the lateral and anterior tracts, intermingled with vacuolization and fissure formation. There were also patches of demyelination in the central grey.

As mentioned before, many vessels showed various stages of thrombosis with thickening of their wall and hyaline degeneration. This was found in both large and small vessels. From observation in man and experimental studies by various authors on the effect of deep X-ray treatment, it can be assumed that the vascular changes seen in this case were, if not completely, at least partly the results of the repeated X-ray therapy.

Vertebral haemangiomatosis causing paraplegia is rather rare. Their localization is mainly in the thoracic and lumbar areas. The X-ray of a solitary haemangioma affecting one vertebra shows more marked radiolucency of the vertebral body than normally associated with coarse striations. The prominence of vertical trabeculae is best demonstrated on a lateral X-ray and there may be bulging of the cortical outline of the vertebra on either side in the a-p X-ray. In some cases the vertebral body may show collapse. If the epidural space is involved this may result in spinal cord compression and more or less severe paraplegia. Myelography will reveal a complete block at the level of the compression. Two illustrative cases of vertebral haemangionatosis at T6 and T9 vertebral level respectively were recently published by Harandi et al. (1975) and previous reports included those of Rand (1960), Dahlin (1967), Gutierez and Spjut (1972).

CHAPTER 9

SPINAL CORD ISCHAEMIA
—ANIMAL EXPERIMENTS

There are numerous clinical reports about spinal cord infarction resulting in complete or incomplete paraplegia following thoracic and abdominal surgery for intact or ruptured aortic aneurysm (Adams & van Geertruyden, 1956; Hara & Lipin, 1960; Gump, 1969; Pasternak *et al.*, 1972; Scher & Healy, 1971; Ferguson *et al.*, 1974) or progressive vascular myelopathy as a result of spinal cord arteriosclerosis (Jellinger, 1976).

Extradural or extramedullary intradural benign tumours causing gradual compression do not, as a rule, directly destroy the anatomical compartments of the spinal cord. In spite of long lasting compression, considerable functional recovery may occur following removal of the tumour (Guttmann, 1936). The degree of functional recovery depends on the size, extension and location of the tumour and its effect on the vascular supply of the cord, i.e. the degree and duration of the occlusion of the vascular supply of the cord at the site of the tumour. However, additional acute traumatization of the vertebral column at the site of an extramedullary tumour exhibiting no previous clinical symptoms may lead, after a free interval, to a rapidly increasing transverse spinal cord syndrome due to haemorrhage or anterior spinal artery thrombosis at the site of the tumour, as reported in this book in a case of neurofibroma following a car accident (see page 161).

ANIMAL EXPERIMENTS ON ISCHAEMIA
AND SPINAL CORD CONTUSION

Numerous animal experiments have been published in recent years on the problem of ischaemia and anoxia in relationship to the development of paraplegia and its treatment. These experimental studies can be conveniently divided into 3 groups.

I. ASPHYXIA—AORTIC OCCLUSION (TUREEN, 1936, VAN HARREVELD AND MARMOUT, 1939; TARLOW, 1953/54)

Van Harreveld & Marmout (1939) found histologically severe destruction of the cells in the grey matter of the cord in cats asphyxiated for 55 minutes. On the other hand, Tarlow (1953) taking up Tureen's (1936) experiments in cats, found that occlusion of the thoracic aorta for 50 minutes in a dog showed paralysis of the hind limbs, not with areflexia but with marked extensor rigidity; histological sections later revealed only selective degeneration of the grey matter, sparing some of the anterior horn cells peripherally. However, he concluded that longer periods of aortic occlusion would destroy all ganglion cells, resulting in flaccid paralysis. He proved this in another dog with thoracic aorta occlusion where, in addition, a transection of the cord at the upper thoracic level was carried out, thus interrupting the blood supply from the anterior spinal artery. From this evidence, it is difficult to understand why Tarlow excluded local ischaemia as a significant cause of paralysis following local spinal vascular occlusion in man, resulting in various degrees of destruction of neuronal elements of the spinal cord. While Tarlow's conclusions regarding the need for early laminectomy in compressing extramedullary spinal tumours are shared by all neurosurgeons, they cannot be applied indiscriminately to immediate and early laminectomy of traumatic paraplegia and tetraplegia following fracture-dislocations, as their mechanism of an acute violence is so very different from that of a gradual spinal cord compression of benign extramedullary tumours (Guttmann, 1973).

2. EXPERIMENTAL SPINAL CORD COMPRESSION (TARLOW, 1957, TATOR, 1971; RICHARDSON & NAKAMURA, 1971)

Of special interest are experimental studies on acute and gradual compressions of the cord. Tarlow (1957) reported on 42 experiments of acute compression of the thoracic cord and 11 of the cauda equina in dogs, using large, medium-sized and small balloons. The duration of compression varied in accordance with the size of the balloons.

Tator (1971), using circumferential compression injuries in monkeys by an inflatable silastic cuff, found that a force of 350 mmHg of 5 minutes' duration produced permanent complete paraplegia in 5 cases but in 6 the initially complete paraplegia showed functional recovery. He found the threshold for immediately complete but reversible paraplegia at 250 mmHg of 5 minutes' compression. However, in two animals a force of only 150 mmHg of 5 minutes duration also resulted in severe neurological deficit and even more in 2 other animals with a compression force of 250 mmHg.

The important conclusions emerging from these compression experiments in animals may be summarized as follows:

(i) There is definite proof of a fundamental difference between the effects of acute compression of the spinal cord in producing irreversible damage of the neural elements as compared with gradual compression. In confirming clinical experiences in man, acute impact of a large compressing force of only 2–5 minutes' duration in animals resulted almost invariably in complete destruction of the cord at the site of the compression which extended to segments above and below the injury (Tarlow's cases 34, 35). Only 1 in 14 dogs exposed for 5 minutes to a large compressing balloon showed functional recovery, starting within 10–18 days after injury, and the histological examination revealed an incomplete anatomical lesion. Conversely, acute impact of a medium sized compression force in spite of longer duration (30–60 minutes) produced permanent destruction of the cord in about 50 per cent only, and a small sized acute compression did not prevent full functional recovery in all but one case (Case 78) following compression of 120 minutes, but the animal recovered and showed only a slight limp.

Cauda equina showed more resistance to a large compressive force than the cord, in spite of long lasting duration of the compression (27 hours), which is also in accordance with the clinical experience in man.

(ii) Tator (1971), amplifying Tarlow's experiments by using circumferential compression and measuring more accurately the varying weights of compressing forces in monkeys, found that a compressing force of 350 mmHg of 5 minutes' duration produced complete and permanent paraplegia in 5 out of 11 cases but 6 made some, although incomplete, recovery (Grade 2–3) which, moreover, started late—4, 5 and 8 weeks—after injury. This is in accordance with clinical experiences in man, in particular with regard to some functional recovery in initially complete lesions of the cervical cord following fracture-dislocation. Tator found that the threshold for immediately complete but reversible paraplegia was 250 mmHg of 5 minutes' duration. However, in two cases a compressing force of only 150 mmHg lasting 5 minutes also resulted in severe neurological deficit.

From these interesting experiments, it would appear that the size of a compressing force and the acuteness and weight of its impact on the spinal cord are decisive factors in producing either almost immediately complete or severe, incomplete destruction of the neural elements and the blood supply and, in particular, of the grey matter at the site of the injury. However, even in these circumstances, neuronal elements may escape the violence of the impact and, in due course, functional recovery although usually of minor degree, may occur.

(iii) In contrast, gradual compression leading to initially complete paralysis did not prevent full functional recovery, in spite of 7, 51, 72 and 84 hours continuous compression resulting in no or moderate histological changes of the cord. This underlines the experiences gained in man with gradual compression of benign extramedullary tumours (Guttmann, 1936).

Richardson and Nakamura (1971), in their electron microscope studies on spinal cord oedema, used a different technique of compression in cats. Spinal cord compression was produced vertically against the longitudinal axis of the cord by a steel rod, the tip of which was fitted into a 6.8×9.2 mm polythylene plate curved sufficiently to fit the convexity of the exposed dura. Various compressive weights were studied but the optimal lesion to avoid large haemorrhage into the spinal cord was produced by 80 gm of weight producing a pressure calculated to be 128 gm/cm. The results of this study will be discussed later (see chapter on chemical prevention of post-traumatic damage to the cord, page 159).

3. SPINAL CORD CONTUSION PRODUCED BY WEIGHT-DROPPING TECHNIQUES

Early crude experiments inflicting blunt injuries by violent blows to the vertebral column in animals, resulting in damage to the spinal cord of various degrees (Schmaus, 1890; Kirdgasser, 1897; Spiller, 1899 and others), have been abandoned and replaced by more sophisticated weight-dropping techniques on the exposed spinal cord, allowing quantitation and standardization of spinal cord lesions. They were originated by Allen (1911, 1914), who developed a technique of dropping a known weight through a perpendicular tube from a calculated height on to the exposed spinal cord with an intact dura in dogs, thus producing an anticipated degree of spinal cord contusion. Freeman & White (1953) and Ducker et al. (1971) confirmed Allen's concept that the amount of pathology in the central grey and white matter of the cord is directly proportional to the severity of trauma. Daniell *et al.* (1975) introduced a modification of Allen's technique to standardize the weight to be dropped to measure accurately the extent of trauma. This method consisted of a weight which was dropped down a centre shaft onto a strain gauge arch assembly which transferred the force to a teflon impounder resting on the exposed dura. The force transferred from the weight to the impounder was recorded by a strain gauge and the force curve was displayed on a storage oscilloscope. The forces induced to the cord were photographed and measured. These studies were carried out on 50 cats and 6 Rhesus monkeys. It was found that a 100 g weight dropped from 5 cm height produced a force curve of less magnitude but greater duration than that produced by 50 g dropped from 10 cm height.

There is, however, no universal agreement amongst experimental workers as to the standard weight and height from which the weight is to be dropped onto the exposed spinal cord. Dohrman *et al.* (1971), studying fine structural alterations in transitory traumatic paraplegia (T10) following experimentally inflicted contusion of the spinal cord in 23 Rhesus monkeys, used 300 g/cm^2 force, and Wagner *et al.* (1971) in their studies on spinal cord oedema following weight-dropping on the exposed spinal cord on 36 cats (T9 to T11) used 400 g/cm^2.

Yeo and Hinwood (1975) in their experiments on sheep, used a weight of 50 g which was dropped through a vertical teflon tubing from a height of 20 cm onto an impounder positioned over the exposed spinal cord at T10 level. These authors studied the following aspects:

(1) The validity of the reproducible contusion injury.

(2) The resulting pathological changes in the moderately contused cord.

(3) The use of isotope myelography to define the degree of spinal cord damage following moderate contusion.

A very important result of these experimental studies was the fact that the degree of contusion occurring within 120 minutes varied considerably, even though the impact injury was standardized at T10 level. Moreover, macroscopic as well as microscopic differences in the degree of congestion, extravasation and axonal swelling were evident in the white and grey matter. The earliest pathological changes in neurones were evident within 15–30 minutes and intramedullary congestion and extravasation of blood initially in grey matter and later in white occurred at 10–15 minutes.

There was also variation in the motor response following applied electrical stimulation of the exposed spinal cord below the level of the trauma immediately after injury. In this connection, the studies of Campbell *et al.* (1971) may be mentioned, who found in cats that, if action potentials were present within three hours after injury, recovery would follow.

Lumbar puncture was found by Yeo and Hinwood to be of little diagnostic value, which is in accordance with the generally accepted views of clinicians.

The authors also confirmed the views held by many experienced clinicians that contrast myelography exposed the recently injured patient to a painful and hazardous manipulation. Conversely, isotope myelography was found to be a more reliable means of elucidating degree and extent of spinal fluid block and by inference the degree of cord swelling. Within 2 hours after injury, the degree of cord oedema varied with the same injury in different sheep. According to the authors, post-traumatic oedema is due to neuronal swelling. Within 4 hours, there was a wide variation in the degree of paraplegia. These findings emphasize how difficult it is to establish a reproducible degree of contusion. Isotope myelography also revealed that even intensively swollen cords rapidly reduced in size over 48 hours. Isotope myelography with a simple portable counter can now be used to assess the degree and extent of spinal fluid block in the recently injured spinal patient.

CHAPTER 10

REGENERATION OF THE SPINAL CORD

The problem of regeneration of the spinal cord following transection in man and animals has for many years been the subject of intensive clinical and experimental research (Müller, 1864–65; Caporoso, 1889; Harte & Stewart, 1902; Fowler, 1905; Marinesco & Minea, 1906; Allen, 1911, 1914; Cadwalader, 1920; Cajal, 1928; Minea, 1928; Freeman, 1952, 1954; Windle, 1955; Hamburger, 1955; Babbini, 1956; Tarlow, 1957; Street, 1967; Campbell, 1967 and others). Windle's book on 'Regeneration in the Central Nervous System', in particular, gives a comprehensive review of the experimental work in animals. From these experiments, it would appear that anatomical regeneration and functional recovery were found in amphibia, reptiles and fish. However, this problem is still unsolved in species of higher phylogenetic scale such as mammals, including man. In view of the histological findings, it is not denied that regenerating nerve fibres may penetrate the glial and fibrous scar barriers under favourable conditions, but functional recovery through regeneration of the severed spinal cord is still unproven. Moreover, animal experiments producing traumatic lesions of the exposed spinal cord by varying pressures of weight in relation to the duration of pressure cannot be accepted as proof of the mechanism and pathology of spinal cord lesions due to fractures and fracture-dislocations of the spine in man. The fact that spinal animals, such as cats and dogs, are able to stand and to learn to walk is not the result of re-innervation of the paralysed muscles but is due to combined action of static and kinetic reflexes elicited below the level of the transection and the compensatory function of back muscles which have their innervation in segments above the transection but have their anatomical attachment below the transection, thus forming a connection between the paralysed part of the body with the normal ones. As pointed out before, in the spinal man it is in particular trapezius and latissimus dorsi and in lower lesions also the abdominal muscles which are responsible for the recovery of the upright position of the body following transection of the cord.

In 1902, Harte & Stewart reported about recovery of motor and sensory function as well as function of bladder and bowels in a female patient with transection of the cord following gunshot injury in whom these surgeons had performed a suture of the cord. This patient was examined 18 years later by Dr Cadwalader (1920) who, however, found a complete paraplegia and considered the previous result of the examination by these authors as a mistake. Other cases of suture of the spinal cord following transection were recorded by Fowler (1905); Babbini (1956); Thomeret (1960) and Street (1967), but no functional recovery occurred over a period of 6 to 11 years. In three cases of complete transverse lesions described by Street (1967), one of the thoracic and two of the distal spinal cord, a resection of the damaged vertebra and resection of the damaged segment of the cord was carried out in operations lasting 6 and 9 hours respectively. The unstable spine was fixed in one case by metal clamps, in the two others by wiring and screws.

A control X-ray 9 months after metal clamp-fixation revealed a considerable deformity of the spine with lateral dislocation of the lower part of the vertebral column. The complete paraplegia in these cases remained unchanged. Street's conclusions on account of his own and other surgeons' experiences are: 'Concerning the technique for suturing the cord, we are quite in the dark, since to date the attempts have been unsuccessful'.

Most unfortunate are sensational reports which sometimes appear in the Press or Television of unproven functional recovery as a result of such operations just mentioned, which raise false hopes amongst traumatic paraplegics and tetraplegics. This happened just a few years ago in the case of a Canadian surgeon who claimed functional recovery in a traumatic tetraplegic and other patients with spinal cord injuries resulting in paraplegia, following an alleged resection of the damaged vertebra and the traumatized section of the spinal cord followed by resuture of the cord. An immediate investigation by the medical authorities concerned revealed that this claim was entirely without foundation. This case aroused considerable publicity through Press and Television in various countries, and it took some time to convince paralysed people all over the world, all hopeful of a miraculous cure, of the fallacy of this claim.

Whether regeneration of the conducting neural elements within the spinal cord followed by functional recovery is possible in certain types of cord lesions where the organization of the anatomical compartments at segmental level is not disrupted but preserved, is still a matter of conjecture. For instance, in a case of complete transverse lesion caused by a long standing neuro-fibroma or meningeoma, at operation the spinal cord may be found to be considerably flattened at the site of the tumour: however, to a greater or lesser degree functional recovery will occur in time, following careful extirpation of the tumour. Foerster (1936) described a case of extramedullary tumour in the mid-thoracic region, who for several years was confined to bed with all symptoms of a complete transverse cord syndrome. At operation, the cord was found to be compressed by a hard extramedullary tumour into a flat thin strand. For a full year after operation, the complete transverse syndrome remained unchanged, but then very gradual recovery of both motor and sensory functions of the lower limbs occurred, which over a period of more than four years became almost complete, apart from residual impairment of posterior column sensibility. Foerster ascribed the functional recovery to a probable axon regeneration of the cord for the following reasons: the very late beginning of the recovery, its progression from proximal to caudal direction and the gradual development of the functional recovery.

In these cases of benign extramedullary tumours, there is no clear relationship between the degree of cord compression as revealed at operation and the time of recovery of axonal conductivity and extent of recovery of the clinical symptomatology following removal of the tumour or other compressing causes. In the writer's monograph on 'X-ray Diagnostic of Brain and Spinal Cord by Contrast Techniques' in Vol. VII (2) of the German *Handbook of Neurology* (Guttmann, 1936), a case of calcified meningeoma in a woman, aged 62, was described. The patient had a very severe though not complete transverse spinal syndrome below T4. At operation, I found the spinal cord to be most severely compressed and after careful removal of the hard tumour the compressed part of the cord did not expand, which was suggestive of long-lasting pressure. Yet, within 6 months after operation she made a complete recovery of all clinical symptoms, could do full house work and take long walks. In another case of meningeoma removed by the writer, the patient—a woman, aged 41—had an almost complete paraplegia below T4. At operation, the matrix of the tumour was found on the anterior surface of the dura developing shaft-like posteriorly and with its main bulk compressing the cord to a thin band which was riding on top of the tumour. However, following total removal of the tumour, the cord expanded, even during the operation, almost to its normal size and the patient made a complete functional recovery within a few weeks and in due course resumed mountaineering.

In this connection, the case of a traumatic paraplegic woman may be mentioned which the writer reported at the 1966 Annual Meeting of the International Medical Society of Paraplegia during the discussion on a paper by Wolman on axon regeneration after spinal cord injury. This patient had a complete transverse cord syndrome following fracture dislocation at T5 level of 27 years duration. During the last few years, the patient had complained of pain in her lower back radiating into the left leg. On examination, I found that she had definitely some appreciation to deep pressure with correct localization in the left leg. I had known her symptomatology for many years, but it was the first time that this appreciation to deep pressure on the left side only was discovered. Wolman (1966) found evidence of well-developed axon regeneration in or near the damaged segments in 12 out of 76 patients with traumatic paraplegia, the time lapse after injury ranging from 12 months to 32 years. The regenerating axons occurred in small bundles both above and below the level of the maximal cord damage in three cervical, five thoracic and four lumbar cases. A very frequent site of bundles of regenerated nerve fibres was in the pia arachnoid on the dorsolateral aspects of the cord above the level of the maximal damage and in the dorsolateral quadrant of the cord near the dorsal root entry zone. The origin of these nerve fibres was clearly in the posterior nerve roots and ganglia. Although there is no proof as yet of true motor and sensory recovery in man following transection of the cord, the now greatly increased life expectancy of traumatic paraplegics and tetra-plegics, as a result of the advances made in the treatment during the last 25 years, has opened new opportunities to study this important problem in man by a close co-operation between clinicians and neuropathologists. The preconditions are detailed clinical records of the initial stage of the cord lesion and careful and systematic neurological check-ups with special reference to motor and sensory functions over a period of many years. Only then will a proper correlation between such histological findings, as described by Wolman (1966) and others, and the clinical symptomatology be possible.

C · Fractures and Dislocations of the Vertebral Column

CHAPTER 11

MECHANISMS OF SPINAL FRACTURES

The vertebral column may be subjected to a wide variety or combination of stresses resulting in dislocation, fracture and fracture-dislocation. Mechanism and classification of injuries of the spinal column, with and without cord or spinal root involvement, have been repeatedly discussed in the old and recent literature (Wagner & Stolper, 1898; Jefferson, 1920–40; Böhler, 1937, 1963; Barnes, 1948, 1961; Taylor & Blackwood, 1948; Watson-Jones, 1950; Taylor, 1951; Schneider *et al.*, 1954; Roaf, 1960; 1971; Kahn, 1959; Witley & Forsyth, 1960; Zettel, 1962; Brocher, 1965–66, 1971; Forsyth & Winston-Salem, 1964; Guttmann, 1931–71; Holdsworth, 1963; Petrie, 1964; Munro, 1966; Kuhlendahl, 1966; Bedbrook, 1969, 1971; Frankel *et al.*, 1969; Cheshire, 1969; Burke, 1971; Mayer & Peters, 1971; Braakman & Penning, 1971). However, views still differ on various aspects. This is understandable, as the forces generated by the impact of the violence causing vertebral and cord injuries produce not merely displacement of the spine in one direction but often any combination of upward, forward, backward, lateral and rotational movements. This is particularly true in accidents where the injured is hurled violently from some position and finally lands against hard surfaces (hurling mechanism).

STABLE AND UNSTABLE FRACTURES

There is still disagreement in the definition of stable and unstable fractures, and the criteria used differ considerably. This, inevitably, has its consequences on the initial management of spinal fractures and dislocations. The recent introduction of the term 'Potential Instability' (Bedbrook, 1970) may not contribute to diminish the confusion. In fact, it may give 'dynamic' or inexperienced surgeons an excuse to rush immediately into unnecessary and useless operative procedure for internal stabilization. Beatson (1963), in his excellent review, showed how difficult it is in the cervical spine to be certain of cases which will prove pathologically unstable. Data given in the literature on instability vary considerably. Gallie (1939), Ellis (1946), Durbin (1957) and others report 10–12 per cent. In Cheshire's series (1969) of 257 cervical fractures, the late instability rate varied between 4·8 and 7·3 per cent in all main groups. The high percen-

97

tage (21 per cent) of instability in his series of 19 cases of anterior subluxation is unusual. In Bedbrook's cases (1970), the late instability was 6 per cent. In 37 cervical injuries, published recently by Burke & Berryman (1971), three (8 per cent) showed late instability following conservative treatment requiring surgical fusion. None showed neurological deterioration because of the delay in fusion.

Talbot (1971) confirmed the low incidence of instability requiring surgical stabilization. Reviewing 600 patients of his spinal Centre he found that in only 21 out of 600 some type of fusion was indicated. Some 20 out of the 600 had had so-called stabilization procedures done before admission to his Unit and more than half of those still presented the same indication for further stabilization which, however, has not been done and 'they are not worse off'.

Burke and Tiong (1975) in a series of 175 cases admitted between 1968 and 1973 have lowered their previous statistics to only 4·2 per cent of the patients requiring spinal fusion for late instability after a conservative treatment. Professor Del Sel, a very experienced orthopaedic surgeon, did not find late instability amongst 150 patients with cervical injuries. (See also chapter on Spinal Fusions, page 170.)

In a series of 612 fractures of various levels of the Stoke Mandeville group of workers (Frankel et al., 1969), the late instability was only 4 (0·65 per cent). These figures of low late instability speak for themselves (see page 151). Some surgeons try to prove instability of a reduced fractured vertebra by control-X-rays in extensive and retro- and forward flexion of head and neck at an early stage. I consider this as much an unnecessary as it is an hazardous procedure, for a fibrous or not yet fully mature bony union may be easily broken by such extreme movements. This control, unless indicated by the development or progression of neurological symptoms, should not be carried out before 6 months after alignment of fracture-dislocations. Bedbrook (1971) from his extensive experience came to the conclusion 'we should never say that a fracture disloca-tion is unstable under at least eight weeks, and probably between eight and twelve weeks, In McSweeney's view (1969) the majority of neck injuries are stable after 4 months. He advocates, however (1975), bony fusion in a small group of patients with bilateral facetal dislocations and no or minimal bony injury and with no consequential neurological impairment, provided stability of the spine is not achieved in a reasonable time. This applies in particular in young people with certain flexion injuries of the cervical spine with widening of the inter-spinous space and partial overriding of the posterior facetal joints, as demonstrated under the X-ray image intensifier. This type of injury 'almost invariably progresses to gross angular deformity and requires surgical fusion' (McSweeney, 1975). It must be noted that these are very exceptional cases. However, indiscriminate spinal fusion following discography in the immediate or early stages after fractures of the cervical spine, especially simple compression-wedge fracture, is inexcusable. By such a procedure not only will the already affected vertebra be destroyed but the two adjacent vertebrae will also be damaged in order to insert the bone graft. The inserted bony block may not prevent further dislocation at its distal margin as I found recently in such a patient who, aged 21, was fused elsewhere on the day of accident (see also Fig. 81). All these observations to which more can be added, do not confirm the enthusiasm of Cloward, Verbiest and others and their radical views are unacceptable.

RETRO-HYPERFLEXION—ANTERO-HYPERFLEXION INJURIES

Another subject of dispute is the term 'Hyperextension Injuries', generally accepted for certain fracture-dislocations, in particular of the cervical spine due to facial or frontal injuries, which, however, was recently criticized by Roaf (1971) as being inaccurate. True hyperextension of both vertebrae and spinal cord may actually occur in vertical direction as a result of excessive skull traction by pull-weights which are too heavy (iatrogenic hyperextension) (Figs. 44, 45). However, the mechanism of certain cervical fractures and fracture-dislocations resulting from a fall or blow on the forehead or face, for instance, following diving into shallow water, is, in fact, that of a retro-hyperflexion of the head and cervical spine, with or without rotation. The violent retroflexion of head and neck forces the spinous and articular processes of the mid-cervical vertebrae (C4–C6) together, and these, now acting as a fulcrum, cause a separation between the vertebral body and the adjacent lower intervertebral disc, which results in dislocation. According to the intensity and speed of the driving force, the separation may still continue and rupture the anterior longitudinal ligament. Moreover, the posterior ligament may then be dislodged from the vertebral body below, become buckled up and thus, squeezing the spinal cord backward against the lower vertebra, cause partial or complete transection of the cord. This squeezing effect also explains the spinal cord damage often found in segments well above and below the fractured vertebra. This mechanism of cervical fracture, first described by Taylor & Blackwood (1948), explains well the spinal cord damage commonly called hyperextension injury, but which is actually due to a retroflexion injury of the spine. Fig. 41a (p. 100) is an example of a retro-hyperflexion injury of C6 on C7 in a man aged 43 who was involved in a motor accident on 6.8.58. As shown, this injury resulted in over-riding of the articular facets of C7 but was reduced by head traction. Moreover, as can be seen there is a narrowing of the processus spinosi between C6 and C7 which disappeared after full reduction. Clinically the patient had a complete tetra-plegia below C7 which was first flaccid but later became spastic. He is still living. This man suffered a lung embolie with cardiac arrest from which, however, he recovered (see page 200).

Sometimes the violent retroflexion which forces the spinosus and articular processes together may produce a fracture of one or two of these processes as shown in Fig. 41b (p. 101) (see also Fig. 49). In some cases with this type of injury occurring in ankylosing spondylitis of the cervical spine, the separation was not found between the body and its adjacent cartilagenous tissues but the vertebral body itself was ruptured and broken in two (Guttmann, 1966) (Fig. 56).

In contrast to the mechanism just described, the mechanism responsible for a different type of injury is caused by ventro-hyperflexion of the head and neck. In such an event, the acting force will not cause a fulcrum at the spinous and articural processes but on the contrary will force together the adjacent vertebrae at the level of maximum stress. Therefore, the gap between the spinous processes will be widened, as shown in Fig. 41c (p. 102). In a man of 20, who was injured on 1.8.67 in a diving accident, the initial ventro-hyperflexion fracture of C3/4 with over-riding articular process was first reduced elsewhere by head traction but on 21.9.67 by internal fixation with a wired graft before the patient's admission to Stoke Mandeville on 14.10.67. After the operation, the initially incomplete tetraplegia temporarily became complete, but in due course the patient recovered the use of the muscles of both hands, he was able to walk and he also fully recovered his bladder function. The urine became sterile.

In this type of ventro-hyperflexion injury, the violent force may drive the anterior-inferior edge of the upper vertebra into the body of the vertebra below, split it into two and may evulse part of it forward or downward (commonly called tear drop fracture). The posterior part of the fractured body will be displaced backwards into the spinal cord and crush it (Fig. 52b).

In both mechanisms, however, the spinal cord above the fulcrum produced by the fracture-dislocation may be stretched upwards in a diagonal direction. Therefore, it would be more accurate to use the terms retro-hyperflexion and ventro-hyperflexion for these two types of spinal injuries.

In a lesser degree of violence in ventro-hyperflexion, the resulting deformity of the spine may be a dislocation in ventro-hyperflexion only.

Vertical stress to the vertebral column, as a result of a fall on the head or seat or neck, may produce a compression fracture with flattening of a whole vertebral body without rupturing the ligamentous complex, but the compressed vertebral body will protrude into the transverse plane anteriorly and/or posteriorly, resulting in more or less destruction of the cord.

Various other factors have to be considered to understand the great varieties of spinal injury.

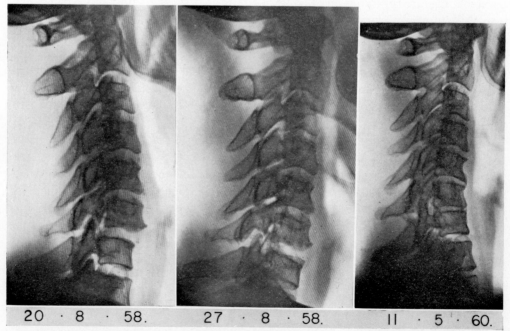

20 · 8 · 58.   27 · 8 · 58.   11 · 5 · 60.

FIG. 41a. Retro-hyperflexion injury with overriding and locking articular facet of C7. Reduced by head traction. Note the narrowing between interspaces of spinous processes C6 and C7 widened after complete reduction.

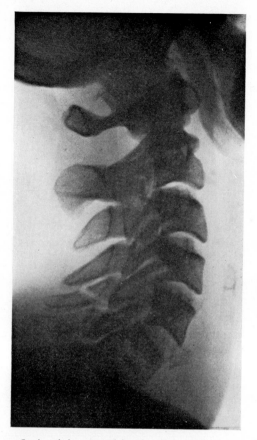

FIG. 41b. Retro-hyperflexion injury resulting in slight dislocation of C6 with destruction of the disc between C5 and C6. Disc material pushed out anteriorly. Note the narrowing of the interspaces between the spinous processes C4–C6, and fracture of C5 spinous process at the level of maximum stress.

(I) CONGENITAL ANOMALIES OF THE SPINE

Congenital and acquired anomalies may influence type, extent and severity of spinal injuries. Congenital anomalies occur in particular in the most proximal (atlanto-axial) and distal (lumbo-sacral) parts of the spine. In the atlanto-axial region, fusion of the atlas to the occiput (atlanto-occipital assimilation) may be combined with platybasia and Arnold–Chiari abnormality of the brain stem and cerebellum. Moreover, there are congenital defects of the arch of the atlas either unilaterally or bilaterally. Furthermore, there may be congenitally complete or partial absence of the odontoid process or separate odontoid process (os odontoideum); the four groups of clinical symptomatology of the latter has been described by Rowland *et al.* (1958). Klippel–Feil syndrome consisting of hemivertebrae, and fusion of adjacent vertebrae and scoliosis of the cervical spine are other examples of congenital anomalies in that region.

In the lumbo-sacral region, the most common anomalies are spina bifida, bilateral or unilateral sacralization of the 5th lumbar vertebra and spondylolisthesis. Although the latter cannot be regarded as a congenital anomaly as such, it develops as a result of a structural vertebral defect, usually of the 5th lumbar vertebra, where the interruption of the neural arch on either side at the pars inter-articularis represents the underlying defect. Scoliosis due to vertebral abnormalities and neuropathies may also be mentioned amongst the congenital anomalies as well as narrowing of the spinal canal.

Of the acquired anomalies of the vertebral column which may influence the character of a fracture, mention has already been made of the ankylosing spondylitis. Certain forms of chronic spondylosis of the elderly, as well as scoliosis after poliomyelitis or muscular dystrophy, and the so-called idiopathic scoliosis may affect the type and severity of spinal injuries. Fig. 41d shows a fracture-dislocation of T4 vertebra following a car accident, resulting in profound lateral-upward displacement of the vertebral column below the fracture in a case of idiopathic scoliosis causing an almost complete paraplegia

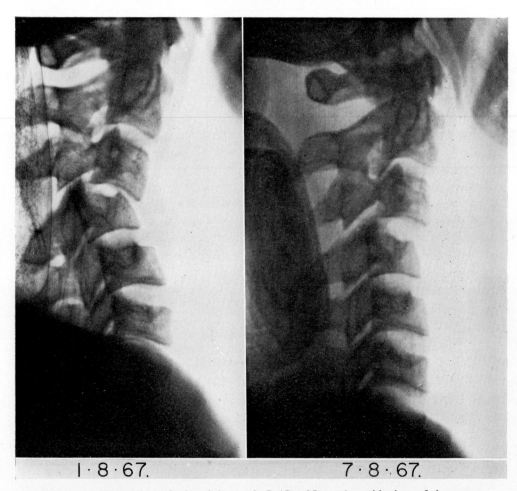

Fig. 41c. Ventro-hyperflexion injury of C3/C4. Note the widening of interspace between C3 and C4 spinous process and overriding of C4 articular facet, reduced at first by head traction. See also Fig. 82, p. 172, demonstrating the end results of wired grafting resulting in return of ventro-flexion in spite of excellent functional recovery.

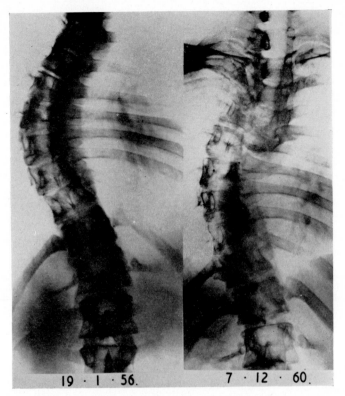

19 · 1 · 56.   7 · 12 · 60.

FIG. 41d.

below T4. The patient, aged 20, sustained a bilateral haemothorax and a spastic paraplegia below T5 but only incomplete sensory loss below T7 with some appreciation to pain in S1 on the right side. He also had sensation of fullness of the bladder and in due course regained some bladder and sexual control in spite of most unusual lateral dislocation of the broken spine.

(2) AETIOLOGICAL FACTORS

Careful history taking and analysis of the accident are essential in clarifying the mechanism. In 1970, I saw a young boy of 7, in the Bihar district of India, who, in a most unique accident, sustained a complete tetraplegia below C7, having been attacked by one of his father's pet lions. X-rays did not show any fracture or dislocation of the cervical spine, nor were there any signs of an external wound on the neck as a result of a bite or claws. The aetiology and mechanism of the injury seemed to be obscure until I found a scar over the boy's forehead. On further questioning the person who saw the accident and came to the boy's rescue, it became clear that the boy had been thrown forward to the ground by the heavy weight of the lion, hitting the ground with his forehead. It was, therefore, obvious that in this case the mechanism of the cervical cord injury was that of a temporary vertebral dislocation, resulting from a violent backward and upward movement of the head and neck, which, however, reduced itself (commonly but wrongly called whiplash mechanism). It is well known that in spinal cord injuries in children, X-rays either do not reveal any bony injury or, if so, these are rarely significant (Guttmann, 1960; Meinecke, 1969). Burke (1971) confirmed this fact on a larger material and explained the mechanism of the cord lesion as a longitudinal traction effect as a result of considerable elongation of the vertebral column, due to its great elasticity in children, which is in accordance with Bedbrook's previous pathological findings (1963–66) in cord lesion following fractures and fracture-dislocations in adults.

(3) DIRECTION OF THE ACTING FORCE

The driving force generated by the impact of the violence may speed in cranio-caudal (vertical), horizontal or lateral directions and be coupled with rotation. As a result, displacement may occur in forward, backward or sideways direction, with compression and with or without rotation of the affected vertebrae.

(4) RELATIONSHIP OF THE ACTING FORCE TO THE POSITION OF THE BODY AT THE TIME OF THE IMPACT OF VIOLENCE

In coalmine or quarry accidents, for instance, the acting force will produce different fractures or fracture-dislocations depending on the position of the body at the time of the impact of falling rocks—i.e. whether the individual had been standing or kneeling in a stooping-forward position or lying in semi-lateral position. It is also important to know whether parts of the spine had been fixed by external supports at the time of accident. In this connection, special mention should be made about the mechanism of spinal cord injuries in the upper thoracic region after 'plane crash landings, as they demonstrate the importance of the position of the body at the moment of injury as an important factor in determining the level of the spinal cord lesion. As Watson-Jones (1941) pointed out, the special fixation of the pilot in the cockpit by his harness over the front of both shoulder joints holds the pilot in his seat and thus prevents the violent forward movement of the trunk, which would otherwise occur at the moment of the crash. Consequently, it raises the site of angulation from the thoraco-lumbar junction to the upper thoracic level—hence the resulting fracture occurs not at the thoraco-lumbar junction (jack-knife mechanism), as commonly found in coalmine and other industrial injuries, but at the upper thoracic or cervical spine. Experience gained at Stoke Mandeville on spinal cord injuries following air-crash landings is in accordance with this conception.

Spinal injuries may also occur as a result of the ejection force from aircraft. Recent research carried out at the R.A.F. Institute of Aviation at Farnborough, Hants. and reported by Reader, Barwood & Griffin (1975) defined the factors which govern human tolerance to rapid acceleration and the levels of human tolerance in relation to ejection acceleration. The modern ejection escape system can recover air crews from a crippled aircraft, and the tolerance to the forces of ejection may be increased by efficient restraint of a suitable harness which also functions as a parachute harness. The telescopic ejection gun is fixed by pulling a handle at the front of the seat pan or by an upper handle which pulls a face blind over the head. Fixing the gun unlocks the seat resulting in its separation from the aircraft and by exploding secondary cartridges the thrust of the gun is sustained. Barwood found that with the face-blind system the incidence of fractures was 38 per cent but became 69 per cent when the seat pan handle was used, the difference being attributable to the push adopted at the time of ejection. The face-blind system allows time to adjust the restraint harness and induces extension of the spine if the urgency is not too great, while the pan handle method, which is used in acute emergency, allows no time for harness adjustment and promotes slight flexion of the spine. The introduction of the rocket-assisted ejection seat results only in slight diminution of incidents (50 per cent).

Incorrect posture and imperfect restraint of the harness result in spinal injuries, and the common landing injuries are crush fractures of the spine, the vast majority being simple compression fractures of one or more vertebrae. The anterior superior part of the vertebra is the most frequently involved. One pilot acquired four fractures the first time following ejection, and two at the second and he also suffered a spondylolisthesis of L5 on S1. Two pilots of the older age group suffered injury of the dorsal vertebrae including burst fractures and marked displacement of anterior fragments.

The average annual incidence of spinal fractures due to ejection according to Griffin is 47 per cent. Hunter, Canberra and Buccaneer showed a high incidence, while Gnat the lowest. However, when the total of ejections was related to the total number of sorties per aircraft, the risk of ejection injury from a Hunter was the lowest.

The standard treatment in the R.A.F. for these fractures is conservative, consisting of bedrest for a minimum of 3 weeks. Following regaining of full spinal extension, the pilot is returned to his Unit but remains in a non-flying capacity for 3 months.

Ewing reported on 69 U.S. Navy aircrew who suffered fractures following ejection, of whom 16 per cent were retired from flying duties and a further 7·2 per cent were restricted to limited flying (Ninow, 1971). It was considered that these figures might have been reduced if the harness had incorporated an anti-G strap.

Fitzgerald & Crotty (1971) found that 13 per cent of RAF pilots aged between 20 and 50 years experienced backache every time they flew; and up to 40 per cent experienced pain at least once during the course of a month of normal flying. Crooks (1970) reviewed RAF aircrew who had ejected in the previous 10 years. One interesting finding in his survey was a high radiological incidence of cervical spondylosis (75 per cent, compared with an incidence of 50 per cent in those who had not ejected). The relation of this high incidence to the ejection sequence requires further investigation.

(5) THE RESULTING ANATOMICAL LESION OF THE SPINAL CORD OR CAUDA EQUINA

Post-mortem examinations of patients with vertebral fractures resulting in paraplegia or tetraplegia have greatly clarified the mechanism involved by demonstrating the relationship of the bony, cartilagenous and ligamentous lesions with the spinal cord or cauda equina lesion. As a rule, the cord lesion is only rarely confined to the point of impact on the vertebral body, although there will be the maximal destruction of the neural elements and vascular supply, but through stretching or pressing effects the cord lesion continues beyond the bony or cartilagenous protrusion and may involve numerous segments above and below, confirming clinical observations of ascending cord lesions in the early stages following vertebral injuries (Guttmann, 1963; Frankel *et al.*, 1969).

CHAPTER 12

CLASSIFICATION OF SPINAL FRACTURES

From the author's experience on more than 2,500 spinal injuries, the following main varieties of fracture of the vertebral column are described in some detail:

(A) FRACTURES OF VERTEBRAL PROCESSES

These are fractures of lateral, spinous and articular processes. They can occur singly, but in the majority of spinal injuries, they occur in combination with fractures of the vertebral body. Fractures of the lateral and spinous processes are sometimes the result of a strong, sudden muscular contraction, such as the clay- or coal-shoveller fracture of the spinous process of the 7th cervical vertebra. Lonnerblad (1934), Mathes (1935) and Hall (1940) reported numerous fractures of spinous processes in shovellers as a result of the sudden jerk in throwing clay when the clay stuck to the shovel. While fractures of spinous and lateral processes do not need special treatment, unless they cause continuous pain and have to be removed, fractures of the odontoid process always require specialized management. Fig. 42 shows fractures of lateral processes of the lumbar vertebrae on the left side, and Fig. 49 demonstrates a fracture of the 6th spinous process.

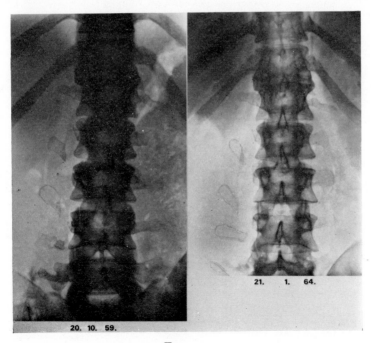

FIG. 42.

107

(B) FRACTURES OF VERTEBRAL BODIES AND THEIR ARTICULATIONS

(1) Cervical spine

The cervical spine is the most movable part of the vertebral column and, although the vertebrae are locked together to form a very stable column, extensive movements in extension, flexion, rotation and sideways tilting are possible.

(a) FRACTURES, DISLOCATIONS AND SUBLUXATIONS OF THE ATLAS

Jefferson (1920) described a type of fracture of the atlas now called Jefferson fracture, caused by a fall on the head or the head striking the ceiling of a car, or an object striking the top of the head. The resultant force, causing a thrust in bilateral direction, usually produces fractures at the weakest points of the atlas ring where the posterior arch connects with the lateral masses, thus the atlas is split into three parts, enlarging its circumference, and consequently the spinal canal. Therefore, damage of the cord is, as a rule, absent or incomplete or only temporary.

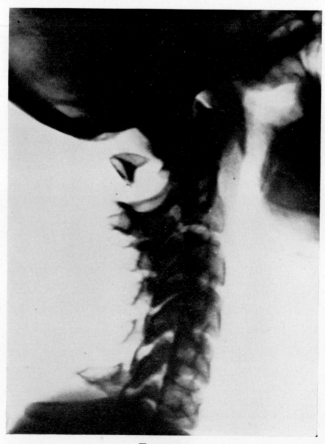

FIG. 43.

Isolated dislocations of the atlas against the axis are not very common, but gross forward or retro-dislocation and rotation may result in immediate death. Forward dislocation of one lateral mass may cause a marked rotatory movement of the head to the opposite side, resulting in a torticollis and neck stiffness. Braakman & Penning (1971) have recently given instructive examples of atlanto-axial rotation dislocation in children resulting in torticollis, and posterior atlanto-axial dislocation without fracture of the odontoid process has been described by Horalson & Boyd (1969), and Wadia (1967) reported a great incidence of congenital atlanto-axial dislocation in India. Sometimes fractures of spinous process or dislocation of the atlas against the axis not producing any cord or root damage may be overlooked if they are associated with a fracture of the distal parts of the vertebral column which causes the paraplegia, as shown in Fig. 43 demonstrating a fracture of the posterior arch of the atlas in such a case.

Wackenheim (1974) now differentiates the following subluxation of the upper cervical spine: (1) Transverse atlanto-condylar subluxation which was found in cases of spasmodic torticollis. Malgaigne (1855) found upper cervical luxation as a fatal catastrophe. (2) Transverse atlanto-axial subluxation with lateral displacement of the atlas on the axis. These patients found rotation of the head painful. (3) Atlanto-axial rotation and

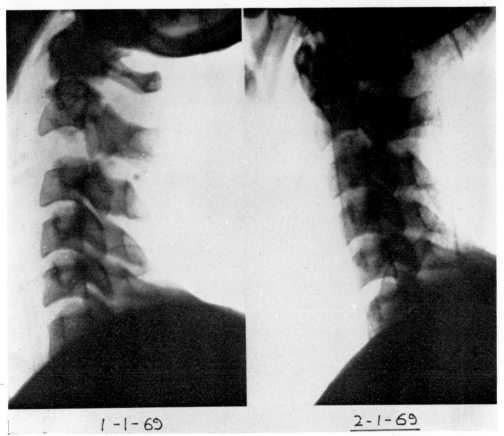

1-1-69   2-1-69

FIG. 44. Over-distraction (vertical hyperextension) of spine and spinal cord resulting from the pull of head traction.

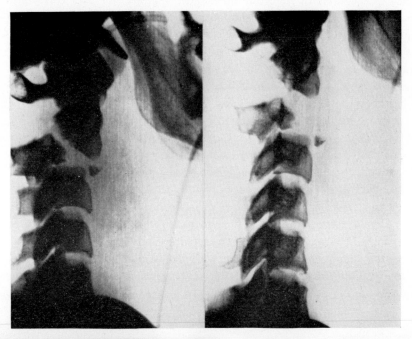

FIG. 45a (Above). Effect of over-distraction following head traction.

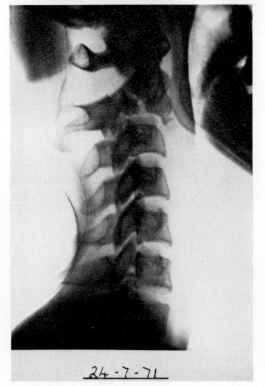

24-7-71

FIG. 45b (Left). Same case following reduction of the pull-weight.

subluxation with rotation of the occiput upon atlas and atlas upon the axis. (4) Antero-superior and antero-inferior subluxation of the atlas by tilting, possibly produced by rupture or stretching of the posterior atlanto-occipital ligaments. Naturally, such detailed differentiation is only possible by highly specialized X-ray techniques.

(b) FRACTURES OF THE ODONTOID

Fractures and dislocations of the odontoid are also produced by forces acting in vertical direction or combined with retroflexion caused by a direct blow, falling on the head or being thrown through a windscreen of a car. They may be associated with fractures of the jaw, as shown in the following case:

A 19-year-old apprentice electrician, while passenger in a bubble car, was involved in an accident on 27 December 1968, and was thrown through the windscreen. Apart from lacerations on skull and chin and a fracture of the right mandible, he sustained a fracture-dislocation of the odontoid with downward displacement of its processes, resulting in a complete motor, but incomplete sensory tetraplegia below C3 with areflexia. He was unconscious for several hours. Following skull traction with 7 lb weight he was at first able to move all limbs and pass urine, but deteriorated later, and 2 days after injury tracheotomy had to be performed and an indwelling catheter inserted into the paralysed bladder in the hospital of his first admission.

On admission to Stoke Mandeville 7 days later, the first X-ray of the cervical spine showed a separation and marked vertical over-distraction of the fractured odontoid from the third cervical vertebra, obviously as a result of the pull of the skull traction (Fig. 44). The weight was immediately reduced and the two vertebrae joined together, with the result that the motor paralysis started to improve and a few days later bladder function also gradually returned. In due course, he made an excellent neurological recovery and control X-rays in marked retroflexion and ventroflexion showed excellent stabilization of the fractured odontoid. He was discharged home on 21 May 1969, about 6 months after injury, being able to walk and having good control of bladder and bowels. Urine remained sterile throughout, following intermittent catheterization (Guttmann, 1949, 1963; Guttmann & Frankel, 1966). On the last clinical check-up on 27 November 1970, the muscle power of all muscles in upper and lower limbs was practically normal, but he still had sensory disturbances of the spino-thalamic tract and upgoing toes to plantar stimulation. He was quite independent and his sexual function had also returned.

Another example of unstable fracture-dislocation of the odontoid, resulting in an incomplete tetraplegia which deteriorated temporarily following vertical hyperextension through excessive skull traction, is shown in Figs. 45a and b. I saw this patient, aged 20, at the Spinal Injuries Centre of the Robert Jones and Agnes Hunt Orthopaedic Hospital, Oswestry, and I am indebted to Mr Sweeney and Dr Jones for letting me have the photo-graph of the X-rays of this case. A weight of 40 lb had been initially used in the hospital where the patient was first admitted. Following reducing the pull weight of the skull traction to 4 lb, the patient made a considerable recovery of his tetraplegia, is able to walk without any support, but still shows some patches of hypoalgesia on the left side. He

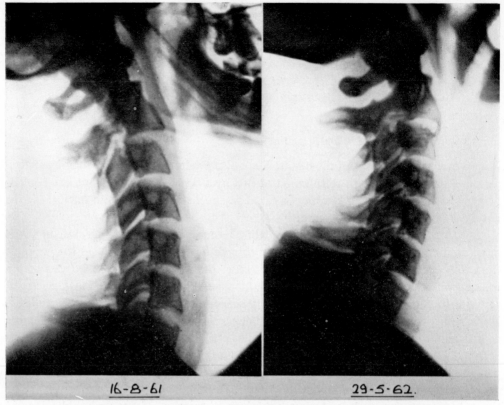

16-8-61   29-5-62.

Fig. 46a.

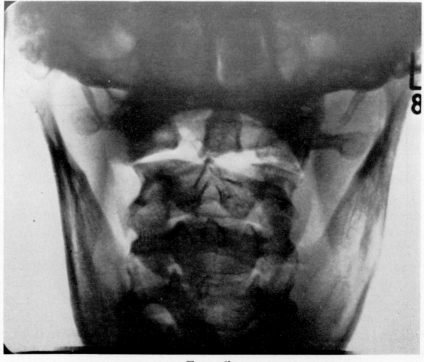

Fig. 46b.

has returned to his job. These are two classical examples of true (iatrogenic) hyper-extension in cephaled vertical direction.

However, especially in retroflexion injuries of the odontoid combined with rotation, the fractured processes may be driven into the spinal cord by the acting force, and may lead to immediate death. An unusual case of fatal dens-fracture of the axis has recently been reported by Mayer & Peters (1971):

A woman, aged 51, while working in a stooping-forward position, received a kick on the buttocks. She was thrown forward, hitting a concrete wall with the vertex of her head, the cervical spine being retro-flexed and the head rotated to the right. Death occurred immediately. The autopsy revealed a fracture of both upper articulations of the odontoid with rupture and displacement of the dens of the axis. The spinal cord showed profound squeezing effects with destruction of the neural elements and haemorrhages mainly at the level of C3/4 segments, but extending upwards to C1 and downwards into the 6th cervical segment. This fracture is commonly called hang-man fracture.

On the other hand, in one of our own patients aged 20, who sustained a fracture dislocation of L1 vertebra and fracture of transverse processes L2 resulting in an incomplete cauda equina lesion with considerable recovery of motor, sensory, bladder, and sexual functions, a fracture of the odontoid process with separation through the pedicles and rotation of the atlas was found. There were no motor or sensory disturbances in the upper limbs or part of the body above the cauda equina lesion—only the arm reflexes were found exaggerated without interfering with the isolated movements of the muscles. Conservative treatment without skull traction was applied and the C2 fracture consolidated satisfactorily with a spontaneous anterior fusion between C2 and C3. Figs. 46a and b demonstrate the severe fracture of the odontoid with separation of the dens axis (a–p picture).

(c) DISLOCATIONS AND FRACTURES OF C3–C7 VERTEBRAE

(i) *Subluxation*

Subluxations without fracture may be unilateral resulting in rotation or tilting of the head to one side (Stimson & Swinson, 1934). This has been confirmed by Watson-Jones (1955), Braakman & Penning (1971) and Wackenheim (1974). According to Watson-Jones, the only feature distinguishing a subluxation from a complete dislocation is that the articular processes have not actually overridden. Braakman & Penning, however, found that in 26 of their patients an initial diagnosis of 'subluxation' was made, while the essential feature of interlocking of the articular processes was overlooked. Fig. 47 demonstrates a subluxation of the mid-cervical spine on the 5th cervical vertebra with forward flexion in a man, aged 51, following a fall down from the top of a flight of stairs while under the influence of alcohol. The X-ray also shows a congenital fusion of the 2nd and 3rd cervical vertebrae. The neurological symptomatology was that of a traction lesion of the 5th cervical roots on the right side only with paralysis of the deltoid and partial paralysis of the biceps and sensory loss over the 5th cervical root distribution. Full anatomical reduction and complete recovery of the root lesion occurred without skull traction following bed rest with retroflexion of the cervical spine produced by a supporting small semi-hard cushion underneath the neck, followed by the application of a cervical collar.

(ii) *Cervical sprain*

Cervical sprain or strain has been interpreted differently (Watson-Jones, 1955; Braakman & Penning, 1971). Braakman & Penning define cervical sprain as partial and temporary disruption of the normal contact between the articular surfaces. In their opinion, there is no real difference between self-reducing dislocations and cervical sprain. Conversely, Watson-Jones (1955) interprets sprain as strain of the interarticular ligaments, as a result of a sudden twisting or jerking movement of the neck without actually displacing or dislocating the joints, and he stresses that such a sprain of the joint must be carefully differentiated from subluxation and self-reducing, momentary dislocation. The main clinical difference between self-reducing dislocation and true sprain of the interarticular ligaments seems to be, in my view, that sprain, apart from producing pain and temporary stiffness of neck movements, does not cause any damage to the spinal cord resulting in incomplete, let alone complete, tetraplegia, while self-reducing dislocations can certainly do so.

(iii) *Dislocations*

In this type of injury of the whole vertebral body, caused, as a rule, by retro-hyperflexion of head and cervical spine, the interspinous, anterior and posterior ligaments may be

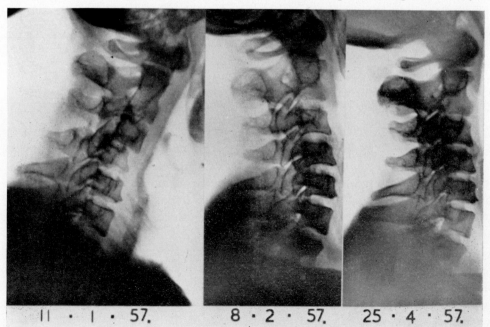

F I G. 47. Subluxation of mid-cervical spine. Full recovery of traction lesion of right 5th cervical root following bedrest and pillow support in retroflexion.

ruptured, the lateral articular capsules torn and the intervertebral disc more or less disrupted. As a result, instability of the spine occurs, unless the articular facets are locked by overriding of the inferior articular facet on the adjacent superior facets. Fig. 48 shows a pure dislocation of the 6th cervical vertebra over the 7th with locking articular facets of the 7th on the 6th and disruption of the intervertebral disc between C6 and C7 vertebrae. Unlocking of the articular processes and full reduction with anatomical alignment were achieved by skull traction combined with a support underneath the dislocation.

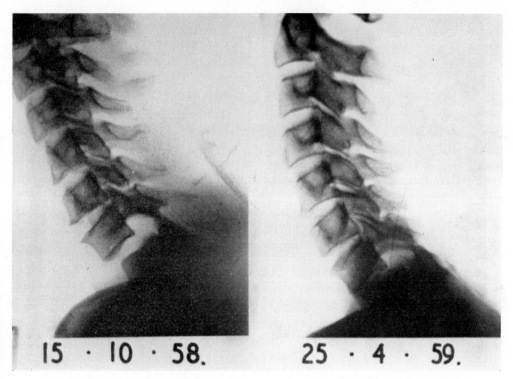

FIG. 48. Dislocation with locked articular facet.

Another example of dislocation of the cervical spine with locking articular process and associated with a fracture of posterior process is shown in Fig. 49 demonstrating a dislocation of C6 on C7 with fracture of the spinous process of C6. Following unlocking of the articular process an excellent reduction was accomplished by skull traction and the broken spinous process fused with the 5th spinous process in due course.

It is well known that dislocations of the vertebral bodies can reduce themselves unless there is interlocking and overriding of the articular facets. This may occur in adults as well as in children. In these cases, the X-rays will not reveal any fracture or dislocation, yet the injury to the cord caused by the momentary jarring effect of the violence may have resulted in an incomplete or even complete transection of the cord. Although such an injury may result in disruption of the ligaments, normal relationships of the bony and ligamentous tissues are re-established following self-reduction.

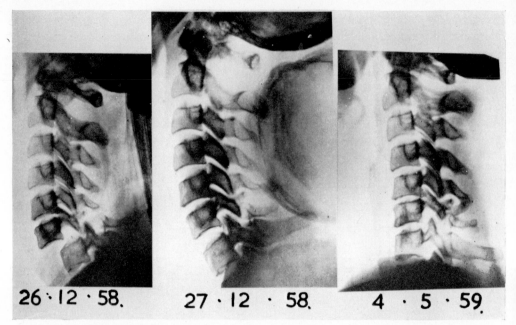

26 · 12 · 58.   27 · 12 · 58.   4 · 5 · 59.

FIG. 49. Dislocation with locked articular facets and fracture of spinous process. Retro-hyperflexion injury.

(d) COMPRESSION FRACTURES AND COMPRESSION-BURST FRACTURES

Vertical stresses may produce compression fractures of cervical vertebrae of varying degrees, including compression-burst fractures with avulsion of parts of the vertebral body. Fig. 50a shows a compression-burst fracture of C7 vertebra with forward avulsion of half of the vertebral body, as a result of a motor bike accident in a man, aged 24. Skull traction achieved good re-alignment of the fractured segments of the body, which, however, still remained protruded anteriorly. A firm bony fusion developed between the fractured 7th vertebra and its neighbouring 6th cervical and 1st thoracic vertebra. Neurological symptomatology: incomplete tetraplegia below C6, complete below T1. He made considerable recovery of hand and finger muscles, including extensors and flexors of the fingers, extensor pollicis longus left and flexor carpi-radialis. Triceps returned to full power. There was also sensory return down to T5. Last seen 23 March 1970. Has become considerably independent.

(e) FRACTURE-DISLOCATIONS

The great majority of injuries of the cervical spine are fracture-dislocations, as a rule, resulting from road, industrial and also sport accidents, in particular diving into shallow water, trampoline, rugby and vaulting sports. The mechanism of the fracture-dislocation may be produced either by retroflexion of head and cervical spine (usually but inaccurately called hyperextension fractures) or ventroflexion of head and neck (ventro-hyperflexion fractures). These injuries may produce most bizarre deformities of the cervical spine due to a combination of various factors.

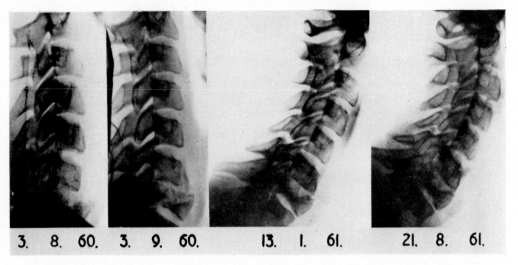

3. 8. 60.   3. 9. 60.   13. 1. 61.   21. 8. 61.

FIG. 50a.

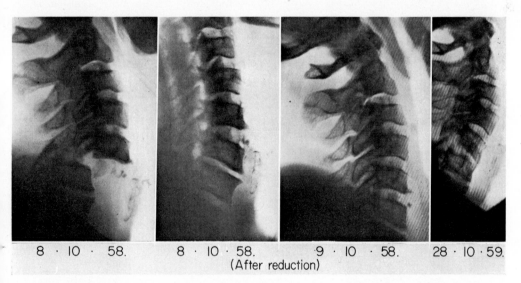

8 · 10 · 58.   8 · 10 · 58.   9 · 10 · 58.   28 · 10 · 59.
(After reduction)

FIG. 50b. Unstable, grotesque retro-hyperflexion dislocation with overriding facets and destruction of the disc between C5 and C6. Immediate reduction by head traction and neck support.

Fig. 50b shows a grotesque dislocation with fractures of the articular process and over-riding facets in a man of 38 following a·diving accident. The inter-vertebral disc between C5 and C6 vertebrae is completely destroyed and the fracture was unstable. The following photos show the results of reduction by head traction. This man had a complete tetraplegia below C5/6 which remained permanent.

Fig. 51 is an example of a profound ventro- or antero-hyperflexion injury. The first three upper cervical vertebrae are hyperflexed forward over the fractured 4th cervical, which is split into two pieces by the impact of the sharp anterior inferior edge of C3

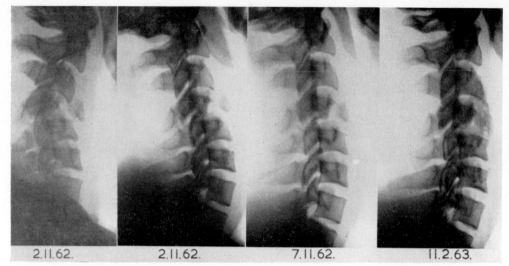

FIG. 51. Antero-hyperflexion injury; burst-compression fracture with evulsion of anterior part of the vertebral body.

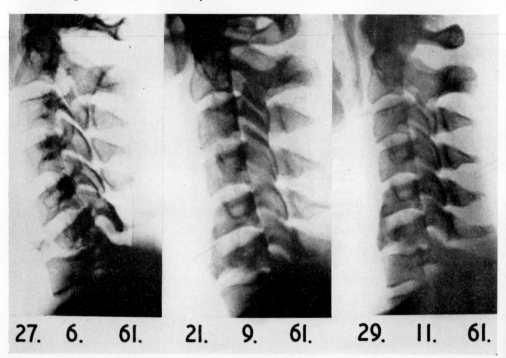

FIG. 52. Antero-hyperflexion injury as in Fig. 51.

vertebra which itself was deformed by the impact of violence. Two-thirds of the body of C4 vertebra are displaced backwards into the spinal canal while one-third is avulsed and displaced forward. Skull traction and small support behind the 4th vertebra resulted in reduction and very satisfactory re-alignment including fusion of the rejoined, initially anterior piece with the adjacent C3 and C5 vertebrae. No change of the tetraplegia.

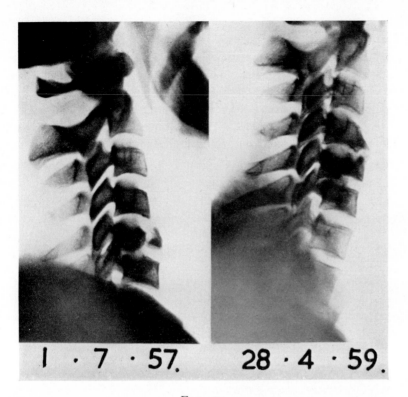

FIG. 53.

Fig. 52 showing a fracture-dislocation of C6 is an example of retro- or dorso-hyper-flexion injury with backward displacement locking articular facets and disruption of the intervertebral disc. A piece from the anterior part of the body was evulsed forwards and upwards. The upward displacement of the chipped off piece demonstrates the inaccuracy of the often wrongly used term 'tear-drop fracture'. Skull traction did not achieve a completely anatomical reduction of the posterior margin of the body. The chipped off piece rejoined the body forming in due course a firm bony fusion with the adjacent C5 vertebra. The initially blocked spinal canal was freed. In another case of this type of burst fracture-dislocation with locked articular facets, a piece of the anterior-inferior part of the fractured C5 vertebra was chipped off upward and rejoined later the upper margin of the anterior part of the vertebra forming a firm bony junction with the adjacent C4 vertebra (Fig. 53). The initially almost complete tetraplegia recovered with mild residual spasticity in the legs. The patient is full-time employed.

Marked discrepancy in the severity between bony and neurological damage is frequently found in cervical injuries, as shown in the case of a 21-year-old girl who was involved in a motor-car accident. As a result, she sustained, through a retroflexion mechanism of head and neck, a profound backward dislocation of C6 vertebra with avulsion of a piece of the roof of its body; in addition, a severe compression-burst fracture of the C7 vertebra occurred with flattening and protrusion of the whole vertebral body, both anteriorly and posteriorly, and locked articular processes. The spinal canal between these two fractured vertebrae was narrowed to about 50 per cent (Fig. 54). Yet miraculously, the spinal cord escaped any damage and there was not the slightest sign of spinal cord or root symptoms. Conservative treatment with a cervical collar was instituted for several months. I happened to see this lady again $3\frac{1}{2}$ years later on the occasion of the second Pan-Pacific Rehabilitation Conference in Hong Kong, where she was employed full time at the information office of the Hilton Hotel. She agreed to be demonstrated at the session on paraplegia. There was no deterioration in her condition whatsoever.

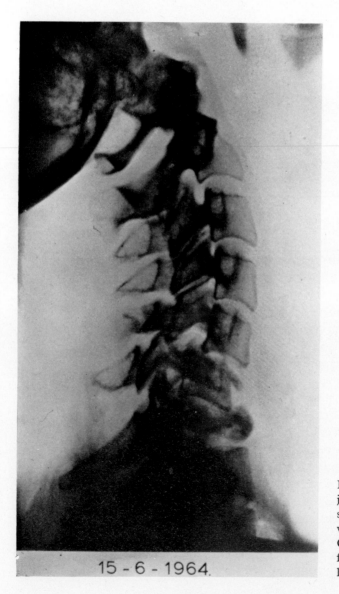

15 - 6 - 1964.

FIG. 54. Retro-hyperflexion injury; avulsion of roof of C6 and severe compression burst-fracture with flattening and protrusion of C7 vertebra; locked articular facets. Not the slightest neurological abnormality.

(f) CERVICAL FRACTURES IN ANKYLOSING SPONDYLITIS AND SPONDYLOSIS

Fractures of the ankylosed servical spine have been repeatedly reported in the literature (Stiasny, 1933; Bergmann, 1949; Howorth & Petrie, 1964; Guttmann, 1966; Brackman & Perring, 1971; Burke, 1971). The mechanism in this condition is mainly one in retro-version of head and cervical spine and fractures may occur due to even mild accidents, such as falling on even ground as a result of losing balance, resulting in tetraplegia. In one case (Fig. 55a), the body of C7 vertebra was broken from its articulations, dis-placed forward and rotated. Reduction of the body and alignment with the body of C6 was achieved by skull traction. As seen in Fig. 55b, the body of C7 has not rejoined its

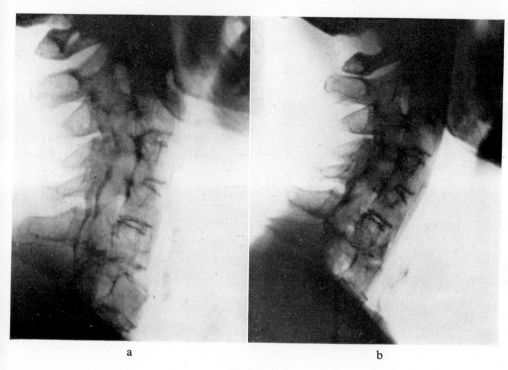

a   b

FIG. 55.

articulations but stability occurred by fixation of the calcified anterior ligament and bony fixation between the bodies of C6 and C7.

In a second case of retro-version, the ankylosed and obliterated intervertebral disc between C6 and C7 caused a rupture through the bodies of these vertebrae with rupture of the calcified anterior-posterior ligamentous complex and upward and anterior separa-tion of the C6 vertebra (Fig. 56). As in this case skull and cervical spine formed a rigid block, the acting force resulted in backward displacement of C7 and its neighbouring upper thoracic vertebra. Further experience will show whether backward displacement of the distal cervical and upper thoracic spine following fractures of C6 represents the characteristic mechanism in ankylosing spondylitis below the fractured C6 vertebra (Fig. 56).

Individuals suffering from chronic cervical spondylosis, in particularly elderly people, can also easily be involved in spinal injuries due to falls. Fig. 57a demonstrates the X-ray of a 74-year-old man with an extensive general spondylosis of the cervical spine, who fell backwards from a haystack and sustained a fracture dislocation of C6 vertebra and locked articular facets and backwards displacement together with C7 vertebra. He

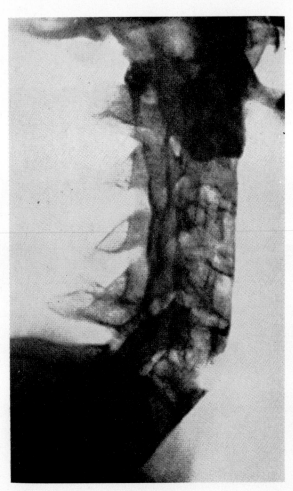

FIG. 56.

sustained a very severe, although not absolutely complete, tetraplegia below C6/7. The motor paralysis at first was almost complete with the exception of the toes of the left foot. Bladder and bowels were paralysed. Skull traction was applied and as seen in Fig. 57b resulted in an anatomical realignment of the spine and fusion between C5 and C6. The patient made a considerable neurological recovery of both motor and sensory function but no restoration of bladder function in spite of two transurethal resections. He was able to walk short distances with the aid of a stick. Last seen on 15 July 1971 at the age of 80.

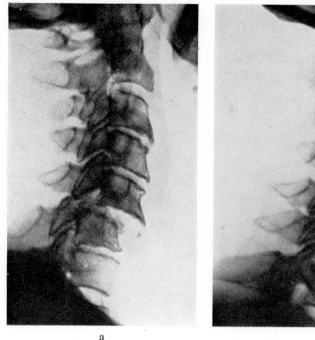
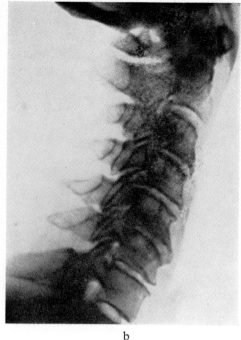

a   b

FIG. 57.

(2) Fractures and dislocations of the thoracic and lumbar spine

SUBLUXATION—DISLOCATION

Subluxations without fractures resulting in cord or cauda equina lesions are rare, but they are often associated with compression-wedge fractures.

Dislocations may occur without fracture of the vertebral body, resulting in more or less severe lesions of the neural elements and blood supply. Fig. 58 demonstrates a marked forward dislocation of the 12th thoracic on the 1st lumbar vertebra in a man, aged 25, following a motor-bike accident. He also sustained associated injuries of long bones and internal haemorrhages, which necessitated immediate laparotomy. He was transferred to Stoke Mandeville Spinal Injuries Centre the day after injury with a complete transverse spinal syndrome below T12, but following postural reduction he made a considerable recovery of motor and sensory functions and partial recovery of bladder function. He was able to walk unaided and returned to his occupation. X-ray taken $7\frac{1}{2}$ years after injury showed satisfactory reduction, although not absolutely anatomical re-alignment of the dislocation. Repeated lumbar punctures showed complete subarachnoidal block, in spite of progressive functional recovery.

In some cases of dislocation associated with a certain degree of rotation, a small piece of the anterior part of the body may be avulsed, as shown in Fig. 59, where an anterior, superior piece of the backwards dislocated vertebra was sheared off and displaced distally in front of the inferior portion of the vertebral body (true tear-drop fracture). Such a

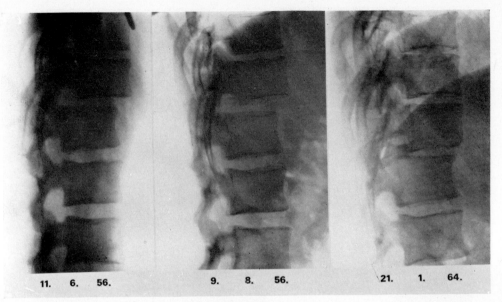

FIG. 58.

dislocation of L2 vertebra was sustained by a man, aged 46, when several bags of malt weighing 112 lb each fell on his back, forcing him to the ground. Conservative treatment by postural reduction and gradual extension resulted in full reduction. The chipped off piece rejoined the upper anterior border of the body and formed a spontaneous fusion with the upper adjacent vertebra. Note the narrowing of the intervertebral space between the previously dislocated vertebra and its adjacent upper neighbour. A later X-ray showed a good anterior bony fusion between the reduced vertebra and its upper neighbour, forming an exostosis at its anterior distal margin to join the upper anterior border of the

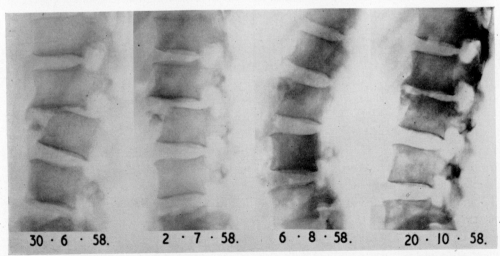

FIG. 59. Tear-drop of L2 vertebra. The chipped off piece rejoined the upper anterior border of the body forming fusion with upper adjacent vertebra following postural reduction.

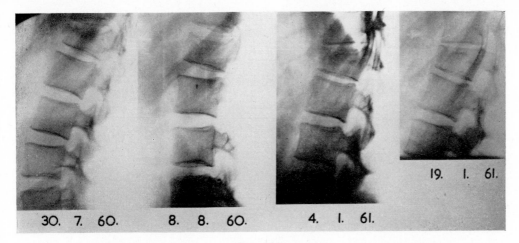

FIG. 60.

damaged vertebra. This is another example of the activity of the natural forces of repair so inherent in the human organism. Neurological symptomatology: the initially complete motor paraplegia below L2 with some patchy sensory paralysis below T12 greatly improved. On last check up on 27 September 1970 ileopsoas, quadriceps and adductors were strong, biceps, gluteal muscles weak. Walks with calipers. Employed in light engineering.

COMPRESSION FRACTURES

There are great varieties of compression fractures ranging from slight or moderate compression of the superior and/or inferior plates of the vertebral body as shown in Fig. 60 of a case with compression of the superior plate. Moreover, there may be more or less

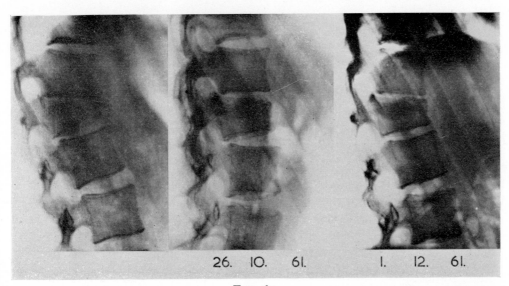

FIG. 61.

marked anterior wedging (Fig. 61), with or without rotation, or complete flattening of
the whole body, resulting in anterior-posterior protrusion (Guttmann, 1963). Compression fractures due to sudden violent antero-hyperflexion such as occur often in quarries
or coalmines result, as a rule, in wedging of the anterior part of the vertebral body to
varying degree with more or less marked posterior subluxation. They are most common

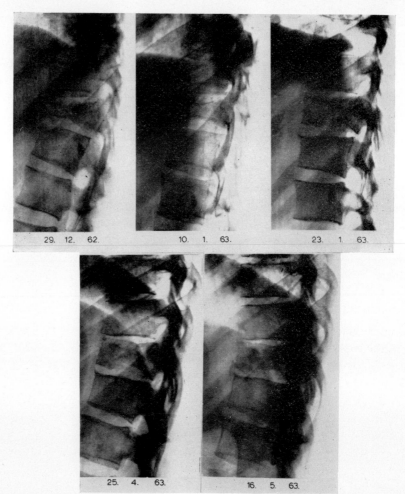

FIG. 62. Vertical compression fracture with flattening and anterio-posterior protrusion
of T12 vertebra. Good expansion and consolidation of the fractured vertebra following
postural reduction.

in the thoraco-lumbar junction (T12–L1/2), the most movable part of the thoraco-
lumbar spine, and produce, as a rule, conus–cauda lesion of flaccid type (Fig. 61).

Fig. 62 is an example of compression fracture with flattening and anterior-posterior
protrusion of the whole body of T12 vertebra as a result of vertical (cephaled-caudal)
impact of violence. Control X-rays demonstrate the effect of postural reduction. The
whole compressed body is re-expanded, and the X-ray $5\frac{1}{2}$ months later shows some
calcification of the anterior longitudinal ligament between the compressed vertebra and

its adjacent lower neighbour, indicating some damage of that ligament. The calcification of the anterior longitudinal ligament may extend over several vertebral bodies and may act as an internal 'corset' in preventing the collapse of the re-expanded compressed vertebra (Fig. 63).

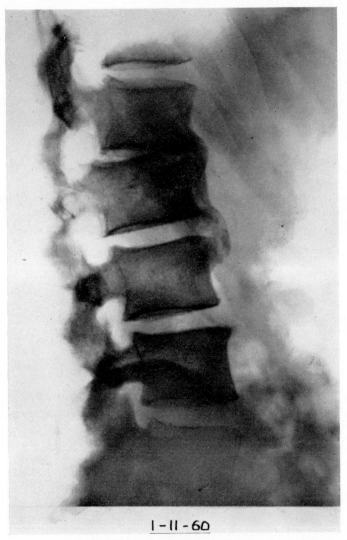

1 - 11 - 60

F IG. 63. Final stage of Fig. 59. Calcification of anterior longitudinal ligament.

FRACTURE-DISLOCATIONS

These are most common at the thoraco-lumbar junction and may involve all parts of the vertebral body, its articulations, pedicles and the whole ligamentous complex. Moreover, they may be associated with fractures of spinous or lateral processes, and may be unstable or stable due to locked articular processes or (in lateral dislocation) by the

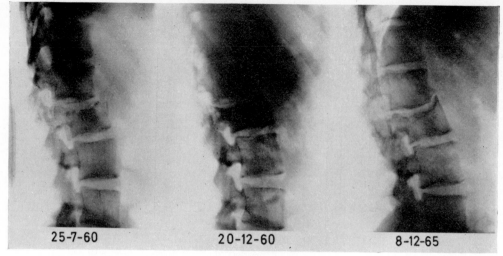

25-7-60   20-12-60   8-12-65

FIG. 64.

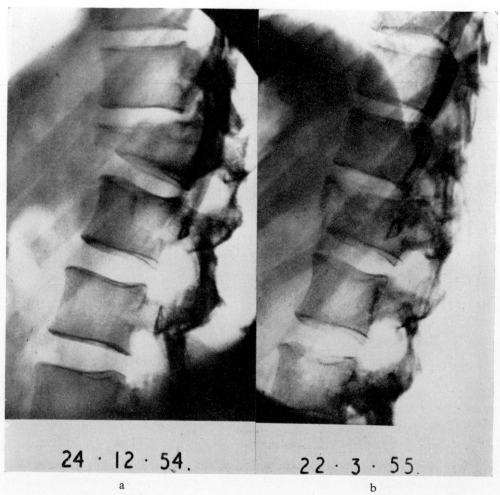

24 · 12 · 54.   22 · 3 · 55.

a   b

FIG. 65. Severe unstable fracture-dislocation with fracture of pedicles and marked distraction of the vertebra. Good alignment and stabilization following postural reduction. Paraplegia unchanged.

interlocked bodies themselves. The dislocation may occur in anterior, posterior and lateral directions, with or without rotation. Of the many varieties which may occur, the following types are described:

Fracture-dislocation with anterior displacement

Fig. 64 shows an anterior displacement of the lumbar spine with fracture-dislocation of L2 vertebra, fracture of the articular processes, destruction of the intervertebral disc and compression and disruption of the superior plate of the body. The injury was a result of a motor-bike accident of an 18-year-old boy who also sustained a fracture of the left

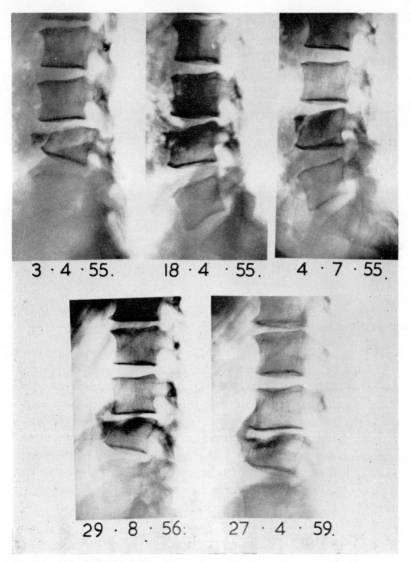

FIG. 66. Unstable fracture-dislocation of L1 with fracture of pedicle. Excellent alignment and stabilization with spontaneous anterior fusion following postural reduction.

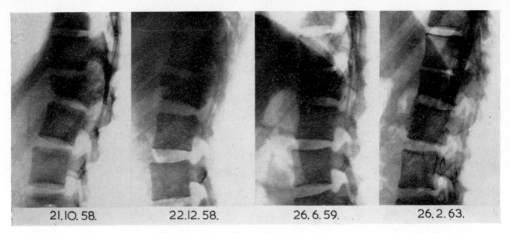

21.10.58.   22.12.58.   26.6.59.   26.2.63.

FIG. 67a.

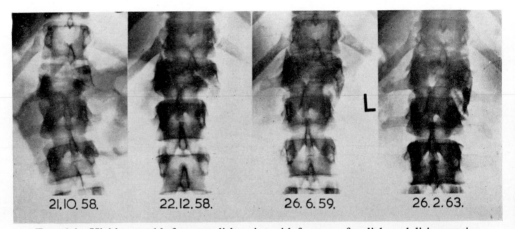

21.10.58.   22.12.58.   26.6.59.   26.2.63.

FIG. 67b. Highly unstable fracture-dislocation with fracture of pedicle and disintegration of L1 vertebra. Satisfactory consolidation and fixation following postural reduction. Paraplegia unchanged.

pubic ramus, subluxation of the left sacroiliac joint and wide separation of the symphysis. The quite unstable fracture-dislocation of L2 became stabilized by postural reduction and the fracture of the articular process consolidated. Of special interest is the growing upwards of the anterior tip of the superior plate, joining a triangular exostosis which developed from the inferior anterior part of the adjacent 1st lumbar vertebra. A–p X-ray showed firm long bridge formation between L1 and L2 vertebrae. Neurological symptoms: incomplete cauda equina lesion below L4. Finally good recovery of quadriceps, hip flexors and adductors, especially on right, sensory loss complete below L4 on left and L3 on right. Able to walk on elbow crutches. Some return of bladder and sexual functions. Returned to his former job as articled clerk with chartered accountant.

FRACTURE-DISLOCATIONS WITH POSTERIOR DISPLACEMENT

Fig 65a is an example of fracture-dislocation of the 1st lumbar vertebra with profound posterior dislocation and fracture of the pedicle. The anterior part of the body is compressed and a large piece of its superior plate sheared off forward. This unstable fracture became stabilized by postural reduction. The compressed body re-expanded, the chipped off piece rejoined the body in its proper place and the fracture of the pedicle healed (Fig. 65b). Neurological symptoms: complete flaccid paraplegia below T10/11 which did not change following reduction.

Fig. 66 demonstrates a fracture-dislocation of the 4th lumbar vertebra in a man, aged 50, causing backward dislocation and rotation, fracture of the pedicle, destruction of the superior plate and avulsion anteriorly of a piece of the anterior superior part of the body. The following X-rays show the various stages of reduction and alignment of the body and its chipped off anterior-superior part, which, in due course, formed an excellent bony fusion by the natural forces of repair between the damaged vertebra and its adjacent upper vertebra. This man, who initially had a complete cauda equina lesion below L4, made a considerable recovery including bladder and bowel function. He is able to walk unaided.

A further variety of fracture-dislocation of L1 vertebra with backward displacement and complete disintegration of the body is seen in Fig. 67a. The body is broken transversely into two slices, as seen in the a–p X-ray (Fig. 67b), the anterior part pulled off and the posterior part with its articulations shattered into fragments and the pedicle broken (lateral X-ray). However, postural reduction and fixation of this quite unstable fracture achieved full restoration and excellent alignment of the fractured vertebra and fusion with its neighbouring vertebrae, as seen in a–p and lateral X-rays $5\frac{1}{2}$ years after injury. The patient, a girl, aged 20, who sustained a motor-car accident resulting in complete flaccid paraplegia below T11, which remained unchanged, made a very satisfactory rehabilitation, married and is the mother of two children.

Fracture-dislocations with lateral displacement

A soldier, aged 33, was involved in a motor-car accident and sustained a severe cauda equina lesion as a result of a fracture-dislocation of L3 vertebra. As seen in Fig. 68 the body of the 3rd lumbar vertebra was split vertically and diagonally into two parts and the larger part of the broken body, together with the 4th and 5th lumbar vertebrae, displaced laterally. Conservative treatment resulted in firm re-union, but with some considerable degree of scoliosis of the distal lumbar spine. The patient made a practically complete functional recovery and returned 6 months after injury to the Army.

An even more dramatic case of fracture-dislocation with complete lateral displacement is shown in Fig. 69. A young girl was involved in a motor accident and sustained a complete paraplegia. X-rays in an orthopaedic department, where the patient was first admitted, showed a profound lateral displacement of the fractured L1 vertebra, together with the whole distal lumbar vertebral column. Attempts made to reduce the fracture-dislocation were unsuccessful as the fractured L1 vertebra was completely interlocked with the T12 vertebra. During the following weeks the patient made a considerable recovery of her paraplegia. About 6 weeks after injury a long bone graft was inserted which, although useless in view of the already interlocked fixation and stable fracture-dislocation, did not interfere with continuing neurological recovery. The final disability,

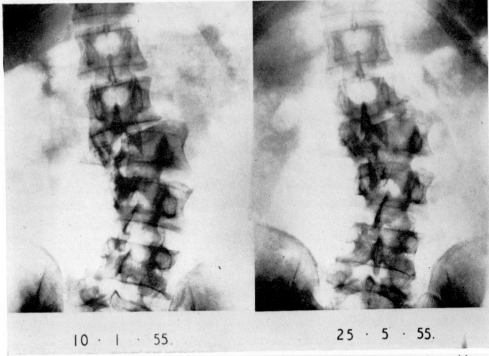

FIG. 68. Fracture-dislocation of L3 with lateral displacement. Firm re-union with some considerable scoliosis but practically complete neurological recovery. Postural reduction.

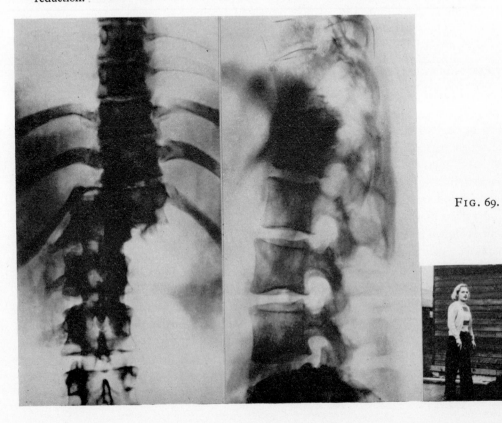

FIG. 69.

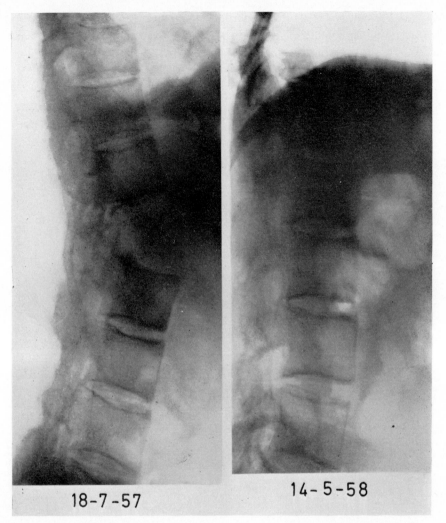

18-7-57   14-5-58

FIG. 70. Retro-hyperflexion injury in ankylosing spondylitis. Profound separation of vertebrae. Good alignment following postural reduction. Paraplegia unchanged.

after admission to Stoke Mandeville, was weakness of the distal muscles of the feet, which did not prevent restoration of walking capabilities with the aid of one stick (Fig. 69). Bladder and bowel functions also returned.

Fracture-dislocation in retro-hyperflexion in ankylosing spondylitis

Fig. 70 shows a retro-hyperflexion fracture-dislocation of the first lumbar vertebra resulting in profound separation of this vertebra from the vertebral column above in a man suffering for many years from ankylosing spondylitis, who was involved in a motor-bike accident. Postural reduction in ventroflexion resulted in re-alignment of the distraction deformity of the fractured vertebral column. The complete flaccid paraplegia below T10 remained unchanged.

Fig. 71a–c demonstrates a retro-hyperflexion fracture-dislocation of the 4th lumbar vertebra, resulting in spondylolisthesis in a man of 60 with long-standing ankylosing spondylitis. This man, whose hip joints were ankylosed in extension, fell at home and

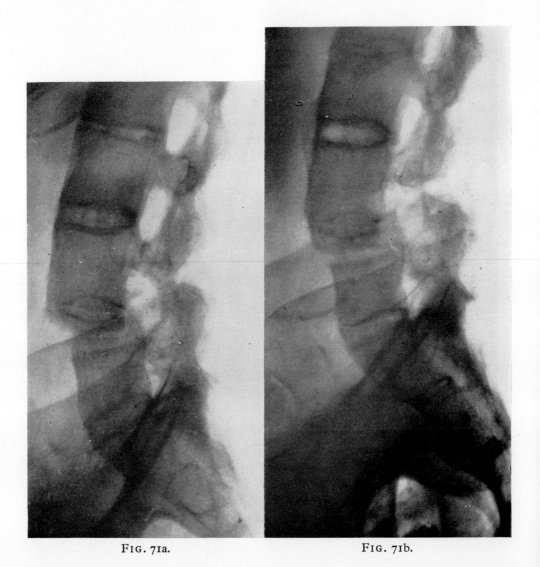

FIG. 71a.   FIG. 71b.

developed severe pain in his back and an incomplete cauda equina lesion below L5 with paralysis of bladder and bowels. Conservative treatment achieved good reduction and almost anatomical re-alignment of the broken spine, and he recovered from his cauda equina lesion including return of bladder and bowel function and was able to walk with the help of walking aids.

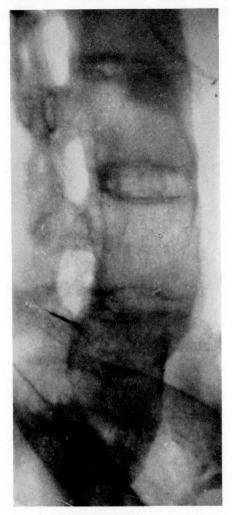

FIG. 71C.

Conclusions

From all these observations, classifications of fractures and dislocations of the vertebral column can be summarized as overleaf.

Classification of fractures and dislocations

A. Fractures of spinous, lateral and/or articular processes

B. Fractures and dislocations of vertebral bodies and their articulations

I. Cervical spine

a. Fractures, dislocations and subluxations of atlas and odontoid
b. Fractures and dislocations of 3rd–7th cervical vertebrae
    1. Subluxation—dislocation—cervical sprain
    2. Compression—compression-burst fractures
    3. Fracture-dislocations due to retro- or dorsal hyperflexion (usually but wrongly called hyperextension injuries)
    4. Fracture-dislocations due to ventro- or antero-hyperflexion
    5. Iatrogenic true vertical hyperextension of fractures due to overdistraction by skull calipers
    6. Cervical fractures in ankylosing spondylitis and spondylosis

II. Thoraco-lumbar spine

a. Anterior compression (wedge fracture) with or without subluxation
b. Vertical compression
    1. Upper and/or lower plates of vertical body
    2. Total compression of body with anterior-posterior protrusion
c. Fracture-dislocations
    1. Anterior or posterior dislocation of the whole vertebral body
    2. Burst-fracture with anterior or posterior displacement and rotation
    3. Lateral dislocation (partial or total)
d. Fracture-dislocations in ankylosing spondylitis.

CHAPTER 13

MANAGEMENT OF SPINAL FRACTURES

FIRST AID AND TRANSPORTATION

The initial management of the spinal cord injured must start at the place of accident (Guttmann, 1968). Proper first aid of a casualty with a suspected vertebral fracture involving the spinal cord not only can reduce the broken vertebra at the place of the accident and thus remove immediately pressure from the spinal cord, if this is the only cause of the paraplegia (extremely rare), but can also prevent a primarily partially damaged spinal cord from becoming a complete lesion. Recently, Geisler, Wynne-Jones & Jousse (1966) reported 29 patients with traumatic lesions of the spine who developed further paralysis through faulty handling during first aid.

As the great majority of paraplegics and tetraplegics are conscious after the accident the following rules should be strictly observed by the first aiders.

1. The injured should be immediately warned not to move at all.

2. All activities of the first-aiders must be carried out slowly and with the greatest gentleness. Any undue haste or rough handling may instantaneously increase the damage to the spinal cord.

3. At least three, but better still four or five people, are needed to move such a casualty from the site of the accident to a more convenient place to await the arrival of medical aid and ambulance.

4. When lifting the injured, greatest care must be taken not to twist or bend the patient either backwards or forwards. If an injury to the neck is suspected any twisting of the neck is particularly dangerous.

5. All movements should be carried out simultaneously by members of the first aid party so that the patient is turned, lifted or shifted in one piece.

6. Every casualty who is conscious should be placed onto his back—i.e. in supine position if found in any other position. This is essential in injuries to any part of the spinal cord as such a casualty may also have sustained additional injuries to other parts of the body, in particular the chest, abdomen or long bones. The prone position, which is still advocated by some workers, would in these cases be very hazardous, particularly in cervical lesions where the respiratory muscles of the chest are paralysed. Only those casualties with suspected injuries to the spine who are unconscious should be placed in lateral or semi-lateral position, to avoid blockage of the upper respiratory tract by aspiration of saliva.

7. The most experienced first-aider must take up command and direct all actions. In injuries of the neck, he should take hold of the casualty's head between his hands and care must be taken not to twist or bend the head forwards or backwards. Moreover, when lifting the patient from a car or other vehicle to the ground, the head should be kept in a straight line within the axis of the body. When placing a paraplegic patient on the ground,

an improvised roll—for instance a rolled-up jacket—should be placed under the suspected site of injury to restore the normal curvature of the spine and thus relieve pressure from the spinal cord. It may be emphasized that, by this management, a fracture dislocation can be reduced already at the place of accident, while the patient is in a flaccid state.

8. Hard objects, such as coins, keys, pipes, tins, lighters, and match-boxes must be removed from the pockets of the injured in order to avoid development of pressure sores during transport. While awaiting the arrival of medical aid and ambulance, the patient should be covered to keep warm. However, hot-water bottles must never be used *on any* part of the body.

9. Pads of soft material should be placed between the knees and in particular the ankles. Knees and ankles should be loosely bound together and a soft support should be placed underneath the calves to prevent pressure sores developing on the heels.

TRANSPORT BY AMBULANCE OR AIR

(a) *Preparation of the stretcher*

The traumatic paraplegic should be transported on a rigid stretcher to prevent sagging of the spine into flexion, or, if this is not available, on a board. If the site of the fracture is known, a support should be placed on the stretcher in accordance with the level of the injury so that a moderate hyperextension is accomplished once the patient is placed on the stretcher. If the site of the fracture is obscure, the normal curvatures of the spine should be maintained by placing supports under the small of the back and the nape of the neck. Ambulances should be provided with packs of sorbo-rubber of various sizes and width to be placed underneath the suspected fracture. For the nape of the neck, such support must naturally be small and narrow.

(b) *Lifting the injured on to the stretcher*

If the injured is already lying on a blanket with a support underneath the fracture, the lifting can be done by the first aiders from either side holding onto the blanket. However, the safest lifting is done directly from the supine position by four or five first aiders maintaining hyperextension by holding the support underneath the fracture in position. The person holding the head should be in command and the injured should be lifted at the order 'up' or 'lift' simultaneously in one piece. The team should carry out the lifting preferably from the side opposite to the stretcher, with the exception of the man who is holding the head. Lifting the injured with the aid of webbing bands, as suggested in the manual of the St John's Ambulance Brigade, is, as a rule, undesirable, as it involves turning the injured and unnecessary manipulation and movements which could easily result in further damage to the spinal cord.

(c) *Immediate medical first aid*

Morphine should not be given indiscriminately to these patients, as its administration, in particular in patients with cervical cord lesions and others with suspicion of lung collapse, may prove disastrous. Before transferring the injured to the nearest hospital the first medical attendant should ascertain, wherever possible, the level of the lesion and, in particular, the completeness of the motor and sensory paralysis and a written statement should accompany the patient. The diagnosis of level of the cord lesions is not difficult even for non-medical first aiders if the injured is conscious. The patient very often complains of pain in his back at the level of the fracture. If he can move his arms, hands *and* fingers the cord lesion is obviously in the thoracic region. If he can bend his forearms, and extend his wrist but cannot extend his forearm and has no or greatly reduced finger movements the cord lesion is situated in the mid-cervical region.

(d) *Transfer to a spinal centre*

Whenever possible a traumatic paraplegic or tetraplegic should be transferred to a Spinal Unit as soon as the patient's condition allows transfer, where the most favourable conditions exist for treating all aspects of paraplegia from the start by a specialized staff. This should apply both in war and peace. This has been recognized by increasing numbers of surgeons during recent years and several hundreds of patients have been admitted to Stoke Mandeville within the first 24 hours after injury. Gregg & Wilmot (1964) have organized a Flying Squad from the National Medical Rehabilitation Centre in Dublin, consisting of a doctor, two nurses and two orderlies who are available to go out immediately on request to any part of Ireland to collect and bring in under supervision any acute traumatic case of paraplegia or tetraplegia. The acute case is usually collected from the hospital nearest to the place of accident. If direct transfer to a Spinal Centre is not possible and the patient has to be admitted to the Casualty Department of the nearest hospital, the medical officer in charge of the case should make contact with the nearest Spinal Centre for immediate transfer of the patient. If this is not possible, the medical officer should seek advice regarding the initial management, in particular of the bladder.

(e) *Air transport*

In recent years, a steadily increasing number of patients with spinal cord injuries have been admitted to Stoke Mandeville by helicopter; during 1966, 34 cases. Service cases were flown to the Centre from Germany within 24 or 48 hours and from Singapore, Aden and Christmas Island within a few days of injury. This has proved a life-saving measure, in particular in paraplegics and tetraplegics complicated by associated injuries to other parts of the body. Fig. 72 shows the admission of a tetraplegic patient to Stoke Mandeville by helicopter. He is just being taken out and note how the doctor holds the head traction to keep the head in line with the axis of the body. Recently Ruge (1969) suggested that 'if the transportation is going to require an hour or more an indwelling catheter should be inserted into the bladder'. This extraordinary recommendation really ignores the principles of proper initial management of the paralysed bladder—the more so as Ruge does not give any details how and by whom this catheterization should be carried out. Actually, there is no indication whatsoever for such a procedure, unless transportation by sea would take many weeks or transport by air has to be delayed for several days. Only then should the paralysed bladder, which can be safely left without

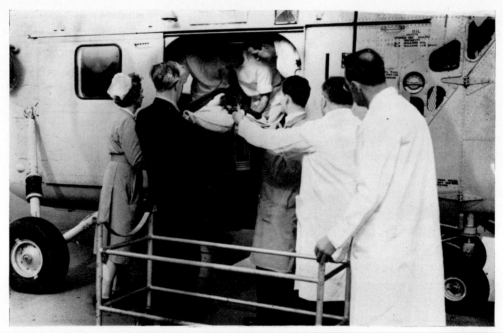

FIG. 72.

any instrumentation for at least 24 hours, especially by a restricted intake of fluid, be emptied. As pointed out in the Chapter on the bladder, this should be effected by intermittent catheterization with the 'non-touch' technique, as described previously, and should be performed by a medical officer and not by para-medical first aiders.

In Switzerland, emergency transportation of acute spinal injuries by helicopter or plane has been organized and highly developed under optimal conditions by Swiss Air Rescue (SRC), under the leadership of an outstanding pilot, Mr Bühler. This is a private organization affiliated officially to the Swiss Red Cross. Acute spinal injury is classified as top-urgent and always given priority assistance (Buergi, 1963; Strange, 1973; Hachen, 1974). Aircraft carrying the sign of S.R.C. may land and take off without restriction in all civilian and most military airports in Europe, Northern Africa and the Middle East.

The SRC squadron comprises 25 helicopters, all specially equipped with up-to-date first-aid material of 300 items including ECG-monitoring unit, defibrillator, respirator, a great many surgical instruments and suture material, laryngoscope for intubation, blood plasma, saline, and 35 carefully selected drugs for the treatment of cardio-vascular and respiratory disorders. The rapid evacuation by helicopter avoids long delays of transportation to spinal units as, in the mountainous regions of Switzerland and on the main highways, especially during weekends, access to the scene of the accident is likely to be blocked (Hachen, 1974).

The rescue programme is continually monitored by radio short waves from RSC Headquarters in Zurich. Therefore, the Swiss Spinal Units are constantly informed about the helicopter's exact location, its flight-plan and the patient's condition on board, so that the rescuers can be given guide lines for special measures by the medical staff of the spinal centre.

THE INITIAL MANAGEMENT OF THE FRACTURED SPINE

Conservative treatment

The methods of conservative treatment as practised in ancient times until the beginning of this century has been discussed in the chapter of Historical Background.

In the 20's and 30's of this century, methods of reduction by hyperextension in prone position were introduced, such as on slings, frames or hammock, as described by Davis (1929) and Rogers (1930) or hanging (Böhler, 1935) and by Watson-Jones' two-table method (1931, 1934). This was followed by application of plaster jackets extending from the symphysis pubis below to the clavicles above. Dunlop & Parker (1933) hyperextended the broken spine in supine position by the weight of head and trunk on one end and pelvis and legs on the other with a padded sling which is placed transversely underneath the fracture and held with a stirrup and lifted with block and tackle. However, Magnus (1931) and his school renounced these methods of forceful reduction and, accepting the spinal deformity, advocated consolidation of the fractured spine by placing the patient flat in his bed in supine position with prolonged recumbency.

All these methods employing plaster cases and prolonged recumbency proved to be unsatisfactory in spinal fractures resulting in paraplegia. There is now general agreement among those with experience of traumatic paraplegia that prolonged immobilization and recumbency is detrimental in these patients, because of the tendency to promote stagnation in the urinary tract resulting in pyelonephritis, stone formation and hydro- or pyonephrosis. Furthermore, it leads to the development of pressure sores and articular contractures. These dangers were greatly increased by plaster fixation, be it jacket or plaster bed. Nissen (1941) advocated plaster beds in view of the disastrous effects of plaster casts in traumatic paraplegia. The idea was that pressure was more evenly distributed in a plaster bed. This concept did not prove to be correct. The volume of the paralysed part of the body, especially the legs, does not remain constant, because there are changes in the degree of vasodilatation as a result of interruption of the spinal vasomotor centres and pathways. In fact, in paraplegic patients who lay in a well-made plaster bed for many weeks or months, not only did this method of fixation prove to be no better than plaster casts, but it greatly promoted the development of sores of the most frightful type. Moreover, this type of fixation caused profound fixed lordosis of the lumbar spine, distortion of the pelvis and atrophy of the normal back muscles, which are so vital for the physical readjustment and the later maintenance of the patient's upright position. In spite of intensive physiotherapy it took many months, if one succeeded at all, to overcome the fixed distortion of the pelvis in those paraplegic patients who were admitted in plaster beds, let alone to heal the pressure sores which had developed as a result of that treatment. This management has been strongly condemned (Guttmann, 1945, 1946; Watson-Jones, 1955; Holdsworth & Hardy, 1953) as utterly contrary to the principles of rehabilitation of spinal paraplegics and as a result it is today hardly ever used, apart from the occasional purpose of transport of traumatic paraplegics. It is fair to say that Nissen himself has abandoned this method.

In contrast to the methods of forceful reduction and long-term recumbency, Sutcliffe Kerr (1956) advocated restoring the vertical position of traumatic paraplegics following fractures within a few days after the injury. He ignored, by this method, the injury to the spine and accepted that there was no hope for recovery of the paraplegia if the paralysis lasted longer than 48 hours after injury. Although this may be true in some injuries of the upper and middle thoracic spine, it is certainly not so in injuries to the thoraco-lumbar part of the spinal cord, where some degree of functional recovery may occur even after weeks. This method, however, did not find acceptance.

Postural reduction combined with regular turning

In 1944 I introduced and developed the method of graduated reduction of fractures and fracture-dislocations of the spine and immobilization on pillow-packs combined with 2-hourly turning of the paralysed patient, day and night. The original pillow-packs were later replaced by the more suitable and more hygienic sorbo rubber packs. The technique is as follows:

The patient is placed by three orderlies, under the supervision of a trained nurse, on the prepared bed, consisting of four sorbo-rubber packs about 40 cm high, which lie on the hard surface of a bed to prevent sagging. An additional pillow or roll is placed underneath the fracture to ensure the normal contour of the spine (Figs. 73a–d). As seen in the figure, the patient's hips, buttocks and sacrum, as well as the heels, are completely free of pressure. From the initial supine position the patient is carefully turned by the orderlies, *in one piece*, at 2-hourly intervals to the sides and later back to the supine position, whereby the hyperextended position of the spine is secured by a heavy sandbag in the lateral positions. The result of the reduction of the broken spine is followed up by repeated control X-rays and the first X-ray controls are taken on the first day or two of this treatment in order, if necessary, to correct or modify the position of the broken vertebra. As a rule the bony stabilization through natural fusion occurs within 6–8 weeks, the fibrous fusion, of course, earlier. Only in the minority of patients was there delayed stabilization and the incidence of late instability was very low (Frankel *et al.*, 1970; Bedbrook, 1971). During the first few weeks, after the patient is transferred to his wheel-chair, a light corset of plastic material is applied to avoid excessive movements and control X-rays may give the indication for discontinuing the wearing of the corset.

From the experience gained on many hundreds of traumatic paraplegics and tetra-plegics following spinal fractures and fracture-dislocations it can be concluded:

1   In compression fractures the compressed vertebral body, whether wedge fractures or those with complete flattening of the whole vertebral body, can be re-expanded and may remain more or less so. I do not share the view that simple wedge fractures do not require reduction and fixation. To leave the impacted anterior part of the wedged vertebra unreduced means ignoring the damage to the anterior longitudinal ligament, which in such a case is crumpled up. If the wedged vertebra is re-expanded by postural reduction the straightened anterior ligament helps to keep the reduced vertebral body, if not

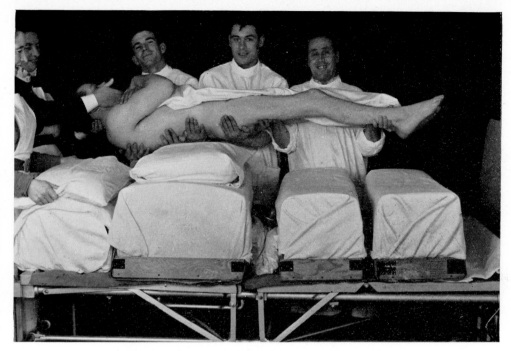

FIG. 73a.

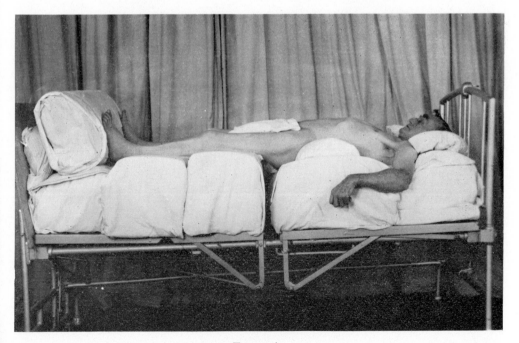

FIG. 73b.

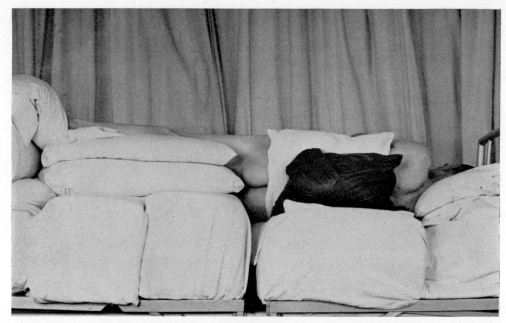

FIG. 73c.

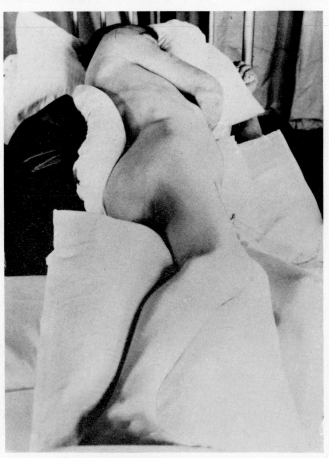

FIG. 73d.

permanently completely expanded, at least in a better position, thus preventing severe angulation later (Figs. 60, 61, 62, 63, 64).

2   Dislocations and fracture dislocations of various types, including those of the most severe burst fractures with avulsion of parts of the vertebral body and regardless whether stable or unstable, can be successfully reduced and stabilized (Figs. 65, 66, 67, 68, 71).

3   Atrophy of the back muscles which is the rule following long-term conservative fixation in plaster casts, plaster beds and following operative procedures, can be absolutely avoided, which is so important for the later physical readjustment of the paralysed.

4   Pressure sores, which hitherto were considered as inevitable, can be completely avoided, thus preventing sepsis and avoiding long-term and costly conservative and surgical treatment afterwards.

5   The continual change of posture counteracts stagnation in the urinary tract, thus preventing the dreaded complications of ureters and kidneys following infection.

6   The constant change of posture has proved beneficial in restoring the disturbed vasomotor control and thus better blood circulation, especially in the high lesions.

All this proves that if nature is given a chance by appropriate conservative treatment and proper positioning of the broken spine, the displaced vertebra and fragments will, in the great majority of cases, find their correct place of re-alignment. It is as much an inherent function of the natural forces of repair to stabilize the broken vertebra as near as possible in physiological alignment as it is to repair defects in other parts of the body.

The disadvantage of this method of management of the broken spine is the great strain to which the nursing staff is exposed, day and night, especially in lifting and turning heavy patients and if several acute cases have to be dealt with, which is the rule in a spinal unit. Therefore, for some years research has been carried out to relieve the strain on the nursing staff by the development of an electrically operated turning bed. With the co-operation of the engineering firm Egerton Ltd., Tower Hill, Horsham, Sussex, such a turning-tilting bed has been constructed, which, by pressing a button turns the bed from the supine position into a 70 degree lateral position. For the turning of traumatic tetra-plegics, I introduced a special skull traction unit, which allows turning of the patient without discontinuing the traction pulley connected with the weight and, thus the head always remains within the axis of the body (Figs. 74a–c). By pressing another button the bed can be tilted head up or down.

This bed has proved very successful and has now been accepted widely in other countries (Guttmann, 1965, 1967).

A modification of the Stoke Mandeville–Egerton Turning bed called Roto-Rest has been made by Dr F.Keane (1966) from the Spinal Unit in Dublin, which is fitted with a silent motor and allows continuous motion of the bed. There are also other turning beds on the market, the best known of these being the Stryker frame and its modifications. This type of turning frame can be changed only from the supine into the prone position and, therefore, has certain disadvantages in the initial treatment of acute patients with fractures and fracture dislocations of the spine:

1   This frame is not electrically operated and needs the attendance of one if not two nurses to operate it.

2   While hyperextension to reduce the fracture dislocation by posture can be easily

achieved in the supine position, this can only be maintained by time-taking and careful manipulation on the part of the nurses when placing the patient into the abdominal position. Otherwise the object of maintaining hyperextension to secure re-alignment and promote stability of the broken spine is defeated.

3   For traumatic paraplegics with associated fractures of the hips, pelvis or long bones, and in particular patients with haemothorax or pneumothorax (let alone those who are unconscious), turning on to the abdominal position is clearly hazardous and, therefore,

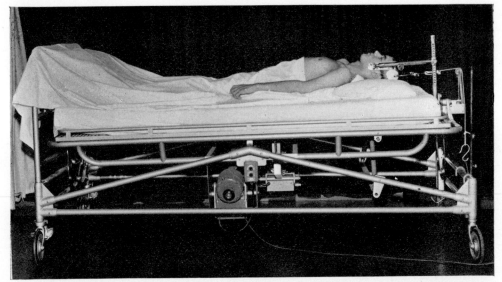

FIG. 74a.

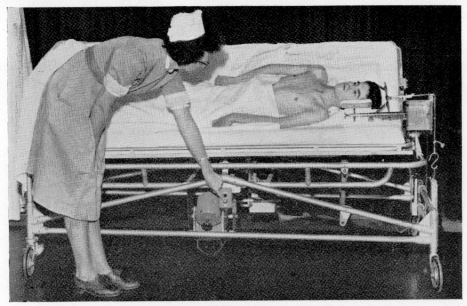

FIG. 74b.

contra-indicated, for such patients have then to maintain their recumbency in the supine position day and night. Owing to lack of regular turning, development of pressure sores is inevitable, as patients have shown admitted to Stoke Mandeville on this frame.

4 Cervical patients placed for long periods in the abdominal position have shown disappearance of the normal contour of their spine.

5 The original Stryker frame was narrow and cumbersome, especially for heavily built patients. Although this has been recently modified by a frame of greater width (Ascoli, 1970), the disadvantages, as mentioned in 1–4, still exist.

Recently, there has been a considerable increase of special bed devices, primarily for the prevention and treatment of pressure sores for geriatric patients and the management of burns and to facilitate nursing. However, they have also been recommended for the treatment of spinal cord injuries. These beds include the Ripple Bed, Air fluidized Beds AFB and IFB (Hargest, 1975) Beaufort-Winchester Flotation Bed (Grahame,

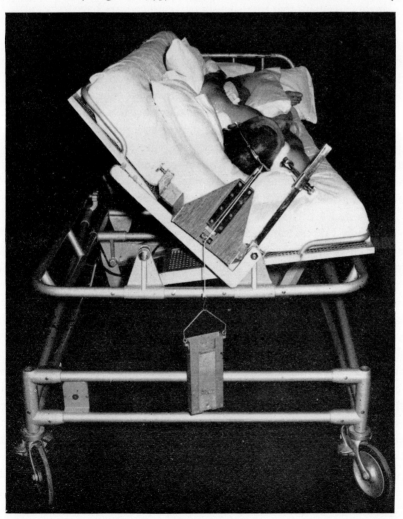

FIG. 74c.

1974), the Low Air Loss Bed, ALBS (Scales *et al.*, 1974), Sand Bed (Stewart, 1970), Rancho Flotation Med Bed (Reswick & Rogers, 1975). From all the data given so far, there is no proof either on theoretical or practical grounds that any of these beds represents an improvement on the turning-tilting beds in the management of fractures and fracture-dislocations of the spine, as mentioned above, nor in the prevention and treatment of pressure sores in spinal paraplegic and tetraplegic patients. If these beds are designed to obviate regular turning of paraplegics and tetraplegics and severely ill patients of other causes, they are unsuitable, as they promote recumbency with its serious effects on vasomotor control and complications of the urinary tract and kidneys, such as ascending infection of the urinary tract and stone formation.

Traction and manipulation in fractures of the cervical spine

There is general agreement that these conservative procedures have to be carried out with the greatest care and gentleness to prevent further damage of the cervical cord.

Traction of the cervical spine with the Glisson sling has been the method of choice before the introduction of skeletal skull traction by Crutchfield (1933), but it is still practised in some countries. In agreement with other workers in the field, I consider this method as unsatisfactory. In the first place, it results more easily in redislocation of the broken spine and cannot be employed in patients with associated injuries of the jaw. Moreover, it causes unnecessary discomfort to the patient, and damage to the jaw and its articulation is by no means unusual, if used for longer periods.

Traction may be combined with manipulation, but forceful manipulation and jerks on the neck can be most harmful to the spinal cord by causing immediately complete or partial tetraplegia and even death (Roger, 1942; Durbin, 1957). Walton (1893) was the first to describe a method of manual manipulation consisting in full rotation to disengage the locked facets followed by lateral flexion to lift the forward facet above the posterior one. This was followed by rotation in the opposite direction, to place the facets in their proper position. This rather forceful method was modified by Taylor (1924) and his method was accepted by other workers in the field. Evans (1961) reported successful manual manipulation in 17 cases of cervical dislocation under anaesthesia combined with a muscle relaxant which greatly facilitates the reduction of the dislocation. However, Harris & Whatmore (1969) reported extreme distraction of atlas and C2 vertebra following manipulation under anaesthesia of a C2/3 fracture-subluxation. In a recent paper Burke (1971) and Burke & Berryman (1971) advocate in view of their experience on 76 cervical cases a policy of conservative management with gentle manipulation in selected cases only, reduction being maintained thereafter by skeletal traction. These authors reserve operation for the few cases which demonstrate late instability or for those even rarer cases in which manipulation fails and the patient has either an incomplete neurological lesion or a double skeletal injury. Their mortality rate was 2 out of 76.

Recently Burke (1975) reported on 28 amongst 175 patients with cervical injuries treated with skeletal traction plus manipulation under general anaesthesia, and Key (1975) reported on 40 patients with unilateral facet interlocking who were treated first with skull traction, but if this failed to achieve reduction within 12–24 hours' manipulation under general anaesthesia was then carried out. Key prefers the term 'increased traction under general anaesthesia with a relaxant and without endotracheal intubation' instead of 'manipulation under general anaesthesia'. In this connection, Jackson (1975) rejects the term 'manipulation' which should be replaced by the term 'manual reduction'. Braakmann (1975) and McSweeney (1975) found X-ray image intensifier of great value in the investigation of neck injuries and in the assessment of instability.

Traction of the thoraco-lumbar spine

Recently, Chalal (1975) introduced a method of continuous lumbar traction in acute thoraco-lumbar injuries with paraplegia. The technique consists of a corset fixed around the pelvis and bilateral strings fixed at the foot end of the bed. Countertraction is applied by lifting the foot end of the bed by 9–12 inches so that the body weight acts as countertraction. However, from the X-rays published in two cases with lateral dislocation, it is obvious that the reduction of the fractures was unsuccessful, and in the third case—a simple compression fracture of Th12 vertebra—this procedure was quite unnecessary. Moreover, Chalal admitted on questioning that two cases developed pressure sores which 'ultimately' healed. This method simply represents a replacement of the long abandoned technique of applying pelvic traction by inserting wire through either side of the pelvis, which in paraplegics invariably broke through the bone and skin. There is no proof that continuous pelvic traction as described by Chalal is a suitable method in the treatment of thoracolumbar fractures, as it is contrary to fundamental principles of the immediate management of traumatic paraplegics.

Neurological results of conservative treatment

It remains now to analyse the effect of the conservative treatment of the spine on the neurological symptoms resulting from fractures and fracture-dislocations. In 1963 I reported about 396 traumatic paraplegics and tetraplegics admitted to Stoke Mandeville within the first 15 days of injury between 1957 and 1963. Of these, 256 arrived within

TABLE 1. Neurological results of conservative treatment

	Fracture-dislocations		Fractures	
	Unchanged	Improved	Unchanged	Improved
Cervical incomplete	18	30	12	23
complete	38	13	5	3
T1–T5 incomplete	1	2	1	3
complete	21	2	4	0
T6–T12 incomplete	4	4	1	9
complete	66	4	17	1
T12 and below incomplete	12	15	2	6
complete	19	5	3	0
Total	179	75	45	45

(3 cases worsened: 30 deaths not included.)

the first 3 days of injury, 194 within the first 24 hours, 113, 28·1 per cent, had additional injuries. Thirty (25 male and 5 female) of the 396 patients (7·6 per cent) died during the early stages of injury, the majority of whom (20) were well over the age of 40, and most of them were cervical injuries. The time between death and injury varied, the majority dying within 8 to 10 days, mainly from pulmonary embolus, other lung complications and head injuries.

344 patients (30 who died are excluded from the statistics) were treated conservatively, the vast majority by the method of postural reduction described above. 254 had fracture-dislocations, and of these 145 (46·86 per cent) had complete transverse lesions, while of 90 fractures without dislocation, 29 (32·2 per cent) produced complete transverse lesions. Table 1 shows the neurological results of the conservative treatment according to the level of the cord and cauda equina lesions and divided into complete and incomplete lesions. The improvement concerns both the motor and sensory function and also, in a number of cases, return of bladder function as described in individual cases in chapter on Classification.

From these statistics, it would appear that initially complete lesions of the thoracic cord show the lowest percentage of improvement. This may be accounted for by the smaller diameter of the spinal canal as compared with its diameter in the cervical and lumbar regions. Therefore, the possibility of the spinal cord escaping the impact of violence is greatly reduced. Conversely, if a cord lesion due to fractures of upper and mid-thoracic vertebrae had initially been incomplete, a remarkably high percentage of neurological improvement was found. This may be due to fixation of the spine through splintage by the rib cage, which more readily prevents additional damage of the spinal cord caused by movements of the patient during transport or by manipulations during X-ray examination, operation, etc., than in injuries of the cervical and lumbar vetebral columns with their infinitely greater mobility.

Of special interest is the high percentage of functional recovery, both motor and sensory, in incomplete, but also, though to a lesser degree, in complete lesions of the cervical cord. It must be stressed that in traumatic tetraplegics, who at first appeared clinically complete, functional recovery may occur as late as 3–5 weeks after injury.

In 1965 Meinecke published a detailed statistic of the conservative management of 134 out of 500 cases of fracture dislocation with spinal cord lesions, who were admitted within 24 hours after injury. There were 104 complete and 30 incomplete lesions. With regard to neurological recovery, the author distinguished 5 groups: 1, very good—i.e. recovery including bladder and bowel functions; 2, good—i.e. recovery of motor function in at least two major joints of two paralysed limbs; 3, moderate recovery of motor function in at least one major joint of two paralysed limbs; 4, little recovery—i.e. recovery of motor function in individual muscles only or recovery of sensory function over at least four segments; 5, insignificant or no recovery. The results achieved in 134 cases showed 60·5 per cent satisfactory vertebral reduction and 49·3 per cent functional recoveries. In the 104 complete lesions, there was 61·5 per cent satisfactory vertebral reduction and 38·5 per cent functional recoveries. In the 30 incomplete lesions, 56·6 per cent showed satisfactory vertebral reduction and 90 per cent functional recovery. Although these two statistics are not absolutely comparable because of the difference in the size of material and, possibly, different type and severity of the vertebral injuries, they demonstrate a remarkable accordance in the high percentage of functional recovery in incomplete lesions following conservative treatment. This fact should always be considered very carefully by surgeons before contemplating the subjecting of traumatic paraplegics and tetraplegics with incomplete lesions to surgical procedures on the fractured or dislocated spine.

A further detailed analysis following postural reduction has been published by my former co-workers at Stoke Mandeville (Frankel *et al.*, 1969) on a total material of 612 patients admitted within the first 14 days of injury between 1950–68. Two hundred and sixteen were cervical, 166 thoracic, 205 thoraco-lumbar and 23 lumbar injuries. These figures include the patients of my own statistic of 1963. The pattern of improvement shown in this large number of patients is in good accordance with that described in my statistic of 1963. However, the percentage of initially complete cervical lesions becoming incomplete following conservative treatment is definitely higher— i.e. 34·15 per cent out of 123 initially complete lesions as compared with 27·12 per cent in my series of 59 complete lesions. Three initially incomplete lesions became complete (2·43 per cent).

With regard to late instability only 4 out of 612 patients (0·65 per cent) developed an instability of their fracture-dislocations after being allowed out of bed. Of these, two had cervical injuries, in one the spine eventually became stable after 6 months in a collar, the other having a fusion performed in another hospital. Two patients had thoraco-lumbar fracture-dislocations. One became stable after an additional 8 weeks in bed, the other finally uniting in increased deformity after 6 months in a plastic corset. The very low incidence of late instability is no doubt due to the fact that the patients have an adequate time in bed, varying between 9 to 13 weeks for the utmost. However, the time, however long, is not wasted and does not delay the patient's rehabilitation, as physio-therapy, psychological adjustment, occupational therapy and teaching prepare the patient both physically and psychologically for the later stages of rehabilitation.

Surgical procedures following fractures of the spine

Already, before the introduction of antisepsis and asepsis, operative procedures for traumatic paraplegia had been advocated by surgeons. In the beginning of the last century it was, in particular, Sir Astley Cooper (1824–27), in England who was the main advocate for surgical treatment of these patients, which brought him in strong controversy with his eminent colleague Sir Charles Bell (1824). The introduction of asepsis and X-ray and the development of orthopaedic surgery and neurosurgery have by no means diminished the discrepancy of opinion regarding time, indication and value of the various methods of surgery. Verbiest (1963) has reviewed the surgical indica-tions for the different types of spinal fractures and their resultant neurological sympto-matology. From this review, it would appear that there is hardly any vertebral damage under the sun which would not be regarded for immediate surgery, whether it be laminectomy, open reduction and stabilization of the spine, by wire, metal plates, bone graft or anterior, antero-lateral or posterior decompression followed by fusion, furthermore whether or not the damage to the spinal cord be complete or incomplete and associated with or without suparachnoidal block. Even psychological considerations were given as indication for decompression by laminectomy (Comarr, 1959). In my and other workers' experience in this field the refusal to carry out any operation on the spine merely on psychological reasons or the resistance to pressure from the patients or their relatives 'to do something' has had not the slightest delay in the patient's rehabilitation, provided the physician or surgeon has properly explained the reason for the futility of such procedure. Moreover, the advocates of this indication are remarkably silent about the psychological effects of an unsuccessful operation, which has resulted in transforming a spinal injury without any or only partial damage of the spinal cord into a complete transverse lesion.

As the main controversy still applies to the indications for the various surgical procedures in the immediate (within 24 hours) and very early stages following spinal cord injuries, they will be discussed individually.

The methods practised in the immediate and early stages are as follows.

Skeletal traction by skull calipers

This method is used for the reduction and stabilization of fractures and fracture-dislocations of the cervical spine. The previously applied method of head traction by the Glisson sling has been replaced by most workers in this field by skull traction with calipers since these were first introduced by Crutchfield (1933). This has been, indeed, a major advance in the immediate and early management of cervical injuries, and striking examples of the great value of this method are shown in figures of the chapters on cervical fractures. Modifications of Crutchfield's original design have been published by Cone & Turner (1937), Barton (1938) and Vinke (1948). Cone has improved Barton's design and the Barton–Cone caliper has the advantage of larger tongs as compared with other designs, and the points of the tongs make an angle of 180 degrees which diminishes the danger of pulling out or penetrating the skull and causing infection or direct damage to the brain. The points are inserted 2 inches above the external auditory meatus—i.e. more distally than with the Crutchfield technique. At Stoke Mandeville, Crutchfield, Blackburn and Barton–Cone calipers were used and we found the latter more satisfactory. Skull traction with wires (Hoen, 1936) and with fishhooks under the zygomatic or zygomatico-molar arches have been described (Neuheiser, 1933; Selmo, 1939; Batchelor, 1946; Soustelle, 1951) but have more or less been abandoned because of the great discomfort to the patient and the obvious danger of infection to the tissues. We admitted two patients with this type of head traction. Both patients felt most uncomfortable and one had a severe infection. This head traction was discontinued immediately. It is generally abandoned.

Laminectomy

This is still the most widely debated and most controversial subject amongst the surgical procedures advocated for the immediate, early as well as late, treatment of spinal injuries. What then are the reasons for many surgeons to justify laminectomy as routine immediate and early treatment in traumatic cord and cauda equina lesions? In the first place it is the ill-conceived idea that compression of the cord resulting from a vertebral fracture is the only or main cause of paraplegia and tetraplegia and that immediate decompression will rectify the damage. It is ignored that the mechanism of spinal cord injury following fracture-dislocations differs fundamentally from that of a slow-growing tumour or tuberculous process of the spine. A vertebral injury producing instantaneous clinical symptoms of complete or partial paralysis is the result of the acute impact of violence on the neural elements themselves, causing concussion, contusion, laceration or transection of the cord. This mechanism is always associated with damage to the vascular supply at, below and above the site of the trauma. In this connection, it must be remembered that, although most severe damage of the spinal cord and roots often occurs in individuals with normal diameter of the spinal canal, this occurs even more readily in individuals with an abnormally narrow spinal canal. In recent years, attention has been drawn to this congenital abnormality of the vertebral column by several authors (Verbiest, 1962; Ehni, 1965; Hinck & Suchdev, 1966; Hancock, 1967).

Secondly, narrowing of the vertebral canal by protruding bone or intervertebral disc alone, as demonstrated by X-rays, or in combination with a subarachnoidal block found immediately after injury, is only too readily accepted as conclusive evidence of the concept of compression, regardless of whether the neurological lesion is complete or incomplete. It must be stressed at once that neither X-ray findings nor the presence of a complete or partial block in the acute stage, are in themselves evidence of compression as the cause of paraplegia or tetraplegia. For it is a well-known fact that, in spite of X-ray evidence of a severe fracture-dislocation with marked narrowing of the spinal canal, the clinical symptoms may be either minimal or even entirely absent, as the spinal cord has miraculously escaped injury. Striking examples of this fact have been previously published (Guttmann, 1954; Meinecke, 1964 and others. See also Figs. 50, 53, 54, 59, 65, 67).

Thirdly, the initially complete block is of no diagnostic value at this stage (Guttmann, 1949), as it is due to temporary oedema or some bleeding into the subarachnoid space which will clear up in due course. Conversely, in spinal injuries resulting in severe damage or transection of the cord, the complete block is due to merging and firm fixation of dura and arachnoidea with the disrupted tissues of the cord and/or the protruding bone which has caused the cord injury. Personal observations at post mortem and those of other workers have frequently confirmed these findings and proved the futility of exploratory or decompressive laminectomy in complete transverse cord lesions with areflexia lasting longer than 24 or 48 hours. This is now generally accepted by surgeons with extensive experience in this field. On the other hand, it was found that considerable recovery of severe cord or cauda equina symptoms may occur in spite of a persistent block and unreduced fracture-dislocation (Figs. 58 and 69). Myelography has also been employed in the acute stage of traumatic paraplegia but has not been found a reliable indicator of the need for decompression.

Many surgeons, especially in the U.S.A., Canada, and in some European continental and eastern countries, still carry out immediate or early decompressive laminectomy in complete and incomplete traumatic transverse lesions of the cord following spinal fracture, regardless of whether there is a sub-arachnoidal block or not, the concept being the prevention of further damage. Moreover, this operation is also advocated in incomplete lesions which do not show or have stopped recovery and even while recovery takes place (Haynes, 1946). From the many tragic results of this 'dynamic' attitude described in the literature and from personal observations, one must ask whether in patients with such disability the risk of immediate or early laminectomy is justifiable in any but the very exceptional cases, as mentioned later in this book. What tragedy the transformation of an incomplete cord lesion into a complete one means for the unfortunate victim needs no further emphasis and is one which no statistics can alter.

If decompression by laminectomy were really so beneficial as is claimed by its advocates, there should be, by now, after the tremendous number of laminectomies carried out throughout the years in many countries, abundant and quite overwhelming statistical proof of the efficacy of this operation and its superiority to conservative management. However, statistics on a large scale have clearly shown the contrary. Comarr (1959) reported 212 amongst 947 paralysed patients who had laminectomies carried out within 24 hours of injury. Only 15·5 per cent showed improvement of symptoms while 304 patients without laminectomy showed 31 per cent improvement.

The detrimental effect of immediate and early exploratory or decompressive laminectomy in traumatic spinal cord lesions, especially of the cervical cord, in increasing cord damage and causing death, is by no means a rare incidence if one considers only those cases reported in the modern medical literature (Taylor, 1929; Merle d'Aubigné, Benassy & Ramadier, 1956; Guttmann, 1949–69; Leimbach, 1962; Carey, 1965; Band, 1963; Harris, 1963, 1971; Holdsworth, 1963; Verbiest, 1963; McSweeney, 1964; Bedbrook, 1970). Special mention may be made in particular of the observations made by Merle d'Aubigné and his co-workers. These outstanding accident surgeons found not the slightest improvement amongst their 54 laminectomized patients and very often increase of the cord lesion. Benassy et al. (1967) published a series of 600 traumatic paraplegics and tetraplegics and came to the conclusion that laminectomy was not helpful in most patients with injuries of the thoracic and lumbar spine. Junghanns (1968) quoted Professor Schmieden in Schmorl's handbook *Die gesunde und kranke Wirbelsaule im Röntgenbild und Klinik* who, from his extensive personal experience and as a result of information gained from questionnaires to other surgeons, came to the following conclusions: The immediate and early laminectomy as routine treatment of severe spinal fractures resulting in paralysis has failed. In particular, it is not suitable to improve most severe cases and does not reduce the mortality rate. This surgical procedure is not indicated in any case of total dislocation with complete transverse lesion and likewise in other cases where a thorough neurological observation has revealed an absolutely definite transverse lesion. In this connection the unsatisfactory results reported by Beneš (1968), an experienced neurosurgeon, as a result of immediate or early laminectomy, particularly in traumatic lesions of the cervical cord, speak for themselves.

Of special interest is a recent detailed study by the American surgeons Morgan et al. (1971) on 230 patients with traumatic spinal cord injuries admitted to Montebellow State Rehabilitation Hospital, Baltimore, from 1953–68. One hundred and twenty-eight patients had complete transection of the cord and none of these at any level benefited from exploratory or decompressive laminectomy. Seventy of the remaining patients had well documented incomplete spinal cord lesions. These cases were selected for the study 'because, in 32 of these patients the loss of function following laminectomy is documented with tragic clarity'. Laminectomy was performed in 42 of these patients. Twenty-two patients (52 per cent) lost neurological function. In contrast, without laminectomy 15 of 28 patients (54 per cent) improved and no deterioration occurred in this group. Only 14 (33 per cent) with incomplete lesions improved neurologically after laminectomy. Unfortunately, no data of time-interval between laminectomy and the resultant neurological improvement is given, which might have clarified how many of the improved cases can really be attributed to the laminectomy. The authors quite rightly acknowledge that the statistic derived from the study cannot be applied to all laminectomies performed for incomplete cord lesions, as other patients who may have made rapid or complete recovery in an acute hospital will not be admitted to a rehabilitation hospital. On the other hand, this statistic is also incomplete in that the authors do not have any data of the number of patients operated in the acute hospital from which they received their cases and how many of them have died in the acute hospital. Sixty-eight per cent of the patients who had laminectomies required stabilization procedures immediately or some time during the course of their rehabilitation. This confirms the well-known fact that the stability of the spine may be profoundly disturbed, the more so as further damage of the muscles at the site of the fracture as a result of the operation adds to their initial traumatic damage and thus helps to promote the development of spinal deformities.

It is significant that even radical advocates of immediate and early laminectomy have changed their attitude in view of their unfortunate results. Covalt, Cooper, Hoen & Rusk (1953) pointed out that laminectomy carries 'a low mortality and morbidity rate'. This is hardly acceptable from either a medical or ethical point of view. Nor is their other argument acceptable by anyone who is familiar with the pathology of the spinal cord following closed injuries of the spine that 'unless it has been determined by surgical exploration that the spinal cord has been transected one cannot conclude during the early weeks after injury that a patient is permanently or irreversibly paraplegic'. Such a statement is surprising as there is general knowledge that no conclusion can be drawn from the macroscopic appearance of the cord as to the prognosis of functional recovery if at operation the continuity of the spinal cord is found intact. For the irreversible damage may be vascular, due either to an anterior spinal artery catastrophy, such as thrombosis or haemotomyelia, or direct squeezing damage of the soft and highly vascular central tissues of the cord up and down the site of the impact of the violence leading to colliquative necrosis (Bedbrook, 1966). Further unfortunate experience of these authors' indiscriminate surgical approach must have changed their views fundamentally, for a later publication of the same institute (Kaplan, Powell, Grynbaum & Rusk, 1966) now frankly admits that development of paralysis following laminectomy is not a rare occurrence and that 'this complication points out the need to be extremely circumspect in exploratory laminectomy, when the degree of paralysis is minimal'. This warning applies, of course, at least as much to incomplete lesions with a greater degree of paralysis.

To what grotesque deformity an early laminectomy following a spinal fracture may lead is strikingly demonstrated in Fig. 75 of a girl, aged 16, who sustained a rather severe incomplete transverse cord syndrome as a result of a compression fracture-dislocation of C5 vertebra. Thirteen days after injury a decompressive laminectomy was performed by a

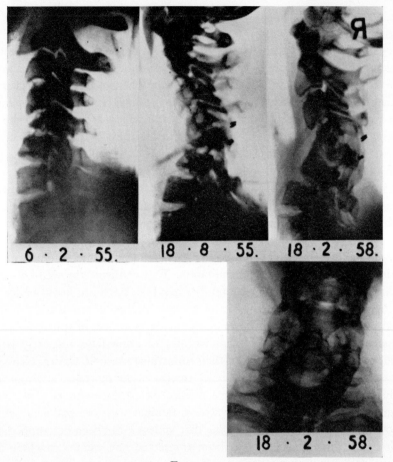

FIG. 75.

highly experienced neurosurgeon elsewhere. From the medical notes it appeared that at operation no stability of the cervical spine was found, and following consultation with an orthopaedic surgeon who was present at the operation it was unanimously decided that there was no indication for a stabilizing operation following laminectomy. Nevertheless, a most profound postoperative deformity of the spine developed as seen in Fig. 75. The laminectomy did not have the slightest beneficial effect on the cord lesion but miraculously the resultant severe vertebral deformity did not increase the preoperative clinical symptoms, a further proof of the adaptability of the spinal cord under certain circumstances to even profound deformities of the spine (see also Figs. 54, 69). In recent years Audic & Maury (1969) gave further proof of deformities of the spine as a result of laminectomy.

From all these observations, to which many more could be added, one cannot escape the conclusion to reject laminectomy as *immediate* exploratory or decompressive procedure in spinal cord and cauda equina injuries following fractures and fracture-dislocations. This was not always the view of the author of this book (see Guttmann, 1930) but, from his own further experiences and the data given from other workers in this field, the risk of laminectomy in causing death, in particular in tetraplegics, or producing irreversible damage of the cord is too great to consider this procedure as suitable in the immediate management of injuries of the spinal cord and cauda equina.

Prevention of post-traumatic necrosis of the spinal cord

(a) Cooling the spinal cord at the site of injury

Longhead *et al.* (1955), Boba (1960), Negrin & Klauber (1960), Kristiansen & Dott (1961) and Ommaya & Baldwin (1963) published observations on the beneficial effect of hypothermia in preventing anoxia resulting from arrest of the cerebral circulation, and this procedure is now widely accepted.

Studies in animals and man have also been reported on the effect of hypothermia in preventing necrosis of the neuronal tissues resulting from ischaemia in traumatic lesions of the spinal cord (Albin *et al.*, 1961, 1968; White, 1972, 1973; Negrin, 1962, 1973; Tator & Deecke, 1973).

The underlying theory is to reverse, at least partially, the effect of cord injury by cooling the cord to prevent the development of post-traumatic necrosis initiated by the trauma. It is assumed that there is a definite time lag before the process of necrosis is fully developed and that during this time the long fibre pathways are mostly intact. Therefore, if this process can be stopped in the acute stage, then useful spinal cord function can be preserved. This theory is contrary to the generally held opinion that the spinal function is immediately and permanently lost following traumatic disruption of the cord. The patient has to be treated within 4 to 6 hours after injury, which in itself seriously restricts the use of this method. The technique consists in performing a standard laminectomy, removing three laminae of the injured site. When the dura is exposed and the cord is found to be so swollen or displaced that it is impinging on the dura, it is recommended that the dura must be cooled for an hour before it is opened. Following opening of the dura, tubes are placed above and below the lesion, which are connected to a heat exchanger and the fluid pumped with an ordinary heart–lung machine. The wound is then slowly filled with ice-cold normal saline until the pump moves the cold fluid through the system to the heat exchanger and back to the wound. A high flow-rate of 500 ccs to 1,000 ccs per minute is established. Temperature measurements in the muscles of the wound near the cord are made and kept to less than 20°C. The cooling is continued for 3 hours, then the dura is left open and the muscles, fascia and skin are closed in the usual way.

Ten patients with cervical cord injuries and tetraplegia were reported by White (1972). However, according to Dr White they were not an 'ideal group'. Five of these patients underwent an emergency laminectomy and were treated with 3 hours of direct cord cooling. Only three had some return of neurological function in the lower limbs and in two of these the return of function was marked. No exact details about the clinical symptomatology before and after cooling were given. Moreover, three of the untreated patients also had some significant improvement in the upper limbs. Dr White himself came to the conclusion that 'Unfortunately no definite study has yet been published that absolutely establishes that direct cooling of the spinal cord is in fact beneficial'. Moreover, in my opinion, the theoretical basis of the theory is not yet proven by systematic histological findings. It must be pointed out—and the three untreated patients are a clear proof—that spinal cord function may not be permanently lost following spinal cord injuries—for it depends entirely on the severity of the initial trauma whether function may recover or not. It has been proved again and again by many patients, both paraplegics and tetraplegics, that the initial complete paraplegia and tetraplegia may recover even to a great extent without surgical intervention, in the stages of reorganization within the damaged area of the cord.

Even less convincing are 3 cases reported by Negrin Jr. (1973). Of these only one case (traumatic paraplegia of the thoracic cord) had a decompression laminectomy about 5 hours after injury. The dura was not opened and post-operative epidural cooling was done for 3 periods of 45 minutes each on the 2nd, 3rd, and 4th post-operative days. There was no improvement whatsoever and a complete flaccid paraplegia has persisted (about 11 years after injury).

The second case (initially incomplete paraplegia) had a decompression laminectomy *one month after injury* (1.7.64) with combined epidural cooling. However, after improvement he became paraplegic again and a second laminectomy on 11.10.64 revealed an epidural granuloma, and, after incision of the dura, arachnoiditis was found. Two weeks later (26.10.64) a re-exploration was done and the dura was found hypertrophic and compressing the cord, reducing its width to about 20 per cent. Subarachnoid hypothermia was performed, moreover the dura was left open. After this decompression the patient improved gradually.

The third case had a spastic tetraplegia and brain stem injury and was in a coma or semi-coma for about 4 months following a car accident in May 1965. A laminectomy *one year later* at the level of C7 to T1 was carried out by subarachnoid cooling of the spinal cord with fluid temperature of $7\,^{\circ}$C perfused to $8\,^{\circ}$C for 45 minutes. Intradural catheters which were left in place for post-operative cooling had to be removed because of staphylococcal infection. This patient improved 3 weeks after a left high thigh subcutaneous tenotomy to reduce the flexion-adduction spasticity.

From the data given, it is quite obvious that these 3 cases are not acceptable as proof of the beneficial effect of hypothermia in traumatic lesions of the spinal cord. In this connection, Richardson & Nakamura's (1971) electron microscope studies may be mentioned, where local hypothermia was started one hour after spinal cord compression, by exposing the dura and irrigating cold Ringer's solution and maintaining temperature between 8 to $9.5\,^{\circ}$C for 3 hours. They found the morphological changes of most structures not very striking, although the swelling of the astrocytic vascular feet was somewhat reduced.

In recent experimental studies, Tator and Deecke (1973) compressed 10 monkeys with the cuff inflated to 350 mmHg for 5 minutes and the cord was perfused at $5\,^{\circ}$C after the dura was opened. A comparison made with 10 monkeys exposed to the same experiment but with the cuff inflated even to 400 mmHg for 5 minutes and the cord exposed at $36\,^{\circ}$C yielded better neurological recovery than with durotomy plus hypothermic perfusion. These findings, if confirmed, may prove that the beneficial effect ascribed to hypothermia by the authors mentioned previously may actually have been due to perfusion alone.

Another experimental approach to study regeneration of the spinal cord following traumatic lesions has recently been made by Wilson and Jagadesh (1976) in cats, by exposing the animals to a pulse electromagnetic field. However, their histo-pathological findings following hemisection of the cord do not allow conclusion on regeneration following complete transection of the cord.

(b) Chemical prevention of post-traumatic damage to the cord

Chemical prevention of cord damage, in particular by minimizing oedema in the immediate stage following injury, has been practised for many years in man by intravenous injection of hypertonic saline or glucose (25–50 per cent) solutions. More recently, Dexamethazone 20–50 mg daily has been said to be more effective. Since Ducker & Hamit (1969) reported improved functional recovery with intramuscular injections of steroids in initially complete cord lesion, this drug has been used by clinicians. At Stoke Mandeville beneficial effects were found in stopping ascending complete lesions or preventing incomplete lesions becoming complete. However, Yeo et al. (1975) reported no significant difference in sheep treated with steroids. The 'depot' form of methyl prednisolone (Depo-Medrol) allows only slow release of the steroids 4 hours after the injection. Therefore, the accumulation of this drug to significant local level may be too late to prevent irreversible damage of the cord.

Osterholm & Mathews (1971, 1972) reported high protective effects of Alpha Methyl Tyrosine (AMT), in an average dose of 160 mg/kg, in preventing irreversible damage in acute traumatic cord lesions in animals, especially of the grey matter. These experiments were based on the assumption that the effects of Norepinephrine, which is four times increased in the traumatic area of cord lesions causing significant neuronal depression and vasoconstriction, can be counteracted by anti-neonephrine drugs. Altogether, 18 drugs and drug combinations were studied in cats. It was found that the highest protection was achieved by Alpha Methyl Tyrosine (97 per cent) and Reserpine (93 per cent). Osterholm found that the animals treated with these chemicals showed invariably smaller necrosis than the controls. However, he admitted that these results are not at all mathematically comparable with each other, as different dosages of drugs were used.

Osterholm's and Mathews' work has doubtless opened a new approach in minimizing acute spinal cord pathology following injuries, but there is still more evidence needed having regard to the conflicting views of other workers in this field (Nafchi et al. 1974; Vise et al., 1974; Yeo et al., 1975). Yeo et al., confirming Osterholm's results on the beneficial effect of AMT, suggested that possibly some of the beneficial effects of AMT may be related to its influence on renal function by causing impressive diuresis, similar to the action of Mannitol on oedema. Richardson & Nakamura (1971), in their electron miscoscopic study of spinal cord oedema, found that intravenous infusion of 20 per cent Mannitol solution (2·5 gm/kg) produced histologically a significant decrease in the volume of the astrocytic vascular feet. The dehydrating action was recognized in the epithelium and astrocyte morphologically, and the swelling of the astrocyte showed the most change in reduction as a result of a change in the water and electrolyte metabolism and not in the blood spinal cord barrier. The authors considered these changes as a temporary effect of Mannitol.

Indications of laminectomy in the early treatment

The question arises whether there is any indication for laminectomy in the early treatment of spinal injuries—i.e. within the first 2 weeks after injury. T.B.Dick (1949)
published a statistic relating to 27 patients subjected to laminectomy more than 7 days
after injury performed at the former Spinal Injuries Centre, Winnick. Twenty-two had
complete lesions before the operation and, although only two proved at operation to be
complete transections, no patient showed evidence of later recovery. Five laminectomies
were performed on patients with incomplete lesions of whom three showed doubtful
improvement which probably, as the author states, was not attributable to the operation.
There are, however, instances, although very rare, where this procedure may be justified
and even indicated.

(1) Ascending neurological deficit in complete transverse lesions

It is not uncommon that in the first few days after injury a complete transverse lesion
may ascend over 1–2 segments. This is due to circulatory disturbances and oedema
around the damaged region of the cord and is in no way justification for laminectomy, for
this increase of clinical symptoms is temporary and will recede spontaneously. However,
an initially complete distal paraplegia may develop ascending symptoms over a great
number of segments within a week or two. This may be due to an intradural but extramedullary haemorrhage at higher level (Foerster, 1929) or a progressive, large localized
epidural haematoma. These are, however, extremely rare incidences, and amongst more
than 2,500 traumatic paraplegics and tetraplegics I have not seen a single case. Laminectomy may be, at least, justified in such an event, but alas—at operation one will find, as a
rule, either signs of a spinal artery thrombosis or a haematomyelia. Frankel (1969) has
given a statistic of 7 patients of Stoke Mandeville with ascending symptoms of at least 4
segments. Six had T11 or T12 fractures with initial symptoms ranging from T12 or L4
rising to T5 and C7/8 respectively. One patient had a fracture-dislocation of T4 and the
initial transverse lesion ascended to C7. All but 2 had a subarachnoidal block, but in one
of these myelography demonstrated a block at the level of the fracture (T12). In this
patient with an initial lesion below L4, the lesion rose to C7/8 and receded eventually
to T1/T3. He was the only patient who had two laminectomies at the admitting hospital
while the lesion was rising, and the spinal cord was described as swollen and pink.
Following the second operation the lesion continued to rise and he was treated with
Heparin, following which there was no further rise. All the other patients were treated
conservatively with Heparin, Dindevan, Rhoemacrodex, Arvine and Prednisolone
respectively and in 6 cases the lesion became static at higher level, and in one case only
the symptoms went down to T11.

(2) Progressive paralysis in incomplete lesions

Progressive paralysis may occur in a case of fracture or fracture-dislocation where initially
there has been an incomplete lesion with no or only minimal signs of cord or cauda equina
involvement. However, it must be stressed again that motor or sensory symptoms in
incomplete cauda equina lesions which have increased in the following days after injury

may recede spontaneously. Therefore, there is no hurry for immediate exploration and the longer one observes such a case by thorough and frequent neurological control the less often will a surgical exploration be necessary. The following case is a good example:

A man, aged 33, was hit by a cement mixer on 23 May 1954, and sustained an incomplete cauda equina lesion. The first X-ray revealed a severe fracture of the fourth lumbar vertebra, apart from multiple fractures of the transverse processes of L1 to L4 on both sides. The lateral third of the right side of L4 was broken off, and there was also a fracture of the pedicles of that vertebra making the whole vertebra extremely unstable. On admission on 24 April 1954 he had a marked weakness of both lower limbs. Knee and ankle jerks and plantar response were absent on both sides and there was sensory impairment below L3 with analgesia in S3 to S5. Bladder and bowels were paralysed. Postural reduction and fixation on sorbo-packs was carried out with regular turnings from side to side every two hours. Four days after admission the motor symptoms increased and gradually all dorsi- and plantar-flexors of the feet and toes became paralysed. However, having regard to the fact that there was no increase in the disturbance of sensation surgical interference was decided against and the conservative treatment continued, as it was felt that the increased motor symptoms were due to oedema or some haemorrhage affecting the anterior roots only which would be absorbed in due course. From 12 May 1954, 19 days after injury and 15 days after deterioration, I was satisfied that the decision not to operate, when the clinical symptoms increased, was correct. The motor function in the toes and feet on the right gradually returned followed by functional recovery of the same muscles as well as the extensor digitorum and peronei on the left side. Bladder control gradually returned. X-rays of 14 June 1954 showed re-expansion of the compressed vertebra and good alignment of the broken-off lateral part, and the fractured pedicles of the fourth lumbar vertebra had become fixed again. In due course, further recovery of muscle function occurred and the patient was discharged home six and a half months after injury, able to walk without support of any kind, and he took up employment very soon afterwards (Guttmann, 1954).

(3) Development of paraplegia after free interval

An extremely rare incidence is the gradual development of paraplegia after a more or less long free interval following acute injury to the back without causing damage to the vertebra and without immediate cord or cauda equina symptoms, in a person with an already existing though asymptomatic pathology of the cord, such as tumour or haemangioma. There is only one case of benign tumour amongst our material where a paraplegia developed after a free interval following injury to the back.

A man, aged 22, was involved in a car accident on 1 November 1959 when the car hit a lamp-post. He was shaken and experienced pain in his back but got out of the car and walked. He was taken to the nearest hospital where no pathological clinical signs of cord involvement was found, nor did X-ray examination of the spine reveal any vertebral injury. He was sent home and went to bed, but he woke up at 6 a.m. because of increasing pain in his back. Some time later, he had paraesthesia in both legs and at 11 a.m. became paralysed and was unable to pass urine. He was taken to the nearest hospital, where a lumbar puncture showed a complete block and myelography a stop at T8 level. The clinical signs were those of an almost complete paraplegia below T8 with sparing of the posterior columns only. At operation on 2 November 1959 a localized neuro-fibroma was found lying in front of T8 level; 'the cord had obviously been damaged and the appearances were suggestive of an anterior spinal artery thrombosis'. The tumour was removed completely but the severe though incomplete paraplegia persisted; the reflexes in the legs did not return for at least 4 weeks and—alas—he developed pressure sores on both heels and sacrum and urinary infection. He was transferred to Stoke Mandeville on 18 December 1959, where the sores were healed, and, in due course, he made some motor and sensory recovery but developed a marked spastic paraparesis. He was discharged on 31 January 1961 and has returned for check-ups ever since. The spasticity was greatly relieved in due course by bilateral iliopsoas myotomy and lengthening of the Achilles tendons. He runs a hairdressing saloon and is married.

Another case of gradually progressive paraplegia following free interval after a back injury was a young boy of 16 in whom an operation and epidural haemangioma was found which had bled.

Holdsworth (1963) reported of 3 cases amongst 150 cervical fractures and fracture-dislocations who had a delayed onset of tetraplegia. In 2 of these patients, there was eventually a complete recovery with conservative treatment. In the 3rd patient the initially partial tetraplegia became rapidly complete. A laminectomy did not produce any improvement.

(4) Pain due to irritation of nerve roots

Pain in the immediate stage following spinal injury is not an indication for immediate operation, but in extremely rare cases excruciating pain due to direct irritation of nerve roots by a splinter may be an indication for operation in early stages (2–3 weeks after injury).

Open reduction and internal fixation

There are several methods advocated for open reduction and internal stabilization of the fractured spine: fixation by bone grafts, wire, metal plates, metal rods with hooks or anterior, antero-lateral or posterior fusion. Moreover, the combination of laminectomy with one of these techniques of artificial stabilization has been frequently practised to counteract instability of the spine following laminectomy. The considerable variety of these methods reveals the discord amongst surgeons regarding the most suitable method for this procedure. Above all, there is still discrepancy of opinion as to indication for and timing of any of these stabilizing procedures. It is the uncertainty of the stability of the fractured spine and the fear that 'potential' instability may cause later damage of the spinal cord or spinal roots or increase the initial neurological deficit resulting from the injury, which still leads many neurosurgeons and orthopaedic surgeons to the dogmatic view that the restitution of the stability of the spine by conservative means is not possible or at least uncertain. Although there is ample proof to the contrary (see Chapter on Classification) many surgeons still advocate immediate or very early open reduction and stabilization procedures. There is also no statistical proof of the view held by some surgeons that these immediate surgical procedures will, as a rule, shorten the rehabilitation of paraplegics and tetraplegics. Some surgeons (Cone & Turner, Rogers, Forsyth and others) consider open reduction under skull traction safer and more effective in cervical injuries than manipulation or traction alone. Here again, there are no comparative statistics available which can prove this assumption. However, other workers in this field give first skull traction an adequate trial and only perform stabilizing operations if traction has failed.

(1) Open reduction and stabilization by metal plates or distracting rods

In 1953, Holdsworth & Hardy, who condemned manipulative reduction, revived Wilson's method of open reduction and internal fixation of the broken spine by bolting two metal plates through one or more spinous processes above and below the level of the fracture-dislocation. In fairness to these authors, it must be stressed that they advocated this method for fracture-dislocations of the spine at the thoraco-lumbar level only, but other orthopaedic surgeons have performed this operation, even in simple compression fractures, at any level of the spine including the cervical spine. This method was described as simple, safe and effective in preventing redislocation and, moreover, that it would promote recovery and prevent further damage. Pennybacker (1953) suggested that this form of stabilization would prevent later angulation. Dick (1955) stated that the spine can be stabilized in this way so securely that 'ordinary' nursing handling is 'absolutely safe' and 'there is no danger of further damage to recovering nerve roots'. However, Hardy (1965) obviously did not agree with this view, as the nursing of his operated cases has been carried out precisely with the same routine and care as in the non-operated cases, much on the same lines as practised at Stoke Mandeville since 1944. From personal observations the author can only warn not to relax the most careful nursing after the procedure.

Since 1953, we have admitted to Stoke Mandeville just under 100 patients in whom open reduction had been carried out elsewhere, and the conclusions which can be drawn from this large material are as follows:

(a)   This operation is by no means simple and safe, especially not in those cases in whom, in addition to the fracture of the vertebral body, the spinous processes and pedicles are broken. Therefore, the difficulties surgeons have to encounter should not be belittled and Holdsworth himself (1954) withdrew his statement of the simplicity of this method.

(b)   This method does not prevent re-dislocation regardless of what kind of metal plate is used. This applies in particular also to that large straight plate propagated by Meurig-Williams (Fig. 76). In fact, this type of plate produced such stiffness and rigidity of the vertebral column associated with excruciating pain that the patient was not able to bend and the plate had to be removed, and this was also necessary after using the Wilson plate. To what tragic consequences an unsuccessful open reduction and fixation with metal plates can lead is best shown by the X-rays and photograph of a young man

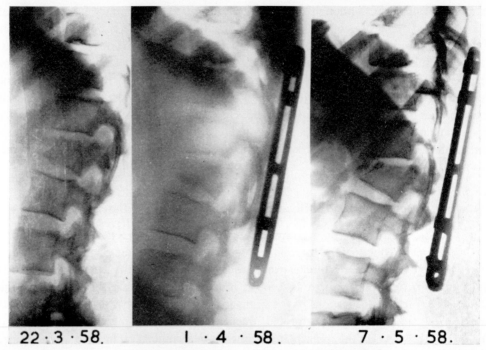

22·3·58.   1·4·58.   7·5·58.

FIG. 76. Failure to maintain reduction by plating.

of 18, who sustained a fracture-dislocation which could have easily been reduced and stabilized by conservative means (Figs. 77a and b).

(c) This method does not prevent later collapse of the initially expanded crushed vertebra (Fig. 78). Consequently, it does not prevent later angulation of the vertebral column of even most profound degrees (Figs. 77, 78).

(d) Plates have been fixed on the wrong vertebra and have either had to be removed

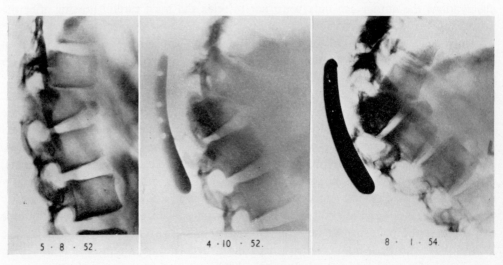

5·8·52.   4·10·52.   8·1·54.

FIG. 77a.

by a second operation or another plate has had to be inserted. What tragic mistakes in this respect can be made is well illustrated in a case of fracture-dislocation of the upper lumbar spine with little displacement. Plates were put at the wrong level—i.e. below the fractured vertebra. When this was discovered after operation, a second operation was carried out and a second pair of plates were fixed at a higher level and uselessly fixed with wire to the lower plates opposite the fractured vertebra. After this operation, the wound broke down and on admission to Stoke Mandeville there was a large gaping wound exposing the metal plates and wire, which were eventually removed and the wound then healed, as also did the large pressure sores over the sacrum and hips with which the patient had been admitted. X-rays and photographs of this case have been published by Sir Reginald Watson-Jones in the fourth edition (Vol. II, 1004–5) of his textbook *Fractures and Joint Injuries* (1955).

(e)   Once the patient is out of bed and mobile, it is not unusual for the plates to become loose so that they cut out of the spinous processes, and have to be removed. This is in accordance with Holdsworth's own experience (Holdsworth, 1963), but in our experience it was not a question that the plates have served their purpose, as claimed by Holdsworth, but that they were detrimental to the patient, causing pain and rigidity of the spine (Figs. 79a and b). Even if they did not, it can hardly be claimed that two operations on the spine shortened the patient's rehabilitation.

(f)   Haematoma and infection following this operation are by no means uncommon.

(g)   Last but by no means least, there is no proof whatsoever that this operation promotes

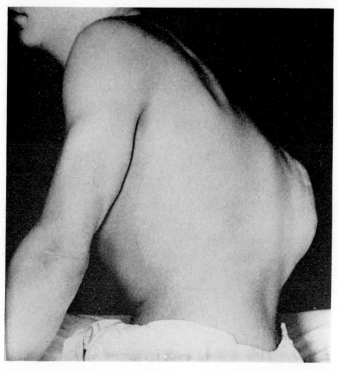

FIG. 77b.

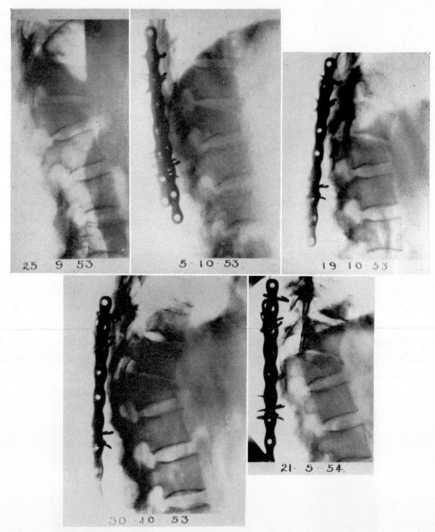

FIG. 78.

more root escape and better neurological recovery than conservative methods. This has been at last clearly pointed out statistically by Hardy himself (1965). In fact there are incidents where the clinical symptoms deteriorated following this operation.

It may be noted that in recent years Holdsworth & Hardy have become very selective by using this method in unstable fractures with the worst displacements, whilst their conservative series includes those with 'relatively less evidence of instability' (Hardy, 1965), and Hardy (1969) stated 'We do have a major conservative regime now'. It seems that these authors have tended to come to the conclusion I expressed in 1954 that 'open reduction in traumatic paraplegics, followed by internal fixation by plating or bone grafts, has its indication, if at all, only in the most excessive types of fracture-dislocation, provided conservative procedures have failed and there is a danger of the dislocated vertebra breaking through the skin. There is only one case in our own large material

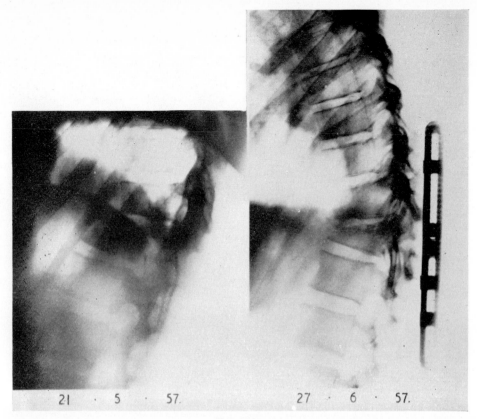

21 · 5 · 57.   27 · 6 · 57.

FIG. 79a.

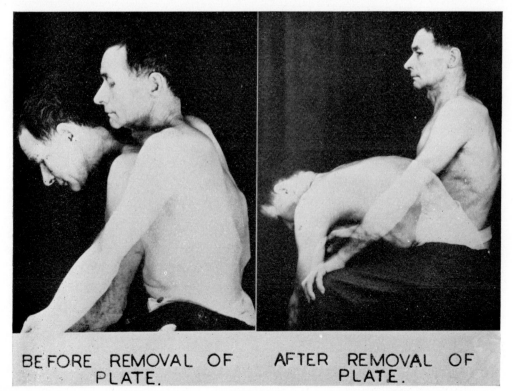

BEFORE REMOVAL OF PLATE.   AFTER REMOVAL OF PLATE.

FIG. 79b.

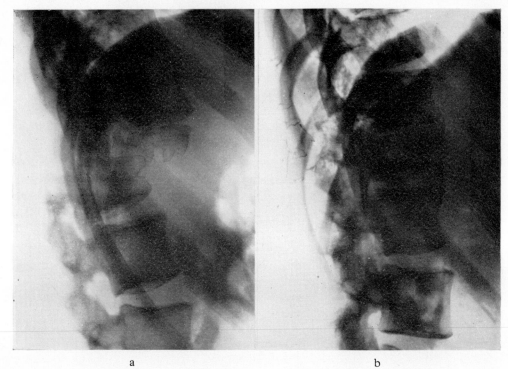

a b

FIG. 80.

of traumatic paraplegics and tetraplegics—a profound fracture-dislocation of the T12 vertebra—necessitating open reduction because of this danger (Fig. 80a). The distal part of the fractured spine was lying right underneath the skin and could not be reduced conservatively. At operation (Dr Walsh) the fracture-dislocation was found to be stable due to firm interlocking of the two ends of the broken vertebra so that the fracture had to be made unstable to be properly aligned. The spinal cord was, as expected, completely transected. At my suggestion, no stabilization with wire, metal plates or other stabilizing material was used to fix the spine, and the patient was treated with the method of postural reduction described previously. Fig. 80b demonstrates the excellent consolidation and stabilization of the fractured spine by the forces of natural repair.

Since Harrington (1962) introduced his system of distraction rods and hooks in the treatment of scoliosis, this method was also used by orthopaedic surgeons for the stabilization of fractured vertebrae, in the hope that this technique would be more suitable than metal plates. Katznelson (1969) reported about 9 paraplegic patients in whom this method was performed. However, the author himself found this series too small to draw conclusions as to the neurological benefit, as not all factors were identical. That this method of internal fixation, however, may not result in solid fusion has been reported by Leidholt et al. (1969). Roberts (1969) reported a series of cases with high incidence of infection, failure of fixation and recurrence of deformity. This author's technique was recently criticized by Lewis and McKibbin (1975). Comparing their own results of 27 plated patients with Roberts' series, they claim that their standard of technical surgery was higher than Roberts', especially with regard to firmness and recurrence of deformity. Moreover, many of Roberts' patients had been in bed for much shorter times and Lewis and McKibbin had themselves experienced increase of deformity in some patients who were mobilized early, i.e. under 12 weeks. Furthermore, complications such as deep sepsis, loose bolts and pain, broken plates causing pain and loose bolts without pain amounted to 9 out of their own 27 patients, in addition to 1 case of deep vein thrombosis and one myocardial infarct—indeed a high percentage as compared with the 12 patients who were treated conservatively with no complications. Out of their 93 patients (64 operated upon, 29 conservatively treated by postural reduction), only 39 (27 plated and 12 treated conservatively) could be evaluated statistically, which, naturally, reduces the validity of the statistics. However, as far as neurological recovery was concerned, Lewis and McKibbin confirmed that there is no proof of Holdsworth and Hardy's original concept that open reduction and fixation by plating has any advantage over conservative methods.

Weiss (1975) from Konstancin reported about a surgical procedure which he calls 'Dynamic Spine Alloplasty' using spring-leading corrective devices, instead of metal plates, to fix the broken spine. He considers the internal fixation of the spine with a spring device more suitable than with metal plates. However, the rationale of his statement that 'dynamic allopathy' can produce 'a steady, gradual correction of the spine in accordance with postural reduction', as described above, is difficult to understand.

From the data produced it would appear that there were 8 deaths amongst 92 patients treated with the spring device. Moreover, wound infection and pressure sores are mentioned as complications. In 3 cases the springs had to be removed 2 months after surgery due to infection and in one case scoliosis was formed due to breaking of the articular processes at one side which also necessitated removal of the 'alloplastic system'. These complications, so far reported, do not justify the claim that the dynamic spine alloplasty with springs is in any way superior to the internal fixation by metal plates.

Spinal fusions

During the last 10 years or so spinal fusion procedures, in particular of the cervical spine, with bone or methyl-metacrylic graft with or without wiring, have been advocated. The main indication for these procedures are the instability of the spine following fractures or dislocations or laminectomy, recurrent deformity following reduction and immobilization and removal of fragments of fractured bone or crushed disc material from the spinal canal. However, timing and type of fusion are still a matter of conjecture—i.e. whether the anterior, antero-lateral or posterior approach is the most suitable in individual cases. Cloward (1961, 1962) propagated the anterior fusion as immediate treatment in fractures and dislocation of the cervical spine, other less dynamic neurosurgeons perform this operation at varying intervals after reduction by skull traction.

Discography has been introduced for the diagnosis of ruptured discs for the lumbar area (Hirsch, 1948; Lindblorn, 1948) as well as for the cervical area (Smith & Nichols, 1957; Cloward, 1958) and has been widely used. However, Smith (1959), following his further experiences, stated that 'relatively few normal cervical discograms are obtained in individuals who have passed the age of 25 or 30 years'. Hirsch *et al.* (1967) abandoned interest in cervical discography because of too many abnormal results in normal individuals. Holt, who in 1964 exposed the fallacy of cervical discography, summarized recently (1975) his views as follows: 'The time has come for a hard and fast moratorium on cervical discography' and later on 'This technique has no diagnostic usefulness'. From all this it seems inconceivable to use discography in fracture dislocations as diagnostic indication of immediate cervical fusion or laminectomy, as is unfortunately still being done.

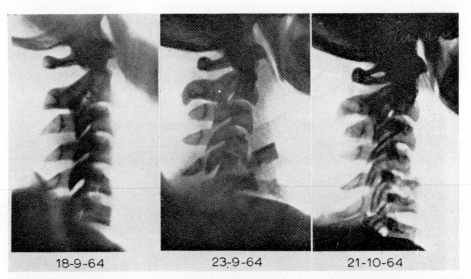

18-9-64   23-9-64   21-10-64

FIG. 81. Note the destruction of three adjacent vertebrae following cervical fusion (see page 89).

While local anaesthesia is possible for the posterior approach, general anaesthetic is, as a rule, necessary, which in cervical patients is administered through a nasal or tracheostomy tube, and, of course, increases the risk of this procedure in cervical lesions with respiratory embarrassment.

It is most important that head and neck are maintained in a safe position during transport to the theatre and to the operating table and throughout the whole operation. Some surgeons (Beckett, Howarth & Petrie, 1964) found a turning frame very helpful in minimizing moving of the patient, and the safe position is best maintained with skull traction of 10 to 15 lb. The operation is carried out in prone position with the head supported on the cerebellar headrest or similar device. Failures of these methods of fusion have been only scantily reported in the literature although I have seen for myself several of these in various clinics. Verbiest (1963) reported such a case and from our own material Fig. 81 shows the disastrous result of an unsuccessful anterior fusion, with the result that following a simple cervical compression fracture, not only the damaged vertebra but two of its neighbours were greatly damaged by this procedure. Beneš (1968) reported 4 patients in whom the anterior approach after Cloward was carried out. One patient died, in the second the reduction was unsuccessful and in the two remaining the clinical symptomatology was unchanged. I have seen several cases demonstrated where the indication for anterior fusion was the stabilization of the fractured spine and the prevention of later deformity. From the control pictures, it was quite obvious that the deformity of the spine after the operation was greater than before. Cloward himself admits quite frankly that in 50 per cent of his patients, an anterior deformity of the cervical spine developed afterwards. Beneš came to the conclusion, from his experience with the Cloward method, that this procedure could hardly be called revolutionary. The case shown in Fig. 81 is a classical example of the results if this operation is carried out indiscriminately as an immediate treatment after fractures of the cervical spine. Beatson (1963) very aptly pointed out. 'Operations are done because surgeons think spines may be unstable and that it is safer to advise fusion. Perhaps it is safer for the surgeon but is such open surgery safe for the patient?' Another experienced orthopaedic surgeon, Mc-Sweeney (1969), had this to say: 'Indiscriminate fusion of the cervical spine in the acute phase is condemned. Apart from open wounds of an initially incomplete lesion, both of which demand exploration, it is difficult to see the need for immediate intervention, much less the indication for immediate fusion.' Del Sel (1975) who also rejects spinal fusion is even more outspoken: 'Our view is that surgical fusion of the spine and particularly of the cervical region for the treatment of traumatic lesions of the rachis, is more an obsession than a real therapeutic need.'

In this connection Kempe's observations (1964) are also of great significance. He reported of 100 patients who had been followed up for a minimum of 12 months after the Cloward procedure. Of the 100 patients 30 had not been given any external fixation after the fusion and no less than 18 developed marked angulation, which developed already in the first month after operation. This statement is of great importance as it is often claimed that this operation greatly shortens the patient's time lying in horizontal position in bed. Kempe described in detail what happened in six cervical cases. In two of them with complete tetraplegia there was no change whatsoever in the neurological deficit and in the remaining four who had various kinds of neurological deficit this anterior decompression did not help in any way the neurological status. In the first two tetraplegics who stayed in the horizontal position the bone graft took very well, and in one who was allowed to sit up after 4 months his bone graft showed perfect healing. Three were allowed to sit up 3 weeks after operation and were given a four-poster neck brace for 10–12 weeks. All three, within 20–24 months, developed severe anterior angulation with the centre of angulation close to the centre of the bone graft. These observations to which others could be added, reveal the fallacy of the claims made that this procedure will stabilize the broken spine unless the patient's post-operative care over long periods in horizontal position is strictly observed until the healing of the broken spine and the bone graft is firmly secured. Myers & Buckley (1967) reported 218 patients of the Neurosurgey Service of Wilford Hall U.S.A.F. Hospital in whom anterior cervical fusions were performed (128 single level fusions, 79 multiple level fusions, 11 block graft fusions). Complications occurred in 60 patients including 6 who had 2 complications each. These complications include primary graft problems such as an obstruction or collapse of the graft, collapse of vertebral body between two grafts, furthermore damage to accessory structures such as damage to the recurrent laryngeal nerve,

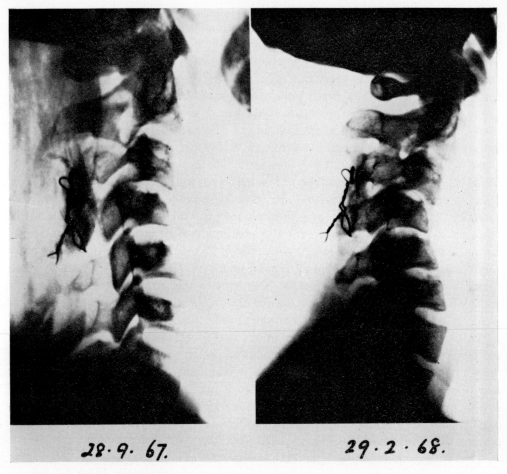

28·9·67.   *29·2·68.*

FIG. 82. This is the same case as described on page 102 demonstrating the unsuccessful results of a wired graft of the processus spinosi.

laryngospasm requiring tracheostomy, dural tears, intermittent dysphagia, neurological complications (Horner's syndrome, transverse lesion), wound infection leading to osteomyelitis and postoperative atelectasis and lung infiltration. The authors admit that the management of the complications delay recovery.

The posterior approach to spinal fusion followed by fixation with wire in patients with dislocations or subluxations is also by no means a guarantee of an improvement of the clinical symptoms or preventing spinal deformity of even marked degrees later, as shown in Fig. 82. Especially tragic are, of course, those patients who, before the operation had no or only mild neurological defects, and who after the operation have become tetraplegics. As an example of an unsuccessful posterior fusion following open reduction of the distal cervical spine the following case may be quoted in detail.

A woman, aged 57, was involved in a car accident in Spain on 22 December 1964, when the car overturned and she hit her head against the roof and was also struck on the back of the neck by a suitcase. She was not unconscious but experienced severe pain in

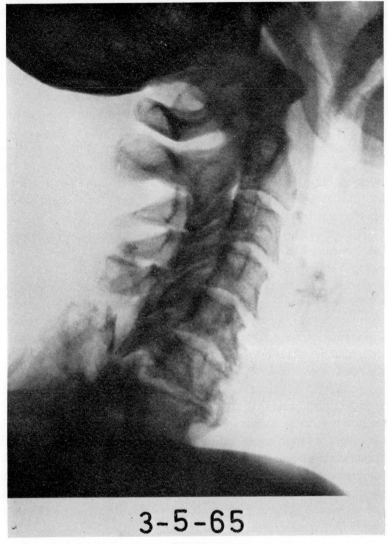

3-5-65

FIG. 83.

the neck, shoulders and arms, especially on the right. She was not paralysed and could walk with help to a car which took her to the nearest hospital where she was detained for 2 weeks, then mobilized for 2 days before being discharged. A week later she returned to England, still walking but still complaining about pain. After she returned home she was seen by an orthopaedic surgeon on 18 January 1965, who found a partial dislocation of the 6th cervical vertebra onto the 7th. There were only minimal and indeed indefinite signs of a cord involvement diagnosed by some weakness in the legs and some sensory impairment. There was no disturbance of bladder and bowel functions of any kind. The X-ray showed only a very slight dislocation of the spine between the 6th and 7th cervical vertebrae and cervical spondylosis (Fig. 83). The surgeon felt that the vertebral injury was unstable and 'potentially' dangerous and advised an operation to fix the broken spine, which was carried out on 21 January 1965 with bone chips taken from the right hip and fixation of the spine by wiring between the 5th and 7th spinous cervical processus. When the patient came round from the anaesthesia she could not move her arms being unable to ring the bell to call the nursing staff and she was generally pretty ill. On the third day after the operation a complete tetraplegia was diagnosed. Although a lumbar puncture did not reveal any sign of a compression a second operation was performed, the wire and bone grafts were removed and the dura opened, but neither haemorrhage nor a compression of the cord was found. The bone chips were reinserted but no fixation by wiring was possible. In due course, following admission to Stoke Mandeville, the patient made a good recovery as far as the function of the upper limbs was concerned, in spite of the fact that the dislocation had recurred, but she is still paralysed in both lower limbs and confined to a wheelchair for the rest of her life.

Munro (1965) reported 28 cases admitted to his department at the Boston City Hospital who, all but one, had been grafted or splinted internally elsewhere. These cases were referred to Munro because of disabling symptoms after these operations. Fourteen bone grafts, 6 wirings, 2 sets of steel screws and one metal plate were removed and this was followed by relief of the symptomatology. Of the bone grafts, eight were united, one was fractured, one was degenerated, two had developed osteomyelitis and one osteoma. Three patients had multiple bone fusions and one multiple wirings. One case was grafted, wired, plated and fastened with metal screws. Munro summed up his views on fusion-therapy as follows:

'Any physician or surgeon who advocates fusion-type therapy for fractures and dislocations of the spine must first ask himself and then answer the following question: Is it good surgical practice to reduce a fracture before fusing or splinting it? If the answer is "Yes", then neither fusion nor splinting of spinal fractures or dislocations until after a period of traction has been employed to make such a reduction. The corollary to this is that the only possible use for fusion is for maintenance, which in turn limits its use, if otherwise suitable to no earlier a period after the injury than one year, and restricts it as therapy to specific, demonstrable, otherwise incorrectable problems inherent in maintenance.

'If the answer is "No" the surgeon thereby goes on record as disagreeing with virtually everybody else's opinion and perpetuates a deformity. He must, therefore, hold himself responsible for any future disability despite any specious arguments or reasons to the contrary.' I entirely agree with the views of Munro, who in the U.S.A. certainly had the greatest experience in the treatment and rehabilitation of traumatic paraplegics and tetraplegics, and McSweeney (1969) an experienced orthopaedic surgeon, also condemned indiscriminate fusion of the cervical spine in the acute phase.

SURGICAL PROCEDURES IN LATER STAGES

The indications for late surgery on the spine and spinal cord following closed spinal injuries are:

1 Persistent or recurring instability of the spine.
2 Restitution of neural function.
3 Treatment of spasticity and contractures.
4 Treatment of pain.

In the following, only items 1 and 2 are discussed as 3 and 4 are dealt with in the respective chapters.

(1) As mentioned before, there are only selected cases where, following conservative treatment of fractures and/or dislocations, late instability of the spine persists or may recur. Although in the majority of these cases stability will be restored eventually by continuing conservative methods, in those cases where neurological symptoms develop or existing symptoms progress the risk of performing stabilizing operations is certainly justified, provided the patients with incomplete lesions are properly informed about the risks. The type of procedures naturally varies according to the type of pathology and the experience and skill of the surgeon.

(2) Laminectomy has been repeatedly performed in both complete and incomplete lesions in later stages in an attempt to restore or improve neural functions. In view of the unsatisfactory results obtained during the Second World War (MacCravey, 1945; Cutler, 1945) the American Army surgeons were instructed to abstain from performing late laminectomies for restoring neural functions. Moreover, there is the danger of increasing the existing deformity or producing instability of the spine as the result of laminectomy.

In incomplete transverse lesions of the cord or cauda equina indiscriminate or routine laminectomy should be condemned. This applies, in particular, to those cases who show spontaneous recovery of neurological symptoms. The demonstration of displacement of bone into the spinal canal (see Fig. 54) or partial or complete suparachnoidal block, as suggested by Haynes (1946) and other surgeons, is in itself no indication for laminectomy as long as there is progressive improvement of the neurological sumptoms. It is in the patient's vital interest to wait at least until the clinical improvement stops. It cannot be emphasized too strongly that the longer one observes such patients and provides them with a fair chance of adequate management, the less one will take the great risk of interfering with the natural forces of repair and healing.

There is general agreement that in progressive increase of the neurological symptomatology a laminectomy may be indicated. The causes of such deterioration can be excessive callous formation at the site of the fracture, osteomyelitis resulting in pachymeningitis, chronic posttraumatic arachnoiditis or muscular thrombosis. Riddoch (1941), Munro (1945), Scarf & Pool (1946) reported satisfactory results of laminectomy in cases with posttraumatic chronic arachnoiditis. On the other hand, Foerster (1929) and other surgeons, including myself, were not impressed with the *late* results of myelolysis in posttraumatic arachnoiditis. Street (1968) also reported only temporary improvement following myelolysis. The irreversible damage of the cord leading to myelopathy is, as a rule, due to progressive changes in the vascular supply of the cord. However, in recent years, Landau, Campbell & Ransohoff (1967) reported a group of 9 patients with incomplete traumatic conus–cauda equina lesions in whom decompressive laminectomy with or without neurolysis of extradural and intradural adhesions was carried out. The interval between injury and surgery ranged from one month to 17 years. There was postoperative improvement in all cases and in 7 the functional recovery was reported as significant.

Conclusions

1   Conservative treatment of postural reduction, as described in this book, has proved to be the safest method in the immediate management of complete and incomplete lesions of the spinal cord and its roots following fractures and fracture-dislocations of the spine.

2   Fractures and fracture-dislocations, even of the worst type, can be successfully reduced and stabilized and functional recovery of the spinal cord and its roots achieved.

3   Conservative treatment is infinitely superior to any immediate surgical procedure in safeguarding the vascular supply of the spinal cord already affected or harmed by the local injury to the spine and spinal cord and general traumatic shock.

4   Indiscriminate exploratory and decompressive laminectomy as routine immediate management of fractures and fracture dislocations is condemned because of the great risk, in particular in incomplete lesions, of transforming these into complete ones. The number of incidents of tragic events after laminectomies are high enough to make any surgeon very circumspect before indulging in any surgical procedure apart from skull traction in injuries of the cervical spine with cord involvement, which in these cases should be the method of choice.

5   There are extremely rare indications for early surgical procedures such as laminectomies, open reduction and spinal fusions.

   There is no statistical proof that laminectomy, open reduction and stabilizing operations by metal plates, etc., or spinal fusions in complete and incomplete lesions of the spinal cord shorten the period of rehabilitation of the patient.

7   Late laminectomy to restore neurological function has proved uncertain and if at all is, as a rule, only temporary.

8   Surgeons of whatever specialty who are engaged in the immediate treatment of spinal paraplegics and tetraplegics should take full account of *all* aspects of the treatment and not merely the spine itself. This applies in particular to the care of the paralysed bladder, which by proper initial treatment—i.e. intermittent catheterization can be kept sterile in the great majority of cases.

9   The surgeon who is contemplating carrying out surgical procedures such as laminectomies or fusions in the immediate stage following spinal fractures with involvement of the spinal cord must be fully aware of the risk he is taking. In incomplete cord lesions, in particular, he should, in his own interest, explain to the patient *and* his relatives clearly and in detail the risks involved. To impress on the patient that he might regret later not having had an immediate or early operation may lead to serious consequences if the operation turned out to be a failure. See also page 155.

D · Gunshot Injuries and Stab Wounds

CHAPTER 14

GUNSHOT INJURIES OF THE SPINAL CORD

Gunshot injuries of the spinal cord are amongst the most dangerous of injuries, the more so as they are so frequently associated with penetrating injuries to other vital organs of the body, the immediate surgical treatment of which often demands priority. This applies in particular to the associate injuries of the chest and abdomen.

There are numerous excellent publications on pathophysiology and pathology of this topic from the First World War (Holmes, 1915; Souques & Mégevant, 1916; Eiselsberg 1916; Collier, 1917; Head & Riddoch, 1917–18; Marburg, 1917; Mingazzini, 1917; Marinesco, 1917; Roussy & L'Hermitte, 1918; Thorburn, 1922; Cushing, 1927; Foerster, 1929). Foerster's experience is based on 395 cases (71 per cent gunshot injuries) and he has given a comprehensive survey of the pathological changes of the spinal cord occurring in complete and incomplete lesions as a result of the various types of gunshot injuries. However, the results of both the conservative and surgical treatment obtained during the First World War and the post-war period reveal a picture of profound hopelessness. Cushing (1927), the leading neurosurgeon of the American Army in that period, very aptly summed up the generally accepted views of the high mortality rate and sad prognosis of these injured as follows: Only patients with partial cord lesions survived. The mortality rate of his own cases was 71·8 per cent, that of the operated cases 62·2 per cent. In the British Army the results were not much better, varying between 47 and 65 per cent (Vellacott & Webb-Johnson, 1919), and according to Thompson-Walter (1927) the mortality rate within 3 years was 80 per cent.

Even in the early periods of the Second World War the prognosis of gunshot injuries of the spinal cord was considered very unfavourable and many physicians and surgeons still adhered to the traditional defeatist attitude towards these unfortunate victims of war. However, in further course of the war a fundamental change at least in the early mortality rate of these patients, took place. This was due to: 1, the great advance in the treatment of traumatic shock in the front-line, in particular as a result of plasma and full blood transfusions; 2, the presence of neurosurgical teams with their special equipment to deal with emergency operations; 3, the introduction of sulfonamides and later penicillin to combat wound infection and also infection of the paralysed bladder; 4, the very early transfer of the wounded from the front to field and evacuation hospitals as well as hospitals at home (greatly helped later by air-transport); 5, last but by no means least the early admission of many patients to Spinal Injuries Centres first set up in various parts of Great Britain.

According to Matson (1948) the overall mortality rate over a 9 months period of 482 patients of the U.S. First Army who reached field and evacuation hospitals was 14·5 per cent. The mortality rate of 93 cases in one individual evacuation hospital was 16·1 per cent and of 85 cases in another was 14·1 per cent.

How greatly the immediate and early mortality rate following injuries of the spinal cord during the later stages of the Second World War decreased as a result of the introduction of a new system of treatment at the Stoke Mandeville Spinal Injuries Centre is shown by a statistic of 351 gunshot injuries admitted during the beginning of February 1944 to 1950 (Guttmann, 1953); 33 patients (9·3 per cent) died and this figure includes patients who died after discharge from the Centre, including 7 patients who died from causes unrelated to their spinal cord lesions, such as tuberculosis, empyema, cerebral haemorrhage and road accident. The corrected figure is, therefore, only 7·4 per cent. The mortality rate of an earlier statistic of 177 patients was 7·3 per cent, the corrected figure 5·6 per cent.

MECHANISM AND CLASSIFICATIONS

It must first be stressed that spinal cord lesions may not be the direct result of a gunshot injury to the cord but may occur as a result of a fall or sudden strong contraction of the back—or neck muscles. Schlagwitz (1920) reported a soldier with a gunshot injury through the heart who by violent retroflexion of head and neck at the moment of injury

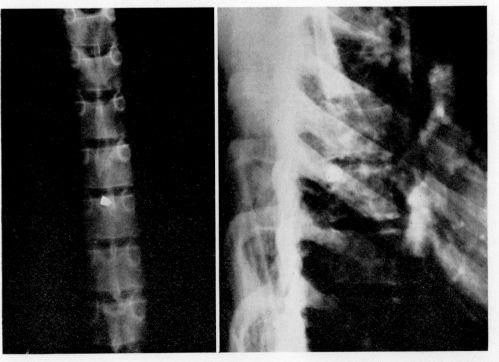

FIG. 84.

sustained a fracture of C7 vertebra. Moreover, vertebral fractures when associated with other injuries may sometimes be overlooked.

A gunshot injury not infrequently produces a complete or incomplete transverse lesion through bone fragments which are driven into the spinal canal. Frangenheim (1916) found bone fragments in 11 out of 58 operated cases following gunshot injuries, which, penetrating the dura, were driven into the spinal cord. Foerster found repeatedly large bone fragments embedded within the roots of the cauda equina. Although bone fragments lead, as a rule, to immediate damage of the spinal cord, in some rare cases they give rise to delayed damage of the spinal cord. Bergmann (1922) reported about a destruction of the 3rd to the 6th vertebral bodies of the cervical spine which, however, only 4 to 6 weeks after the injury produced the first symptoms of spinal cord involvement.

Gunshot injuries of the spinal cord and cauda equina can be classified in the following groups:

(1) *Missile penetrating the cord*

The severance of the cord or its roots may be total or partial but even in a partial severance of the cord the remaining neural elements or their vascular supply may be irreversibly damaged by the force generated from the penetrating missile although the missile itself may be small as shown in Fig. 84 of the patient referred to also in the chapter on phantom sensations.

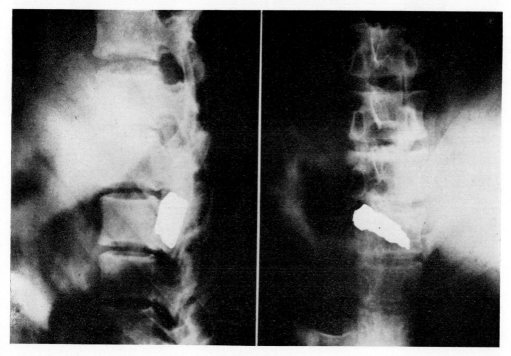

FIG. 85.

(2) *Missile lodged intramedullary*

Such injuries have been described by many surgeons and the symptomatology of the published cases varies. Although a missile of a small calibre lodged intramedullary may cause only partial lesions, larger missiles, especially grenade splinters, usually cause complete transections of the cord and at operation the two stumps of the cord are found to be separated by the missile. Figs. 85 and 86 are examples of cord transection as a result of war injury of my own patients from the Second World War. In the case shown in Fig. 85 a 4 cm long grenade splinter transected the cord at the level of T11 segment causing a complete flaccid transverse lesion below that level. On admission to Stoke Mandeville there was considerable C.S.F. discharge from the wound which was highly infected, but fortunately there were no signs of meningitis. I removed the missile immediately and the wound healed without complications. The other man was shot by a sniper and

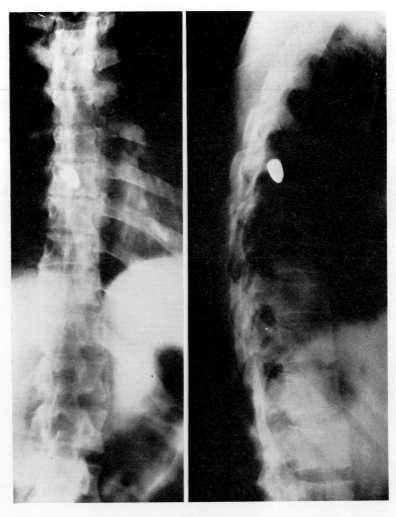

FIG. 86.

sustained a complete transection of the cord below T8. He was admitted several months after injury in a pitiful condition due to sepsis from a huge sacral bedsore which was healed at Stoke Mandeville (Fig. 86). The man made a good rehabilitation but died 10 years later from renal deficiency resulting from ascending infection following supra-pubic cystotomy.

(3) *Missile lodged extramedullary but intradurally*

In this group there is a greater possibility of incomplete cord lesions and immediate removal of the missile may result in more or less improvement of the neurological symptoms (Jourdan, 1915; Marburg & Ranzi, 1917; Foerster, 1929). However, the immediate

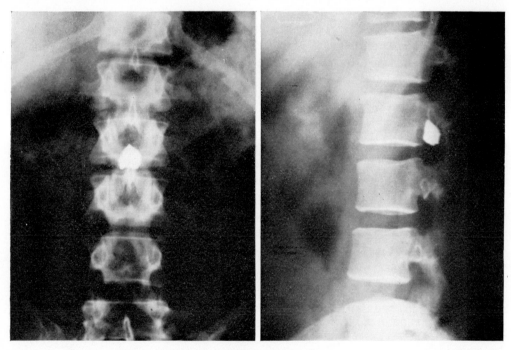

FIG. 87.

removal of the missile may not result in any improvement of the paraplegia as a result of the initial impact of the missile on the cord.

Missiles lodged intrathecally in the cauda equina region may produce only partial root lesion as shown in Fig. 87 of a soldier who sustained an incomplete cauda equina lesion, affecting S2–S5 spinal root. The splinter was not removed and the man has been employed full time for 30 years as a store-keeper.

Wandering of intradural but extramedullary missiles of small size from its original site toward the end of the spinal canal has been repeatedly described (Simmonds, 1915; Heineke, 1917; Selberg, 1917).

(4) *Missile lodged extradurally*

Marburg and Ranzi found this type in 9 cases of cauda equina level and in 20 cases at various levels of the cord amongst a total of 145 operated patients. This injury may occur if the missile has been fired from a great distance and lost a good deal of its power by penetrating other parts of the body.

(5) *Ricochet-injury of the spinal cord*

This type of injury occurs if the projectile hits the vertebral body, spinous or articular processes producing a fracture and injury to the cord or its roots. However, by the impact of the missile on the bone, it is deviated from its original course and ricochets towards the site of its entry into the body. A most unusual case in this respect was described by Foerster (1929). A bullet went through the teeth and mouth to the anterior surface of the cervical spine of a soldier and ricocheted from there to the mouth, was swallowed by the patient who later passed it per vias naturales. As a result of the impact of the bullet on the cervical spine the soldier sustained a tetraplegia.

(6) *Indirect cord damage following gunshot injuries to other parts of the body*

Such cord damage was observed following gunshot injuries to nerve trunks, in particular the arm plexus (Leva, 1915). Reinhardt (1915) described a case where the bullet avulsed a spinal nerve resulting in a tear of the dura and producing a traction lesion of the spinal cord involving the posterior and lateral tracts. Foerster (1929) published an interesting X-ray of a case where the bullet penetrated the thorax anteriorly and struck the 11th rib, bending the nose of the bullet which lodged on the inside of the rib about 8 cm from the spine. There was an immediate complete transverse lesion of the cord following the impact of the bullet on the rib resulting in violent tearing and traction of the rib at its articulation with the corresponding vertebra.

BLAST INJURY OF THE SPINAL CORD

In both World Wars cases of spinal cord injury following exposure to the effects of a detonating high explosives such as mine or grenade were described. Only those cases are considered who were not thrown to the ground. In the First World War Mott (1916) studied the anatomical changes of the brain and spinal cord in two cases who died a short time after a grenade explosion. He found extreme venous stasis in the small vessels of the brain and spinal cord with rupture of their wall and small perivascular haemorrhages; and Marinesco (1918) and Mairet & Durante (1919) found in their experiments in dogs and rabbits in addition to many major and small haemorrhages in internal organs, especially lungs, numerous echymoses and perivascular haemorrhages in brain and spinal cord with enormous dilatation of the lymph sheaths of the vessels. Marinesco found the haemorrhages more marked in the grey matter than in the white tracts of the spinal cord, and in agreement with Mott he also found pathological changes of the ganglion cells in the acute cases. In the Second World War Zuckerman (1940) described haemorrhages in brain and spinal cord as a result of exposure to explosions. These were confirmed by animal experiments (Whitteridge, Krahn & Zuckerman, 1942). In dis-accordance with these authors Greenfield & Russell (1963) have taken the view that blast (Vent d'obus or Vent explosiv of French authors) by itself had little effect on the brain or spinal cord and that lesions in these organs following bomb explosions were due to other factors, especially CO poisoning in the case of the brain and subluxation of the spine in the case of the spinal cord. Wolman (1967) described a case who in 1917 at Passchendale following explosion sustained a paraplegia, which, however, improved within 18 months and who died in 1960. From his histological results of the spinal cord (small cavity in C8 surrounded by dense gliosis and small areas of demyelination in the posterior and lateral tracts of C4 and T5), Wolman concluded that these pathological changes were compatible with an old contusion rather than with a direct effect of the blast.

Various theories have been advanced regarding the mechanism of blast on the spinal cord. Guillain (1920) believed on account of his experiences during the First World War that the pathological changes are the result of the sudden air pressure. Other authors compare the changes following explosion with the effects following Caisson-disease (decompression sickness). In their opinion the mechanism of blast is the development of air bubbles due to sudden reduction in atmospheric pressure followed immediately by increase of atmospheric pressure (Rothman, 1915; Chatelin, 1917; Sollier, 1918). Léri (1918), Foerster (1929) and others assume a contusional effect on the spinal cord as a result of enormous pressure with high speed, and Foerster found the anatomical changes identical with those produced by acute pressure to the cord as a result of gunshot —or blast violence. There is, however, general agreement that death occurs as a result of damage to the lungs.

INITIAL TREATMENT OF GUNSHOT INJURIES

There is general agreement of all authors that as soon as possible an adequate débride-ment of the wound should be carried out in combination with local and systemic anti-biotic therapy. This is of particular importance if the missile has first perforated the bowels before penetrating the spine and spinal cord. The wound should be excised to its depths and all tissues contaminated with pieces of clothing and other external material removed. Early laminectomy may under certain circumstances be necessary to perform a thorough and complete débridement, especially if the missile or bone splinters lying outside the dura appear to be contaminated. This is particularly necessary if the dura is found to be perforated and cerebro-spinal fluid leaks through the wound. Pro-vided that immediate systemic antibiotic therapy is employed, a laminectomy should not be hurriedly performed with inadequate equipment and personnel and the patient should be immediately evacuated as an emergency—if possible, by helicopter—to a place where satisfactory preparations for this procedure exist. The wound should be sprinkled with sulfanomide-penicillin powder but kept open before the transportation.

With regard to the indications for decompressive laminectomy in cases of gunshot injuries, there has been great controversy amongst neurosurgeons (Pool, 1945; Haynes,

1946; Matson, 1948). Matson admitted that decompression is the least urgent of reasons for early laminectomy and Haynes clearly stated that the prognostic difference between laminectomy at 48 hours and 10 days is of minimal difference although he himself was in favour of removal of bone debris and foreign bodies under 48 hours. Matson, although advocating that compression should always be relieved as soon as possible, agreed that incomplete lesions of the cord in whom the neurological deficit has increased were extremely rare during the Second World War 'which lends weight to the belief that the greater part of the physiological loss is due to damage produced at the moment of injury rather than by subsequent compression'. There is, however, general agreement that peripheral vascular collapse demands priority over any other treatment, and there is no doubt that the treatment of traumatic shock by immediate plasma and, even better, full blood transfusions has saved many lives, especially in spinal injuries associated with chest and abdominal injuries.

TREATMENT OF WOUND INFECTION

In spite of all preventive measures, as outlined above, wound infection has occurred following gunshot injuries during the Second World War although infinitely less as compared with the First World War, thanks to the introduction of sulfonamides and, especially, since the discovery of penicillin. Our very first traumatic paraplegic following gunshot injury, admitted after the opening of the Stoke Mandeville Centre on 2 February 1944, developed an epidural abscess which, however, healed after opening and penicillin

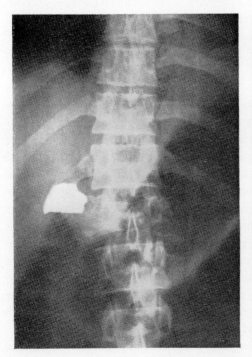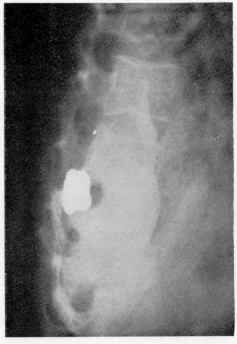

FIG. 88a.

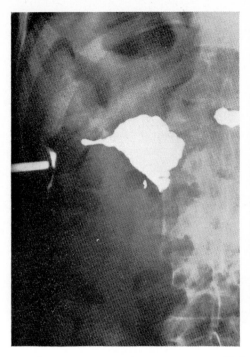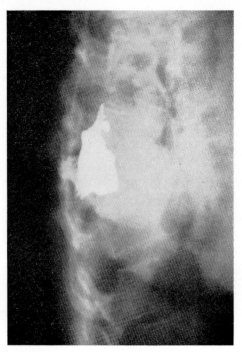

FIG. 88b.

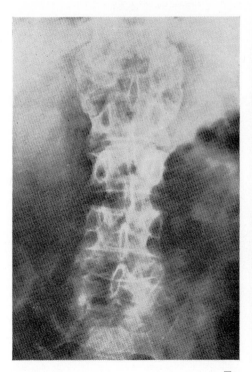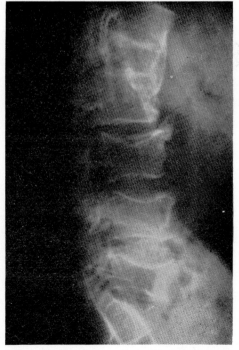

FIG. 88c.

treatment. The paraplegia below L2/3 remained unchanged but the patient made an excellent rehabilitation and was full time employed in his former job in a factory and is still alive.

Spread of the infection may lead to osteomyelitis resulting in disintegration of one or several vertebrae, as described by Frangenheim (1916), Dietlen (1920) and others in the First World War, especially following grenade injury, if the missile had not been removed. One of our own cases who sustained a complete transverse lesion below T8 following grenade injury in the Second World War developed osteomyelitis of the second lumbar vertebra with fistula formation. He was admitted and Fig. 88a shows the large grenade splinter and the osteomyelitic spine. Fig. 88b revealed, following contrast filling, the grenade splinter lying in an abscess cavity. Following removal of the missile, and evacuation of the abscess and antibiotic therapy, the fistula closed and the osteomyelitis subsided. Fig. 88c shows the final result of the healed osteomyelitis and demonstrates the osteoporosis of the vertebral column. The patient took up full-time employment and worked for many years in an office. He lives at present in Italy and returns occasionally for clinical check ups.

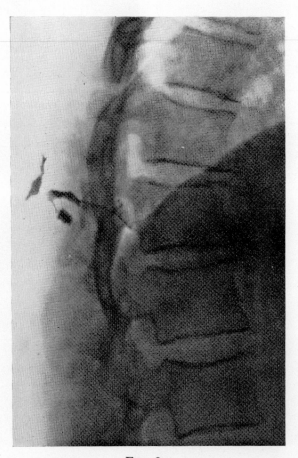

FIG. 89.

Chronic infection of a vertebra resulting in fistula formation may lead to chronic inflammatory reactions of the meninges. Fig. 89 shows the result of a contrast filling of the fistula in the case of a former naval officer who was wounded in the Second World War. There are also two fine branches of the fistula proceeding towards the 11th thoracic vertebra. At operation, following exposure of the fistula and dirty granulation of the osteomyelitic bone, I found a massive chronic pachymeningitis post-traumatica with considerable thickening of the dura. The granulations were removed as far as possible and following antibiotic therapy the fistula closed. There was no change in the incomplete transverse lesion below the mid-thoracic cord.

CHAPTER 15
STAB WOUNDS OF THE SPINAL CORD

Stab wounds of the spinal cord have been repeatedly reported in the literature (Petren, 1910; Rand & Patterson, 1929; Foerster, 1929; St John & Rand, 1943; Rosenberg, 1957; Lipschitz & Block, 1962; Lipschitz & Hagen, 1964; Lipschitz, 1967, 1971; Key & Retief, 1970). Lipschitz, neurosurgeon at Baragwanath Hospital, Johannesburg, has recently (1971) written a review about 252 cases of this type of spinal injury treated by him and his team during a period of 12 years. The fact that this hospital is situated in an area of coloured people living in South Africa under primitive and unsatisfactory social

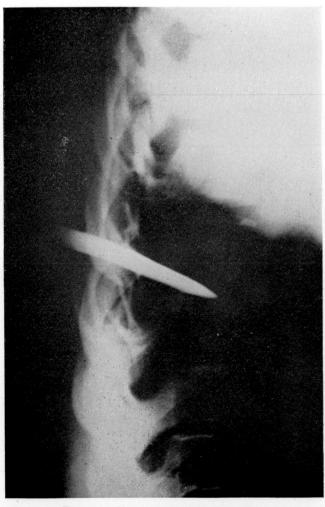

FIG. 90a. By courtesy of Dr Ailie Key.

and economic conditions and, moreover, the shortage of more sophisticated weapons amongst these people, accounts for this very large material of stab wounds. In contrast, there are only 4 cases of stab wounds in our own material over a period of 27 years— three women and one man. The latter was admitted during the war with a bayonet wound of the neck resulting in an incomplete cervical lesion from which he almost completely recovered by conservative treatment. When I visited Lipschitz's spinal unit in 1957 almost every second or third patient had a stab wound of the spinal cord but at the time of my second visit in 1970 the percentage was infinitely lower as a result of improved social and economic conditions amongst Africans. Seventy-three per cent of stab wounds affected the thoracic, 15 per cent the cervical and 8 per cent the lumbar regions. There was a discrepancy between the level of the external wound and the level of the cord injury. In only 4 per cent was there a leakage of C.S.F. through the wound. Key & Retief (1971) of the spinal unit, Cape Town, reported about 70 stab wounds amongst 300 new lesions admitted between November 1963 and January 1967 to the Spinal Unit at Conradie Hospital in Cape Town, which also reveals a high percentage of stab wounds of spinal cord injuries.

The vast majority of victims of stab wounds amongst the coloured people in South Africa are men, the age varying between 15 and 50 years. Various types of knives are

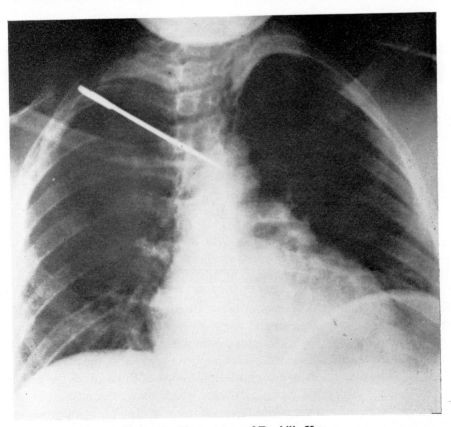

FIG. 90b. By courtesy of Dr Ailie Key.

used as weapons for attack or defence but other sharp instruments are also employed such as screwdrivers and bicycle spokes. While most of the stab wounds in Lipschitz's material are the result of generalized stabbing, in some instances they have been deliberately inflicted with great skill to the spine to produce paraplegia or tetraplegia, particularly when a gang of young detribalized Bantus, called 'zossies', the equivalent of our 'rockers' or 'greasers', wish to take revenge on an opponent (Figs. 90a and b). Stab wounds are often not confined to the spine but may injure other organs in transit, such as major vessels, the brachial plexus, trachea or oesophagus, the lung, heart, diaphragm and abdominal organs which on admission to the hospital need priority treatment to save the life of the victim. Lipschitz found 86 associated injuries in 252 stab wounds of the spinal cord.

Recently Dr Ailie Key, at my suggestion, has given a detailed statistic of 200 cases of stab injuries observed at the Cape Town Spinal Injuries Centre between 1963 and 1970, summarized in Table 2 (personal communication). There were 170 males (85 per cent) and 30 (15 per cent) females, all coloured people, the age varying between 11 and 58 years, the majority between 20–30 (73 per cent) years. The weapons used were mainly knives (188) but also axes, nails in wood, sickle, bicycle spoke, asegai, screwdrivers, wire and scissors. In the majority of cases 115 (57·5 per cent) only a single carefully placed wound was inflicted but in other victims up to 10 wounds or more occurred. In 9 cases haemopneumothorax and in one penetrating abdominal wound were associated injuries, 8 had C.S.F. leakage which stopped spontaneously in 7. One hundred and fifty-two patients were admitted by plane (86), train or ambulance within 48 hours, the majority (111) within 24 hours. The average stay in hospital was 4·75 months.

TABLE 2. Level of the lesions

Cervicals	complete	10	} 48
	incomplete	38	
Thoracic	complete	33	} 104
	incomplete	107	
Lumbar	complete	1	} 12
	incomplete	11	
Total		200	

Ninety of the 156 incomplete lesions were of Brown-Sequard type. The neurological recovery was good in 111, fair in 53 and no recovery in 34 cases. Two (1 per cent) died (1 due to septic meningitis, the blade having been missed for 2 days, 1 due to associated head injury). Twelve patients needed laminectomy for removal of the blade.

While stabbing may result in a complete transection of the cord, in the majority of cases they produce incomplete lesions, amongst which Brown-Sequard types are predominant. However, only in the minority of them is the classical hemisection of cord found, as described by Brown-Sequard.

Two of our own cases are good examples, especially the first one who appeared initially as a complete transverse lesion.

Case 1. M.G., aged 22, while returning home on 31 July 1967 from a public house where she was employed was assaulted and stabbed between the shoulder blades. She was immediately paralysed and following admission to the nearest hospital the stab wound was explored down to T4/5 laminae. She had a complete transverse lesion on the right below T6 and on the left below T11. On admission to Stoke Mandeville on 3 August 1967 she showed an incomplete transverse syndrome below T6 but complete below T8 with flaccid paraplegia of both lower limbs, and areflexia of the abdominals and both lower limbs. The sensory loss below T8 was complete without sacral sparing; bladder and bowels paralysed. Lumbar puncture on 5 August 1967 showed an incomplete block, protein 200 mg per cent 1·2 ml red cells, 360 polymorphs and 220 lymphocytes, bacteriological examination was negative. Haemoglobin 52 per cent. Following blood transfusions her general condition greatly improved and on 15 August 1967, 16 days after injury she showed the first recovery of iliopsoas, hamstrings and quadriceps on the left side only, and the complete sensory loss was now complete below T10. The reflexes in the lower limbs were still absent apart from plantar flexion of the feet on plantar stimulation. In due course the function of all muscles in the left leg returned and by 30 August 1967 there was also recovery of weak function of the proximal muscles of the right leg. Knee and ankle jerks were still absent but plantar stimulation produced up-going toes and withdrawal response. Following intensive physiotherapy she started walking exercises on 5 October 1967. By that time the paresis of the lower limbs was of spastic type and knee and ankle jerks were exaggerated. At the time of discharge on 3 February 1968 she was quite independent, walking with sticks and a BK caliper on the right. The urine was sterile and some bladder control had returned.

Case 2. J.U.R., on 31 January 1966, a married woman aged 28, while in her caravan with her two small children was assaulted by being stabbed in her back with a knife. She immediately fell down and was taken to the nearest hospital where the stab wound was sutured. She was admitted to Stoke Mandeville on 2 February 1966 with an incomplete transverse spinal lesion below T10 on the right with patchy hypoalgesia below L3 and areas of hyperpathia. On the left she had a patchy sensory disturbance below T11/12 with analgesia in L5 and patchy hypoalgesia below that level. There was also impairment of postural sensibility below these levels. With regard to the motor function there was a complete paralysis of the right leg with a flicker of the adductors and hamstrings only, while on the left leg there was only a paresis of all muscles but the power in the iliopsoas, quadriceps, inner hamstrings and dorsi and plantarflexion of the feet was quite strong. The lower abdominal reflexes were absent and so were the knee and ankle jerks on the right side. Plantar stimulation was negative but on the left she had a brisk ankle jerk and a withdrawal to plantar stimulation. The knee jerk was also absent. The bladder and bowels were paralysed and the bladder was treated with intermittent catheterization. On 7 February 1966 she started spontaneous micturition which gradually improved and the urine which was at first infected became sterile. On 24 February 1966 she started getting up and taking part in all activities of the Centre. Bladder and bowel function returned to normal. The muscles of the right leg also improved in particular the proximal muscles and the plantarflexors of the feet, while the extensors still remained paralysed. Through increased spasticity in both lower limbs she developed very marked plantar-flexion contractions on the left which necessitated a lengthening of the Achilles tendon on 23 May 1966 after which her walking capabilities greatly improved and the spasticity greatly decreased. She was discharged on 30 June 1966. On 27 September 1966 and 12 May 1967 check ups, bladder and bowel function were normal. Her gait was spastic but individual muscles on the left were of full power and so were the proximal muscles of the right leg, but the tibialis anterior and peronei were still paralysed. Sensation had also improved but there were still patches of analgesia and hypoalgesia below T10.

These cases show interesting symptoms of scattered injuries to the spinal cord resulting in incomplete lesions of dissociated type.

In certain patients the impact of the weapon may produce a Contre Coup action on the cord. Although the cord at the site of the impact may remain intact by the violence, the spinal cord may be pushed against the wall of the spinal canal and the clinical symptoms may be produced by the damage to the opposite side of the spinal cord.

In 4 per cent of Lipschitz's material, infection occurred either in the form of meningitis or abscess formation. Abscesses may be intra- or extradural and in some patients a chronic granuloma developed, especially when the patient was treated with antibiotics. Both abscesses and granulomas may increase in size and result in an increase of the neurological deficit. In chronic granulomas it may take weeks or even months until signs of compression become apparent.

TREATMENT OF STAB WOUNDS

The initial treatment consists of débridement of the wound and suture in combination with antibiotic treatment. The management of the paraplegia is, of course, the same as outlined in previous chapters. As the stability of the spine is, as a rule, not disturbed, early mobilization of the patient should be instituted. The indications for operations are:

1   Removal of the retained foreign bodies, such as the broken off tip of the weapon, after careful preparation of the patient.

2   Treatment of C.S.F. leakage which does not cease within 3 or 4 days. Lipschitz excised the skin and damaged muscles of the wound which were then resutured. In contrast to Rand & Patterson (1929) and St John & Rand (1953) who carried out laminectomy to reduce the compression, Lipschitz did not find this ever necessary in his own cases and feels that surgical procedure, apart from the indications mentioned above, is as unnecessary as it is hazardous.

3   If the knife, following damage to the spinal cord, has remained embedded in the vertebral body, a Brodie abscess of the vertebra may develop as the result of the broken off tip of the knife. The treatment of this abscess may take several months. The foreign body must, of course, be removed.

4   If a granuloma or late abscess produce increasing neurological symptoms, laminectomy is, of course, indicated.

E · Complications

CHAPTER 16

ASSOCIATED INJURIES

Injuries of the spinal cord, be they caused by fractures, gunshot or stab wounds, are often associated with injuries of other parts of the organism. In the author's statistic of 396 traumatic paraplegics and tetraplegics following closed injuries admitted within the first 15 days following injury, there were 113 (28·1 per cent) with major associated injuries, such as skull injuries with or without cerebral involvement, fractures of the long bones or pelvis, fractures of ribs resulting in pneumo- or haemothorax, fracture of sternum, scapula or clavicle and injuries to the internal organs (Guttmann, 1963). The following case is an example of how multiple and severe these additional injuries can be.

A man of 48 was inside a lead shot blasting machine, when the machine was inadvertently switched on. When taken out of the machine, he had the following injuries: the left arm was avulsed above the elbow and the remaining part of the left humerus was broken; there were multiple fractures of the ribs near the costal margin and laceration of face and left scapula; there was also a fracture-dislocation of the 6th cervical vertebra, resulting in a complete tetraplegia below C6. He was taken to the nearest hospital, and because of severe respiratory distress a tracheostomy was carried out immediately. A metal piece was removed from the axilla and scapular area. The wound was sutured and part of the remaining humerus was amputated. He was transferred to Stoke Mandeville Hospital on the second day after injury. In spite of these severe and multiple injuries, he did not develop a pressure sore and he was discharged to his home 18 months later.

In recent years other authors have described associated injuries to closed injury of the spinal cord (Benassy, 1968; Frankel, 1968; McSweeney, 1968; Meinecke, 1968; Silver, 1968; Tricot & Hellot, 1968). Meinecke reported on 340 associated injuries out of 595 traumatic cord lesions (57·1 per cent), of whom 42·7 per cent were skull injuries, 31·4 per cent thorax injuries and 37·7 per cent injuries to the upper and lower limbs, mainly fractures and dislocation. Harris reported on 90 associated injuries to traumatic cord lesions. On the other hand Tricot and Hallot's statistics show only 28 associated injuries amongst 250 patients with cord damage. Jacobson & Bors (1970) described 67 per cent major injuries in addition to 114 spinal cord lesions of the Vietnam War, the majority of them (43) involving the chest and 26 the abdominal organs. These figures clearly reveal the multiplicity and diversity of problems with which a spinal unit has to deal.

CHAPTER 16

TREATMENT OF ASSOCIATED INJURIES

Although it is realized that the treatment of a number of serious associated injuries will need priority and will have to be dealt with at the hospital to which the paralysed patient is admitted as a an emergency, should immediate transport to a spinal unit not be feasible, it is important that the staff of a spinal unit be acquainted with the principles of the management of the most common associated injuries.

Resuscitation

This has, of course, highest priority to get the spinal injured out of traumatic shock as quickly as possible, especially if the associated injury has resulted in considerable blood loss. Blood transfusions are the method of choice, preferably with fresh packed cells, to restore oxygen-carrying capacity. Intravenous transfusion to restore electrolyte balance should be given with great care to avoid over-transfusion, especially in high thoracic and cervical lesions where the vasomotor control is abolished and the danger of developing oedema of the lung is, therefore, increased. Dialysis procedures have to be considered in cases with anuria which cannot be overcome quickly.

Fractures of long bones

The immediate conservative correction of uncomplicated fractures of long bones in the paralysed area does not differ from that discussed in the chapter on pathological fractures. The author agrees with McSweeney (1968) to delay surgery for fracture of the long bones for at least 3–4 days until the patient's general condition is satisfactory and his vasomotor control has recovered. In our experience throughout the years, fractures which virtually never needed surgery were fractures of the scapula, clavicle, ribs, pelvis, calcaneus and comminuted fractures near the end of long bones unless they produced gross deformity. On the other hand, fractures of long bones in the paralysed limbs resulting in multiple fragmentation or accompanied by pressure on larger vessels, fractures which are not reducible due to inter-position of muscles, unstable fractures of ulna and radius and certain avulsion injuries of patella or olecranon certainly need surgical correction including plating and nailing (Meinecke et al., 1967). Tricot & Hallot (1968) favour early osteosynthesis in fractures of lower limbs.

Abdominal injuries

The absence of bowel sounds, which occurs frequently in complete closed cervical injuries, resulting in meteorism is certainly not an indication for immediate laparatomy. Its management, including treatment of stress gastric and duodenal ulcers, has been discussed in the chapter on intestinal function. Unlike gunshot and stab injuries of the abdominal organs, associated injuries of internal organs to spinal fractures are rare. Meinecke (1968) reported an unusual case of complete paraplegia due to fracture of L2 and L5 vertebrae with multiple associated injuries, who, on admission, was severely shocked. An X-ray showed signs of abdominal complications as a result of a rupture of the diaphragm. At operation 2 hours after admission an 18 cm tear in the diaphragm was found through which stomach, spleen, transverse colon and greater omentum had moved into the thoracic cavity. The entrails were replaced and the rupture of the diaphragm closed. Postoperatively the patient developed haemothorax but recovered and made a good rehabilitation.

Chest injuries

These are relatively frequent, especially associated to thoracic spinal fractures, consisting in fracture of ribs, sternum, haemothorax, pneumothorax and contusion of the lung, heart or aorta. Frankel (1968) mentioned a case of delayed rupture of the aorta who lived for several days after his accident. The treatment of fractured ribs has been greatly facilitated since the introduction of the Stoke Mandeville–Egerton turning bed, especially in cases with multiple rib fractures associated with a sternal fracture resulting in 'flail' chest. The serious complications of rib fractures are haemo- and pneumothorax. Haemothorax may develop gradually and is signified clinically by increasing dyspnoea, and an X-ray will clarify the diagnosis. In our experience, repeated aspiration with a wide bore needle has, usually, proved an adequate treatment. The diagnosis of a pneumothorax is readily diagnosed by X-ray, and should be treated immediately by an intercostal drainage tube connected to an underwater seal. Some of our patients with injuries of the thoracic spine associated with rib fractures were suffering from chronic bronchitis before the accident and, of course, are in danger of lung complication. They have to be watched carefully and, if necessary, a temporary tracheostomy may become a life-saving measure.

Head injuries

Cerebral concussion is a frequent associated injury to many spinal injuries at any level. Harris (1966) found 31 head or facio-maxillary injuries in 43 cervical cord injuries. Cerebral concussion will usually clear up by conservative management in time, varying from a few hours to several days followed by a state of confusion. Harris suggested that the echo encephalography can be helpful in the diagnosis of acute intracranial haematoma. Compound fractures of the skull have to be dealt with immediately. Another indication for surgery in associated head injury can be rhinorroea of cerebral fluid as a result of a fracture of the frontal sinus, if this does not cease spontaneously and an X-ray of the skull reveals a pneumocephalus (Guttmann, 1936).

CHAPTER 17

VENOUS THROMBOSIS AND PULMONARY EMBOLISM

Incidence

Pulmonary embolism has become an increasingly major cause of death following severe injuries and major surgical procedures. According to the Registrar General's Report for England and Wales (Department of Health and Social Services, 1970) there has been a sixfold increase in mortality due to pulmonary embolism during the period 1943–70. Sevitt & Galagher (1959) reported that 65 per cent of patients following major surgery developed deep vein thrombosis and 20 per cent of them had pulmonary emboli, of which four-fifths were of major degree. Earlier, Murley (1950) studying 1,763 surgical cases found the overall incidence of fatal pulmonary embolism to be 1·11 per cent but the incidence of non-fatal embolism five to six times greater. Moreover, the introduction of the fibrin-uptake test (FUT) with ^{125}I-fibrinogen revealed a very high rate of deep-vein thrombosis in immobilized patients, as reported 30 per cent by Kakkar (1970) and 41 per cent by Williams (1970) in general surgery, in 50 per cent by Mayo (1971) in urological surgery, in 54 per cent by Field (1972) in orthopaedic surgery, and in 18 per cent by Friend (1972) in gynaecology.

Deep venous thrombosis and pulmonary embolism also represent two of the most serious complications in traumatic paraplegia and tetraplegia, especially in the acute and early stages following injury.

In 1963, the writer found an overall death rate of 9 (2·27 per cent) from pulmonary embolism in 396 patients admitted to Stoke Mandeville within the first 15 days of injury during the period 1951–63. Amongst the total death rate of 30 (7·6 per cent) from all causes, the 9 patients, 4 of them cervicals, who died from pulmonary embolism represent a high percentage (30 per cent) of the total death rate (Guttmann, 1963). In this connection, a statistic of Tribe (1963) of 150 post-mortem examinations performed at Stoke Mandeville Hospital on patients of the National Spinal Injuries Centre from 1945–62 may be mentioned. Death within two months of injury occurred in 16 patients, of whom six (37·5 per cent) died from pulmonary embolism within 4–18 days after injury. With the exception of one—an elderly lady with an incomplete lesion of C7 and severe hypertensive heart disease—all were complete thoracic lesions between T5–T10 levels. One, (T10), died six days post-operatively following open reduction and fixation of the spine with metal plates carried out elsewhere, three had haemothorax and two associated fractures of the thoracic cage. The site of the venous thrombosis in five were the legs, in one the pelvic veins. No pulmonary emboli occurred in any of the chronic patients.

Since these reports, venous thrombosis and pulmonary embolism have been subjects of considerable discussion amongst spinal specialists (Philipps, 1963; Walsh & Tribe

1965; Guttmann & Frankel, 1966; Watson, 1968, 1974; Hachen, 1974; Silver, 1974; Chahal, Rossier, Weiss, Walsh, Talbot & Frankel, 1974).

Walsh & Tribe (1965) found an overall incidence of venous thrombosis and pulmonary embolism of 13·2 per cent out of 500 patients admitted to Stoke Mandeville within 14 days of injury, of which 3 per cent were fatal within 4–85 days following injury. Watson (1968), of the Sheffield Spinal Unit, reported an overall incidence of venous thrombosis in 54 out of 431 cases (12·5 per cent) and of pulmonary embolus in 22 (5 per cent) patients of whom 7 died (1·5 per cent). In a further statistic of 234 cases during the period 1968–72, Watson (1974) found 42 cases of venous thrombosis (17 per cent) and pulmonary embolism in 24 (10 per cent) with a death rate of $2\frac{1}{2}$ per cent. He attributes this increase over his previous 10-year period to better diagnosis. Rossier (1974) found 7 deaths in 32 acute cases, 5 of them following pulmonary embolism —a very high ratio (46 per cent).

There is no doubt that venous thrombosis and pulmonary embolism are more frequent in complete lesions than in incomplete ones. The levels of the cord lesion with the highest incidence are the thoracic and cervical areas, and death from pulmonary embolisms is highest in the cervicals. Males were more affected than the females. The site of the thrombosis were the legs, especially the left (Philipps, 1963; Watson, 1974), but in some cases of embolism pelvic vein thrombosis was found. The incidence of pulmonary embolism varied in individual years, but in one particular year it was as high as 25 per cent (Walsh & Tribe, 1965). This was confirmed by Watson (1968), and 1965 was the year with the highest incidence of both venous thrombosis (25 per cent) and pulmonary embolism (5 per cent) as well as of death (9 per cent).

In the majority of the acute and early stages, the first 2 months are the critical periods, in particular the first 2–3 weeks. The age group mainly affected by death as a result of embolism are patients between 40 and 65 years of age, although thrombosis and embolism may occur at any age except in children and very young adults.

The incidence of thrombosis and embolism may vary in individual countries and races. Chahal (1974) had only 4 cases of deep-vein thrombosis in 200 patients within the last three years, none of whom died, and Rossier (1974) found the ratio of deep-vein thrombosis during his first 14 months in his Unit in U.S.A. to be much lower than he had experienced in Geneva. Pool (1974), during 9 years in Indonesia, never saw thrombosis of the legs. This considerable difference in the incidence of deep-vein thrombosis and pulmonary embolism in traumatic paraplegics and tetraplegics needs further systematic study, and it will be seen whether this difference is due to inadequate diagnosis, diet, environment, climate (hot and humid temperature) or racial differences.

Pathology and pathogenesis

Deep-vein thrombi form more commonly in calf veins than in thigh veins, at first as small nidi in valve pockets, saccules or at vein junctions, and grow by an additional process of repeated deposition of thrombus-coagulum from the flowing blood, and thus layered structures of platelet-fibrin units are formed. Growth occurs from the original site of the thombus in forward direction, but after venous blockage it may progress in retrograde extension. According to Sevitt's studies (1975), most recent thrombi have two main regions: (1) red areas restricted distally to the venous valve pocket by the vein wall and dominated by red cells with fibrin lamina and (2) larger white regions characterized by platelet-fibrin units, often covered by the red areas. As intimal damage was found to be absent, Sevitt concluded that the nidi are formed on normal epithelium. A few pockets contained tiny circumscribed platelet clumps or masses of deposited leucocytes. In connection with these studies, MacLachlin (1951) may be mentioned, who demonstrated phlebographically that the stagnation of blood occurs in the soleal sinuses, and Philipps (1936) found phlebographic absence of the soleal sign in 28 out of 34 flaccid paraplegic limbs. Gibbs (1957) found in autopsy studies that the same sinuses were the principal site of venous thrombosis.

Several factors are to be considered in the pathogenesis of deep-venous thrombosis. There is general agreement that the most important factor is the stagnation of blood flow, which in the acute state of traumatic paraplegia and tetraplegia is caused by the sluggish venous stream as a result of loss of tone in the tissues of the paralysed limbs during the stage of spinal shock, probably intensified at first by the traumatic shock. This results in a weakening or absence of the calf muscle pump (Dodd & Cockett, 1956). Although Whitteridge (1957), investigating the cardiovascular disturbances in paraplegics, has shown that there is still a significant arterial, capillary and venous tone, this remaining tone in the smooth muscles is obviously not sufficient to compensate for the loss of the muscular tone and the absent muscle pump. Prolonged immobilization of the paralysed limbs and the effect of gravity greatly contributes to sluggish venous stream. Watkin et al. (1948) concluded from their studies on the effect of electrical muscular stimulation in normal and paralysed lower limbs that the blood flow increased by 100 per cent in normal and spastic limbs, but they found no increase in limb blood flow in flaccid paraplegia. This conclusion, however, needs re-investigation, as it is in some discord with findings on the effect of electrical stimulation of denervated flaccid muscles following peripheral nerve lesions, as described by Gutmann & Guttmann (1944), who found in their animal experiments distinct beneficial effects of electrical exercise on the denervated muscles as compared with the untreated ones, which they ascribed to better metabolic conditions of the exercised muscles through improved blood circulation. Jackson (1945) confirmed these results in peripheral nerve lesions in man. Watkins et al.'s negative results may have been due to insufficient electrical stimulation of the flaccid muscles.

Tetraplegics, in addition to their profound loss of vaso-motor control resulting in sluggish venous stream, also have a flaccid paralysis of their intercostal and abdominal muscles in the acute stages following injury and consequently a greatly diminished negative intrathoracic pressure which normally aids venous flow to the heart. Therefore, the negative suction force is diminished.

As in other severe injuries, thrombokinase (Rowdon Foot, 1960) may be released, especially in traumatic spinal paraplegics with associated injuries, which facilitates local clotting.

Diagnostic methods

It is generally accepted that thrombi may be present without clinical signs. On the other hand, clinical evidence of a thrombus is not always supported by objective signs. This applies in paraplegics and tetraplegics to oedema of the feet due to posture. The technical diagnostic methods which in recent years have proved of significance in the early diagnosis of deep venous thrombosis are as follows:

Phlebography has already been mentioned and, no doubt, allows accurate diagnosis of the site of the thrombosis, as shown in Philipps' paper (1963). Hachen (1974) advocates this technique, particularly in all situations requiring enzymatic thrombolysis or thrombectomy.

Cooke and Pilcher (1974) reported a good relationship between the results of phlebography and thermography in acute DVT as there is increase in skin temperature due to inflammatory reaction round the thrombus and the increased blood flow in the skin (Provan, 1965). This has been confirmed in a comparative study of thermography and phlebography on 50 patients by Bergquist *et al.* (1975). The AGA Medical System (AGA 680) was used for thermography and the front of the thigh and the popliteal fossa and calf were studied in all cases and a diagnostic agreement was found in 92·2 per cent.

Fibrinogen-uptake test (FUT) with ^{125}I-fibrinogen is important for early detection of venous obstruction in the calf. After previous blocking of the thyroid with potassium iodide, 100 microli of the radio-pharmaceutical are injected intravenously and a Pitman 235 isotope-localization monitor is used to identify the thrombus. According to Hachen (1974), recordings are usually first made after 24 hours and then daily for a week which provides information of daily changes in the size of the thrombus.

Ultrasound-flow detection is mainly used in screening for femoral thrombosis and results can be read within 3 minutes. However, as the vessels must be blocked by at least 50 per cent this test has its limitation in the detection of the thrombus.

Premonitory signs

The most significant sign of deep venous thrombosis is swelling of the leg, not infrequently combined with low grade temperature. However, in paraplegics this swelling of the leg may be obscured by postural oedema, and the low grade temperature may be mistaken as being caused by active urinary infection. The diagnosis of deep venous thrombosis can be made if by changing the position of the patient the swelling does not soon disappear whether or not raised temperature is present.

However in pulomonary embolism any premonitory sign may be completely absent and the following case is a typical example. It is described in detail as the patient recovered and showed most interesting symptoms during recovery:

C.H., aged 43, was admitted to Stoke Mandeville on 6 August 1958 with a complete tetraplegia below C7/8 following fracture-dislocation below C6/7 sustained on 2 August 1958. He was treated with skull traction and intermittent catheterization and the urine was kept sterile. On 14 September 1958 (43 days after injury) at 9.50 a.m., when treated by a physiotherapist moving his left leg, he suddenly felt 'queer', grew pale and became unconscious. He was seen 1 minute later by Dr Michaelis who found him unconscious with eyes widely opened, slight rotatory nystagmus, pulse very weak and irregular, Cheyne-Stokes breathing, upper chest cyanotic. When I saw the patient 10 minutes later (10 a.m.) he was pulseless, no nystagmus, corneal reflexes absent, respiration stopped. Oxygen and artificial respiration had been started almost immediately and coramin injections were given intravenously and intramuscular.

At 1010: Slow return of colour and irregular pulse. Still deeply unconscious.

1015: Pulse 80, regular, B.P. 130/45, respiration improving, unconsciousness less deep, corneal reflexes weakly positive.

1030: Responding to calling his name, moaning. Oxygen and artificial respiration continued.

1035: Says he 'is feeling not too bad' but cannot see or recognize anybody.

1054: Clearer. Can now distinguish torchlight flashed in front of eyes.

1100: Can distinguish finger movements, speaking coherently.

1105–15: Can recognize light of matches and torch but no objects.

1120: Says he does not know 'what all this is about'.

1125: Saw a match being moved, but no shape; becomes emotional and cries. After a few minutes: 'what made me cry then?'

1135: Recognizes objects, shape and colour (banana, pen, glass, matchbox and flowers with colours).

1145: Holding normal conversation but vision slightly blurred.

1155: Movement in hands and fingers returned as have reflexes and spasms in legs.

It is assumed that in this case a small pulmonary embolism elicited a profound cardio-vascular reflex-response leading to prolonged spasm in the posterior cerebri arteries resulting in blindness. The gradual return of vision with later return of colour vision is indicative of a temporary lesion of the calcarina-posterior lobe area.

This man was discharged home on 19 November 1959 having recovered finger muscles on his right hand. He is still alive and fit (last clinical check up 1974).

Watson (1974) also reported sudden death without any warning in 6 patients with embolism.

Prophylaxis and therapeutic procedures

General nursing

The prevention of pressure to the calves from prolonged recumbency, by frequent turning of the patient to lateral positions combined with elevating the foot end of the bed, is a most essential prophylactic procedure in facilitating venous return (Guttmann, 1973). Electrically controlled turning and tilting beds have proved most useful in this respect, and they greatly facilitate the work of the nursing staff. Breathing exercises should be added, in particular in cervical injuries. Moreover, regular resistance exercises with the aid of chest expanders should be started as early as possible in the absence of haemothorax and fractures of the ribs, to improve the general blood circulation and the venous return (Guttmann, 1973). Recently, Dollfus (1974) has confirmed the great value of head-down position in the Egerton-Stoke Mandeville tilting and turning bed in preventing deep venous thrombosis. He keeps the patients in head-down position at 15–20° for 7–8 weeks, and since introducing this procedure he has not observed clinically any deep-vein thrombosis amongst his paraplegics and tetraplegics. However, he combines this procedure with Calciparin therapy, which he and his colleague are now using immediately after injury.

Measures to improve the blood flow through the leg veins have not been entirely successful. Static calf compression has not been found effective in promoting venous return and preventing deep venous thrombosis. Roberts & Cotton (1975) assessed the effects produced by simulated exercise from passive flexion of the foot, using a motorized foot mover. They found that the venous flow and its pulsatility could be greatly increased. Although their subsequent clinical trials on pre-operative intermittent calf compression in patients with evidence of malignant disease showed beneficial results, this problem needs further studies. The effect of electrical stimulation on blood flow in the calf muscles during the stage of flaccidity in spinal shock and early stages following spinal injury (Watkin et al., 1948) is still uncertain.

Two drugs have been found to decrease platelet aggregation and thus to be effective in preventing DVT: Dextran-70 and recently Hydroxychloroquine sulfate. Lambie et al. (1970) found during gynaecological operations and for 3 days afterwards that dextran-70 reduced the incidence of DVT below that of a comparable group given Warfarin. Weiss (1974) confirmed this beneficial effect by a drop of DVT of 80 per cent. On the other hand, Rinney et al. (1970), administering 500 ml dextran-70 to a group of patients 4 hours before operation and repeated once within 48 hours, did not find reduction of the incidence of DVT with either a control group or a group given intensive physiotherapy.

Carter et al. (1971) found a reduction in the incidence of DVT demonstrated by phlebograms following application of Hydroxychloroquine.

As another preventive measure, blood transfusions should not be given through veins of the paralysed limbs to avoid clotting.

Benassy (1965) emphasized the danger of second transportation from one hospital to a spinal centre, without previous preventive therapy by anticoagulants. This again speaks for the need of immediate admission within the first 24 hours of traumatic paraplegics and tetraplegics to a spinal centre.

Anti-coagulants therapy

There is general agreement that any drug capable of preventing thrombus formation may lead to haemorrhagic complications if incorrectly administered (Guttmann, 1963, 1973; Harris, 1965; Olden Kott, 1966; Fean, 1968; Bell, 1968; Hachen, 1968, 1974; Smith, 1969; Silver, 1974). In this connection, it may be noted that in the event of these complications, Vitamin K in doses 5–20 mg, the antidote to the depressed clotting factors, takes some time to be effective before a protective range of at least 30 per cent has been reached.

In all acute spinal cord injuries, immediate estimation of prothrombine efficiency should be done routinely, and it is agreed that anti-coagulant therapy is most effective at 30 per cent or less of prothrombine efficiency.

The administration of oral anticoagulants as immediate, especially emergency treatment has been abandoned by many clinicians. Hachen (1971) found in acencoumarol an interval of 38 to 42 hours between the administration of its first dose and the development of presumably safe prothrombin levels. Moreover, oral coagulants have a narrow range between effective and safe dosage. Attention must also be drawn to the interference of other drugs with the action of oral anticoagulant either by inhibiting or potentiating them, as shown in a table published by Hachen (1974). Therefore, oral anticoagulants have been replaced by heparin (Heparin-Evans) injections to provide rapid therapeutic effect, either by intravenous injection of 10,000 I.U. which will last 4 hours or by intramuscular injection 7,500 K–10,000 I.U. given at the same time which will cover 8–12 hours after the effect of the intravenous dose has worn off. This treatment should be continued as maintenance dose for at least 36 hours, after which time the treatment is continued by oral Dindevan therapy.

Following the remarkable results obtained by Kakker (1972), Nicoloides (1972) and van Kroumhoven (1974) in the prevention of post-operative deep-vein thrombosis following administration of 5000 i.u. Ca-heparin (Calciparin) or Sodium-heparin (BP in Great Britain and USP in U.S.A.) 12 hours for 7 or 8 days, these drugs have also been employed in the acute stage of spinal cord injuries. Hachen (1974) made a comparative study of oral anticoagulant therapy (Sintrom)/versus low-dose subcutaneous Calciparin (10,000 i.u. 12 hourly) from the second day and continued for 3 weeks and then substituted by Sintrom, the change in medication being effected in 48 hours. He confirmed the striking effect of Calciparin injections found by the authors mentioned above. There was only 6·8 per cent deep venous thrombosis in 44 patients as compared with 21 per cent in 76 patients treated with oral anticoagulants, and no fatal pulmonary embolism as compared with 6·5 per cent in the oral coagulant group. However, Calciparin did not prevent haemorrhagic complications, although they were less (4·5 per cent) than in the oral coagulant group (5·3 per cent).

Recent trials comparing conventional anticoagulant therapy with thrombolytic agents such as streptokinase and monitoring the effects by phlebography before and after treatment are still in an experimental stage and no definite conclusions on the long-term benefit of streptokinase have been made.

Contra-indications to anticoagulant therapy

In a considerable number of traumatic paraplegics and tetraplegics who have associated injuries with profound haemorrhage, immediate anticoagulant therapy is contra-indicated. This applies, in particular, to head injuries with severe cerebral concussion and haemorrhage from ear and nose and also to patients with severe haemo- and/or pneumothorax and haemorrhage of the kidneys. Moreover, in the presence of marked haemorrhagic fluid found in the CSF on the first lumbar puncture, indicating bleeding into the subarachnoid space and/or cord itself, one will have to be very circumspect before starting immediate anticoagulants.

The presence of an acute gastric or duodenal ulcer such as stress ulcer, as we found in some of our paraplegic and especially tetraplegic patients, should also be considered as contra-indicative of anticoagulant therapy. The same applies to *active* chronic gastric and duodenal ulcers already in existence before the spinal cord injury, and careful consideration regarding immediate coagulant therapy should also be given to those patients with an anamnesis of chronic ulcers.

CHAPTER 18

RESPIRATORY DISTURBANCES

Disturbances of the ventilatory function may present most serious complications in the immediate and early stages following spinal cord injuries. This applies to three groups of patients: (1) tetraplegics who are deprived of the function of their main respiratory muscles, in particular intercostals and abdominals; (2) those patients with thoracic and lumbar lesions associated with fractures of ribs and sternum resulting in haemo- or pneumothorax; (3) patients of any level, in particular those of advanced age, who were suffering from respiratory afflictions before their spinal injuries, such as asthma, chronic bronchitis, pneumoconiosis etc. Therefore, all these patients demand the utmost vigilance of both the medical and paramedical staff day and night from the start, as ability to ventilate is greatly reduced in these patients, leading to anoxia, and obstruction in their respiratory tract may occur by aspiration of fluid or tracheal stenosis following tracheostomy. In fact, airway obstruction represents one of the main causes of early death in these patients. Therefore, repeated assessment of the patient's condition is essential. Details of clinical symptoms are given in the chapter on Clinical Symptomatology.

PATHOPHYSIOLOGICAL ASPECTS

(1) Vital capacity

Since Hutchinson (1846) studied measurement of vital capacity, this remained the standard test of pulmonary function. Sturgis *et al.* (1922), searching for a more dynamic index than vital capacity, found that maximum ventilation was achieved in the last minute of exhausting exercise, while Hermannsen (1933) postulated that the highest ventilation was achieved by maximum voluntary effort and that this far exceeded ventilation on exercise or in response to breathing CO_2. This was the start of the maximum breathing capacity test (MBC) or maximum voluntary ventilation test (MVV). Cournand *et al.* (1939) and Baldwin *et al.* (1948) found that airway obstruction reduced MVV.

Research on vital capacity in tetraplegics and paraplegics developed only in recent years. In co-operation with Gilliatt & Whitteridge, we found (1947) that, while the vital capacity in the early stages of tetraplegia was low, in later stages a patient with a complete lesion below C6 lying in supine position had a vital capacity of 2·8 litres and an inspiratory capacity of 2·2 litres, measured while sitting in a wheelchair. This was found to be sufficient to ensure adequate ventilatory function in his daily activities, including sport. In a more recent study on this subject (Guttmann & Silver, 1965), we found the vital capacity in the initial stages of tetraplegia as low as 0·3 litres (in the writer's further experience even 0·1 litre) but increased later to 1·2–3·3 litres. Cameron *et al.* (1955) studied the effect of posture on vital capacity in 11 tetraplegics and found that it was only 65 per cent of a predicted normal, when examined with the patients in supine position, but that it could be increased by strapping the patient to a tilting table and tilting his head down 15°. Conversely, vital capacity was decreased by elevating the head 15° above the horizontal. They attributed these postural effects to the paralysis of the abdominal muscles, which allowed the intestines to bulge through the flaccid abdominal wall, whereby the diaphragm assumed a lower position in the chest resulting in smaller excursions. Talbot et al. (1957) and Wingo (1957) described similar reduction in the vital capacity in tetraplegics.

Hemingway et al. (1958) found the vital capacity reduced in a group of tetraplegic patients to approximately two-thirds of normal and the maximum breathing capacity half of normal. These authors were surprised at the magnitude of ventilating capacity which these patients had retained, since they only had inspiratory muscles. Stone (1962) also found a marked reduction in vital capacity in tetraplegics ranging from 70 per cent to 25 per cent. He made more detailed studies, including determination of expiratory volumes, and found a reduced expiratory reserve volume ranging from 500 to 50 ml; furthermore the maximum voluntary ventilation (MVV) showed a consistent reduction related to the loss of expiratory muscle function, ranging from 75 per cent to about 20 per cent. The residual volume of gas remaining after forced expiration was found to be greatly increased, between 140 per cent to 200 per cent.

Grossiord et al. (1963) studied the action of the shoulder girdle and abdominal muscles during breathing in tetraplegics, using a combination of spirometry and electromyography. They confirmed that the shoulder girdle muscle contracts during expiration.

(2) Auxiliary respiratory muscles

Reflex function of intercostals. There is general agreement that the diaphragm, intercostals and abdominals are the most important respiratory muscles, and in tetraplegia sternomastoid and trapezius are the most important auxiliary respiratory muscles to assist the diaphragm in compensating for the loss of the intercostal and abdominal muscles. In a previous publication on Physiotherapy (Guttmann & Bell, 1958), I put forward the hypothesis that the paralysed intercostal muscles may participate in the act of breathing by reflex action, once they have regained their tone after the stage of spinal shock has subsided and the cord has regained its automatic function. Therefore, the problem of reflex activity of the intercostals was examined electromyographically in a comprehensive study (Guttmann & Silver, 1965) in a total of 19 patients with complete lesions between C4 and C8 following fracture dislocation of the cervical spine (17 men and 2 women). Their ages varied between 17 and 60 years. In these studies, both skin and needle electrodes were used, the latter giving more distinct details of intercostal activity during inspiration. Three groups of tetraplegics were considered:

1   Those examined during the stage of spinal shock and followed up until full reflex activity of the isolated cord developed as shown in Table 3. Figs. 91a–c of case A.P.J. (complete C4/5 lesion) demonstrate the electromyographic findings during and after the stage of spinal shock.

2   Tetraplegics with unilateral paralysis of the diaphragm in addition to the intercostal paralysis. Figs. 92a and b of case M.S.C. (complete C4 on the right, C5 on the left with additional paralysis of the right diaphragm) reveals almost no activity of the 6th right

TABLE 3. Details of four patients examined within eight days of injury

Name	Age	Lesion	Days since injury	Tendon reflexes			Plantars		Electromyography					Vital capacity (litres)
					Right	Left	Right	Left	S.M.	5	6	7	8	
G.R.M.	32	Transverse spinal cord syndrome complete below C5 due to fracture-dislocation C5/6.	3	Knee jerk	−	−	−	−	+	−	−	−	−	1·9
				Ankle jerk	−	−	−	−						
			5				−	I.S.Q.	+	+	+	−	+	1·7
			7				−	I.S.Q.	+	+	+	+	+	1·9
			12				contraction of hamstrings.		+	−	+	+	+	1·9
		Complete below C6 on the right, and C4 on the left. On screening 107 days after injury the diaphragm was contracting equally on both sides.	100	Knee jerk	+	+	↑	+	+	−	+	+	−	2
				Ankle jerk	+	+		+						
A.P.J.	24	Transverse spinal cord syndrome complete below C5 on the left C4 on the right due to fracture-dislocation C5.	1	Knee jerk	−	−	contraction of hamstrings.	−	+	−	+	+	+	1·7
				Ankle jerk	−	−		−						
			2	Knee jerk	−	−	I.S.Q.	−	+	−	−	+	−	1·7
				Ankle jerk	−	−		−						
			10	Knee jerk	−	−	↑ with flexion withdrawal of leg and thigh.	−	+	−	+++	+++	+	1·7
				Ankle jerk	+	+		+						
			15	Knee jerk	+	++	↑	++	+	−	−	+	−	1·7
				Ankle jerk	++	++		++						
			192	Knee jerk	++	++	↑	++	+	−	++	+++	++	2
				Ankle jerk	++	++		++						

J.T. 42 — Transverse spinal cord syndrome complete below C5 due to fracture-dislocation of C5/6. On screening 15 days after injury the diaphragm was contracting equally on both sides.

Case					
4	Fractures of both lower limbs made it impossible to assess the state of the tendon reflexes.	+ + +	1
29		+ −+ +	1·2
40		+ −+ ++	1·9

78 — Transverse spinal cord syndrome complete below C6.

Knee jerk	+	not obtainable	↑	++ −+ +++ ++	2·2
Ankle jerk	+	not obtainable		

M.J.H.O. 18 — Transverse spinal cord syndrome complete below C8 due to fracture-dislocation C6.

Case					
8	Knee jerk	+	+	↑	+ − − (+)	1
	Ankle jerk	−	−	fanning of the toes.	
17	Knee jerk	−	−	↑	+ − + +	1·4
	Ankle jerk	+	+		
21	Knee jerk	−	−	↑ flexion with- drawal of whole limb.	+ − + +	1·4
	Ankle jerk	++	++		
197		Spastic	↑	+ ++ +	3·3

− No activity.
(+) Slight irregular activity.
+ Definite activity.
++ Marked activity.

intercostal space as compared with the left but definitely increased activity 20 days later during recovery of the right diaphragm (Fig. 92b). Fig. 93 shows reduced activity in 7 R.I.S. as compared with L.I.S. $1\frac{1}{2}$ months after complete lesion below C5. There was greatly reduced function of the right diaphragm.

3   Patients studied in later stages only—i.e. 3 months or more after injury. In Fig. 94 of case R.H. (complete lesion below C6 $10\frac{1}{2}$ months after injury) the electromyogram shows marked activity of the sternomastoid and also of the 3rd, 6th and 8th intercostal spaces, and Fig. 95 case J.H. (10 months after complete lesion below C6) shows activity during inspiration over the 3rd and 5th interspaces as well as the abdominal muscles but much more marked expiratory rhythm in the intercostal spaces.

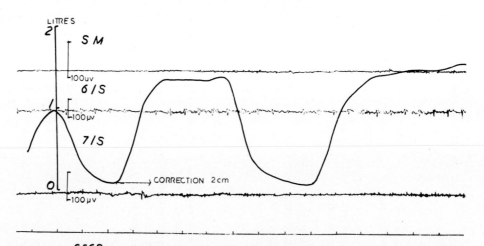

FIG. 91a. A.P.J. 1 day after complete lesion below C4(r), C5(1). S.M.: Sternomastoid; 6/IS: 6th intercostal space; 7/IS: 7th intercostal space. Little irregular activity in all three leads during inspiration. Figs. 91–97 from Guttmann and Silver, 1965 (*Paraplegia*, **3**, 1–22).

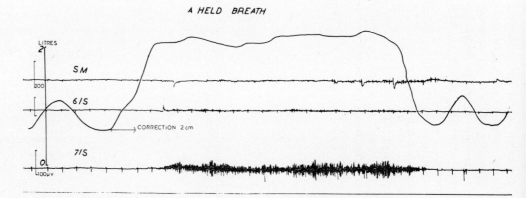

FIG. 91b. A.P.J. 10 days after injury. Increase in the activity in 6th and especially 7th interspaces.

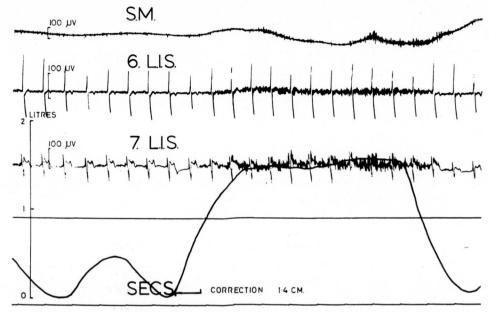

FIG. 91c. A.P.J. 192 days after injury. Further increase in the activity of 6th and 7th intercostal spaces. Activity is elicited by a breath of less than 0·5 litre, which in the previous figures did not produce any activity.

The outstanding feature of the results obtained was the difference in the response of intercostal activity to the stimulus of breathing between the immediate and later stages of traumatic paraplegia. During spinal shock, it was difficult to record action potentials

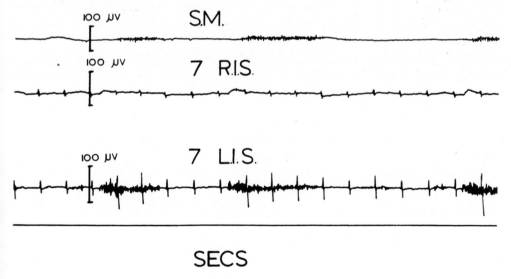

FIG. 92a. M.S.C. 5 days after complete lesion below C4 on right and C5 on left. Screening showed paralysis of right diaphragm. Almost no activity in 6 R.I.S. as compared with good activity of 6 L.I.S.

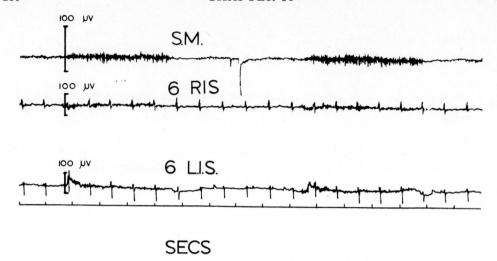

FIG. 92b. M.S.C. 20 days after injury, no apparent difference between right and left side. Right diaphragm recovering.

from the intercostal muscle to the act of respiration. They were of small amplitude and duration and consisted in irregular bursts to maximal inspiration only; moreover, they were only found anteriorly in the 6th, 7th and 8th intercostal spaces. It is likely that the complete lack of action potentials above the 6th intercostal space is due to the greater thickness of the tissues overlying the upper part of the chest. It is known that such electrical inactivity in the upper chest also occurs in normal subjects. Conversely, Campbell (1958) found that in normal females following radical mastectomy including removal of the pectoral muscles, and also in dyspnoic patients with very thin chest walls, the pattern of electrical activity of the intercostal muscles in both upper and lower intercostal spaces was essentially similar. Once the full reflex activity of the isolated cord developed, the increase of the electrical response of the intercostals to inspiration was very conspicuous. The amplitude of the action potentials was larger and they could

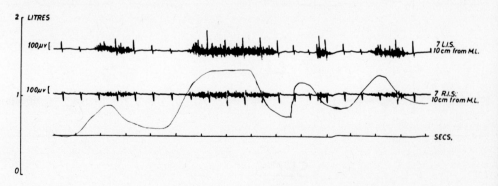

FIG. 93. I.C. 1½ months after complete lesion below C5. Reduced activity in 7 R.I.S. compared with 7 L.I.S. Screening showed greatly reduced function of right diaphragm.

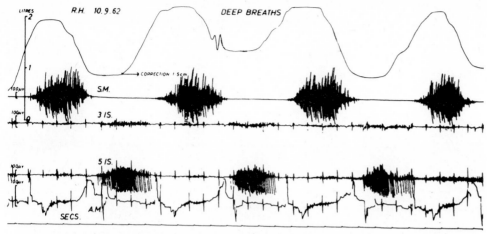

FIG. 94. R.H. 10 months after complete lesion below C6. Activity present during inspiration in 3rd and 5th interspaces and in abdominal muscles, but much more marked separate expiratory rhythm in the intercostal spaces.

be elicited by smaller inspiratory impulses. Moreover, they were detected over a much larger area, as high as the 2nd and 3rd intercostal spaces.

The act of breathing is as much an appropriate afferent stimulus to the intercostals and abdominals evoking a stretch reflex as the distension of the muscular wall of the bladder and bowels or a stroke to the plantar surface of the sole of the foot. During the stages of heightened reflex activity of the isolated cord, an afferent stimulus as distant as that produced by plantar stimulation may elicit contractions in the intercostals in these high lesions. Conversely, a deep breath may evoke flexor or extensor spasms of the legs (Fig. 96).

It was found that the reflex activity of the intercostals showed a rhythm pattern in close relationship to the act of breathing; it commenced in either mid or late inspiration and lasted until early expiration. In two subjects, a separate expiratory rhythm was

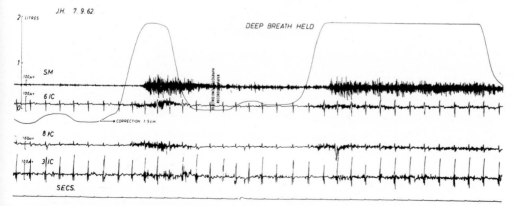

FIG. 95. J.H. 10½ months after complete lesion below C6. The activity in 3rd, 6th and 8th interspaces is identical in timing and increases progressively in amplitude.

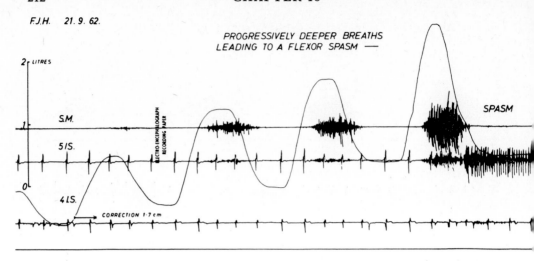

FIG. 96. F.J.H. 4 years after complete lesion below C6. No activity in 5th interspace with breath less than 1 litre. With progressively larger breath there was progressive activity until with the largest breath a flexor spasm of legs developed. Spasm also seen in 4th I.S. which until then had been silent.

detectable. The respiratory rhythm in cervical cord lesions below C5 was maintained in the early stages of tetraplegia almost entirely by the excursion of the diaphragm, which is the principal contributor to the force of inspiration. On descending during inspiration, the diaphragm separates passively the lower ribs on account of its anatomical attachment, thus causing a stretch effect on the intercostal muscles which acts as afferent stimulus of a stretch reflex. This stretch reflex increases in intensity commensurate with the subsiding of the spinal shock and the return of the reflex activity in the spinal cord. It is, therefore,

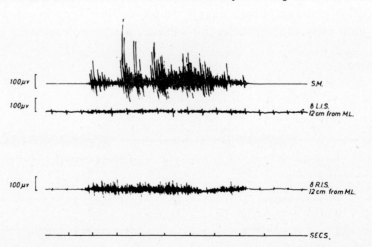

FIG. 97. B.F. 4 months after complete lesion below C3 on left and C5 on right. Diaphragm paralysed on left. The difference between the activity on 8th L.I.S. and 8th R.I.S. is very marked. However, 8 L.I.S. shows reduced activity.

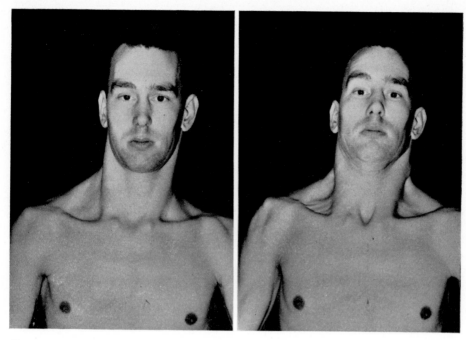

FIG. 98a. Hypertrophy of sternomastoid and trapezius in complete C4 lesion. Note elevation of shoulder and expansion of chest wall on deep inspiration.

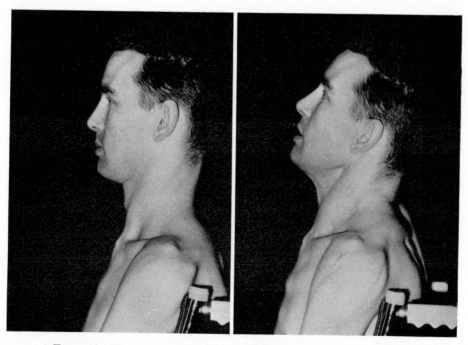

FIG. 98b. The same patient, lateral view at rest and deep inspiration.

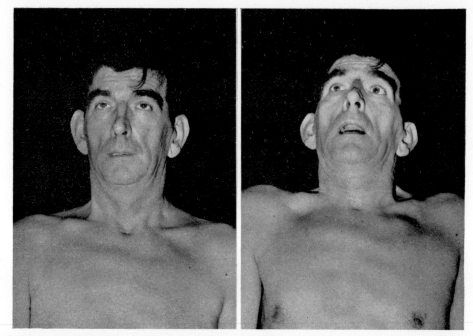

FIG. 99a. Complete lesion below C5. Hypertrophy of sternomastoid. Increase of antero-posterior diameter of the chest on deep inspiration.

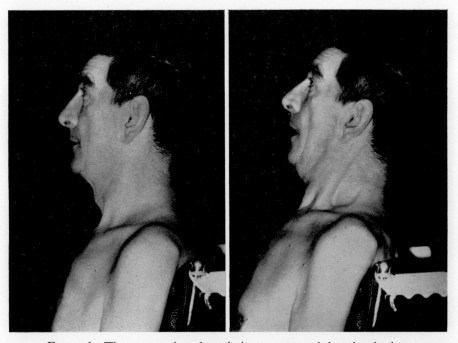

FIG. 99b. The same patient, lateral views at rest and deep inspiration.

not surprising that in a case of unilateral paralysis or impaired diaphragmatic activity in cervical cord lesions, the reflex activity of the corresponding intercostal muscles is greatly reduced as shown in Figs. 92 and 93. However, we found that even in the presence of complete hemi-diaphragmatic paralysis the reflex activity of the intercostals is not abolished, as shown in two of our high cervical lesions. If, as shown in one case, it may at first be absent it will appear, however diminished, in due course (Fig. 97). It may be noted that in cases with unilateral diaphragmatic paralysis the rhythmic respiratory movement is maintained by the function of the diaphragm of the other side, as well as by the function of accessory respiratory muscles, in particular sternomastoid. Moreover, it is likely that the elastic expansion of the lung itself during inspiration acts as a contributory force in stretching the intercostal spaces, thus serving as an additional afferent stimulus to the reflex response of the intercostal muscles.

In the early stage of tetraplegia, the intensity of the compensatory respiratory function of the sternomastoid varies, and its development to full strength as an auxiliary force in the act of breathing, by exerting an upwards pull on the xiphosternum and thus increasing the antero-posterior diameter of the chest and the vital capacity of the lung, may take some time and systemic exercises are needed. Its auxiliary force, also assisted by the trapezius and the scaleni, can be considerable, and may help to improve the negative intrathoracic pressure which is diminished as a result of the paralysis of the intercostals in the early stages following transection. Therefore, by increasing the negative suction force the venous blood flow to the heart may be increased. By training, the sternomastoid may develop a profound hypertrophy as shown in two patients with complete lesions below C4 and C6 (Figs. 98a and b and 99a and b). My studies on the function of the sternomastoid on the upwards movement of the anterior part of the upper thorax have confirmed the findings of that great French clinical physiologist on muscle function, G.B.Duchenne (1866). Recently, Silver & Moulton (1969) using the method of Davis & Moore (1962), have amplified our findings on chest movement in detailed studies on tetraplegics.

Conclusions

Although the diaphragm is the main contributor in restoration of the vital capacity of the lungs, our findings indicate that the co-ordinated reflex function of the intercostal muscles resulting from the rhythmic movements of the chest also plays a part in the process of respiratory recovery. The intercostal muscles by regaining their tone once the spinal shock has subsided help to restore by their reflex contractions the tension and rigidity of the intercostal spaces essential for a more powerful function of the diaphragm.

Meteorism. This is the result of the paralysis of the intestines in the immediate stage following cervical injury and leads to an impairment of the function of the diaphragm and thus increases the respiratory distress, even if the segmental supply of the phrenic nerve is not involved. Therefore, immediate steps have to be taken to restore the intestinal function as quickly as possible, and injections of 0·3 to 0·5 mg Prostigmine every 4 to 5 hours have proved invaluable and even a life saving measure.

(3) Fluid balance (oedema)

As a result of the paralytic vasodilatation following the interruption of the vasoconstrictor fibres in the spinal cord, the fluid balance is disturbed, the more so as in the early days following transection of the cervical cord the renal function is slowed down resulting in oliguria and sometimes even anuria. This results in changes in the hydrostatic and colloid osmotic pressure leading to increased transudation of fluid from the intravascular into the intrastitional spaces and formation of oedema. Therefore, fluid intake has to be considered most carefully. In patients who arrived following routine administration of large intravenous isotonic saline or glucose solutions, the over-infusion resulted in pulmonary oedema, which in turn increased the hypoventilation caused by the paralysis of the intercostals and abdominal muscles in these high lesions. In those cases who died, the post mortem showed large amounts of fluid in the chest cavity indicating that these patients were drowned in their own body fluids. One man, aged 51, with a complete lesion below C4/5 received 3 litres of dextran together with adrenaline before being transferred to Stoke Mandeville. He was dead on arrival and the necropsy revealed a massive pulmonary oedema. Therefore, promoting diuresis in overhydrated tetraplegics is imperative. Intravenous urea has been used as an osmotic diuretic but in recent years mannitol solution (half a litre of 20 per cent solution) has proved the most effective measure (see also chapter on Renal Deficiency).

(4) Nutritional deficiency

Meteorism with loss or impairment of the digestive intestinal function as well as disturbances of the fluid balance may lead to nutritional deficiency, especially if the paralysis of the peristalsis in the initial stage of tetraplegia also involves the stomach resulting in acute dilatation which, in turn, increases the respiratory distress. This is indeed a very serious complication, the more so as vomiting occurs which not only may lead to depletion of electrolytes, but the danger of inhalation of vomit resulting in acute blockage of the airways leading to pulmonary collapse is great. Gastric aspiration through a nasal tube should be instituted as soon as possible and the removed gastro-intestinal secretion replaced with nutrient fluids at a rate of 40–50 ml per hour, gradually increasing the amount of fluid commensurate with the improvement of the function of the stomach. Loss of gastric hydrochloric acid may result in alkalosis and has to be treated accordingly. Failure of absorption from the small intestine as a result of the paralysis of peristalsis and associated with acidosis makes intravenous transfusion necessary, which should be continued as long as the paralysis or impairment of intestinal function persists. Amongst the administered nutrient fluids, fruit juice expressed from grapefruit and oranges rich in vitamins and mixed with glucose, have been found invaluable. Parentrovite, a concentrated B and C complex with glucose in injectable form, is recommended in these cases. Attention must be paid to the caloric requirement of these patients, and the provision of at least 1,800 to 2,000 K calories should be established. To counteract depletion of body protein, intravenous infusion of amino-acid solutions may be necessary as long as oral intake of food is not possible. Cheshire & Coats (1966), in their comprehensive paper on 'Respiratory and Metabolic Management in Acute Tetraplegia' have given a detailed description of the synthetic amino-acid composition of the two Aminofusion Solutions commonly used: Aminofusion 850 and Aminofusion forte and also of the 10–20 per cent Fructose solution combined with 4–6 per cent v/v Alcohol used for intravenous transfusions in acute tetraplegia. The repeated assessment of the electrolytes is essential. In particular, potassium deficit which delays the recovery of smooth muscle function (Marks, 1950) must be restored (see also chapter on Renal Deficiency).

(5) Airway obstruction—atelectasis

A most serious effect of the paralysis of the intercostals and abdominals is the interference with the cough reflex, as the tetraplegic is unable or has greatest difficulty to expectorate collection of sputum. It may be stressed that this is not only an immediate danger for air-way obstruction in the acute stages but also later, should the tetraplegic develop a bronchitis or other infection at any level of his respiratory tract. In the acute stages, the fluid dysbalance increases the secretion which is accumulated in the bronchioles and this is enhanced by keeping the patient in supine and head up position. The resulting obstruction of the airways leads to atelectasis. As a result the mediastinum will be pulled to the side of the collapsed lung, as shown in the X-ray, due to the difference in the intrathoracic pressure. Moreover, the diaphragm is pulled upwards, thus increasing the respiratory distress. If the bronchial obstruction can be relieved by immediate suction through an endotracheal tube, the atelectasis is reversible. It is obvious that the airways must be kept clear by assisted respiration (see chapter on Physiotherapy) and by liquifying the bronchial, tracheal and pharyngeal secretion by steam inhalation. For some time, we have been using the Marshall–Spalding blower humidifier. This apparatus, used in conjunction with a tracheostomy box, provides a steady stream of warm saturated air or oxygen thus preventing crusting in the air-ways. A dust filter is fitted at the air-intake to the blower to ensure a clean air intake by the patient. This unit can be incorporated in the East–Radcliffe Respirator which we have used at Stoke Mandeville for some years. Another humidifier is the Devill–Bliss nebulizer, marketed by the British Oxygen Company. According to Sara (1965), adequate humidification at the optimum temperature can be best achieved by nebulization of warmed water, and the Puritan nebulizer incorporating a heating coil and a thermostat has been found satisfactory and can be used in conjunction with the Bird intermittent positive pressure respirator (Cheshire, 1964; Cheshire & Coats, 1966). We have not used sodium bicarbonate or proteolytic enzymes (Taylor, 1960; Bremner, 1962), as we were satisfied with postural drainage and humidification by nebulization. A new drug with mucolytic action is Bisolvon (Bromhexine hydrochloride, Boehringer), which has proved effective in decreasing sputum viscosity, especially if signs of bronchitis are present. It can be given together with tetracycline (8 mg) as Bisolvomycin in capsules of 250 mg (Burgi, 1964; Hamilton et al., 1970).

Bronchodilator drugs can be of great relief to the patient with respiratory distress. Adrenaline, which is an effective bronchodilator, can be administered by inhalation with a nebulizer containing 1 per cent solution of adrenaline or adrenaline and atropine compound. Alternatively, the drug can be given subcutaneously of 0·1 per cent solution in doses of 0·2 ml to 0·5 ml. Isoprenaline is another drug for immediate effect, which can be given by inhalation of a nebulized solution of 1–2 per cent isoprenaline sulphate but may also be given by mouth in doses of 10–20 mg tablets which are dissolved under the tongue. However, undesirable side effects of this drug are tachycardia and dizziness. Recently, Lustman (1970) and Choo-Kang *et al.* (1970) found Salbutamol (Ventolin-A and H) more effective than Isoprenaline. The bronchodilator action of 200 mcg of Salbutamol was found to be equal in effect to 1,000 mcg of Isoprenaline without its tachycardia. Aminophylline (neutrophylline) is either administered as suppository per rectum or is most effective as intravenous infusion in doses of 250–500 mg. Finally, corticosteroid drugs (prednisone by mouth in doses of 10 mg every 6 hours) are also used but should be controlled by repeated measurements of the forced expiratory volume.

In patients with tension pneumothorax and haemopneumothorax, thoracocemtesis, which has to be repeated, especially in haemopneumothorax, is indicated and has proved a life saving procedure. The technique adopted at Stoke Mandeville for the treatment of pneumothorax is intercostal drainage connected to an underwater seal, and we found the risks of tube drainage slight. Haemothorax is usually treated by aspiration through a wide bore needle which can be repeated if necessary. This procedure was found to be a lesser risk of infection than an intercostal drain. Needle aspiration can be repeated if at the first session all blood could not be removed.

Tracheostomy—tracheal stenosis—strictures. There is no doubt that tracheostomy has proved a life saving measure, both in patients with severe head injuries and cervical injuries suffering from respiratory distress, and this applies also to thoracic lesions with associated injuries such as fractures of ribs, xiphosternum and haemopneumothorax. However, it should not be used indiscriminately, having regard to the great advances made in physiotherapy. If, in certain cases with airway obstruction, tracheal catheterization is contemplated, intubation with a naso-tracheal tube should be tried first, in the technique of which an experienced anaesthetist could be of great help. However, prolonged intubation must be avoided as it may lead to excoriation and ulceration in the cricoid region. This has been found to occur, especially in children. Fearon (1966) reported an incidence of 8 per cent in 72 children who had been intubated for more than 8 hours. Pressure sores involving the cartilage may occur within 30 hours (Hardcastle, 1966), especially through constant movement by intermittent positive pressure ventilation (IPPV) occurring between the tube and the mucosa.

There are many observations of serious risks reported following tracheostomy, the most important being the laryngeal and bronchial stenosis resulting in strictures with dense fibrosis. A variety of stenosis may occur following insertion of a non-cuffed and, in particular, a cuffed tube which has recently been reviewed by Harley (1971) who has given a classification of air-way obstruction following tracheostomy with assisted ventilation. It is true that, as a result of Jackson's work (1921, 1954), high tracheostomy has been abandoned because of the danger of producing laryngeal stenosis as a result of perichondritis and cartilage necrosis, but infracricoid and, in particular, tracheal stenosis still not infrequently occur, and many workers consider stenosis after tracheostomy and intermittent positive pressure ventilation as the commonest type (Johnston *et al.*, 1967; Cooper & Grillo, 1969; and others). The stenosis at cuff level is of circumferential type, leading to dense fibrous strictures. Tube-tip stenosis is the result of a long tracheostomy tube impinging the lower portion of the trachea. This may result in ulceration of the carina or affecting the right main bronchus leading to collapse of the right upper lobe or collapse of the left lung. The backward inclination of the trachea and the curvature of the tracheostomy tube may produce ulceration of the anterior wall and may lead to perforation of the innonimate artery (Watts, 1963), while ulceration of the posterior wall of the trachea may result in tracheo-oesophageal fistula.

It must be remembered that, in the acute stages of cervical lesions, as a result of the paralysis of the vasoconstrictors the tone of the tissues in the trachea is lowered as it is in other parts of the body, such as the urethra and bladder. Therefore, the vulnerability of the tracheal mucosa is increased, especially if an inflatable polythene-type tracheostomy tube is used which is not deflated frequently. This has the risk of damaging the mucosa and developing a pressure sore, which soon becomes infected, resulting in tracheal stenosis (Guttmann, 1970). Gibson (1967) considered over-inflation of the cuff, movement of the tracheostomy tube with each stroke of the respirator and secondary infection as the main causes of stenosis, and Bannister and Braver, 1969, blamed the relatively hard 'Portex' tracheostomy tube for this complication. Frankel (1970) described in detail 4 patients of tracheal stenosis in whom the plastic 'Portex'—cuffed tube was used in recent years, contrary to the soft rubber tubes which were used before at Stoke Mandeville with satisfactory results. Two of the patients were C5 and C6 lesions, one encephelomyelitis and one L1 fracture with associated chest injury. The patient with encephelomyelitis was operated 15 months after tracheostomy by Mr G.Grimshaw, chest surgeon in Oxford, who dissected out the dense fibrotic stricture and approximated the cut end of the trachea with interrupted sutures, but the patient died 5 days later due to rupture of the innominate artery into the trachea. In another case (C6), the excision of the stenosis one year after injury was successful. In the two remaining cases, dilatation of the stenosis proved unsuccessful and a long term use of size 34 Chevalier-Jackson had to be inserted, which in both cases was eventually successfully removed. Following these experiences, the 'Portex' tube was abandoned and only rubber cuffed tubes are used as a routine. The conservative treatment consists of repeated dilatation of the stenosis. However, this should be carried out with greatest care and gentleness, as there is the great risk of eliciting undesirable autonomic hyperreflexia leading to cardiac arrest, which will be discussed in detail in the following paragraph. How far Wolf *et al.* (1973) special method of controlled cuff filling, which allows accurate adjustment of the cuff and this avoids pressure against the tracheal wall, will prove a method of choice remains to be seen.

Surgical and mediastinal emphysema. An unusual complication following tracheostomy was found in one of our patients with a complete C4 lesion following gunshot injury. During his transfer from Aden by plane he was on positive pressure respiration. However, during the journey the tracheostomy tube became displaced

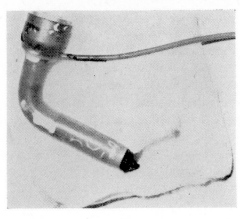

a

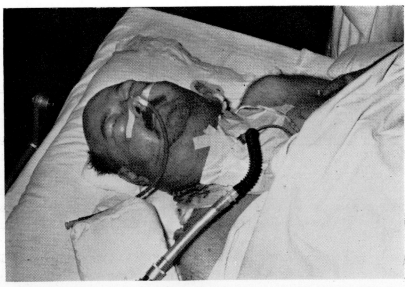

b

FIGS. 100a and b. Traumatic paraplegia below C4. Patient admitted with profound
surgical emphysema of the face due to displacement and blockage of the tracheostomy
tube. From H. Frankel, 1968 (*Paraplegia* 5, 228).

and when the patient arrived he was deeply unconscious and face and neck showed a
profound surgical emphysema, which expanded with each stroke of the respirator.
Following replacement of the tracheostomy tube, the surgical emphysema subsided
within a week. This case was described by Frankel (1968) and Figs. 100a and b shows
the patient with his surgical emphysema after his admission to Stoke Mandeville.

   Flexer (1970) and Rabuzzi & Reed (1971) described mediastinal emphysema in
children following tracheostomy in 15 per cent and 43 per cent respectively. Bergström
& Diamant (1960) performing routinely X-ray controls in tracheostomized children
found mediastinal emphysema in 25 out of 60 cases.

Pneumothorax. Although this complication and its pathogenesis has first been described by Wilks (1860), it was Neffson (1949) who found that 25 per cent of patients with unilateral and 80 per cent with bilateral pneumothorax following tracheostomy proved fatal. This was caused by a displaced tube resulting from an opening placed too low in the trachea. Reading (1958) suggested that many cases previously diagnosed as dying from broncho-pneumonia may have died from pneumothorax. Salmon (1975), in a comprehensive paper on tracheostomy, discussed the indications, techniques, including the various tubes, and complications of this procedure. He stressed that the correct site of the incision in the trachea is through the second, third and fourth rings and that to perform this operation below the fourth ring should be considered as surgical mal-practice.

Pressure and ulceration of the anterior tracheal wall. The very important danger sign of ulcerating the anterior tracheal wall, as a result of pressure from the tip of the tracheostomy tube affecting the inominate artery, is the pulsating cannula, for the pounding artery against the tube creates the fistula eventually damaging the arterial wall, resulting in late fatal haemorrhage as mentioned above. Therefore, the medical, nursing and physiotherapy staff of a spinal unit must always be alert to this most serious complication. Mathog *et al.* (1971) published a comprehensive review on this subject.

Cardio-vascular reflexes. Another serious complication in tracheostomized patients are cardio-vascular reflexes elicited by endotracheal suction and inflation of endotracheal cuffs. These have been reported by several authors as occurring in non-paraplegic patients, consisting of arrhythmias caused by suction and inflation of endotracheal cuffs (Reid & Brace, 1940), and sudden death has been reported by Davis *et al.* (1953), Nelson (1957), Green (1959), and Stephenson (1958) reviewed reports of death from cardio-vascular reflexes. Dollfus & Frankel (1965) reported these reflexes in a tracheostomised case with a complete lesion C4/6, in whom attacks of cardiac arrest were elicited by inflating the cuffed tracheostomy tube and endotracheal suction to keep the airway free. From the electrocardiographic findings, it is quite clear that before the cardiac arrest started there was a profound brachycardia identical with that observed in visceral distension and hyperactivity in other internal organs (Guttmann & Whitteridge, 1947; Guttmann, 1953–54, 1965, and others).

All this shows how circumspect one has to be when contemplating tracheostomy in spinal injured patients.

Discontinuing artificial respiration

As soon as respiratory power has improved and the vital capacity is adequate—i.e. 500–800 ml, the patient should be weaned off the respirator. He is gradually disconnected from the respirator and is encouraged to breathe spontaneously for short periods which are gradually increased without exhausting the patient. Electrical stimulation of the phrenic nerves to exercise the diaphragm may be useful and accelerate the return of spontaneous respiration but it was not found to be necessary in our patients. When the spontaneous respiration is satisfactory during most hours of the day attempts should be made to let him sleep without the respirator for a certain period of the night. During that period many patients need reassurance that they will wake up if the respiration becomes inadequate and will not die in their sleep, which is their anxiety. Sleeping tablets are, of course, contra-indicated.

The cuff of the tracheostomy tube can be permanently deflated once it is ascertained that he can swallow food by mouth easily.

Healing of the tracheostomy wound is not infrequently delayed but only in the minority of cases may surgical closure or plastic repair be necessary.

CHAPTER 19

METABOLIC DISTURBANCES OF THE
SKELETAL SYSTEM

In recent years, intensive research has been undertaken on biochemical and biophysical problems of the catabolic and anabolic phases following transection of the spinal cord. The spinal man offers, indeed, infinitely better possibilities in this respect than the spinal animal, provided there exists the closest co-operation between the clinician and biochemist and the patient is kept under scientifically comparable conditions. For a proper analysis of data, it is absolutely essential that the patient be kept on a standard diet and that in series investigations the timing of taking blood samples and the hourly or 24-hourly collection of urine be strictly observed.

Osteoporosis—'spontaneous' fractures

Bone formation and bone absorption are continuous reciprocal physiological activities throughout life, although the rates of exchange vary with age and differ in various parts of the skeleton. Bone formation consists of two processes which are under cellular control: (a) laying down of a cellular matrix (osteoid) and (b) deposit of bone salts. Bone formation is controlled by the single nuclear osteoblasts and their function is to lay down calcifiable collagen fibrils in a suitable ground substance and produce alkaline phosphatase, but the precise role of this enzyme in bone formation is still obscure. The collagen has the capacity to promote the formation of crystals on the surface of its fibrils. The bone absorption is regulated by the multinuclear giant osteoclasts. The physiology and pathology of these ground elements of the skeletal system, osteoblasts, osteoclasts, osteocytes, collagen matrix and their relationship to the calcium, phosphate and protein metabolism have been studied repeatedly in recent years (Bartelheimer, 1956, 1962; Fourman, 1960; Glinebe, 1962; Norrdin, 1962; Eger, 1962; Paeslack, 1965). Although there are still gaps in our knowledge of the complex mechanism, it is now a well-established fact that prolonged bedrest, in particular when combined with immobilization, results in changes of the mineral metabolism associated with atrophy of soft tissues, especially muscles, as well as of the skeletal system. This has been proved even in non-paralysed individuals following fractures (Howard et al., 1945; Dietrick, 1948) as well as in healthy volunteers. In spinal paraplegics this is the rule in the parts below the level of the lesion, be it complete or incomplete (Guttmann, 1953, 1971). The level of the lesion is of importance in so far as the immobility of the motor apparatus in high lesions involves larger parts of the body. Age plays a subordinate part and the writer has seen considerable degrees of osteoporosis in spinal cord paralysed young children. It is also agreed that chronic infections of the urinary tract or caused by osteomyelitis as a result of pressure sores accelerate and greatly increase osteoporosis in paraplegics and tetraplegics. Even if these complications and other factors are absent it is still a matter of

TABLE 4

Patient	Injury	Completeness	Serum alkaline phosphatase (K.A. units)		Urinary calcium mg/24 hr		Urinary hydroxyproline mg/24 hr	
			Min.	Max.	Min.	Max.	Min.	Max.
F.W.	C4, 5	C	3·6	15·8	144	276	28	158
D.W.	C4, 5	C	9·4	10·3	84	675	44	121
A.W.	C5, 6	C	3·5	12·1	112	490	21	100
J.S.	C5	C	3·7	6·4	213	486	88	144
E.W.	C6	C	3·7	6·8	160	566	25	118
J.P.	T6	C	6·7	11·8	121	666	80	180
V.G.	T6, 7, 8, 9	I	2·8	8·2	216	518	57	92
R.W.	T7	C	5·7	20·3	304	613	60	107
D.MacB.	T10	C	2·5	8·5	289	603	42	94
D.E.F.	T11, 12	C	2·7	4·8	143	302	49	58
C.M.G.	T12, L1	C	7·0	12·0	107	456	50	82

C—Complete.
I—Incomplete.

conjecture whether the osteoporosis is primarily due to diminution or inhibition of bone formation (osteoblast–osteoporosis). X-rays do not give any information about the degree of the osteoporosis in the early stage of cord lesions. However, changes of protein, especially loss of albumin, demonstrating the disturbance of the nitrogen balance, and increased calcium and hydroxyproline excretion in the urine as well as the increased serum alkaline phosphatase, indicate the processes of decomposition in bone and muscles. The increased calcium excretion is independent of the diet of the patients. In recent years, attention has been paid to hydroxyproline excretion in transverse lesions of the cord (Klein, Van den Noort & De Jak, 1966), following introduction of hydroxyproline-estimation in the urine, as an index of the collagen metabolism by Ziff *et al.* (1956) and Dull & Hinnemann (1963). Our own results (Guttmann, Edwards & Mehra, in press) from series investigations on spinal paralysed patients in the immediate and early stages following spinal injuries at various levels are in accordance with those of Klein *et al.* in so far as they show close correlation between calcium and hydroxyproline excretion, but our total values of these two parameters were higher as compared with

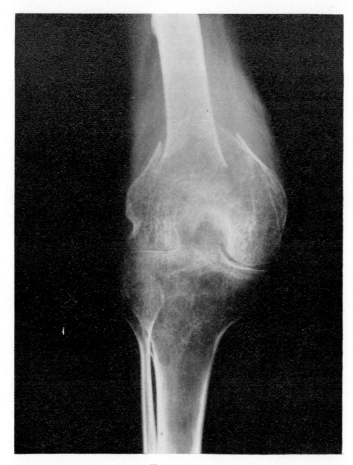

FIG. 101a.

those of these authors (Table 4). The serum alkaline phosphatase showed marginal values in 3 cases and only in 3 cases raised values.

Various factors may accelerate the development and increase the intensity of osteoporosis. Infections and toxaemia resulting from pressure sores, pyelonephritis and renal deficiency are the most important factors. Plaster casts and, in particular, plaster beds play a great role in this process of decomposition. How far hormonal factors or lack of nutritional components to the matrix as a result of disturbances of blood circulation following cord injuries play a role in this process still needs clarification. In particular, the question may be raised whether or not the slowing down of the blood circulation as a result of the paralytic vasodilatation caused by the interruption of the vasoconstrictors in complete transverse lesions of the cord may promote or accelerate this process of demineralization.

Although osteoporosis may develop in all skeletal parts below the cord transection, as a rule the parts most afflicted are the pelvis, the upper third and the supracondylar region of the femur. The osteoporotic bone with its rarefied spongiosa becomes easily

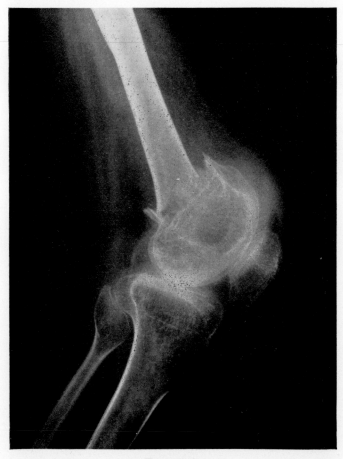

Fig. 101b.

brittle and often slight movements of the body during turning of the patient or passive movements of a leg by a physiotherapist may produce a fracture of the femur, usually called a 'spontaneous' fracture. The impacted supracondylar fracture is the typical fracture sustained by paraplegics, from falling out of the wheelchair on to the knee (Figs. 101a and b). Fractures of the femur may occur as sport injuries in paraplegics. This was seen in two untrained paraplegics who were engaged in basketball games. In 1953 the author described 7 cases and he later collected with his colleagues Michaelis and Melzak 100 cases of fracture due to osteoporosis in paraplegics. Comarr *et al.* (1962) also reported these pathological fractures.

TREATMENT OF OSTEOPOROSIS

The aim of the treatment is to discontinue the immobilization of the patient as soon as possible by frequent and regular changes of his position. In recent years, this has been greatly facilitated through the introduction of the electrically controlled Stoke Mandeville–Egerton turning bed. Furthermore, frequent passive movements of the paralysed limbs and active resistance exercises of the non-paralysed upper limbs with chest-expanders have proved invaluable to improve the blood circulation. Of great importance is the restitution of the disturbed nitrogen balance, especially in patients suffering from pressure sores and osteomyelitis. This can be best achieved through repeated blood transfusions whereby the oxygen carrying erythrocytes are essential for the tissue metabolism. High protein diet combined with vitamins is essential, especially vitamin D

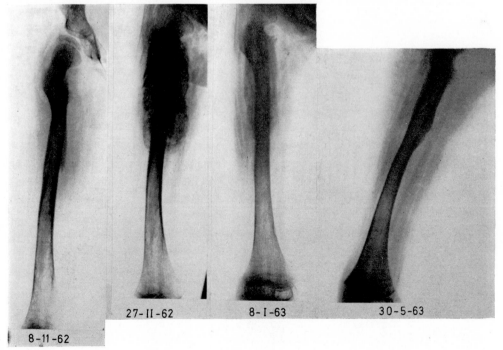

27-II-62   8-I-63   30-5-63

8-11-62

FIG. 102a.

which increases calcium and phosphate absorption from the intestine and promotes calcification by direct action on bone. As soon as the paraplegic is up in his wheelchair, intensive physiotherapy, including standing and, in particular, sportive activities have been invaluable in combating osteoporosis.

DIAGNOSIS AND TREATMENT OF PATHOLOGICAL FRACTURES

The diagnosis of a pathological, so-called spontaneous fracture may be difficult due to the loss of sensation in the paralysed area. As a rule, the patient will just complain of a swelling in the trochanteric area in the case of a pathological fracture of the femur or above the knee in the case of a supracondylar fracture. It is important that the member of the nursing staff who discovers such a swelling inform the medical officer in charge of the case immediately, and an X-ray will easily reveal the fracture. Occasionally, the patient or his physiotherapist carrying out passive movement may hear a click which indicates a fracture or dislocation.

The treatment of pathological fractures is, as a rule, conservative, by applying very well bolstered splints which have to be inspected frequently to prevent pressure sores.

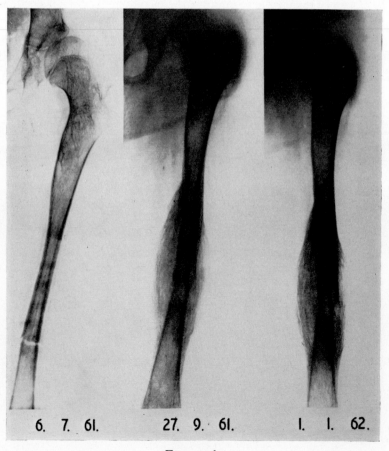

6. 7. 61.   27. 9. 61.   1. 1. 62.

FIG. 102b.

In fractures of the femur, we have been using modified Thomas splint. Freehafer & Lawry (1963) use a form of cushion-splint. Healing and consolidation of this fracture occur relatively rapidly, at a certain stage with considerable periosseous calcification around the fracture (Eichenholtz, 1962). However, alignment and consolidation, in particular of fractures of the mid-shaft of the femur, may be difficult or even impossible due to marked spasticity. In one of our patients with a comminuted fracture of the right mid-femur, I had first to eliminate the profound spasticity by an intrathecal alcohol block before the fracture could be explored surgically and united by plating (Dr Michaelis).

More or less large haemotomata with excessive extraosseous calcification occur frequently following fractures of long bones, especially if an extensive haematoma has developed surrounding the fracture. However, these calcifications decrease in later stages of the healing process and are eventually absorbed. This was seen, in particular, in children as seen in Figs. 102a and b.

CHAPTER 20

SOFT TISSUE CALCIFICATIONS AND OSSIFICATIONS

Periostal and extraosseous calcifications of soft tissues are a common result of pressure sores, if the infection penetrates into the deepest tissues including the bone, producing osteitis and osteomyelitis. They are discussed in more detail in the Chapter on Pressure Sores.

Repeated trauma of moderate degree to muscles, such as pressure and squeezing, may lead to the development of circumscribed ossification in non-paraplegic individuals. The most well-known examples are the 'Riderbone', which develops in the adductors and the ossification in the deltoid muscle of soldiers from recoil of the gun during firing practice.

Para-articular ossifications

A special form of para-articular ossification exclusively of non-infectious or traumatic aetiology has been repeatedly observed in both complete and incomplete paraplegics and tetraplegics below the level of the lesion. Although Riedel (1883) and Eichhorst (1895) described this condition, it was Mme Klumpke-Déjérine and her co-workers (1918–19) who made a detailed study on this subject in spinal paraplegic soldiers of the First World War. Statistical data of the frequency of this condition vary considerably. Déjérine & Ceillier (1919) found para-articular ossifications in 48·7 per cent, Soule (1945) in 37 per cent, Abramson (1948) and Abramson & Komberg (1949) in 41 per cent, Liberson (1953) in 37 per cent, Damanski (1961) and Hardy & Dickson (1963) in 16 per cent, Paeslack (1965) in 40 per cent, and Freehafer & Yurick (1966) in 17 per cent of their patients. However, in some of the publications pathological ossifications of different aetiologies (infection, osteomyelitis, fractures) are included, which may account for the high percentages. In our own material, where local infection, pressure sores and fractures are excluded as aetiological factors, the percentage is not higher than 5 per cent.

The predilection places of para-articular ossification are the medial border of the femoral condyle, upper third of the femur, anterior part of the hip, middle and upper part of the pelvis, medial and lateral aspects of the knees and the surroundings of the elbow joint. The joints themselves remain unaffected, in contrast to their involvement and destruction as a result of infection due to pressure sores. However, the para-articular ossifications can become so massive, especially around the hip joints, that an extra-articular ankylosis develops which, in due course, may prevent the patient from sitting or, in the case of the elbow-joint its movement may become impossible. Since the Second World War there has been an increase of publications on this subject (Brailsford, 1941; Soule, 1945; Heilborn & Kuhn, 1947; Wonns & Gougeon, 1947; Miller & O'Neil, 1949; Poppe, 1953; McNear, 1954; Storey & Tegner, 1955; Finkle, 1956; Finkelman, 1956;

Skotnikov, 1958; Rosak, 1961; Bénassy *et al.*, 1960, 1963; Michaelis, 1964; Freehafer & Yurick, 1966; Couvee, 1971; Rossier, 1972). A more detailed statistic was published by Wharton & Morgan (1970). They found 90 patients amongst 447 cases with heterotopic ossifications (20 per cent). Twenty patients (3 per cent) had serious articular restrictions.

In spite of the numerous publications, there is still discrepancy of opinion regarding the classification and terminology of this process, and different descriptions are used in the literature such as para-articular ossification (the term adopted by the writer), para-osteoarthropathia, osteosis neurotica para-articularis, heterotopic ossification, dystrophic ossification, neurogenic ossifying fibromyopathy, neurogenic ossifying fibromyositis and myositis ossificans circumscripta traumatica.

The aetiology and pathogenesis of the para-articular ossification is still obscure. However, there is general agreement that the transformation of the connective tissue into osteid tissue, leading to ossification, always develops below the level of the spinal cord lesion. All stages of ossification from collagen into bone containing Haversian systems may be demonstrated.

Various hypotheses have been advanced to explain the aetiology of para-articular ossifications in spinal cord lesions. On the one hand, lack of passive and active exercise has been considered as the cause for promoting this condition, but one should then

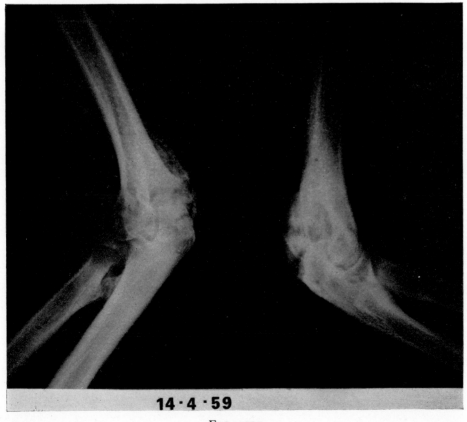

14·4·59

FIG. 103a.

expect an infinitely higher incidence amongst paraplegics. On the other hand, vigorous passive movements, carried out by physiotherapists in the immediate and early stages following transverse lesions, especially forceful hip flexion and abduction of the legs resulting in small haemorrhages and stress to the muscles and connective tissues, were thought to be aetiological factors in developing this pathological process. In the writer's view, this could be acceptable at least as an additional factor to account for changes in the protein-mineral metabolism, set up as a result of the transverse lesion of the cord. In this connection, it is worthwhile mentioning that chronic trauma to paralysed muscles such as quadriceps, as a result of pressure due to continuous lying in prone position, may produce lamellated ossification of the connective tissue between the muscle fibres,

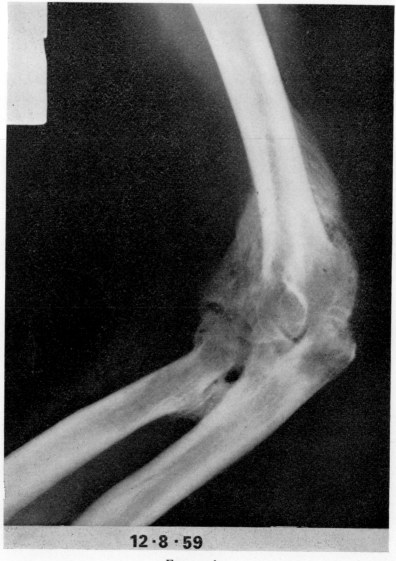

12·8·59

FIG. 103b.

generally called myositis ossificans. Bénassy *et al.* (1960, 1963) suggest changes of the O_2 and CO_2 exchange in the proximal blood circulation of the paralysed limbs as an important factor in the pathogenesis of the para-articular ossification. How far this process of para-articular ossification has the same or similar underlying aetiology (constitutional calciogenic diathesis) as the rare disease of myositis ossificans progressive of non-paralysed, mainly young individuals, which affects in early stages neck and back muscles, in particular latissimus dorsi and trapezius, is still unknown. The onset of this disease is characterized by attacks of stiffness, swelling and tenderness. There is hyperplasia of the intermuscular connective tissue with deposits of calcium between the muscle fibres. The eventually ossified connective tissue lies lamellated or in flat sheets within the axis of the muscles. There is no doubt about the (constitutionally) increased capacity of the connective tissue for ossification (calciogenic diathesis); however, the underlying cause of the anomaly of the mineral metabolism is unknown.

In the development of para-articular ossifications in transverse lesions of the spinal cord, three stages can be distinguished:

1 Stage of swelling and induration of soft tissue within the areas of pelvis, upper thigh or above the knee-joint and in cervical lesions outside the elbow joint. This condition may develop already in the early stage following cord lesion, and the passive mobility

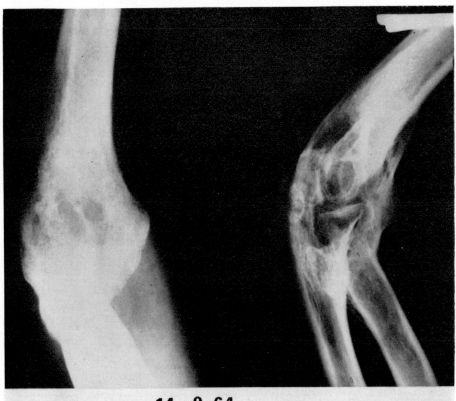

14 · 9 · 64

FIG. 103c.

of the paralysed leg or forearm is diminished. X-ray investigation at this stage reveals cloudy, streaky or patchy densities in the muscles involved.

2   Stage of calcification. This can develop within a few weeks and even within a few days (Rosak, 1961). The X-ray shows irregularly shaped calcareous deposits within the para-articular tissues.

3   Stage of ossification. The process of ossification is finalized and has led to dense ossification of ligaments, fasciae and muscles surrounding the joints, resulting in extra-articular ankylosis. At operation, the bony mass is often found to be quite eburnean.

The para-articular ossifications occur, as a rule, bilaterally. Figs. 103a–c demonstrate para-articular ossification around the left and right elbow joints in a man, aged 50, who on 5 January 1959 sustained a severe though incomplete traumatic tetraplegia below C5, with paralysis of triceps, pronator teres, brachioradialis and all hand and finger muscles. The function of deltoid and biceps was present but greatly reduced. All muscles of the lower limbs were functioning but reduced. The reflexes in the lower limbs were present and Babinski was positive while the arm reflexes were absent. There was complete sensory loss below C5 and no control of bladder function. Twenty-three days after injury, swelling of the left elbow area was noticeable, followed soon by swelling of the right elbow. Within the following weeks, the mobility of the elbow joints decreased and eventually they became ankylosed, in spite of intensive physiotherapy and recovery of function in hand and finger muscles. On 8 March and 25 March 1960 respectively the para-articular ossifications were removed (Dr Michaelis) but soon recurred, resulting again in contractures of the elbows. Fig. 103c shows the severe para-articular changes 4 years after operation.

Figs. 104a–c shows stages 2 and 3 in the development of bilateral para-articular ossifications around the hip joints and also the result of successful removal of the greater part of the ossifications and restoration of movement of the hip joints (Dr Michaelis) in the case of a nurse, aged 22, who sustained a complete paraplegia below T6, following fractures of 4th–7th thoracic vertebrae on 12 July 1963. In her case, there was considerable difficulty in passive hip flexion about 3 months following injury and an X-ray of 14 October 1965 showed early patchy calcification around the trochanters and pelvis on both sides. A control X-ray of 2 May 1965 following readmission to the Centre revealed dense ossifications around the hip joints, producing complete ankylosis, and any passive flexion of the hips was impossible. Partial excision of the ossification on 11 June and 6 August 1965 respectively (Dr Michaelis) resulted in restoring hip flexion to 90°, which remained permanent. In other cases in which excision was not possible, osteotomy at the upper third of the femur just below the distal end of the ossification established hip flexion and restored sitting position of the patient. In 8 cases operated by Dr Michaelis, lasting good results were achieved in 50 per cent. However, all workers in this field (Michaelis, 1964; Freehafer & Yurick, 1966; Gregono, 1966; Ebel, 1966) agree that excision of the ossifications, once the ossification process is finalized, or osteotomy are the methods of choice to eliminate the extra-articular ankylosis, but recurrences are not uncommon. Operations before the process of ossification has been finalized have proved unsuccessful and recurrence invariably occurred.

The problem of the determination of maturity of the heterotopic ossification is

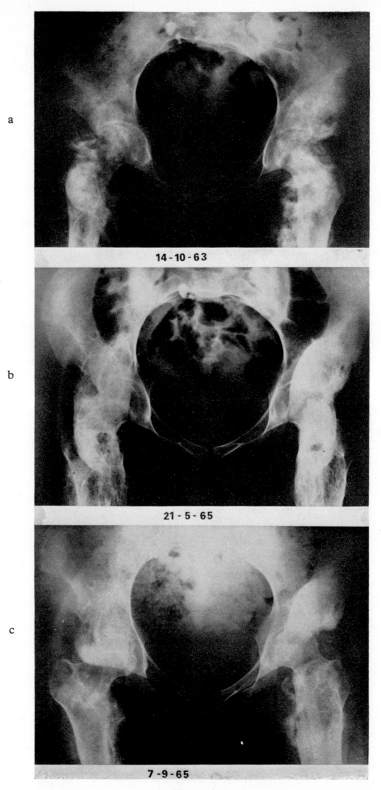

a

b

c

14 - 10 - 6 3

21 - 5 - 65

7 - 9 - 65

FIG. 104.

still unsolved in spite of comprehensive studies carried out in recent years. Rossier *et al.* (1973) found, amongst the many parameters they examined, serum alkaline phosphatase and serial bone scans essential in determining maturity of the heterotopic ossification. Although normal alkaline phosphatase values are not absolute proof of stabilization of the osteogenic process, there is no doubt that increased serum phosphatase is indicative of bone growth and immaturity of the ossifying process, and should be considered as contraindication to surgery. According to Rossier *et al.*, serial bone scan with decreasing isotope uptake over a period of time seems to be a reliable parameter in determining approaching maturity of ossification, thus indicating the most suitable time for surgery.

Recently Stover *et al.* (1976) found disodium etidronate, one of the diphosphonates effective in the prevention of post-operative recurrences of heterotopic ossification in spinal cord injury patients. The patients were started on this drug with approximately 20 mg/kg/day 2 weeks before the operation and continued on the same dosage after operation for 6, 30 and 39 weeks respectively. Medication was administered orally 1 hour before breakfast with a glass of fruit juice. As side effects of disodium etidronate elevation of serum phosphate (Recker *et al.*, 1973), mild nausea and abdominal discomfort were observed which were controlled by giving this drug in divided doses. The authors consider Disodium Etidronate safe for clinical use as it has also been found in clinical trials with Paget's disease (Russel *et al.*, 1974). From the data given by Stover *et al.* of seven patients with heterotopic ossification, there is evidence that Disodium Etidronate delayed post-operative recurrence with maintanance of good range of motion as long as the drug was administered up to 39 weeks, while the controls developed recurrences, shown radiologically, within 3 weeks. However, following withdrawal of this drug recurrence developed. Therefore, further trials with longer treatment periods will be necessary.

F · Neurophysiological and Clinical Aspects of Spinal Cord Injuries

GENERAL

The pathophysiological effects of any kind of injury to the spinal cord or cauda equina have to be considered from four main standpoints:

1   The level of the lesion. The higher the lesion the more extensive is the loss of motor, sensory and autonomic functions and, moreover, the greater are the metabolic changes of the organism.

2   The extent of damage to the spinal cord in the transverse plane. This may involve the whole cross section of the cord at any level, resulting in a complete transverse spinal syndrome, or the damage may be partial, involving some of the long tracts or central grey matter and its synapses, resulting in a great variety of incomplete transverse syndromes of more or less dissociated type.

3   The extent of damage in the vertical—i.e. longitudinal plane. This may occur as an entity in itself, as is the case in haematomyelia, syringo- or hydromyelia. On the other hand, it may be associated with a transverse lesion involving either a few or all segments of the isolated cord—i.e. the part below the transverse lesion.

4   The time factor which is important in determining the damage to the cord and the resulting symptomatology—i.e. whether the onset of the cord lesion was sudden or gradual.

The term generally accepted for transverse lesions of the spinal cord involving thoracic, lumbar and sacral region, is paraplegia. Tetraplegia is the Greek term used by the writer and other authors for transverse lesion of the cervical cord. There is no clinical or scientific reason why the term tetraplegia should not be universally accepted instead of the often confusing, combined Greek and Latin, names: quadriplegia, quadraplegia, or quadruplegia. It is not uncommon for the writer to be asked in court and on other occasions to explain the 'difference' between tetraplegia and quadriplegia, and it is really time that we brought our terminology in order.

CHAPTER 21

THE ACUTE COMPLETE TRANSVERSE SYNDROME

This may be caused either by transection or severe lesion in continuity or purely by transient physiological interruption. As a result, there is complete interruption of the function of the anterior and posterior neuronal elements and their synaptic and root connections at the level of the lesion. In addition, there is also a complete interruption of the conductivity of all long tracts descending from cortical or subcortical centres of the brain as well as of the main afferent pathways conducting impulses arising from skin, muscles, tendons, ligaments, joints and viscera.

The various pathologies resulting in an acute transverse syndrome can be divided into:

(a) Transection of the cord

This may occur as a result of gunshot or stab wounds or fractures and fracture-dislocations of the spine and may involve one or several segments according to the type of injury. All ganglion cells and axonal elements are destroyed at the site of the severance and the organization of their anatomical compartments is disrupted. The severed dura, arachnoidea and pia, as well as the segment of the cord, are replaced by a dense fibrous scar or by a piece of bone or, as in the case of stab and gunshot injuries, by a metal body.

(b) Lesions in continuity

In this condition one has to distinguish between disruption and preservation of the segmental anatomical arrangement. In the former case, the meningeal coverings and the outer shell of the cord at the level of the injury remain intact but the anatomical arrangement and organization including ganglion cells, axons and synaptic connections at segmental level are disrupted and replaced by glial or fibrous tissue. This may occur following crush injuries of the spine, transverse myelitis necroticans or a vascular catastrophy.

In the case of preservation of the segmental anatomical organization, the ganglion cells and their synaptic connections may lose their function due to the pathological process but the axonal anatomical arrangements of the long ascending and descending tracts within the spinal cord are not as disorganized as described above. Therefore, a greater or lesser degree of functional recovery is possible after the cause is removed. This may occur in certain types of pathological conditions causing gradual compression, such as extra-medullary tumours, furthermore collapsing osteomyelitic or tuberculous vertebrae or vascular thrombosis. This problem has been discussed previously in the Chapter on Regeneration of the Spinal Cord.

(c) Physiological interruption (commotio spinalis)

In this condition, the anatomical structures of the neural elements at the level of the lesion have not suffered any definite damage and their anatomical arrangement is not disorganized; only their conductive power is temporarily cut off, but this will recover completely within hours or a few days. (See also Chapter on Regeneration.)

CHAPTER 22

PATHOPHYSIOLOGY OF THE MOTOR
SYSTEM

The loss of voluntary function of the skeletal muscles is one of the main symptoms of transverse spinal cord lesions. The paralysis of the muscles at segmental level of the lesion differs fundamentally from the motor paralysis below the level of the transverse lesion.

Motor paralysis at segmental level

The muscles innervated by the affected segment or segments at the level of the lesion show the classical signs of a flaccid paralysis of lower motor neuron type as a result of the destruction of their anterior horn cells and anterior roots. There is loss of reflex function and tone of the muscles and their electrical excitability undergoes changes (degenerative reaction, RD), and the electromyogram reveals a curve characteristic for a lower motor neuron lesion. Moreover, there are alterations of their blood supply and trophic condition resulting in muscular atrophy. These changes are found at any level including conus and cauda equina.

Motor paralysis below the level of the lesion

In contrast, the motor paralysis below the level of the transection is of upper motor neuron type provided that the segments below the transverse lesions are intact. Although the motor paralysis as the immediate effect of the sudden onset of a transverse lesion is at first also of flaccid type with areflexia (stage of spinal shock), in due course muscle tone and reflex function of the muscles will return (stage of reflex automatism) and the motor paralysis is of spastic type. However, the paralysis of the skeletal muscles below the level of the transverse spinal cord lesion will also be of lower motor neuron type if in addition to the cord damage in the transverse plane destruction of the cord in the vertical plane has occurred. This will also affect the reflex function of the isolated cord resulting in hypo- or areflexia of skeletal muscles.

CHAPTER 23

PATTERNS OF REFLEX DISTURBANCES

In the following, both the stage of spinal shock and the various stages of reflex automism will be discussed in detail:

A. Stage of spinal shock

Since Marshall Hall (1841) introduced the term 'spinal shock' for the state of a transient in—or hypoexcitability of, the isolated cord which exists immediately and in the early stages following partial or complete transection of the spinal cord, this phenomenon has been the subject of very extensive clinical and physiological research and discussion. While the majority of modern investigators hold the view that spinal shock represents a dysbalance of the function of the internuncial neurons and not of the motor neurons, the intrinsic mechanism of this phenomenon and its variations amongst the various species in the evolutionary scale is still not fully understood. One of the reasons for this is the fact that experimental workers in this field adopted different technical procedures and modes of investigation, including different types of anaesthesia. This is in particular the case when the functions of the spinal cord have been studied in preparations of animals of higher grade in the evolutionary scale. Koley's & Muckerjee's (1964) comments on the techniques used are as follows:

1 Sherrington's preparations were not a spinal preparation, but a decapitate preparation.
2 The technique of pithing the cord used by Goltz (1869) is suitable only in small animals such as frogs and guinea-pigs. His theory that spinal shock is due to stimulation of the cut stump of the cord was challenged by Sherrington as unproven and is now generally rejected.
3 Treat's technique (1941) used in cats by blind puncture and cauterization, avoiding traumatic effects of laminectomy, has the uncertainty of complete separation of the cord.
4 McDowall's technique adopted more or less by Downman, McSwiney and Muckerjee himself is a preparation which converts the preparation into 'decerebrate with cordotomy'. Artificial respiration was always required to maintain the life of the animal.

To the techniques of these workers may be added that of Barnes et al. (1962) who measured the resting potential of cells in the lumbar segment of the spinal cord of the cat before, during and after the cord was functionally blocked by cooling with 0C brine passed through a copper tube surrounding the cord at mid-thoracic level. They came to the conclusion that the physiological derangement in spinal shock is a hyperpolarization of motor neurons. The authors consider this as a result of random synaptic bombardment by nerve endings, either directly or indirectly activated from more cephalad regions, which normally keep the cells in slightly hypopolarized state.

However, whatever the techniques and the experimental results in animals may have been, the modern concept of spinal shock is based on the work of Sherrington and his school, which suggests that the transient reflex depression in the segments below the spinal cord transection is the result of the sudden withdrawal of a predominantly facilitating or excitatory influence of descending supraspinal tracts, resulting in a disruption of transmission at the synapse and thus rendering the process of conduction impossible or difficult. In recent years, thanks to the work of Eccles and his colleagues (1964), much of the research was concerned with the mechanism of synaptic excitation and inhibition, whereby the importance of the peripheral organs in the muscle system has been more and more recognized in the process of transmission. It has been concluded that a primary factor in the tendinous areflexia in spinal shock is the reduced discharge of spindle receptors, produced by relaxation of intrafusal muscle fibres through the acute deficit of the fusimotor control from the gamma-motor neurons. There are other factors involved in the mechanism of spinal shock, and McCouch (1964) postulated three as probably significant.

1   Loss of facilitation from descending tracts.

2   Persisting inhibition from below acting upon extensor reflexes. It has been shown that if in a decerebrate animal a transection of the spinal cord is performed in the mid-thoracic region, the extensor rigidity of the fore-limbs resulting from the decerebration is intensified as a source of inhibition arising from the lumbar enlargement if the cord has been removed from its effect upon extensor reflexes of the cervical and upper thoracic spinal segments (Ruch, 1956). On the other hand, I found in the spinal man with cervical lesion resulting in intractable spasticity of both lower and upper limbs that elimination of the thoraco-lumbar portion of the spinal cord by intrathecal alcohol block decreased rigidity and spasticity in the upper limbs.

3   Axonal degeneration of interneurons. Axonal degeneration is more severe where the axon is cut near the cell body. This accords, according to McCouch, with the greater severity of spinal shock from lesions at lower levels.

Neurophysiological research in recent years through new developments in electro-myography and combination of new methods of testing spinal reflex pathways has provided further information in the complex process of reflex behaviour of the isolated cord both in spinal shock as well as in later stages of established spasticity (Brown *et al.*, 1967; Eklund, 1971; Burke *et al.*, 1972; Delwaide, 1973; Hagborth, 1973; Lance *et al.*, 1973; Desmedt, 1973; Ashby *et al.*, 1975). Recently, Ashby, Vevrier & Lightfoot (1975) made a comprehensive study on segmental reflex pathways in spinal shock and spinal spasticity in six normal subjects and 10 patients with spinal cord lesions—10 physiologically complete—using the Achilles Tendon Reflex (ATR) to estimate transmission in the Ia monosynaptic pathway and the Tonic Vibration Reflex (TVR) in the Ia polysynaptic pathway to motoneurones. The percentage of the motoneurone pool (M-response) which can be activated by these pathways was used as a measure of transmission. The ratio of the H reflex (vibration) to reflex (control) was used to estimate the degree of presynaptic inhibition of the Ia monosynaptic pathway. The studies were carried out with the subject in prone position, the leg to be examined being mobilized in a padded frame with padded clamps gripping the malleots and the angle joint fixed at 90°.

Based on their findings, the authors propose an hypothesis which postulates that the motoneurone pool may be activitated by a monosynaptic pathway which is presynoptically inhibited while the polysynaptic pathway is not and that the interneurones of the polysynaptic pathway require supraspinal facilitation.

'In spinal shock the presynaptic inhibitory mechanism appears to be capable of blocking the whole traffic in the monosynaptic line. The Ia monosynaptic pathway excites only 5 per cent of the motoneurone pool. This may be attributed to depressed fusimotor drive (Weaver et al., 1963), an increase in presynaptic inhibition (demonstrated by the authors) and a decrease in the excitability of the motoneurone (Barnes, 1962; Diamontopoulos and Olsen, 1967). The Ia polysynaptic pathway is incapable of exciting the motoneurone pool. This may be attributed to the loss of vestibulo-spinal facilitation of interneurones (Gillies et al., 1971).

In established spasticity the presynaptic inhibitory mechanism is less effective than normal. The Ia monosynaptic pathway now excites about 40 per cent of the motoneurone pool. This could be due to an increase in fusimotor drive (Dietrichson, 1973) but Delwaide (1973) has suggested that the decrease in presynaptic inhibition may be one of the most important factors. Even though the monosynaptic pathway is hyperactive the Ia polysynaptic pathway still appears incapable of exciting the motoneurone pool, suggesting that supraspinal facilitation of interneurones is of primary importance for the transmission of activity in this pathway.'

In the following various problems concerned with the reflex behaviour of the skeletal muscles during the stage of spinal shock in man are discussed:

(1) *Spinal shock and traumatic shock*

In spite of a certain superficial similarity, as far as fall of blood pressure (in high lesions) is concerned, there are fundamental differences between spinal shock and traumatic shock, and these two phenomena should not be confused. While in transections above the sympathetic outflow (T5), especially cervical lesion, there is initially a marked fall of blood pressure, this returns to normal very soon, while the reflex depression as a result of the spinal shock remains unchanged for more or less long periods. Furthermore, in distal cord lesions, spinal shock is severe while the blood pressure may remain normal immediately after injury. If the traumatic shock results in fall of blood pressure, this is readily restored by blood transfusion but this has no effect on the intensity of the spinal shock. Moreover, it does not make any significant difference to the degree of reflex depression due to spinal shock whether the anterior spinal artery is severed or not. (Hunter & Royle, 1924).

(2) *Latent period between time of cord transection and spinal shock*

In analysing various factors involved in spinal shock in man, there is first the question whether the sudden withdrawal of the innervatory influence from supraspinal centres as the result of partial or complete cord transection disrupts the transmission at the synapse in the segments caudal to the lesion immediately or whether the ganglion cells at the synapse still retain their charge of energy and excitability for a short period and are thus capable of maintaining for a while the process of conduction. I have found the ankle jerks, plantar response and, in particular, anal sphincter and bulbo-cavernosus reflexes to be still present immediately after cord transection and they may disappear only after a certain latent period, while the anal reflex may not disappear at all. It is well known that immediately after decapitation in man by guillotine, as practised not long ago in France, the knee jerks are still elicitable for several minutes (Barré, 1915). In this connection, it may also be remembered that Collier (1916, 1917) succeeded in the first days following cord transection in eliciting the initially abolished knee jerk following faradization of the quadriceps for 5–15 minutes. These observations of clinical neurologists of the old school are today of particular interest in the light of modern physiological research on spinal shock, as they indicate that the sudden withdrawal of the excitatory influence of supraspinal centres and their descending tracts on the transmitting synapses in the stage of spinal shock can be temporarily obviated by strong peripheral afferent impulses. Conversely, Foerster (1908, 1911) proved the importance of the afferent system on the reflex activity of the spinal cord by dividing the posterior roots resulting in distinct though, according to number of divided roots, variable degree of reflex depression. All these observations have been invaluable in furthering our knowledge in the mechanism of spinal shock in the spinal man. There is no doubt that neurological examinations at frequent intervals by the same examiner during the immediate and early stages following complete as well as incomplete traumatic lesions of the spinal cord are of utmost importance in determining intensity, duration and site of spinal shock as well as evaluating the intricacy and variability of reflex return in the spinal man. Therefore, the need for accurate records cannot be overstressed, the more so as the modern student can now approach this subject with more sophisticated methods of investigation than the investigator of the past.

(3) *Intensity and duration of spinal shock*

It is now generally agreed that intensity and duration of spinal shock increase commensurate with the vertebrate scale, especially in the primate species. The higher the cerebral development the deeper the spinal shock. A comparison of different species reveals a striking parallel between the degree of development of suprasegmental structures and their descending tracts and the intensity and duration of the spinal shock resulting from the cord transection. Sherrington found it impossible to elicit the knee jerks for about a month in the case of a monkey, whilst in a rabbit its absence lasted only 10 to 15 minutes. In lower species, reflex activity may even occur without delay after severance of the cord. Fulton & McCouch (1937) found that in the Erythrocebus group of monkeys all reflexes are depressed but none of them abolished, while reflex depression in the macaque, baboon and especially the chimpanzee may be almost as great as or even greater than in man.

The duration of spinal cord depression in man varies considerably, and reflex activity of skeletal muscles may appear within a period from 3 or 4 days (this occurs in particular in young individuals) and up to 6 weeks after injury. Septic conditions resulting from pressure sores and infection of the urinary tract play an essential part in delaying reflex automatism of the spinal cord. The physiological derangement in the isolated cord during spinal shock naturally also affects the onset of automaticity of bowels and bladder, which may be considerably delayed, as may also be the dysbalance of temperature regulation, in transections of the cervical cord. This will be discussed in the respective chapters concerning these problems.

(4) *Caudal and cephalad direction of reflex depression*

It is generally agreed that the direction of reflex depression is from proximal to caudal— i.e. the reflex depression is more severe and lasts longer in the segments of the isolated cord situated more proximal to the transection, and the distal segments follow later. Thus, in complete transverse lesions of the cervical cord, the arm and finger reflexes as well as the abdominal reflexes are abolished immediately, while the reflexes of the distal parts of the paralysed legs, such as ankle jerks and, in particular, reflex responses to plantar stimulation (plantar or dorsi flexion of the toes and weak withdrawal response of one or both legs) as well as bulbo-cavernosus and anal reflexes may be present or disappear only after some latent period, a proof of the dysbalance of the afferents and efferents at various levels within the isolated cord.

From experimental studies on cord transection in animals, it was for many years accepted that the transient depression of the excitability of the cord in the stage of spinal shock manifests itself in caudal direction only. Sherrington mentioned, as an example of the absence of headwards spread of depression due to spinal shock, the fact that, in spinal animals after transection of the 5th cervical segment, the respiratory activity of the phrenic motor cells is hardly affected and in transection behind the brachial enlargement he found the reaction of the upper limbs little if at all disturbed. However, this concept was not confirmed by Ruch & Watts (1934), who described distinct changes in reflex activity following post-brachial transection or cold block of the spinal cord. Earlier, Monakow (1914) who introduced the term 'diaschisis' (meaning dissolution of neural function) postulated that diaschisis is operative not only in the downward direction but also upward. From my personal experience in traumatic complete lesions in man, an upward spread of transient depression of cord function in the initial stages of spinal shock is by no means unusual. For instance, the transient impairment of finger movement and loss of reflex of the forearm may occur in upper thoracic lesions as low as T4. This transient impairment representing a concussional effect of the cord above the transection may disappear within a few hours or few days after injury.

B. Stage of reflex return—reflex automatism of the isolated cord

Once the stage of spinal shock subsides and the synaptic relays are released from the resistance imposed upon them through the process of spinal shock, afferent impulses arising from peripheral stations of the nervous system in skin, tendons, muscles, ligaments, joints, and viscera begin to elicit their excitatory influence on the neural elements within the isolated cord. Conversely, the cord reacts, now unrestrained from supraspinal inhibitory influences, with complex efferent responses (Mass Response). The reflex automatism of the isolated cord thus established, is characterized by hyperreflexia, rigidity and spasticity of the muscles.

In recent years, the excitatory and inhibitory function of synapses, which act as devices for the transmission of information from one neuron to another by a chemical transmitter mechanism, has been the subject of intensive research by cell physiologists, and electron microscopy has contributed much information on the monosynaptic and polysynaptic connections of the spinal cord, pre-eminently through the work of Eccles and his school (Eccles & Lundberg, 1959; Eccles, 1964; Lundberg, 1964; Granit, 1966; Eccles & Schadé, 1964). Synapse, a term originally proposed by Sherrington (1897), now embraces the presynaptic terminal with its synaptic vesicles, synaptic cleft and the subsynaptic membrane with its special receptive and reactive mechanism. Moreover, the important part which peripheral receptor organs, such as Golgi's tendon organ and especially the muscle spindle, play in the complex mechanism of the spinal cord has also come to light. Although Sherrington (1897) recognized the muscle spindle as a sensory organ, the detailed organization of this encapsulated organ in nuclear-chain and nuclear-bag fibres and their innervation by group I and II sensory and gamma I and II motor nerve fibres has only recently been elaborated. Cooper & Daniel (1956), Boyd *et al.* (1964) and Rushworth (1960, 1964) found the muscle spindle contribution to the afferent influx dominant in the majority of clinical states of either rigidity or spasticity of the skeletal muscles in the paralysed limbs. Whitteridge (1966), Rushworth (1966) and Phillips (1970) have given excellent reviews on this problem. In this connection, it may be remembered that it was the realization of the importance of afferent impulses on motor reflex response in the treatment of spasticity and rigidity which many years ago led Foerster (1911) to introduce the posterior rhizotomy in the treatment of spastic conditions.

As a rule, reflex return is in headward direction. The reflexes appearing first in the spinal man are anal and bulbo-cavernosus reflexes and responses to plantar stimulation such as plantar and/or dorsiflexion of the toes and the ipsilateral flexor reflex of the leg. Actually, the ipsilateral flexor reflex of the leg may be elicitable before a significant reflex response of the toes or tibialis anterior or return of the knee and ankle jerks is noticeable (Fig. 105). At first, a strong stimulus or summation of several stimuli to the sole of the foot is necessary to elicit any reflex response of muscles of the leg and there is fatigue in their reflex-responses. Moreover, there are differences in onset and intensity of reflex recovery between the two sides of the lower and (in cervical lesions) upper limbs indicating a difference in the intensity of spinal shock within the two halves of the isolated cord. In later stages of reflex automatism, the receptive field increases and various reflexes can be elicited by light stimulation of cutaneous areas. Although the early crossed reflex is also flexion of the contra-lateral leg associated with adduction, this is followed later by the development of extension synergy. It has been suggested that the persistence of the flexor reflex response (one phase reaction) signifies a complete transection of the cord, while the return of the leg following withdrawal to its original position in extension (two phase reaction) is characteristic of an incomplete lesion. The writer's observations did not confirm this theory. The clinical significance

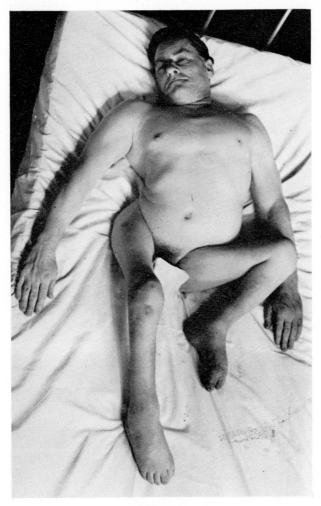

FIG. 105.

of the change in reflex pattern will be discussed later. In the following, a few examples may be given to demonstrate the variability of reflex patterns on the recovery from spinal shock:

Case 1. A soldier aged 23 sustained a gunshot injury on 2 July 1944 of the 10th thoracic vertebra, resulting in complete transverse spinal syndrome below T9 with flaccid paraplegia. The medical notes stated that he was very shocked but he recovered following blood transfusions. Twelve days after injury, he was examined by Dr George Riddoch, no doubt the most experienced British neurologist on spinal injuries. The patient then still showed a complete flaccidity of both lower limbs and areflexia, with the exception of the ankle jerks which showed just a flicker. Eighteen days after injury, he was admitted to Stoke Mandeville Spinal Centre. There was still a complete transverse spinal syndrome below T9, and Table 5 demonstrates the return of reflex function.

TABLE 5. Complete transverse lesion below T9

	20.7.44		12.8.44		28.8.44		20.11.44		14.5.45	
	R	L	R	L	R	L	R	L	R	L
Abdominals	+	++	++	++	++	++	++	++	++	++
Cremasterics	-	-	-	-	-	-	-	-	-	-
K.Js	-	-	+	+	+	+	++	+	++ (clonus)	++ (clonus)
							(clonus)	(clonus)		
A.Js	((+))	((+))	(+)	(+)	(+)	(+)	++	++	+	++
							(clonus)	(clonus)		(clonus)
Plantars	→	→	←	←	←	←	←	←	←	←
Withdrawal	-	-	(+)	(+)	+	+	++	++	++	++
					(flexion synergy)		(flexion)		(extensor synergy prevalent)	

In this case, recovery of reflex function from spinal shock occurred within 6 weeks after accident, and it may be noted that although the ankle jerks returned earlier, the intensity of reflex response became more marked in the knee jerks once these returned. Moreover, while at first the flexion synergy of the lower limbs was predominant, it gradually diminished and was replaced by the prevalent extension synergy.

Case 2. Another example is a young soldier aged 19, who sustained a complete tetraplegia below C7 as the result of a fracture dislocation of C6 following diving into shallow water.

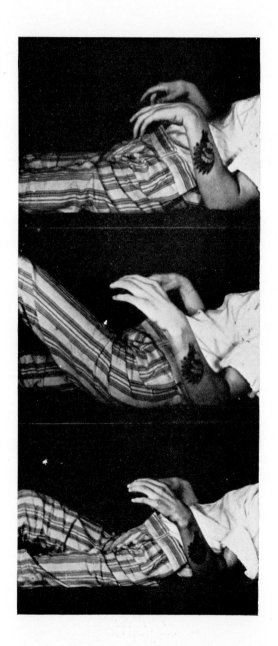

FIG. 106. Increased reflexogenic spread in complete tetraplegia on plantar stimulation.

TABLE 6. Complete transverse lesion below C7

	13.8.44 R	13.8.44 L	14.8.44 R	14.8.44 L	16.8.44 R	16.8.44 L	19.8.44 R	19.8.44 L	24.8.44 R	24.8.44 L	4.10.44 R	4.10.44 L	25.10.44 R	25.10.44 L
B.Js	+	(+)	+	+	(+)	(+)	+	+	+	+	+	+	+	+
S.Js	(+)	(+)	(+)	+	(+)	(+)	+	+	+	+	+	+	+	+
T.Js	−	−	−	−	−	−	−	−	−	−	−	−	−	−
Abdominals	−	−	−	−	−	−	−	−	−	−	−	−	−	−
Cremasterics	−	−	−	−	−	−	−	−	−	−	−	−	−	−
K.Js	−	−	(+)	+	((+))	((+))	+	+	+	+	+	+	++	++
A.Js	(↓)	(↓)	(↓)	(↓)	((↓))	((↓))	(↓)	(↓)	(↑)	(↑)	←	←	←	↑
Plantar resp.	−		−	−	−	−	−	−	(flexion)	(flexion)	flexion	flexion	++	++
Withdrawal resp.													increased reflexogenic zone	
Priapism	+	+	+	+	+	+	+	+	+	+	+	+		
Rectal sphincter	+		+		+		+		+		+		spreading upper limbs	

respiratory distress (weakness of diaphragm) abdominal distension extensor Carp. rad. weaker

He was seen on the day of injury on 13 August 1944 by a neurologist who reported complete paralysis below C8 of flaccid type with areflexia including the triceps jerk. There was, however, a plantar flexion response to plantar stimulation on both sides. There was also priapism. On admission to Stoke Mandeville one day later, he had a bilateral Horner's syndrome, marked vasodilatation in face and neck with obstruction of the naso-pharyngeal passages, paralysis of both triceps and of all finger and hand muscles with the exception of the extensors of the wrist and the radial portion of the extensor digitorum on the left. There was complete sensory loss below C8 but also marked sensory impair-ment in C7. The pattern of reflex return in this case is shown in Table 6, which also shows a gradual reflex recovery in the cephalad direction. At the end of October 1944 a marked increase of the reflexogenic zone over the whole paralysed area of the body was noted. Plantar stimulation on either side not only set up marked flexion synergy of the ipsilateral paralysed leg but also resulted in contraction of the ipsilateral trunk and abdominal muscles and marked response of the paralysed extensors of all fingers and thumb on the same side. This extensive reflex response of the fingers and thumb on stroking the sole of the left foot could be elicited bilaterally (Fig. 106) but only ipsilater-ally on stroking the right sole. In due course, this exaggerated reflex response gradually diminished in intensity but was still elicitable. Moreover, the profound flexion synergy of the lower limbs gradually decreased and in the middle of 1946 was replaced by a prevalent extensor synergy.

In contrast to this group of patients with early return of the ankle jerks, there are other complete transverse lesions where the return of the tendon reflexes nearer to the transection, such as the knee jerk, may precede that of the ankle jerk, as shown in the following example.

Case 3. A soldier aged 20 sustained a complete transverse lesion below T8 with a right haemo-pneumothorax as a result of a gunshot injury on 25 June 1944. On admission to Stoke Mandeville 11 days after injury, he showed flaccid paralysis of both lower limbs with a complete sensory loss below T8 and loss of control of bladder and bowels. The pattern of reflex return is shown in Table 7. While in this case the extensor response of the big toe to plantar stimulation appeared much earlier than either knee or ankle jerk, the knee jerks returned before the ankle jerks and it may be noted that there was not only a definite delay in the return of the right ankle jerk but the intensity of the withdrawal response was also less marked on the right side indicating a difference in the intensity of the spinal shock between the two halves of the spinal cord below the level of the lesion.

Case 4. A further case in this group is a soldier aged 19, who sustained a gunshot injury to the 7th cervical vertebra resulting in a complete transverse lesion below T1/2. He was operated upon one day later and the spinal cord was found almost completely severed by a foreign body, which was removed. A suprapubic cystostomy was performed on the same day, a procedure which was also done in the other cases described leading to infec-tion. There were also pressure sores in the last two cases. On admission to Stoke Mande-ville 3 days later, there was a complete flaccid paraplegia below T1 with paralysis of the abductor pollicis longus and brevis and slight weakness of the long finger flexors on the

TABLE 7. Complete transverse lesion below T8

	6.7.44		18.7.44		31.7.44		25.8.44		6.9.44		20.12.44		15.3.44	
	R	L	R	L	R	L	R	L	R	L	R	L	R	L
Abdominals	+	+	+	+	+	+	+	+	+	+	+	+	+	+
Cremasterics	−	−	−	−	−	−	−	−	−	−	−	−	−	−
K.Js.	−	−	−	−	−	+	(+)	+	+	+	++	++ (clonus)	++	++ (clonus)
A.Js.	−	−	−	−	−	−	−	−	(+)	(+)	+	+	+	+
Plantars	←? ←	−	←? ←	−	(↑)(+) ←+	− ←	(+) ←+	− ←	(+)← +	(+)← +	←+ ←+	←+ ←+	←+ ←	←+ ++
Withdrawal	−	−	(pyrexia)		(flexion synergy)		(flexion synergy)		(flexion synergy)		(flexion synergy)		(extension synergy more marked than flexion synergy)	

right side which later recovered completely. The paralysis of the lower limbs and trunk was flaccid and there was a complete sensory loss below T1 on the right and T2 on the left with an incomplete Horner's syndrome on the right. The pattern of reflex return in the lower limbs and abdominals is shown in Table 8.

TABLE 8. Complete transverse lesion below T1/2

	1.11.44		27.11.44		19.12.44		26.2.45	
	R	L	R	L	R	L	R	L
Abdominals	—	—	—	—	—	—	—	—
	—	—	—	—	—	—	—	—
	—	—	—	—	—	—	—	—
Cremasterics	—	—	—	—	—	—	—	—
K.Js.	—	—	+	+	++	++	++	++ (clonus)
A.Js.	—	—	—	—	+	+	++	++ (clonus)
Plantars	—	—	—		↑	↑	↑	↑
Withdrawal response	—	—	—	—	+ (flexion synergy)	+	++ (flexion adduction synergy)	++

These cases demonstrate the variability of reflex return following spinal shock. It may be noted that the cremaster reflex has been absent throughout and remained so. The absence or late return of this reflex, which I confirmed again and again, is not in accordance with other authors who claim that the cremasteric reflex usually returns early (McCouch, 1964).

Varieties in reflex-pattern

Four groups may be examined, in which certain muscles or muscle groups become dominant in the reflex synergy.

1. Preponderance of the extensor hallucis longus and tibialis anterior

The contraction of the extensor hallucis longus on plantar stimulation represents one of the original components of both extensor and flexor synergies. It is indeed one of the very early signs of any reflex activity of the isolated cord. Although this reflex was first described by E.Remark (1893), it was Babinski (1896) who realized the clinical significance of the phénomène du gros orteil which is generally accepted as Babinski's sign. It is well known that the extent of its reflexogenic zone and the intensity of its motor response varies. Sometimes the reflex response of the extensor hallucis longus either alone or in combination with spreading of the toes (signe de l'eventail) may show a profound preponderance over any other muscles of the lower limbs, and in some patients the contraction of this muscle may be very violent and permanent, resulting in subluxation of the terminal phalanx of the big toe, as described in a case of complete paraplegia below T4 (Guttmann, 1953).

In the same group of reflex response belongs the tibialis anterior. The reflex contraction of this muscle, either in combination with the extensor hallucis longus or isolated, may become so preponderant that finally a contracture of the foot in dorsiflexion and inversion occurs (spastic pes varus). This will be particularly profound if, during the stage of spinal shock, a pressure lesion of the superficial branch of the external popliteal nerve has occurred due to faulty position of the leg, resulting in peripheral paresis or paralysis of the peroneal muscles. On the other hand, in the rare case of a peripheral lesion of the anterior tibial branch of the external popliteal nerve leading to paralysis of tibialis anterior and extensor hallucis longus the resulting unrestrained reflex activity of the peronei will lead to profound eversion of the foot (spastic pes valgus).

2. Preponderance of plantar flexors of feet and toes

In several patients with complete and also incomplete lesions resulting in marked spasticity of the paralysed legs, a profound preponderance of the plantar flexors of the feet and toes was found. Slightest stroking of the sole and tapping against the plantar surface of the toes (Rossolimo's sign) or the capitulum of the 5th metatarsal (Mendel-Bechterew's signs) produce brisk plantar contractions of the toes. This may occur in one leg only, though it was usually seen bilaterally. This may become exaggerated as a result either of keeping the feet and toes in plantar flexion during the stage of spinal shock, instead of at the right-angle, or as a result of a pressure lesion of the external popliteal nerve at the level of the head of the fibula through faulty position in the early stages following transection of the cord, resulting in peripheral paralysis of the antagonists of the plantar flexors, namely the dorsiflexors of foot and toes. This peripheral nerve lesion additional to the upper motor neuron lesion of the cord, can be diagnosed by the absence of any reflex response to cutaneous stimuli within the area of cutaneous distribution of the external popliteal nerve—for instance by pricking or stroking with a pin. Reflex responses to nociceptive cutaneous stimuli are obtained only at the border of the cutaneous distribution of this nerve. Moreover, electrical examination of the muscles in question and an electromyogram will reveal complete or incomplete R.D. of the muscles supplied by the external popliteal nerve.

3. Preponderance of crossed reflexes

These are very common in the spinal man but develop at a later stage of reflex return following spinal shock, when excitability and responsiveness of the reflex arcs have greatly increased and ankle and knee jerks as well as ipsilateral flexion reflex are well established. They occur in both complete and incomplete transverse lesions. The most common crossed reflex resulting from plantar stimulation of the foot is the extensor thrust of the contralateral leg, consisting of contraction of contralateral extensors of the hip, adductors, quadriceps and plantar flexion of the foot and toes. Fig. 107 demonstrates the crossed reflex-response of the feet and toes following plantar stimulation of the

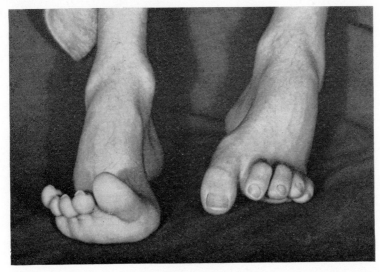

FIG. 107.

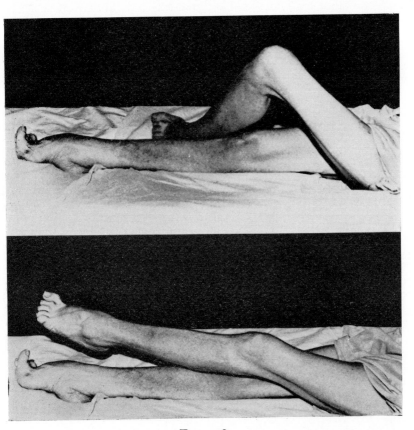

FIG. 108.

right foot. In cases with high degree of spasticity, alternating withdrawal contractions on one side and extensor thrust on the other may occur spontaneously or with only slight extrinsic stimulation and may become most disturbing to the patient, especially at night. On the other hand, the crossed extensor contractions of the legs associated with adductor contractions to unilateral stimulation may be the earliest true crossed reflex-response (Fig. 108). It has already been mentioned that in tetraplegics below C6/7, once the receptive field is extended over the whole area below the level of the lesion, strong unilateral plantar stimulation of the foot may result in ipsilateral and contralateral contraction of the paralysed extensors of the fingers (Fig. 106).

4. *Alternating and synchronous rhythmic contractions*

Rhythmic, alternating flexor and extensor contractions of the paralysed lower limbs have been previously described by Riddoch (1917) and Foerster (1936), and special mention may be made of the coitus reflex described by Riddoch as an example of rhythmic alternating flexion and extension synergies of the hips.

Rhythmic contraction confined to single muscles or muscle group may also occur synchronously. One of my patients, a young soldier with a complete lesion below T3 whose paraplegia since his injury in 1944 gradually developed from a flexion into an extension synergy, showed interesting rhythmic synchronous contractions occurring simultaneously only in the tibialis posterior on both sides (Fig. 109). These rhythmic contractions occurred spontaneously at rest in bed, but the intensity and rate could be increased by various stimuli including change of posture. Rhythmic continuous contrac-

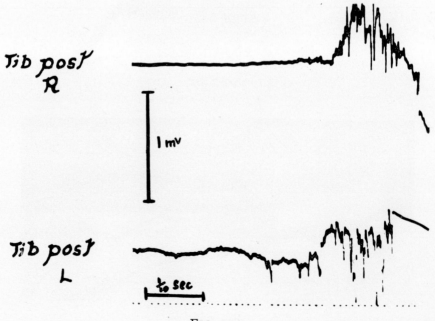

FIG. 109.

tions also may occur, although rarely, in the extensor group of the trunk erectors in complete and incomplete cervical lesions. They may become very troublesome to the patient and make his life miserable. In one of the writer's tetraplegics, these rhythmic contractions of the trunk erectors leading to spasmodic retroversion movements (opisthotonic reflex response) of the body could be eliminated following intra-thecal alcohol block at the level of the thoraco-lumbar junction, thus eliminating a considerable amount of volleys of afferent impulses to the heightened reflex activity of the isolated cord.

Superficial (cutaneous) reflexes

In cord transection above T5, abdominal and cremaster reflexes are, as a rule, abolished. However, this is by no means consistent, and in several complete lesions at high level these reflexes, although greatly diminished and easily exhaustible, were found to be present.

Failure of reflex return

Failure of reflex return will occur if the transverse lesion is associated with a lesion in the vertical plane. This may involve either only those muscle groups supplied by certain segments or all muscles below the level of the lesion, according to the extent of the longitudinal lesion. The areflexia will persist and involve the entire paralysed region and the muscle groups will show all signs of a lower motor neuron damage indicated by atrophy and reaction of degeneration to electrical test. In such instances, the grey matter of the isolated cord has sustained a definite damage either through haematomyelia or ischaemic necrosis, as a result of vascular occlusion.

As already mentioned, septic and toxic conditions leading to anoxia, in particular due to severe infection of the urinary tract or pressure sores, may profoundly affect the reflex activity of the isolated cord and may lead to hypo- and even areflexia, the latter in the final stages of life. On the other hand, it must be remembered that the onset of toxic conditions may lead first to an increase of spasticity. This was not infrequently found as the first symptom of a recurrence of urinary infection or even of an infected ingrowing toenail.

Clinical significance of paraplegia-in-flexion or -extension

FACTORS INFLUENCING REFLEX-SYNERGIES

Riddoch (1917), studying the activities of the flexor and extensor reflex arcs of the paralysed lower limbs advanced the theory that it is frequently possible to say whether conduction of the spinal cord has been completely destroyed or not. This has led to the conception that paraplegia-in-flexion is pathognomonic of complete transection of the cord while paraplegia-in-extension is pathognomonic of incomplete lesions. Moreover, Fulton, Liddell & Rioch's animal experiments (1930a, b) indicated that the extensor hypertonus depends on the transmission of postural reflexes along intact vestibulo-spinal and probably also ventro-reticulo-spinal pathways to the cord centres below the level of the lesion and only destruction of these tracts results in a preponderance of the flexor reflexes and paraplegia-in-flexion. However, experimental and clinical experiences have shown that Riddoch's theory is no longer tenable.

Sherrington found a variability in the order of recovery of the various spinal reflexes from spinal shock in the dog, following complete transection of the cord, and in some individuals a preponderance of extensor rigidity was evident: 'The limbs are kept extended at knee and ankle to a degree that it is difficult to break through by the inhibition accompanying elicitation of the flexion reflex stimulation of the foot'. Sherrington's explanation was that 'some incidental circumstances determining the preponderance of some passive attitude of the limb during the early days succeeding the lesion may, by its influence on the interaction of the recovering spinal arcs, impress an unwanted reflex habit about the limb'. Denny Brown & Liddell (1927, 1928) found that the predominant flexor reflex-activity in the stage of reflex automatism of the isolated cord following transection in the cat and dog was replaced in time by such strong extensor spasticity and rigidity that the animals were able to stand. In this connection, it may be remembered that Riddoch (1917) himself had found that, in later stages of heightened reflex activity of complete lesions, the difference in the tone of the extensor and flexor groups (the latter being predominant) becomes less marked. Foerster (1936) reported two cases of transection of the cord of over one year's duration, with preponderance of extension reflex synergy. In one of these cases, the extensor reflex of the legs could be elicited in both legs by stimuli applied to the ano-genital region. Further proof of the great variability in the reflex activity was given by Elkins & Wagner (1946), Scarff & Poole (1946), Scarff (1952), Dick (1949) and Kuhn (1950). The latter author found 19 amongst 28 patients with complete transection at levels between T2 and T12 who had extensor spasms predominant over flexor spasms.

The great number of traumatic paraplegic survivors from the First World War prompted me to study the important problem of factors influencing the patterns of reflex function in the spinal man (Guttmann, 1946, 1952, 1953, 1954, 1970). There is no doubt that septic conditions due to pressure sores and urinary infection as well as contractures of muscles and joints maintain and increase the predominant flexor synergy. Moreover, there can be no doubt about the great influence which the positioning of the paralysed limbs during the early stages of paraplegia has on the development of the patterns of reflex synergies in later stages, in both complete and incomplete lesions of the spinal cord. In particular, prolonged fixation of the paralysed limbs in adduction and semi-flexion, as is so often produced by the habit of nurses placing a pillow or other support under the knees, invariably promotes predominant flexor synergy and consequently paraplegia-in-flexion (Guttmann, 1946). The explanation is that the constant approximation of the insertion points of the flexors of hips and knees in such cases causes facilitation (Bahnung) of their stretch reflex, and at the same time the constant over-stretching of their antagonists, the extensors of hips and knees, result in a weakening of the stretch reflex of the latter. Conversely, in paraplegics with complete lesions who did not develop flexion contractures of legs and hips during the early stages through faulty positioning but remained free from septic conditions, the initially pre-dominant flexor reflex synergy gradually decreased in later stages and the extensor reflex synergy became predominant. Factors which have proved effectual in facilitating extensor activity are:

1   Placing the paralysed limbs during spinal shock in abduction and extension at hips and knees and keeping feet and toes in dorsi-flexion while the patient lies in supine position.

2   Placing the patient in prone position, which, particularly in high thoracic and cervical lesions, as in babies whose pyramidal tracts are not yet developed, promotes the extension reflex of the body.

3   Early passive movements of the paralysed limbs.

4   Restoration of the upright position of paraplegics and tetraplegics—in particular standing in parallel bars.

It has already been pointed out that prolonged overstretching of the skeletal muscles by faulty positioning of the paralysed limb causing structural damage of the muscle and resulting in unrestrained action of its antagonist represents an important factor in determining the reflex pattern of the paralysed limb. Another common cause of structural damage of a muscle and its peripheral nerve supply is pressure produced by plaster or splint. In this connection, the constant pressure against the capitulum fibulae, causing damage to the popliteal nerve and thus resulting in additional peripheral nerve lesion of the tibialis anterior and the dorsi-flexors of the toes, is one of the frequent causes of the predominance of the plantar flexors of the toes and feet.

CHAPTER 24

SYMPTOMATOLOGY

A. COMPLETE TRANSVERSE SPINAL SYNDROMES AT DIFFERENT LEVELS

HIGH THORACIC AND CERVICAL LESIONS

Certain symptoms are common to all complete cervical and upper thoracic lesions. These are:

1 Areflexia or hyporeflexia of both motor and autonomic systems during the stage of spinal shock;
2 Hyperreflexia of skeletal muscles in later stage;
3 Postural hypotension;
4 Automatic bladder and bowel function;
5 Autonomic hyperreflexia due to visceral distension and visceral hyperactivity.

UPPER CERVICAL SEGMENTS, C1–C4

Traumatic lesions of the upper cervical cord following fracture-dislocations of the atlas or epistropheus may be confined solely to C1–C4 segments, while, on the other hand, pathological processes such as tumours originating from these segments may ascend and involve also cranial nerves of the oblongata. Conversely, tumours originating at the level of the foramen magnum may first manifest themselves by the symptomatology of upper cervical cord compression. Pain in the neck and occipital region, intensified by movements of the head, combined with paraesthesia over the C2 distribution and followed by paraesthesia such as sensation of intense cold and spastic weakness of the upper and lower limbs, either unilaterally or bilaterally, are early symptoms of such a cord involvement (Naffziger & Brown, 1933; Symonds & Meadows, 1937; Bennett & Fortes, 1945). Involvement of one or both vertebral arteries may lead to disturbances of their distal branches, resulting in atrophy of muscles of the forearm and hand and thus simulating amyothrophic lateral sclerosis. Involvement of the unilateral spinal trigeminal tract may cause sensory disturbances in the face of lamelliform type. Tapping of occiput or mastoid process may produce reflex contractions to greater or lesser degree of the upper cervical muscles (trapezius and sternomastoid).

In complete transverse syndromes of the upper cervical segments, splenius capitis, recti and obliqui, sternohyoideus, geniohyoideus, and thyreohyoideus are paralysed, and only trapezius, sternomastoid and platysma are still acting owing to their innervation by the accessory and facial nerves respectively. The greatest complication in traumatic lesions is the paralysis of the diaphragm resulting from the interruption of the segmental innervation of the phrenic nerve. As all other respiratory muscles below the transection are also paralysed, this respiratory paralysis will lead to death within the shortest time, unless tracheostomy and artificial respiration are carried out immediately. However, in transverse lesions confined to C4—for instance, following stab wounds—the segmental innervation of the phrenic nerve by C3 may be sufficient to ensure good function of the diaphragm, once the post-traumatic oedema of the cervical cord above the transection has subsided.

Below the transection, all voluntary movements in both upper and lower limbs as well as trunk are abolished and, as soon as the stage of spinal shock is over, spasticity and rigidity of these muscles develops. The spastic paralysis of the arms is one in extension. Furthermore, all forms of sensibility, control of bladder, bowels and sexual function as well as vasomotor control and heat regulation are abolished.

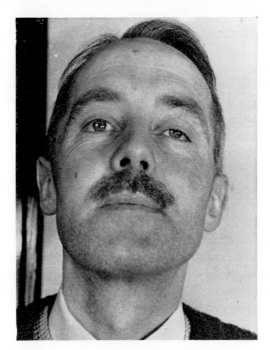

FIG. 110.

One of the classical symptoms is the unilateral or bilateral Horner's syndrome as a result of the interruption of the oculopupillary fibres, which originate in the hypothalamus and descend in the anterolateral tract to the ciliospinal centre which is situated in the intermediolateral horns of C8, T1 and T2 (Fig. 110). There may be dissociation in the paralysis of the three components of Horner's syndrome: dilator of the pupil, involuntary superior palpebral muscle (Müller's muscle) and the hypothetical orbital involuntary muscle (Landström's muscle). Furthermore, as a result of the vasoconstrictor paralysis there is at first a marked paralytic vasodilatation involving also the face and resulting in blockage of the nasal air passages (Guttmann's sign), and without tracheostomy the patient's mouth is almost permanently open to enable shallow respiration in these cases.

The patient has difficulty in talking and speaks with a low and nasal voice in a rather staccato fashion. He also has difficulty in swallowing. The respiratory rate is increased and the patient uses the few remaining auxiliary respiratory muscles, trapezius, sterno-mastoid, platysma and alae nasi. The vital capacity may be practically nil or as low as 50–100 ml. The patient is unable to cough and even with a tracheostomy tube *in situ* cannot bring up mucus; his respiration becomes bubbly if the mucus is not removed by suction or tilting the patient down. His colour may become cyanotic owing to obstruction of the air passage resulting from accumulated secretion and collapse of a lung may occur. He may become increasingly irrational and finally lose consciousness as a result of anoxia.

The sensory loss in complete lesions involving C2 and C3 segments affects the whole body, including the occipital area, the ear and submental region of the face. In lesions at C4 the sensory loss reaches up to the middle of the neck but leaves the ear and sub-mental area free.

Until recently, tetraplegics with transverse upper cervical lesions were doomed to death within a few hours or days, but with the modern means of management they can survive for a considerable time and can even become wheelchair bound. There is an improvement in the vital capacity of the lung, due to strong compensatory action of trapezius and sternomastoid, the latter sometimes becoming hypertrophic. They are able to move about in an especially adapted electrically driven wheelchair, which they control by movements of the head. However, these patients will remain liable to lung collapse and, particularly, pneumonia, especially in the age group over 40. As a rule, the life expectation of these very high tetraplegics is greatly shortened.

C5 SEGMENT

In the acute stage of a complete transverse lesion at C5, the function of the diaphragm is greatly impaired if not completely abolished as a result of post-traumatic oedema. Moreover, meteorism as a result of the initial intestinal paralysis will aggravate the respiratory distress, as described in upper cervical lesions, and tracheostomy may become imperative. However, in due course the diaphragm will regain its full function, once the segmental innervation of the phrenic nerve has fully recovered from its initial shock. Moreover, as levator scapulae (C3–C5) and rhomboids (C4–C5) are only partially dener-vated and trapezius and sternomastoid are intact, the vital capacity of the lung will, in due course, be definitely better than in the upper cervical lesions. Supra- and infraspinatus (C4–C5) will also be only impaired and some outward rotation of the arm will be possible. The muscles deprived of their segmental innervation are deltoid, biceps, brachialis internus, brachioradialis and supinator brevis. The deltoid, biceps and supinator reflexes are either abolished or greatly diminished. The arms lie motionless alongside the body (Fig. 111). The shoulder may be markedly elevated due to the uninhibited action of levator scapulae and trapezius, as a result of the paralysis of the depressors of the shoulders. In recent years, it has been suggested that the segmental innervation of the biceps is somewhat higher than that of the deltoid (Grossiord *et al.*, 1963). I cannot confirm this from personal experience. The reflexes below the level of the lesions become exaggerated and this applies also to the spastic finger flexion reflex. Moreover, a tap on

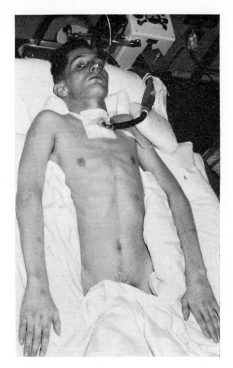

FIG. III.

the distal end of the radius may elicit exaggerated finger flexion (inversion of the radius reflex).

The loss of sensibility involves the body, including the arms, but leaves the neck and a triangular area of the anterior aspect of the upper arm free.

C6 SEGMENTS

Although at this level the segmental innervation of the diaphragm is well above the level of the lesion, its function may be interfered with initially by the ascending oedema of the cord or by the meteorism as a result of the intestinal paralysis, and a tracheostomy may become a life-saving measure. Tetraplegics at that level exhibit a very characteristic abnormality of posture of their arms. As a result of the segmental paralysis of the depressors of the shoulder and adductors of the arms (pectorals, C6–C8), latissimus dorsi (C6–C7–C8), internal rotators of the arms (subscapularis, C5–C7), and extensor of the forearm (triceps, C6–C8), the shoulders are elevated, the arms are abducted and the forearms are flexed due to uninhibited action of deltoid, biceps and brachioradialis. Furthermore, the segmental paralysis of lower motor neuron type also involves the extensor carpi radialis longus. All other hand and finger muscles innervated below C6 are paralysed as are all muscles of trunk and lower limbs.

Of utmost importance from a practical point of view is the avoidance of permanent flexion of the forearm due to overaction of the flexors resulting from paralysis of the triceps. This easily leads to flexion contractures of the elbow joints—indeed a very serious complication greatly aggravating the disability of the tetraplegic (Fig. 8). It must be remembered that the degree of segmental innervation of the triceps by the 6th, 7th and 8th cervical segments shows individual variations. In certain cases, the segmental innervation of C6 may be strong enough to compensate to some degree the loss of C7 and C8. Therefore, the degree of functional recovery of the triceps due to this remaining innervation of C6 depends largely on the efficiency of the early management of the upper limbs in tetraplegics. If the triceps during the stage of denervation is allowed to become overstretched by faulty positioning of the forearms in permanent flexion, its functional recovery, if it occurs at all, will be very poor. Therefore, in transverse lesions of C6 attention must be paid to keeping the forearm in extension and the arms in adduction.

The deltoid and biceps reflexes are often exaggerated but the triceps reflex is absent. Tapping of the triceps produces contraction of the biceps (inversion of the triceps reflex). The degree of spasticity of all muscles below the level of the lesion varies and the paralysis of the lower limbs may be one in flexion or extension. With regard to the extent of the reflex responses to extrinsic and intrinsic stimuli see page 249.

The sensory loss in the upper limbs involves the forearms, hands and fingers including the thumbs. The sensibility over the lateral aspect of the arms including the dorsolateral aspect of half of the forearm is intact as this is supplied by C5.

C7 SEGMENT

As a rule, the function of the diaphragm and auxiliary respiratory muscles is strong enough to compensate for the paralysis of the intercostal and abdominal muscles, and tracheostomy is indicated in selected cases only when complications develop. The posture of the arms is still one of abduction and external rotation although sometimes less pronounced than in C6 lesions since the adductors and internal rotators (subscapularis, pectoralis major, teres major and latissimus dorsi) are only partly paralysed. The forearm is kept in flexion due to overaction of the biceps. However, as already pointed out, in a considerable number of complete lesions at C7, especially when confined to its more distal part, the C6 innervation of the triceps is strong enough to compensate for the loss of the C7–C8 innervation of this muscle and, in due course, may ensure its function against resistance and sometimes even against gravity, provided faulty positioning of the forearm in permanent flexion has been prevented from the start. This experience is not in accordance with Foerster's (1936) view, who found the triceps always totally paralysed in complete lesions at C7. The more the transverse lesion is confined to the distal part of C7 the stronger the function of the triceps.

In contrast to complete lesions at C6, the extensor carpi radialis longus is functioning and the hand shows radial deviation. However, if the lesion involves the more distal part of the nuclear part of C7, the extensor carpi radialis brevis is also functioning and the hand shows less radial deviation. Moreover, in such an instance, there is also some, though reduced, function of the extensor digitorum communis, especially of the extensor indicis proprius. The function of the pronator teres and flexor carpi radialis is reduced and so is the function of the flexors digitorum sublimis and profundus and also flexor pollicis longus.

Biceps and radius reflexes are present, the triceps reflex may still be of paradox type. The finger flexion reflex is exaggerated once the isolated cord develops its automatic reflex function.

The sensory loss involves, apart from the body, the inner side of the arms and fore-arms as well as the ulnar side of the hands including the 5th–3rd fingers, sometimes also to some degree the index finger.

C8 SEGMENT

There is no longer that abnormal posture of the upper limbs as described in C6 and C7 lesions, for the adductors and internal rotators of the arms are strong enough to counter-act the overaction of their antagonists. The same applies to the triceps which can now definitely extend the forearm against gravity and in due course regains full power. The latissimus dorsi in co-operation with trapezius becomes strong enough to ensure the upright position of the tetraplegic. The pronator teres can equalize the overaction of the supinators of the hand, and the action of extensor carpi radialis brevis prevents the radial deviation of the hand, caused by the extensor carpi radialis longus, the more so as the extensor carpi ulnaris and flexor carpi ulnaris are also functioning; the long finger flexors are now stronger. Moreover, the flexor pollicis longus and brevis, extensor pollicis longus and abductor pollicis longus muscles are also working. The extensor pollicis brevis, interossei and opponens are still greatly reduced in power or paralysed, and abductor pollicis brevis is still completely paralysed as this muscle is mono-segmen-tally innervated by T1. The paralysis of the interossei and lumbricals results in a claw-hand due to overaction of the extensor digitorum communis and flexor digitorum sublimis and profundus. This, however, does not prevent the tetraplegic at that level from writing, feeding himself, typing and taking up sport such as table tennis and archery (see chapters on Physiotherapy and Sport).

Bilateral or unilateral Horner's syndrome and disturbances of sweating involving face, arms and upper part of the trunk are present. The triceps reflex is either still absent or diminished and so is the finger flexion reflex. The sensory loss includes the 5th and 4th finger and hypothenar eminence and medial side of arm and forearm.

The respiratory distress is, as a rule, less pronounced. However, the loss of vasomotor control is still apparent when the patient is raised from the horizontal to the upright position but this can be overcome by training (see chapter on Physiotherapy).

In the past, life expectancy of tetraplegics involving even the distal cervical segments was considered as very short—as a rule, no longer than a few months. Advances made in the initial treatment of these patients has changed this dramatically (Guttmann, 1964). Therefore, the problem of tetraplegia has become a social problem of increasing import-ance from year to year.

T1 SEGMENT

Flexor digitorum profundus and sublimis, flexor policis longus and brevis, extensor pollicis longus and brevis, abductor pollicus longus and opponens are functioning and triceps has its full power. However, there is partial paralysis of the adductor pollicis, interossei and lumbricals. The abductor pollicis brevis is still paralysed. Foerster has always emphasized that this muscle is the only monosegmentally innervated muscle of the upper limbs and my own experience is in accordance with his view in the great majority of cases. C8 may also take part in its innervation in individual cases.

There is also a nuclear Horner's syndrome and anhidrosis in face, neck and arm (Fig. 110). The triceps reflex is present. The sensory loss in the upper limbs involves the medial side of the forearm and distal part of the upper arm. Figs. 115a and b demonstrate the sensory loss of touch, pain and temperature sensibility following resection of the posterior root of T1. The loss or marked impairment of the interossei and lumbricals in C8/T1 lesions is a handicap in the adduction phase of the arms during swimming competitions!

T1–T5 SEGMENTS

While in transverse lesions at T1 the respiration is still of some diaphragmatic type, the inspiratory function of the lungs increases the lower the level of the upper thoracic lesion, commensurate with the increase of function of the intercostal muscles. Therefore, in lesions at T5 the inspiratory function of the lung is already very strong. Moreover, the extension of the upper thoracic spine is also much stronger as compared with that of higher thoracic and cervical lesions.

The common symptom of complete transverse lesions above T5, especially in T1 and cervical lesions, is the loss or impairment of the vasomotor control resulting in postural hypotension leading to syncope when raising the patient from the horizontal to the upright position.

The sensory loss in T2 lesions extends up the whole body to the inner side of the upper arm, in T3 lesions it includes the axilla, in T5 lesions the nipples.

T6–T12 SEGMENTS

In complete transverse lesions from T6 downwards the individual segments of the rectus abdominis and of the lateral abdominal muscles are spared. In lesions T6–T9, the supra-umbilical segments of the rectus abdominis are functioning and on voluntary action the umbilicus is pulled upwards. A simple test to provoke this action is the so-called 'kit-test', whereby with the sudden forced expiration on calling the word 'kit' the umbilicus is pulled upwards in these lesions. In transverse lesions below T10 the infra-umbilical segments of the rectus are acting and the upward pull of the umbilicus disappears, but the distal lateral parts of the abdomen are forced out on abdominal pressure on account of the paralysis of the lower fibres of obliquus internus and transversalis abdominis. In lesions below T12 all abdominal muscles are functioning with full power.

All abdominal reflexes are abolished in T6 lesions, while in lesions at and below T10 the upper and middle abdominal reflexes are present. In T12 lesions, all abdominal reflexes are present, but the cremasteric reflexes are absent. Knee and ankle jerks become exaggerated and, as in all transverse lesions above the thoraco-lumbar junction, the paralysis of the lower limbs is of spastic type.

The sensory loss in T6 lesions extends to the xiphoid, in T7/8 to the lower costal margin, in T10 to the umbilicus and in T12 to the groin.

TRANSVERSE LESIONS OF THE LUMBAR CORD (EPICONUS AND CONUS)

These may still be of spastic type below the transection if the lesion is confined to the lumbar segments. While the knee jerks are reduced or absent as a result of the involvement of L2–L4 segments, the ankle jerks are present and may be exaggerated, including ankle clonus. If L4 has escaped, the knee jerks may be present, though diminished, but plantar stimulation may provoke withdrawal response, and Babinski's sign and its modifications (Oppenheim, Gordon and Chaddock) are positive. In lesions also involving L5, knee jerks and Babinski's sign are absent but ankle jerks are still positive and so are Rossolimo's and Mendel-Bechterew's signs. However, not infrequently, traumatic lesions of the 12th dorsal and the first two upper lumbar vertebrae result in destruction of the distal thoracic and lumbosacral cord, resulting in areflexia and paralysis of lower motor neuron type. This applies in particular to the epiconus syndrome affecting L4–S2 segments.

With regard to the disturbances of bladder, bowels and sexual functions in these distal lesions, see the chapter dealing with these functions. In the following, only the paralysis of the muscular system, reflexes and sensory functions are discussed.

L1 SEGMENT

The quadratus lumborum is still reduced in power and all muscles of the lower limbs are paralysed, including cremasterics, iliopsoas and sartorius. The cremasteric reflex is absent. Knee and ankle jerks are exaggerated and the pyramidal signs, as mentioned above, may be present.

Sensory loss involves all areas of the lower limbs and extends to the groins and to the back above the buttocks.

L2 SEGMENT

All distal abdominal muscles and cremasterics are intact and there is also some, although reduced, function of iliopsoas and sartorius. Sometimes the sartorius may be the only muscle present at this level and its contour is clearly visible underneath the skin on voluntary contraction. There is also a flicker of the gracilis. The cremasteric reflex is positive.

Sensory loss involves the lower limbs with the exception of the upper third of the anterior aspect of the thighs.

L3 SEGMENT

There is better hip flexion, due to increased function of iliopsoas and sartorius, and the adduction of the legs is also increased, due to action of the adductor longus, pectineus and gracilis. The legs are outwards rotated. The function of the rectus femoris is reduced. The knee jerks may be absent or greatly reduced.

Sensory function is present over two-thirds of the anterior aspect of the thighs, otherwise there is a complete sensory loss over the lower limbs, including the saddle area.

L4 SEGMENT

Hip flexion and adduction is quite powerful and the outwards rotation of the legs is more marked as the presence of the obturator externus adds to the function of the iliopsoas in this respect. Sartorius is strong enough to produce some flexion of the knee. Extension of the leg is also increased due to greater power of the rectus femoris which is now supported by the function of vastus lateralis and medialis. The patient is able to stand and walk slowly on even ground by stabilizing the knees fairly well but is not able or has greatest difficulty to walk upstairs. Moreover, as a result of the paralysis of the gluteus medius the oscillation of the pelvis in the frontal plane is impeded during walking and the gait is of wobbling type which is similar to the insufficiency of the abductors in congenital dislocation of the hip. The knee jerks are absent.

Sensory function is present over the whole anterior aspect of the thighs, extending distally to the upper medial aspect of the knees, otherwise there is complete sensory loss in legs and saddle area.

L5 SEGMENT

Hip flexion and adduction is of full power and so is extension of the leg. The quadriceps is of full strength and, as the main flexor of the knee, the biceps femoris is still paralysed and the inner hamstrings are not strong enough to counteract the strong action of the quadriceps, this results in hyperextension of the knee during walking and may lead, without appropriate caliper preventing hyperextension, to a genu recurvatum. Although the tensor fasciae latae and gluteus medius are functioning, their power is not strong enough to prevent the wobbling gait, although this is less pronounced than in L4 lesions. Below the knee the tibialis anterior and posterior are functioning, and, as the segmental innervation of the former is almost entirely by L4, its action is very powerful resulting in equino-varus position of the foot as its antagonists, the peroneal muscles, are still paralysed. Knee jerks are elicitable.

Sensory function is present over the whole anterior aspect of the thighs and the medial aspect of the legs, including inner ankle and innerside of the soles, while the dorsum of the feet, outer aspect of the legs and ankles and posterior aspect of the lower limbs and the saddle area are anaesthetic.

S1–S2 SEGMENTS

The S1 syndrome is characterized through the position of the foot in dorsiflexion (pes calcaneum), as a result of the paralysis of the triceps surae and flexors of the toes, and, therefore, there is overaction of the extensor digitorum longus, extensor hallucis longus and tibialis anterior. The foot is no longer in extreme supination as the peronei are of good power. Flexion of the foot in pronation is possible by action of the peroneus longus through its insertion on the first metatarsal. The function of semitendinosus and semi-membranosus is increased but biceps femoris may still be paralysed or show only weak function. The ankle jerks are absent and may be paradox (dorsiflexion of the foot); plantar stimulation does not produce any response.

Sensibility is lost over the whole sole and outer aspect of the foot below the outer ankle, heel and middle aspect of the calf as well as posterior part of the thighs and saddle area. However, the hollow of the knee is sensitive due to overlap from L3, L4 and L5 segments.

In S2 lesions the pes calcaneum is no longer present, as gastrocnemius and soleus

TABLE 9. Segmental innervation of the muscles of the upper limb

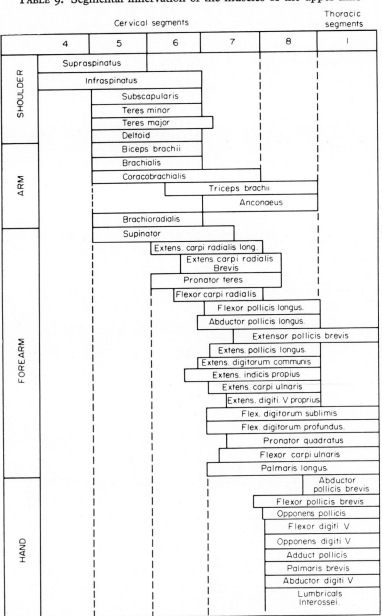

TABLE 10. Segmental innervation of the trunk muscles

	Cervical segments								Thoracic segments												Lumbar segments					Sacral segments					Coc.
1	2	3	4	5	6	7	8	1	2	3	4	5	6	7	8	9	10	11	12	1	2	3	4	5	1	2	3	4	5		

Short deep neck muscles

Deep long muscles of the back

Splenius muscles

Latissim. dorsi.

Trapezius

Levat. scap.

Rhom- boids

Longus colli

Longus Capitis

Scalenes

Pectoralis major

Pectoralis minor

Sub- clavius

Serrat. ant.

Diaphragm

Serrat. post. sup.

Serrat. post. inf.

Rectus abdominis

Ex. oblique, abdom.

Transverse abdom.

Int. oblique, abdom.

Quadratus lumborum

Intercostal muscles

Levator, sphinc-ter ani, perineal, and coccyg. m's

TABLE II. Segmental innervation of muscles of the lower limb

Region	Muscle	Th12	L1	L2	L3	L4	L5	S1	S2	S3
HIP	Iliopsoas		X	X	X					
HIP	Tensor fasc. lat.					X	X	X		
HIP	Glutaeus medius					X	X	X		
HIP	Glutaeus minimus					X	X	X		
HIP	Quadratus femoris					X	X	X	X	
HIP	Gemellus inferior					X	X	X	X	
HIP	Gemellus superior					X	X	X	X	
HIP	Glutaeus maximums						X	X	X	X
HIP	Obturat. int.						X	X	X	
HIP	Piriformis						X	X	X	
THIGH	Sartorius		X	X	X					
THIGH	Pectineus			X	X					
THIGH	Adduct. longus		X	X	X					
THIGH	Quadriceps femoris			X	X	X				
THIGH	Gracilis		X	X	X					
THIGH	Adductor brevis			X	X	X				
THIGH	Obturator ext.				X	X				
THIGH	Adduct. magn.				X	X	X			
THIGH	Adduct. minim.				X	X				
THIGH	Articularis gen.				X	X				
THIGH	Semitendinosus					X	X	X	X	
THIGH	Semimembranosus					X	X	X	X	
THIGH	Biceps femoris						X	X	X	X
LEG	Tibialis ant.					X	X			
LEG	Extensor halluc. long.					X	X	X		
LEG	Popliteus					X	X	X		
LEG	Plantaris					X	X	X		
LEG	Extensor digit. longus					X	X	X		
LEG	Soleus						X	X	X	
LEG	Gastrocnemius						X	X	X	
LEG	Peroneus longus					X	X	X		
LEG	Peroneus brevis					X	X	X		
LEG	Tibialis posterior					X	X			
LEG	Flexor digit long.						X	X	X	
LEG	Flexor hallucis longus						X	X	X	
FOOT	Extensor halluc. brevis					X	X	X		
FOOT	Extensor digit. brevis					X	X	X		
FOOT	Flex. digit. brev.						X	X		
FOOT	Abduct. hall.						X	X	X	
FOOT	Flexor hall. brevis						X	X	X	
FOOT	Lumbricals						X	X	X	X
FOOT	Adduct. hall.							X	X	
FOOT	Abduct digit. V							X	X	
FOOT	Flexor digit. V							X	X	
FOOT	Opponens digit. V							X	X	
FOOT	Quadrat. plant.							X	X	
FOOT	Interossei.							X	X	X

are functioning, but the patient is not able to stand on his toes due to the paralysis of the long flexors and intrinsic muscles of the toes. There is full extension and abduction of the hip, as the gluteal muscles are of full power, and so is flexion of the leg as the biceps femoris is intact. The ankle jerk may be weakly positive. Plantar stimulation may produce dorsiflexion of the toes (peripheral Babinski), due to the paralysis or weakness of the plantar flexors of the toes. The foot shows claw-toes formation as a result of the paralysis of the intrinsic muscles of the toes.

Sensibility is lost over the upper posterior aspect of the calf the postero-lateral aspect of the thigh and the saddle area.

S3–S5 SEGMENTS

There is no paralysis of any leg muscles. The paralysis is confined to bladder, bowels and sexual functions. The knee and ankle jerks are present but the anal and bulbo-cavernosus reflex is abolished. The loss of sensibility involves the saddle area, including the posterior and the two distal thirds of the anterior aspects of the scrotum, the glans penis, perineum, the anal area and extends to the upper third of the posterior aspect of the thighs.

Various authors have published charts of the segmental innervation of individual muscles (Bruns, Lazarus, Flatau, Edinger, Bing, Villiger). My own muscle chart is mainly in accordance with that of Foerster (1927) with certain modifications arising from my own experience on spinal cord injuries (Tables 9–11).

B. INCOMPLETE LESIONS OF THE SPINAL CORD

There are great variations in incomplete cord lesions depending on aetiology, level of the lesion and degree of damage to the various components of the neural elements. They can be conveniently divided into two main groups, viz. (1) pathological processes affecting diffusely more or less all the neurons as well as the efferent and afferent tracts at any level but not resulting in complete interruption of their functions, and (2) circumscribed processes affecting distinct parts of the cord and resulting in incomplete lesions of dissociated type.

As far as the peripheral neurons of the anterior horns and their synapses are concerned, either there may be paralysis of lower motor neuron type of all muscles innervated by the segment or segments at the level of the lesion, or some muscles supplied by the same segment have escaped damage completely or are only slightly damaged.

In acute incomplete lesions following vertebral fractures affecting the supranuclear pathways, namely the pyramidal and extrapyramidal tracts, there is at first hypo- or areflexia during the stage of spinal shock, but, as a rule, the reflexes below the level of the lesion will soon return and become exaggerated. However, in severe though incomplete traumatic lesions of the cord both at high level and, in particular, below T10, T11 and T12 level, reflex return below the level of the lesions may be considerably delayed. In the majority of cases, provided the initial positioning of the paralysed legs was correct, there may be preponderance of extension synergy rather than flexion synergy, but the contrary, namely flexion synergy, may occur if the legs were kept in continuous flexion. The flexor–withdrawal reflex in incomplete lesions may be one-phased—i.e. the extremity may not return to its original position—or it may do so (two-phase reaction). Therefore, these reflex responses are not indicative of a distinction between complete transverse lesions (one-phase response) and incomplete lesions. If not all supranuclear pathways are interrupted and, especially, if the extrapyramidal tracts remain intact, voluntary function below the level of the lesion is more or less preserved. The paresis is of spastic type in extension.

Various observers have drawn attention to the occasional development of atrophy of the hand muscles, in particular in the intrinsic muscles of the fingers in high cervical or atlanto-axial lesions, which may lead to misinterpretation and diagnosis of amyotrophic lateral sclerosis or syringomyelia. The cause of this phenomenon lies in an impairment of the blood supply at high cervical level. It must be remembered that most of the vascular supply to the cervical cord runs down the anterior spinal artery originating from the vertebral arteries. Therefore, very high cervical or atlanto-axial lesion, caused by tumour or fracture, may block the arterial supply in these areas, resulting in impairment of the descending blood supply to the distal parts of the cervical cord and giving rise to clinical symptoms of lower cervical level.

There exists a lamellar arrangement of the fibres within the pyramidal tracts (somatotopic division) which accounts for the variations in extent of the supranuclear paralysis affecting individual areas of the body. This is particularly conspicuous in incomplete lesions of the cervical cord, where the pyramidal fibres for the upper limbs are situated medially within the pyramidal tract area while the fibres for the lower limbs lie eccentrically and those for the trunk in the middle of the tract. This anatomical arrangement explains the variations in spastic paresis involving various parts of the body, especially in extramedullary tumours of the cervical cord. Symonds & Meadows (1937) described in detail the clinical symptomatology of tumour compression of the cervical cord in the neighbourhood of the foramen magnum. They found in four of their cases, where the compression of the tumour was to one side of the midline, that the spastic paresis was first noticeable in the ipsilateral upper limb followed by weakness of the ipsilateral lower limb. However, in two of their cases they found, in confirmation of Elsberg's (1929) experience, that the weakness of upper motor neuron type developed in the contralateral lower limb. Moreover, in one of their cases, the weakness developed after lumbar puncture and was confined to the upper limbs and affected both equally, although the tumour was situated laterally.

Such lamelliform arrangement also exists, as mentioned before, in the afferent tracts, both the spinothalamic and posterior column tracts, which is also particularly apparent in the cervical cord.

Incomplete lesions of the spinal cord may also affect autonomous mechanism. In cervical lesions, fibres concerned with oculopupillary activity and originating in the hypothalamus pass to the cilio-spinal centre of T1 and T2 segments through the anterolateral tracts, in close relation to the pyramidal tracts. Unilateral cordotomy carried out above T1 always results in Horner's syndrome of the ipsilateral side associated with disturbances

of vasomotor and sudomotor function and the same may occur in incomplete lesions of
the cervical cord as a result of fracture dislocations of the spine or tumours. There may
be dissociations in degree of involvement between the various components of the autonomic mechanisms. Disturbances of sweating in cervical lesions may be patchy and involve
only certain segments or areas of the body below the level of the lesion. As the
Horner's syndrome at that level is of central—i.e. supranuclear type—the reflex response
of its components to afferent impulses, especially the dilator pupillae, is increased and
may lead to spasmodic pupillodilation or constriction (called by Pierre Marie in 1892 miosis
à bascules). Cocaine applied to the conjunctiva dilates the pupil in these supranuclear
lesions in contrast to its negative effect in peripheral lesions of the oculopupillary system.

Bladder, bowel and sexual function may more or less be affected in incomplete
lesions, and there may be considerable dissociations in the degree of involvement in
these functions depending on the level, type and acuteness of the lesion. Incomplete
lesions may be so light as to result in slight precipitate micturition only, on the other hand
they may for all practical purposes produce the same total retention as a complete
transection of the cord. Sexual disturbances may vary from ejaculatio praecox to complete impotence.

Manifestations of distinct incomplete cord lesions

It has already been pointed out that symptoms or syndromes of incomplete lesions
resulting from injury or disease depend on the degree of damage affecting the various
sections of the grey or white matter of the cord. The main syndromes which may occur
either separately or in combination are listed below.

Anterior horn syndrome

Destruction of the ganglion cells in the anterior horns leads to muscular paralysis of
lower motor neuron type. The affected muscles are atonic and there is areflexia, reaction
of degeneration and atrophy. Virus infections, in particular poliomyelitis, are the main
causes, but vascular processes such as atherosclerosis and meningovascular syphilis may
also lead to amyotrophy without affecting the pyramidal tracts. Anterior horn lesions
may involve all muscles of the extremities as well as the trunk, but as a rule spare muscles
or muscle groups scattered over a considerable area of the body resulting in dissociated
types of lower motor neuron paralysis.

Anterior horn lesions are not infrequently combined with vasomotor disturbances,
such as cyanosis and coldness as a result of an associated damage to the lateral horns.
Moreover, disturbances of sweating may also occur as studied in detail during a polio
epidemic in Silesia, Germany, in 1932 (Guttmann, 1933).

Pyramidal tract syndrome

There is a variety of intrinsic (congenital, hereditary) and extrinsic (syphilis, avitam-
inosis) degenerative processes resulting in selective degeneration of the pyramidal tracts
which are grouped together under the collective term 'Spastic Spinal Paralysis'. Amongst

the congenital varieties a spinal form of Little's disease may be mentioned which is practically confined to the lower limbs. The same applies to a certain form of disseminated sclerosis. Isolated damage to the pyramidal tracts following acute injury of the spinal cord is very rare but it is not uncommon as residual syndrome following rcovery of incomplete traumatic lesions and following removal of extramedullary tumours of the spinal cord.

Combined anterior horn and pyramidal tract syndrome

The clinical picture is characterized by muscular paralysis of peripheral type, combined with pyramidal signs such as exaggeration of reflexes and pathological reflexes such as spastic finger-flexion reflex, Babinski, etc. Corresponding to the number of affected muscles of lower motor neuron damage, the hyperreflexia may disappear in later stages. Amyotrophic lateral sclerosis is the classical representative of this combined anterior horn and pyramidal tract involvement. Fibrillations and fasciculation of muscles are the early manifestations of degenerative changes of the anterior horn cells.

Combined anterior horn and anterolateral tract syndrome

This is a relatively frequent syndrome in incomplete lesions of the cord, characterized by segmental muscular paralysis of lower motor neuron type and, below the level of the lesion, by bilateral spasticity and dissociated sensory loss—i.e. analgesia and thermo-anaesthesia—while touch and posterior column sensibility remain intact. This syndrome is caused by damage to the anterior spinal artery following fracture dislocations of the spine, anterior spinal artery thrombosis or compression of extramedullary tumours. Bladder, bowels and sexual functions are also involved.

Combined posterior column and lateral tract syndrome

Loss of posterior column sensibility resulting in ataxy combined with spasticity due to pyramidal tract involvement is the clinical symptom. This syndrome may be due to impairment of the posterior spinal arteries supply, toxic and degenerative processes, deficiency disease, traumatic lesions or tumours compressing the posterior aspect of the cord. Subacute combined degeneration of the cord (posterior lateral sclerosis) associated with progressive pernicious anaemia is the classical example of this syndrome due to a deficiency disease, while Friedreich's ataxia represents the hereditary degenerative form of this syndrome. The degeneration is most marked in the posterior columns, especially the fasciculus gracilis, being more pronounced in the lower part of the cord, although the pyramidal and dorsal spinocerebellar tracts as well as Clarke's column are also involved. Brown (1892) described a variety of hereditary ataxy in five successive generations of the same family. While the histological examination revealed degeneration of the cells of Clarke's column, the posterior columns and the dorsal spinocerebellar tracts, there was practically no degeneration of the pyramidal tracts.

Central syndromes

The two classical representations of a central damage or destruction of the spinal cord are haematomyelia and syringomyelia. While the former is characterized by an acute onset and rapid progression caused most commonly by traumatic influences, with or without fractures of the vertebral column, the latter is of very insidious onset and slow progression. In both afflictions the cervico-thoracic area is the commonest site of the lesion. The initial symptom of haemotomyelia is pain or paraesthesia in the neck radiating into one or both arms followed by rapid development of muscular weakness or paralysis of peripheral type due to damage or destruction of the anterior horn cells. The sensory disturbances are due to destruction of the sensory fibres in the grey matter. When the destruction is limited to the posterior grey commissure affecting the sensory fibres at their decussation, analgesia and thermoanaesthesia over a greater or lesser number of segments result. When the haemorrhage is large enough to affect or compress the spino-thalamic and posterior column tracts, impairment or loss of all forms of sensibility in one or both lower limbs will occur. There is also spastic paresis or paralysis below the level of the lesion due to involvement of the pyramidal tracts. Bladder, bowel and sexual functions are also involved and show various types of impairment.

In syringomyelia the commonest early symptoms are wasting and weakness of the small muscles of the hands. As a result of the elongation of the syringomyelitic cavity, most frequently situated at the base of the posterior horns, the decussations of sensory fibres derived from the posterior roots are damaged, and pain and temperature sensibility is impaired or abolished (dissociated sensory loss). When at a later date the spino-thalamic tracts are compressed, pain and temperature sensibility is impaired or lost over the greater part of the body and the lower limbs, but this sensory disturbance may be of patchy or segmental type. The same applies to the disturbances of sweating (Guttmann & List, 1928). When the syringomyelitic process advances to the upper cervical area, the spinal trigeminal tract may be involved, resulting in a concentric type of dissociated sensory loss of the face. The posterior column sensibility is, as a rule, the last to be involved and is most pronounced in the lower limbs. Trophic changes in syringomyelia are often very striking and osteoarthropathy (Charcot's joints) is part of the classical symptomatology. As in haematomyelia, bladder, bowels and sexual function are involved.

Schneider et al. (1954) have drawn attention to a syndrome of acute central cervical cord injury caused by simultaneous squeezing of the cord anteriorily and posteriorly resulting from severe retro-hyperflexion (wrongly called hyperextension) injuries of the cervical spine. This central damage may occur without apparent damage to the vertebrae and, according to the authors, is caused by an inward bulge of the ligamentum flavum during retro-hyperflexion of head and neck. This central cervical cord syndrome is characterized by a dissociation in the degree of motor paralysis or weakness between the upper and lower limbs, the upper limbs being more affected. There are also varying degrees of sensory disturbances below the level of the lesion, as well as bladder, bowels and sexual disturbances.

My own observations on the traumatic cervical central syndrome are in accordance with Schneider and his colleagues. However, this syndrome is not confined to so-called hyperextension (retro-hyperflexion) injuries but may also occur in antero-hyperflexion injuries and also in intramedullary as well as extramedullary tumours.

In explaining the anatomical arrangement underlying the relative sparing of the legs in the cervical central syndrome, Schneider and his colleagues confirm Foerster's views (1936) of a somatotopic division of the cortico-spinal fibres within the lateral pyramidal tract in the cervical cord area where the cortico-spinal fibres within the lateral pyramidal tract descending to the lumbar-sacral areas lie laterally in the pyramidal tract (eccentricity of the cortico-spinal fibres of the lumbar-sacral areas). Hopkins & Rudge (1973) in their paper on 'hyperpathie in the central cervical cord syndrome' seem to accept Nathan and Smith's view based merely on a review of the literature that there is no evidence of such lamelliform somatotopic division in the pyramidal tract. Their argument is that 'although somatotopic organization is absent, as the cortico-spinal tract descends the length of the cord some segmental organization must take place as fibres pass medially to their termination. They form axosomatic or axodendritic synapes chiefly on neurones in the nucleus proprius, basal part of the posterior horns, intermediate zone and central horn. These fibres, as they pass medially, must be more susceptible to a central medullary lesion. A lesion of this type in the cervical area would thus damage a large proportion of the cortico-spinal fibres destined for this segment'. This argumentation is hardly convincing to disprove the lamelliform somatotopic division in the cervical cord. For it is well known that the descending cortico-spinal fibres do not connect directly with the segmentally anterior horns but through their axodendritic synapses within their respective segments of the cord. Moreover, histo-pathological and clinical findings are not in accordance with Hopkins' and Rudge's statement that 'the fibres passing to the lumbar neurones are randomly distributed'. In the most severe cervical lesions, the sacral sparing, in particular of the most distal sacral segments, is not uncommonly the only sign of an incomplete lesion which cannot be explained by a random distribution of the descending cortico-spinal fibres. They are indeed the most eccentrically situated fibres at the level of the cervical cord.

Unilateral transverse lesion (Brown–Sequard's syndrome)

The syndrome of hemisection of the cord has been described in detail by Brown-Sequard in 1850. However, it is, in its classical form, a rare occurrence in most countries, with the exception perhaps of South Africa where spinal cord injuries due to stab wounds are common amongst the coloured population. More commonly, a stab injury of the cord may not only sever one half of the cord but may somewhat encroach on the other half, thus producing bilateral symptoms. The typical hemisection of the cord is characterized by ipsilateral motor paralysis of supranuclear type below the level of the lesion due to interruption of the pyramidal tract. The deep reflexes are exaggerated and there are all the pathological signs (Babinski, etc.) once the initial spinal shock has subsided. There is also some motor paralysis of peripheral type due to destruction of the cells of the anterior horn of the segment at the level of the lesion. This is particularly conspicuous in hemisections of the cervical cord. In addition, there is vasomotor paralysis, hypo- or anhidrosis and loss of posterior column sensibility on the ipsilateral side. There may be some cutaneous hyperpathia on the same side. On the contralateral side, pain and temperature sensibility is lost. The upper level of this sensory loss is likely to be a few segments below the level of the lesion, as fibres entering the spino-thalamic tract do not cross the cord for a few segments. On

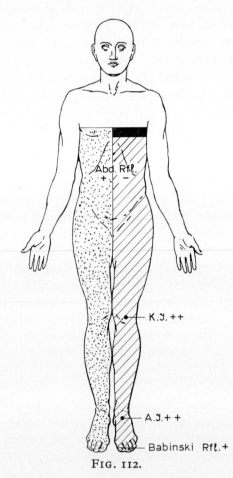

Anaesthesia
L.M.N. paralysis
{ U.M.N. paralysis
{ Loss of post. col. sensibility
Loss of spino- thal. tr. sensibility

Abd. Rfl.
+ / −

K.J. ++

A.J. + +

Babinski Rfl. +

FIG. 112.

the other hand, the fibres entering the cord just below the lesion are caught before they cross and thus cause a small zone of analgesia and thermoanaesthesia just below the lesion on the ipsilateral side (Fig. 112). Touch sensibility is not affected. Unilateral cord transections are most common in the thoracic region but do not give rise to Brown-Séquard syndrome in the lower lumbar and sacral area.

INCOMPLETE CONUS–CAUDA EQUINA LESIONS

Differentiation between purely incomplete conus lesions and cauda equina afflictions is often very difficult. The symptomatology of incomplete lesions of the cauda equina largely depends on the site of the lesion and the number of anterior and posterior roots affected by the pathological process. These lesions are often of dissociated type. It is not unusual that tumours involving the cauda equina, such as neurofibroma or ependymoma, may produce for some considerable time, as do prolapsed intervertebral discs, radiating pain of sciatic type before disturbances of bladder, bowels and sexual functions as well as numbness or weakness in certain muscles become manifest. Angiomatous malformations involving the conus and cauda equina may also produce a symptomatology of dissociated type. A classical example of incomplete cauda equina lesion of specific involvement of posterior root resulting in their degeneration occurs, of course, in tabes dorsalis, leading to ataxy and dribbling incontinence due to distension of the bladder as a result of the sensory loss.

Great varieties of incomplete conus–cauda equina involvement also result from traumatic lesions due to fracture dislocations of the lumbar vertebrae. The abnormality of the gait, as a result of the paralysis of the gluteal muscles especially gluteus medius, has already been described in the section on complete conus–cauda equina lesions. In a certain type of incomplete lesion due to polio or fracture of the lumbar spine, the paralysis may involve the quadriceps while the gluteal muscles are more or less intact, enabling the patient to stand and walk, although the abnormality of the gait is of different type as compared with that of cauda equina lesions affecting the gluteal muscles.

The stabilization of the knee joint in patients with paralysis of the quadriceps is ensured by the function of the gluteus maximus in combination with that of the soleus; therefore, the walking capability is maintained. The stabilization of the knee joint is only in danger when the line of gravity falls behind the knee joint axis. Per contra, the characteristic feature of the gait in patients with paralysis of the gluteus maximus, but intact quadriceps, is the backward thrust of the trunk causing the line of gravity to fall behind the joint centre and thus preventing the jack-knifing of the hip joint (see chapter on Physiotherapy).

CHAPTER 25

DISTURBANCES OF SENSIBILITY

(a) Disturbances below the transverse lesion

Distinction has to be made between the sensory disturbances in the immediate and early stages of complete transverse lesion and those in the later stages. In complete lesions, the conduction of all afferent impulses subserving the various modalities of superficial and deep sensibility mediated by the posterior columns, anterior and lateral spino-thalamic or ventro- and dorso-spinocerebellar tracts are interrupted at the level of the transection. The resulting loss of sensibility in the paralysed areas involves appreciation of touch, superficial and deep pressure, pain, itching as well as pleasurable sensations, temperature, position and movement (kinaesthesia), vibration (pallaesthesia), two-point discrimination, and appreciation of writing figures or letters on the skin (graphaesthesia). The border line between the sensitive and insensitive parts of the body is at first sharp to all forms of sensation. However, once the spinal segments above the transverse lesion nearest to the transection assume their compensatory overlapping sensory function, the areas of anaesthesia, analgesia and thermo-anaesthesia become dissociated, and the area of analgesia, unlike its distribution in peripheral nerve lesions, exceeds the area of anaesthesia (Fig. 113). The photographs also show the relationship between disturbances of sensibility and sweating (see chapter on Sweating).

(b) Disturbances above the level of the lesion due to tendinous or articular contractures

Pain and parasthesia are especially conspicuous in shoulders and arms in complete lesions of the cervical cord. Although the traumatized cervical roots may have initially produced some root irritation, there is no doubt that the pain above the level of the lesion in most of the cases we have seen was caused by tendinous or articular contractures in shoulders, elbows and fingers, due to faulty positioning of the upper limbs in the early stages following injury. In particular, in complete lesions below C6 where the triceps is paralysed, flexion contractures of the elbow as the result of overaction of the normal biceps are relatively common and are produced by continuous flexion of the forearms. Fig. 8 shows the agony in the face of a young soldier, who was admitted 4 months after a cervical injury below C6, when the sister tried to extend the forearm. Articular contractures in the hips, also in the small joints of the vertebra caused by long fixation in plaster casts and plaster beds, were also found to be the cause of nerve irritation above the lesion in cauda equina injuries. It was most striking that in those patients where these contractures were the only or main cause of pain the pain gradually disappeared commensurate with the relief of the contractures by regular passive and active movements as shown in Fig. 8.

(c) Disturbances at and above the transverse lesion due to root or segmental irritation

Nociceptive border zone reactions. Patients with complete transverse lesions, especially of the mid-thoracic and thoraco-lumbar cord, not infrequently develop an hyperpathic zone at the border and above the lesion which may involve one or more dermatomes. In some cases, this border zone hyperpathia may become a dominant clinical symptom, and the patient usually complains of a feeling of band-like tightness and pain of burning character. The slightest touch may become very unpleasant and the simplest pressure of the bedclothes may elicit great discomfort. The irritation of the sensory elements in these segments above the transection may lead to muscular reflex responses consisting of irregular fascicular twitching or cramp-like contractions of the muscles supplied by the border zone segments. It may also lead to hyperactivity of autonomic mechanisms in this area, such as band-like vasodilatation, piloerection and sweating. Moreover, the triple response as described by Lewis (1927) may be exaggerated in this hyperactive border zone, which shows how the intensity of this local reflex response may be influenced by the state of the segmental reflex activity of the spinal cord (see chapter on Vasomotor Control).

Pain and paraesthesia occur frequently in cauda equina lesions, especially partial ones. The root irritation is caused either by peri-radicular adhesions, as a result of post-traumatic arachnoiditis, or by post-traumatic changes in the damaged roots themselves. In these cases, the pain is often of a more spasmodic character described as 'shooting pain' and can be exaggerated by various extrinsic and intrinsic factors, such as atmospheric changes, noises, and acute infection of the body, especially of the urinary tract, etc.

(d) Phantom sensations

Paraplegics and tetraplegics with complete transection of the cord or cauda equina may complain of distressing burning and tingling sensation below the level of the lesion. These sensations may be diffuse in character and are usually imperfectly localized. In numerous cases, they are associated with phantom sensations and are referred either to the lower limbs generally or to some specific area in the completely insensitive lower limbs, such as feet, toes, or the ano-genital region.

During the First World War, Riddoch (1917) observed the occurrence of phantom sensations in patients with transection of the spinal cord and, since the Second World War, several reports on this subject have been published in traumatic paraplegics (Schulte, 1947; Becker, 1959; Beck, 1949; Bors, 1951b; Pichler, 1954; Heye, 1956; Pollock *et al.*, 1957; Guttmann, 1957, 1969). Phantom sensations are often experienced immediately and in the initial stages following spinal cord injuries and are described as 'feeling as if my legs were blown off', or 'swelling to twice their size'. However, unlike phantom sensations after amputations, the phantom sensations in paraplegics do not, as a rule, represent a dominant symptom and may gradually disappear, except in cauda equina lesions where they can remain more or less permanent and troublesome.

In analysing certain phenomena appearing in connection with these phantom sensations, the following may be mentioned:

1. *Posture of the phantom limb*

Varieties of posture of phantom limbs have been repeatedly described but the most common posture is one of flexion, although the paralysed limbs may actually be lying extended on the bed. Riddoch's case of complete lesion below T9 had the feeling 'as if someone were pulling my legs, trying to get them straight. The more they pulled the tighter the strings became and soon I had to cry out with pain.' Other postures described are 'my legs are floating in the air' or 'curled underneath me'. The intensity of phantom sensation may be influenced by change of posture. Furthermore, the posture of a phantom limb may be influenced by the position of the limb immediately prior to the occurrence of the paraplegia, if the pre-paraplegic's posture was associated with an experience of violent stress and emotion, as shown in the following observation of one of our patients with a complete lesion below T11 due to gunshot injury.

In 1943, a soldier at the age of 28, when leaving his tank during a battle in Italy, sustained a gunshot injury of his right knee and fell to the ground. He noticed that the right leg was lying useless in an extremely internally rotated position and he experienced a violent cramp-like sensation in this leg around the knee. A few minutes later, he received a gunshot injury in the back and immediately became paralysed below his waist. Soon after admission to hospital, his right leg was amputated at mid-thigh level. For the following six months, he had phantom sensation in the paralysed, amputated side only, and the position of the phantom limb was always the revivification of the position of the right leg as experienced immediately after his primary injury, before receiving his spinal injury. The phantom sensation gradually disappeared. It may be noted that this patient, who, since 1948, has been full-time employed in his former job as a bank clerk, was readmitted in June 1951, with a fracture of his left tibia below the knee, which occurred when his caliper gave way and he fell to the ground. This fracture did not elicit any sensory effects nor were phantom sensations of any kind experienced.

2. *Effect of late amputation on phantom limb*

An interesting question is whether a phantom sensation occurring as a result of paraplegia may be influenced by a later amputation, and the following case may be quoted.

An A.T.S. girl, aged 25, sustained a complete spinal cord lesion below T8 following fracture dislocation of the spine in May 1945. After the injury, she had phantom sensations and felt her legs to be lying in extended position. It may be noted that, in this case, the intensity of the phantom sensation increased when the patient was changed from the supine on to the lateral position. This phantom sensation did not alter, although she developed a septic bedsore in another hospital, penetrating into the left knee-joint and leading to a profound internal rotation of the left leg, resulting in contracture.

In May 1949, the left leg had to be amputated above the knee. No change of phantom sensation was experienced after the amputation. It still persisted on both sides, as before.

This is in accordance with Pollock and his colleagues (1951), who also found persistence in the character of phantom sensation in paraplegics, following amputation of a paralysed limb. These authors stressed the point that burning pain which had been present in both paralysed limbs persisted after amputation. Furthermore, they found persistence of pain in the paralysed legs following spinal anaesthesia below the level of the lesion, although all spasms and reflex activity were suppressed. On the other hand, the burning pain disappeared following spinal anaesthesia above the lesion. In accordance with this observation I found in such cases permanent disappearance of the painful phantom sensation following intrathecal alcohol block above the cord or cauda equina lesion, when the alcohol block below the level of the lesion had been unsuccessful.

From these observations, it can be concluded that painful phantom sensations localized in the paralysed limbs, experienced by patients with complete cord lesions, originate from the distal end of the segments proximal to the spinal cord transection and that this pain sensation is comparable to the pain referred from a neuroma of an injured peripheral nerve.

3. *Telescoping*

Telescoping of phantoms in spinal cord lesions have not been observed in our cases, in contrast to such development resulting from neuroma formation following amputations in non-paraplegic patients.

4. *Extinction of phantom limbs*

It is well known that a phantom limb following unilateral amputation of a leg or arm is abolished by a lesion of the parietal lobe of the contralateral side of the brain occurring later. No observations on this problem are available in complete or incomplete lesions of the spinal cord.

(e) Local and remote sensory disturbances due to visceral hyper-activity in the paralysed area

The problem of referred pain, in relation to the activity of hollow, muscular walled viscera, in non-paraplegic individuals has a literature too vast to review here.

Since Sturges' (1883), Ross' (1888), Lennander's (1903) and Mackenzie's (1909) work, there has been controversy relating to pain and discomfort originating from pathological visceral conditions amongst many authors. Sir Thomas Lewis (1941), in his book *Pain*, has given an excellent review about the theories held by various workers in this field. In more recent years, investigators have been concerned with research on sensations with specific visceral action pattern, such as hunger, nausea and abdominal dread ('butterflies in the stomach'), in relation to their mediation by afferent pathways (Grossmann & Stein, 1948; Wenger, 1950; James, 1957; Wright, 1965). Crawford & Frankel (1971) compared 60 (42 complete) cervical lesions with 23 thoracic, lumbar and sacral lesions as to their awareness of abdominal hunger, dread and nausea before and after their spinal lesion. They came to the conclusion that these sensations arising from the abdomen are mediated by the vagus and not the sympathetic supply.

In analysing my own observations on pain and other nociceptive, subjective pheno-mena arising from visceral activity, particularly pain, below the level of a spinal cord lesion due to distension or reflex activity of bladder, urethra, uterus and colon, various types of responses can be distinguished:

Following distension of the bladder the first is discomfort or a throbbing sensation, which is localized by most patients with complete lesions in the lower abdominal region (more or less distinctly in the suprapubic area), occasionally spreading to the lateral aspect of the thighs. This local effect of bladder distension may be found in patients with complete lesions at any level, including complete lesions of the cervical cord. It was observed during routine bladder washouts and cystometric studies or as a result of blockage of a urethral or suprapubic catheter. Blockage of a ureter by a stone, resulting in violent ureteric contractions and acute hydro- or pyonephrosis, may also be accompanied by local pain and discomfort in these patients. The local sensation may not necessarily be painful. This was found before or during ejaculations, as a result of intrathecal injection of prostigmine in patients with complete traumatic lesions of the mid-thoracic and lower cervical cord, who experienced some pleasurable sensation in the penis.

The other subjective response observed following bladder distension is not closely related to the area of the distended organ but occurs after a certain latent period as a result of cardio-vascular effects following reflex vaso-constriction in the paralysed area elicited by the distension of the bladder. The patient experiences a throbbing or some-times 'quivering' or shivering sensation, which extends upwards in the midline of the body to the throat, sometimes associated with tightness in the chest, and progresses to the back of the neck, causing a feeling of fullness or heat (or both) in the head, which is followed by frontal headaches, the latter being especially marked behind the eyes. These sensations are very conspicuous in lesions above T5 and cervical lesions.

The mechanism of these remote nociceptive sensory responses, some of which have been described by previous authors (Bowley, 1890; Riddoch, 1917) has been studied in detail by me, in co-operation with Whitteridge (1947), and is described in the chapter on Bladder Disturbances.

Another mediator of afferent impulses arising from abnormal visceral activity in the anaesthetic area, in complete spinal cord lesions of higher level, is the phrenic nerve. In one of our patients—a girl of 24, with a complete lesion below T2/3—the initial sign of an acute perforation of a duodenal ulcer was a violent pain first in the right then in the left shoulder. When seen immediately after by the M.O. in charge of the ward, she showed signs of a vasomotor collapse. The spasticity in both legs was greatly increased and, in particular, the abdominal muscles were quite rigid. Having regard to the pre-paraplegic history of a duodenal ulcer in this case, a perforation was diagnosed and confirmed at operation carried out immediately. She made an excellent recovery and satisfactory rehabilitation.

This case raises another important point—namely, whether, in a paraplegic of high level who, in his pre-paraplegic life, had been suffering from pain and discomfort, as a result of gastric or duodenal ulcer, these sensations may persist or recur if the ulcer becomes active again. The patient mentioned above actually experienced, on occasions, her old ulcer complaints, though less intense, after she became a paraplegic with a high thoracic lesion. In this connection, another case may be mentioned: a war pensioner with a complete traumatic lesion below T5 had a duodenal ulcer before his injury, and recurrence of this ulcer was accompanied by the same, though somewhat clouded, pain in the anaesthetic upper abdominal region, mainly on the right side, which he had before his injury. During one of his regular check-ups, a marked deterioration of his general condition was noted. Detailed examination revealed that not only had his discomfort in the upper abdominal region increased during the last two weeks before admission, but there was no doubt whatsoever about a local tenderness to pressure in the right abdominal region, appreciated as a dull ache. He deteriorated further in the following few days, and, as the X-ray showed a small patch of air in the upper abdominal region, a slight perforation was diagnosed and confirmed at operation. This patient's life, too, was saved. He made a good recovery and returned home, where he continued his business.

In summarizing the pathways of conduction of the afferent impulses, arising from abnormal, visceral activity in the anaesthetic area in complete spinal cord lesions, the following routes may be considered:

Directly related to the affected viscera (such as urethra, bladder and colon):

a. Along autonomic nervous pathways, travelling extramedullary below the transection, until the pathways connect with nerve fibres, which are themselves connected with spinal segments above the transection.

b. First via posterior roots and spinal cord, as far as the level of the transection, and continuing extramedullary, as described in (a).

Indirectly related to the affected viscera:

a. Along the phrenic nerve and referred as pain in the shoulder. This may occur in the event of an abdominal catastrophe, caused by perforated gastric or duodenal ulcers, affecting ramifications of the phrenic nerve in the diaphragm.

b. Along the perivascular nerve supply, in the form of ascending sensation in the midline of the body, resulting in headaches, etc., and associated with vasodilatation, rise of blood pressure, etc.

It may be assumed that, in patients with high spinal transection, who were suffering from gastric or duodenal ulcers in their pre-paraplegic life, persistence or recurrence of the local pain and the appreciation of localized tenderness to pressure are transmitted (more or less distinctly) through the auxiliary, afferent, extramedullary pathways, once the main route through the corresponding posterior roots and spinal segments is cut off by the transection of the cord.

Control of pain

The analysis of the various patterns of painful sensations observed in paraplegics and the better understanding of the underlying mechanisms naturally have their bearing on the management of pain.

However, it must be admitted that the details of pain mechanism are still obscure, as so many nervous pathways, relay stations and chemical transmitters are involved which may act not only as mediator but also as modulator of nociceptive responses. Keele (1957) believes that there are at least three chemical substances involved in the production of pain. There is also the problem of pain inhibition by centrifugal tracts or at segmental level. The question of relationship of the unmyelinated 'C' fibres to burning pain and that of small myelinated delta fibres of the 'A' group to pricking (fast) pain is still a matter of conjecture (Bishop, 1946; Landau & Bishop, 1958; Jones, 1956). The same applies to the question where 'A' fibres and 'C' fibres synapse within the spinal cord.

With regard to the problem of control of pain in the spinal man, it must be stressed that, for a proper evaluation of these sensations, full consideration must be given to the pre-paraplegic personality of the individual and his habitual pattern of reaction to painful stimuli. It must be kept in mind that, while the threshold of pain perception is relatively uniform in man, the expression of the individual's response to pain varies widely not only from individual to individual in accordance with his whole psychological make-up, but also in the same individual under different circumstances. Moreover, there are psychological factors, which, on the one hand, lower the pain reaction threshold, such as anxiety, apprehension, fatigue, fear and frustration, and on the other there are those which raise the reaction threshold and act as pain depressors or inhibitors. Therefore, it must be the task of everyone concerned with the management of pain in paraplegics, be he physician or surgeon, to take all these factors into account and to mobilize, from the beginning, those readjustment forces in the nervous system which promote the development of the suppressor mechanisms to sensory irritation. I have found that, from the early stages of clinical treatment, distraction of the patient's attention from his affliction and diversion and mobilization of his concentration to regular work and early pre-vocational training, as well as sport, is most helpful in the control of pain in paraplegics. In this connection, it is of utmost importance to be very circumspect in prescribing heavy pain killers, in particular opiates, and sleeping drugs in the immediate and early stages of paraplegia. Their action on the central nervous system, especially if given routinely and prolonged, have very undesirable side effects.

From the beginning of our work on paraplegics, we have been extremely reluctant and selective in the administration of barbiturates and, in particular, opiates, for the control of pain in these patients and have discarded them very early, as these drugs no doubt act adversely on the mobilization of the natural inhibitors to sensory irritation and the concentration of the patient on his readjustment to his disability. I feel that the thoughtless and indiscriminate prescription of heavy drugs, in which I also include pethidine, valium and librium, has no more place in the management of these patients than the hasty and early cordotomy or posterior rhizotomy, let alone sympathectomy. In the very few instances of intractable, nociceptive border-zone reactions at and above the level of complete spinal cord lesion, I have been satisfied with the intrathecal alcohol block above the spinal cord lesion (the same could also apply to phenol), which is infinitely less destructive than the operative procedures mentioned above.

Disturbances of sensibility in incomplete lesions

Although an anatomically incomplete cord or cauda equina lesion may initially reveal a complete sensory loss below the level of the lesion, sooner or later certain if not all modalities of sensibility may recover in accordance with the functional return of the posterior column or spinothalamic tracts. It is well known that the various modalities of sensibility have separate representations in both the posterior column and spino-thalamic tract. Moreover, there exists a lamelliform arrangement of a somatotopic division of the various areas of the body within these tracts which is particularly con-spicuous in the cervical cord. In the spino-thalamic tract, the fibres conducting pain, itching, tickling, libidinous sensation, and temperature sensibility for the cervical seg-ments are situated medially, while the fibres of the tract conveying impulses from the

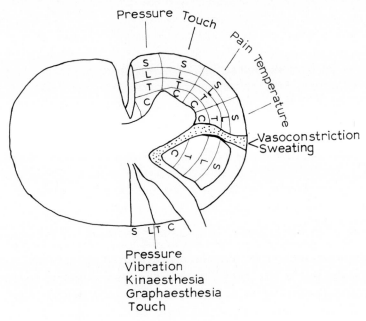

FIG. 113.

trunk lie intermediately and the sacral segments are represented laterally (rule of the eccentricity of the long fibres) (Fig. 113). This anatomical arrangement accounts for the fact that, in extramedullary pathological processes of the cord, such as meningioma or neurofibroma, compressing the lateral aspect of the cervical cord, the first disturbances of pain and temperature sensibility may occur in the lower extremity and trunk. Moreover, in such afflictions of the cord it is exceptional to find that appreciation to pain, heat and cold is equally affected. Sometimes cold or heat stimuli, although not appreciated as such, may evoke unpleasant sensation. Moreover, there is some segregation of the repre-sentation of the various modalities of spino-thalamic sensibility, whereby pain and, in particular, temperature conducting fibres lie nearest the pyramidal tracts.

In the posterior column tract, the fibres for the cervical area lie nearest to the posterior horn area, while those for the sacral segments are situated closest to the dorsal medium septum. In the cervical cord, there is also a clear division of the posterior column into two parts demarcated by the posterior intermediate sulcus. The medial part, fasciculus gracilis (Goll's tract), is composed of the long posterior root fibres for the lower part of the body (T4 and below), while the lateral part, fasciculus cuneatus (Burdach's tract), contains the fibres for the upper parts of the body (from T3 upwards). There is also some segregation of the various modalities of posterior column sensibility (pressure, vibration, position sense, kinaesthesia, touch). The predominant symptom of posterior column involvement is ataxia, resulting in a positive Romberg's sign, if the disturbance of postural sensibility affects both lower limbs. Knowledge of these anatomical arrange-ments, as shown schematically in Fig. 113, facilitates the understanding of the dissocia-tions in the clinical symptomatology of incomplete lesions of the spinal cord. All this explains the often irregular and dissociated disturbances of sensibility in the later stages of incomplete and in particular recovering cervical lesions (Fig. 132). This applies not only to dissociation between pain and temperature sensibility but also to pain, tickling and libidinous sensations and the various components of postural sensibility. In lesions with interruption of the spino-thalamic tracts, the sensation of vibration, which is mediated by the posterior column tract, is intact but the accompanying tickling sensation conducted by the spino-thalamic tract is abolished. Moreover, it may be stressed that immediately after injury certain types of sensibility may be spared in areas below the level of the lesion, even in only a few dermatomes, which allows the correct diagnosis at once. Such sparing occurs not infrequently in the lower sacral segment in incomplete lesions of the cervical cord. Therefore, repeated sensory tests—preferably by the same investigator—in the state of spinal shock and in the early days and weeks after injury are essential.

Sensory disturbances in lesions of posterior spinal roots

The area innervated by a single posterior root is termed dermatome. Detailed studies have been carried out in the past in animals and man, following resection of single posterior roots (Sherrington, 1898; Foerster, 1933, 1936; Keegan, 1943), by clinical observations in herpes zoster or afflictions of internal organs (Head, 1893, 1901), strych-ninization of the root entry zone in the cat (Dusser de Barenne, 1935), vasodilatation following electrical stimulation of the peripheral end of a divided posterior root (Bayliss, 1901; Foerster, 1933, 1936), and hyperaesthesia induced by injection of 5 per cent or 6 per cent saline solution (Kellgren, 1939; Lewis, 1942). As a result, charts of a derma-tomal pattern of the whole body have been mapped out by various authors, the most well known are those of Head (Fig. 114a) and Foerster (Fig. 114b). While giving a rough orientation of the metameric cutaneous arrangement and being sufficient for clinical diagnosis, they do not give details of the true distribution of individual posterior roots and their overlap with their neighbours, nor do they show the different areas of distri-bution of the various modalities of sensibility, in particular the relationship of the areas of anaesthesia and analgesia. Although following resection of a single posterior root in man, especially in the thoracic area, there is an immediate sensory loss for all qualities, the area of sensory loss will shrink and altogether disappear within a very short time, not

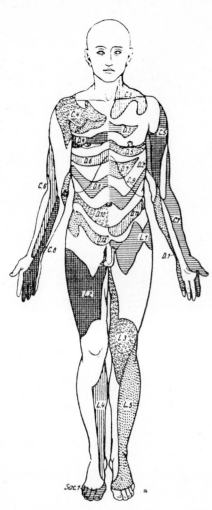

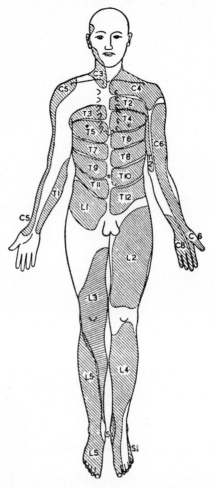

FIG. 114b. Dermatomes described by Foerster (1936) as redrawn by Lewis (1942). Determined by the method of 'remaining sensibility' following root section on human cases carried out by Foerster.

FIG. 114a. Human dermatomes as evolved by Head (1920) on the basis of herpes zoster in man.

infrequently within a few days, as a result of the overlapping function of its adjacent roots. Only if the function of these roots is impaired by a pathological process, such as compression by an extradural or extramedullary tumour, will the resection of a single posterior root have a long lasting effect. There are dissociations in the extent of the loss in the various modalities. In contrast to the size of the area of anaesthesia (touch sensation), which is larger than the area of analgesia in complete lesion of peripheral nerves, in root lesion this is the reverse—i.e. the zone of analgesia being larger than that of anaesthesia. The area of loss of temperature sensibility is, as a rule, the largest in both peripheral nerve and root interruption. Figs. 115a and 115b demonstrate the loss of touch, pain and temperature sensibility after the resection of the first thoracic posterior root following removal of a benign tumour (Professor Cairns, Oxford). The hatched line shows the

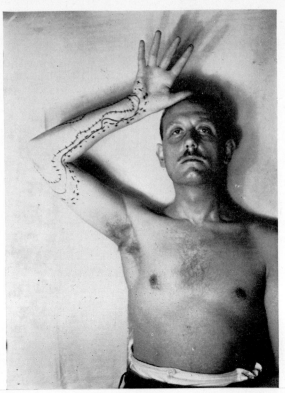

FIG. 115a. Sensory loss following resection of ThI root. ——————— touch, — — — — — — — — — — pain, × · × · × · × · × cold and warm sensibility, —/—/—/—/—/— shrinkage of sensory loss 10 days after resection.

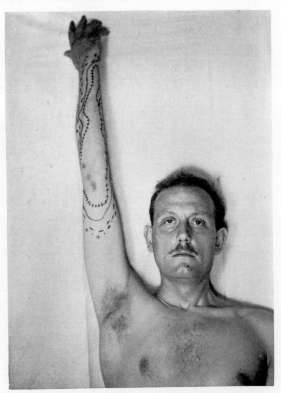

FIG. 115b. Same as 115a—different position.

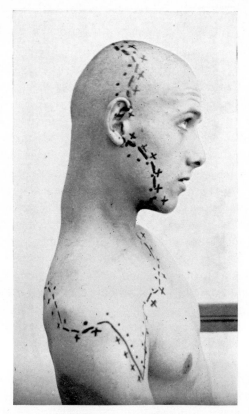

FIG. 116. ——— touch, ... pain, × × × temperature.

shrinkage of the area of sensory loss 10 days after the operation. Only if at least two to three adjacent posterior roots are resected in man will a permanent sensory loss result. However, in later stages following resection of several posterior roots, the difference between the extent of the areas of anaesthesia and analgesia may be less distinct, as I sometimes found in man. Fig. 116 demonstrates the residual sensory loss following resection of C2 to C4 posterior roots which I carried out in a case of torticollis spasticus. The area of analgesia in this case was found to be larger only over the vortex of the skull and back of the shoulder.

The body image

In connection with the disturbances of sensibility, the body image may be discussed. The presentation of the body to consciousness and the relationship of one part to another, known as body scheme (Schilder), body image, postural scheme (Head), l'image de notre corps (l'Hermitte), is constantly reinforced by afferent impulses from all parts of the body, including labyrinth and visual impulses. While disturbances of the body image in cerebral lesion, especially of the parietal lobe and thalamus, are frequent and have been widely discussed in the neurological literature (Head & Holmes, 1920; Gerstman, 1924;

Van Bogaert, 1934; Schilder, 1935; l'Hermitte, 1939; Critchley, 1949; Russell Brain, 1951; and others), there is little known about this problem in the spinal man. Heilporn & Noel (1968) made a thorough study on 40 traumatic paraplegics and tetraplegics (C4 to L4) during the acute stage after injury and found that the body image remains unchanged at least during the acute phase. This is certainly true in the majority of cases. However, as we have shown, phantom sensations in paraplegics represent positive disorders of the body image. In later stages, however, the sensory extinction of the body below the transection may result in a gross disturbance of the body image as an entity, and the patient, especially when standing for the first time between parallel bars, supported by his arms and calipers, may have the illusion that the body above the transection is somehow suspended in the air, especially when visual impulses are abolished by closing the eyes (negative disorder of body image). However, in due course, the entity of the body image will return even when the eyes are closed. In this connection, it is interesting to note that some patients in their dreams have the full body image when walking or standing, either dreaming that they are walking normally without calipers or in some cases with calipers. One female patient with congenital paraplegia due to spina bifida, who never could walk properly, always walks with a 'wobbly' gait in her dreams. Of special interest is another female patient with a complete lesion below T5, who has a full body image while awake, having phantom sensation in both legs. She volunteered the observation that in her dreams she loses the body image and feels that the part of the body above the level of the lesion is suspended in the air, when in her dream she is in upright position.

Another female paraplegic reported four types of dreams. She sustained her paraplegia at the age of 14 as a result of a riding accident. She repeatedly had dreams of riding as she did before her accident. She also had dreams of walking normally but only appreciated her body above the level of the lesion. Thirdly, she had anxiety dreams of opening her bowels, which woke her up. This has always been her fear when at work or when engaged in sport. She has been for many years one of our outstanding sportswomen, especially in fencing, and has taken part in all international Stoke Mandeville Games. She was, at the age of 32, engaged to a teacher who incidentally has been her fencing coach. Both had no previous practical sexual experience, but recently she had dreams of sexual desire and love play on various occasions, in which her fiancé was lying on her. Her previous anxiety dreams mentioned above have not recurred since.

These are a few examples of the paraplegic's dream-world but there is still much to be learned on this subject.

Sexual day dreams and sleep dreams amongst both sexes of paraplegia are not uncommon and they might also be accompanied by orgastic sensation. Morey (1960) described phantom orgasm in the dreams of paraplegic men and women.

POSTURAL CONTROL

Reorientation of sensory function

In complete lesions above the 12th dorsal segment, postural sensibility in the hip joint is abolished, and as a result the paraplegic when raised from the horizontal to the upright position has difficulty in keeping his balance. The higher the transection of the cord the more profound is the disturbance of posture, and this applies in particular to upper thoracic and cervical lesions. In the past, such a person was, as a rule, confined to bed or had to be transported in lying position in a spinal carriage. If the upright position in such cases was attempted, it was achieved by propping them up with artificial aids such as heavy leather and steel corsets. Moreover, the postural disturbances in lesions above T5 are greatly aggravated by the loss of vasomotor control as the result of the interruption of the splanchnic innervation (see chapter on Vasomotor Control).

Experience in the last 25 years on the spinal man has shown that the sensory disconnection between the paralysed and normal parts of the body does not remain permanent (Guttmann, 1946, 1953a, 1967, 1969). In later stages of complete transverse lesion, afferent impulses arising from paralysed parts of the body are mediated centrally and new connections with afferent pathways above the cord transections are established and thus some reorientation of sensory function and a reorientation of the postural control take place. Such transformation of function of afferent mechanisms in the human body is of immense importance for the rehabilitation of the spinal man.

In analysing the pathways conducting afferent impulses arising from paralysed parts of the body, the following routes have to be considered:

It must be remembered that in all transections of the lumbar, thoracic and up to the middle cervical cord, there still exists a bridge between the paralysed parts of the body and the central nervous system above the level of the transection, provided for by nature through the anatomical arrangements of certain muscle groups, which have their segmental supply above the cord transection but their anatomical insertion points are attached to areas below the transection such as the lower part of the spine, and, most important of all, to the pelvic girdle. These are, in particular, the trapezius (supplied by the accessory nerve as well as the upper cervical segments), which has its insertion points distally to the 12th dorsal vertebra, and, especially, the latissimus dorsi (supplied by C6, C7 and C8), with its anatomical attachments on the lumbar fascia and posterior rim of the pelvis. In more distal lesions, say below T10, these connections of the back muscles are intensified by the rectus abdominis (segmental supply T5–T12) which is also attached to the pelvis. Through their attachment to the pelvis, these muscle groups, innervated above the level of transection, play an essential part in the reconditioning of the afferent system in complete transverse lesions in restoring postural control in the spinal man. For, proprioceptive impulses arising from any movement of the pelvis are transmitted centrally along the afferent nerve fibres of these normally innervated muscles and thus reconnect the insensitive part of the body with the cerebral and cerebellar centres and their connections with the labyrinths and their arcs subserving postural control, promoting appropriate efferent postural responses to the paralysed area. Eventually, a new pattern of postural sensibility develops along the nerve supply of the trunk muscles, which enables the paraplegic even of higher level to regain his postural control and restore his upright position without the aid of artificial support by corsets. This is first accomplished under visual guidance by balancing exercises in sitting position in front of a mirror, during which the patient raises his arms in various directions, whereby he learns to compensate by visual control for the unsteadiness of the trunk resulting from the loss of postural sensibility. Gradually, in due course, commensurate with the development of the new pattern of postural sensibility, he will be able to sit with his arms raised and eyes closed and keep his equilibrium (Guttmann, 1945, 1946, 1953a, 1962, 1967). The lower the transection of the cord the less time it will take to establish the new pattern of postural control. On the other hand, spinal paraplegics suffering from additional labyrinthine affliction will have greatest difficulty in regaining their postural equilibrium.

Further details of the reorientation of posture are discussed in the Chapter on Physiotherapy.

CHAPTER 26
DISTURBANCES OF VASOMOTOR CONTROL

POSTURAL HYPOTENSION

It has been known for a long time that change of posture from the supine to the erect position or from sitting to standing in non-paralysed subjects is accompanied by changes in systolic and diastolic blood pressure, which in certain individuals may be considerable, and this phenomenon has been a subject of clinical and experimental studies (Bradbury & Eggleston, 1927; Stead & Ebert, 1941; Jeffers et al., 1941; Bridgen, Howarth & Sharpey-Schafer, 1950; Verel, 1951; Johnson et al., 1966, 1971; Spalding, 1969; and others).

Hill (1895) studied the circulatory changes occurring as a result of passive tilting in spinal dogs and demonstrated the importance of the splanchnic system in maintaining homeostasis in the vertical position. Since 1945, I have carried out systematic studies on this problem with my colleagues, to analyse the effects of postural changes on the cardio-vascular system with a view to re-establishing vasomotor control in the spinal man, and results have been published elsewhere (Guttmann, 1946, 1953; Jonasson, 1947; Guttmann, Munro, Robinson & Walsh, 1963).

The studies were carried out on patients with complete and incomplete lesions at different levels of the spinal cord. The subject to be studied remained on a tilting table in the supine position for about 30 min before being tilted into the vertical position. During this time an E.C.G. record was taken and blood pressure and pulse rate measured. Moreover, a blood sample was taken to determine plasma catecholamine levels before, during and after the tilting experiment. My co-workers Munro & Robinson (1960) have shown that spinal subjects with high cord lesions have a significantly lower level of adrenaline and noradrenaline in the peripheral plasma than have normal controls. Therefore it was of interest to examine also the effect of postural changes on plasma catecholamine levels in relationship to the vascular changes during and after tilting. Continuous E.C.G. recordings were made, starting from the time when the subject was tilted vertically and continuing until he was tilted back to the horizontal and had recovered from the effect of the vertical posture. The time elapsing before the plasma sample, indicating the response to the vertical tilting, was taken depended upon how long this position could be maintained without fainting occurring. If fainting did not occur, the subject was held vertically for about 15 min before blood sampling and then returned to the horizontal. The final blood sample was taken about 15 min after he had resumed the horizontal position. The subject was encouraged to describe his sensation during the procedure, in particular the premonitory signs of failing consciousness.

It was found that, while paraplegics with lesions of the distal cord and cauda equina did not differ from other non-spinal convalescent patients, those with lesions above T5 showed a profound vascular maladaptation to the postural change from the horizontal to the vertical tilting, as a result of the interruption of their splanchnic control. This

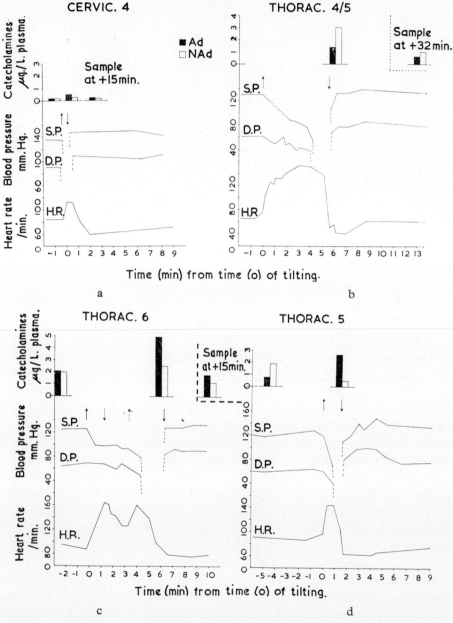

FIG. 117. Shows heart rate (H.R.), systolic pressure (S.P.), diastolic pressure (D.P.) and catecholamine changes in paraplegic subjects before, during and after being tilted vertically on a tilt table. The arrows indicate tilt to the vertical (↑) and return to the horizontal position (↓). Plasma adrenaline values are shown ■ and noradrenaline □. Fig. 117a: Male aged 25 with complete C4 lesion, sustained 13 weeks earlier: fainted in upright position. Fig. 117b: Male aged 20 with complete T4/5 lesion, sustained 8 weeks earlier: fainted in upright position. Fig. 117c: Male aged 18 with complete T6 lesion of 17 weeks' duration: fainted in upright position. Fig. 117d: Male aged 24 with complete T5 lesion of 17 weeks' duration: fainted in upright position.

vascular maladaptation to the vertical position in complete lesions above T5, particularly in cervical lesions, manifests itself in rapid and uninhibited accumulation of blood in the abdominal area and lower limbs due to the inability of the blood vessels in the viscera to contract, due to deprivation of control of the roots of the splanchnic nerves. This results in decrease in the supply to the central veins and insufficient return of venous blood and consequently insufficient cardiac output. The blood pressure shows rapid and steep fall, the pulse rate is raised to the highest level and syncope follows in a few seconds or minutes.

Figs. 117 and 118 demonstrate the results on B.P., pulse, Figs. 119 and 121 catecholamine levels and Fig. 120 shows the E.C.G. findings.

The invariable, premonitory symptoms of syncope after vertical tilting are blurring and finally loss of vision. Giddiness, buzzing and ringing in the ears were less frequently mentioned. Tingling in the hands, headaches and nausea may also occur, but vomiting never occurred. Those who fainted became paler whilst held in the vertical position but on being returned to the horizontal showed flushing in the face, which was particularly marked in subjects with cervical lesions.

The response of blood pressure and heart rate to vertical tilting depended on whether consciousness was retained in the vertical position. In patients who fainted, there was an immediate increase of heart rate in the vertical position and this usually persisted after consciousness was lost; systolic and diastolic pressures fell and became unrecordable. After return to the recumbent position, a sustained bradycardia occurred and was invariably associated with blood pressure above the normal. When consciousness was

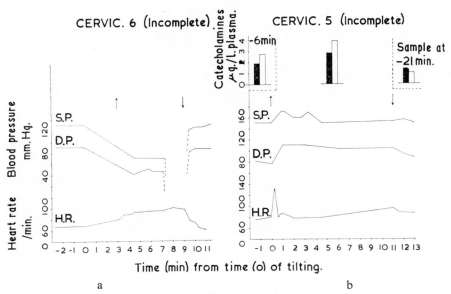

FIG. 118. Symbols as in Fig. 117. Fig. 118a: Female aged 24 with incomplete C6 lesion but extensive paralysis: lesion of 17 weeks' duration: did not faint in upright position. Fig. 118b: Male aged 19 with incomplete lesion at C5/1: moderate paralysis of 13 weeks' duration: did not faint in upright position.

retained, there was either a transient or slight retained increase of heart rate and systolic pressure and a maintained rise in diastolic pressure.

The changes in heart rate were recorded by the E.C.G. during and after tilting procedures. Only occasionally was irregularity associated with the cardiac acceleration in the vertical position, and the main changes observed in the vertical position were found in the P and T waves, due to the cardiac acceleration. Depression of ST segment occurred in 4 patients, when consciousness was lost.

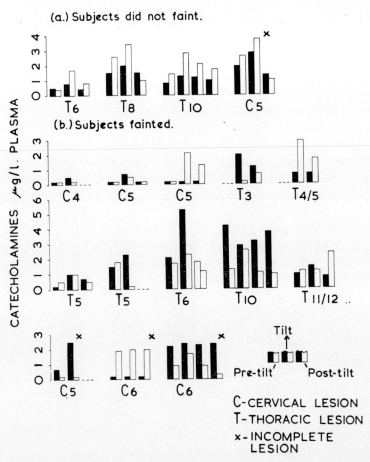

FIG. 119. Shows the adrenaline and noradrenaline values in the peripheral plasma of paraplegic subjects in response to movement vertically on a tilt table. Adrenaline values are shown ■ and noradrenaline □. Fig. 118a shows the response of subjects with complete or incomplete lesions tilted and retained in the vertical position for 15 min without fainting. Fig. 118b shows the response of subjects with complete or incomplete lesions tilted to the vertical and fainting. ■ A ■ B ■ C represent the adrenaline and noradrenaline plasma levels in the horizontal pre-tilt position, the vertical position and the post-horizontal position respectively.

Thorac. 5 lesion

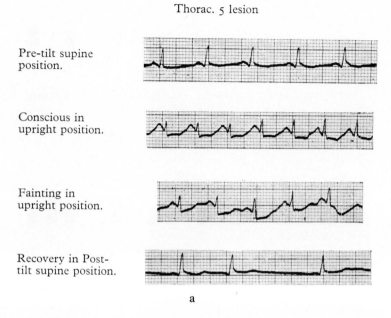

Pre-tilt supine
position.

Conscious in
upright position.

Fainting in
upright position.

Recovery in Post-
tilt supine position.

a

Thorac. 4 lesion

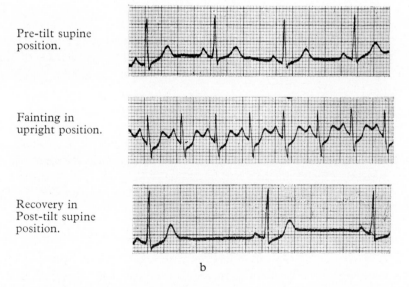

Pre-tilt supine
position.

Fainting in
upright position.

Recovery in
Post-tilt supine
position.

b

FIG. 120. Shows the ECG records (leads 1) from two spinal subjects who fainted
when tilted upright. a, Male patient, aged 20, with T5 lesion for 25 weeks; b, Male
patient, aged 20, with T4 lesion for eight weeks.

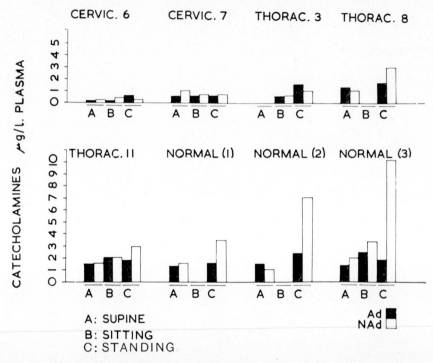

FIG. 121. Shows the adrenaline and noradrenaline values in the peripheral plasma of normal and paraplegic subjects with different levels of lesion (A) supine, (B) seated and (C) standing or held vertically for 2 min. Adrenaline values are shown ■ and noradrenaline □.

The plasma catecholamine changes in patients who fainted after tilting to the vertical showed a marked degree of inconsistency. It was found that the increase of adrenaline was much greater than noradrenaline in the plasma, and the total catecholamine values were increased.

It is obvious that these disturbances of vasomotor control to change of posture from the horizontal position in cord lesions above T5 can be more easily elicited the more recent the cord transection. This was found by Silver (1971) in the acute stages of tetraplegia during tilt-up experiments ranging from 15° to 45° with maximum duration of 350 sec, by measuring blood pressure and heart rate.

Reconditioning of postural hypotension

Attention was paid to means of overcoming the postural circulatory disturbances in these high spinal cord lesions. It was found that regular and frequent change of posture from the supine to the lateral position in the early stages following transection represents in itself an important stimulus in setting up vasoconstrictor responses in the isolated cord to restore the crippled vasomotor control.

TABLE 12

Case	Segmental level of lesion		Sweat test	Response to extrinsic stimuli		Response to deep inspiration		Response to bladder inflation	
	Right	Left		Finger	Toe	Finger	Toe	Finger	Toe
1	C6/7	C6/7	Not done	Nil	Nil	Vasoconstriction	Nil	Vasoconstriction	Vasoconstriction
2	T1/2	T1/2	Few pin-points of sweat on nose, lips, chin only	Nil	Nil	Vasoconstriction	Vasoconstriction	Vasoconstriction	Vasoconstriction
3	C8/T1	C8/T1	Not done	Nil	Nil	Vasoconstriction	Vasoconstriction	Vasoconstriction	Vasoconstriction
4	T3	T1	Few pin-points on right side of nose	Nil	Nil	Vasoconstriction	Nil	Vasoconstriction	Vasoconstriction
5	T4	T4	Not done	Poor vasoconstriction	Nil	Poor vasoconstriction	Vasoconstriction	Not done	Vasoconstriction
6	T5	T5	Level of lesion confirmed	Poor vasoconstriction	Nil	Poor vasoconstriction	Nil	Not done	Not done
7	T6/7	T6/7	Level of lesion confirmed	Vasoconstriction	Nil	Vasoconstriction	Nil	Vasodilatation	Vasoconstriction
8	T6/7	T6/7	Not done	Vasoconstriction	Nil	Vasoconstriction	Nil	Vasodilatation	Vasoconstriction
9	T8	T7	Level of lesion confirmed	Vasoconstriction	Nil	Vasoconstriction	Nil	Not done	Vasoconstriction
10	T10	T10/11	Level of lesion confirmed	Vasoconstriction	Nil	Vasoconstriction	Nil	Vasodilatation	Vasoconstriction

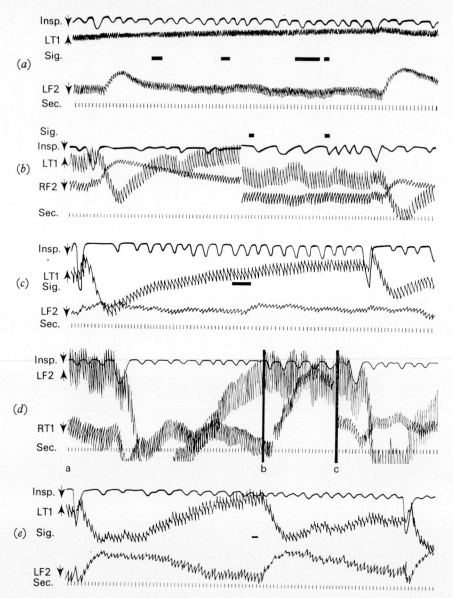

FIG. 122a. Case 1. From left to right: responses to a deep inspiration, four pin-pricks on face and a further deep inspiration. From above downwards: *Insp.* ↓ = respiratory record inspiration downwards: *LT*1 ↑ = left big toe volume, dilatation upwards; *Sig.* =signal for pin-pricks; *LF*2 ↓ = left index finger volume, dilatation downwards. Finger vaso-constriction accompanies deep inspiration but not pin-pricks. b. Case 2. Two sections of record to show responses to (*a*) deep inspiration, and (*b*) two auditory stimuli, shown by signal, followed by deep inspiration. Symbols as in Fig. 122a. Finger and toe vaso-constriction accompanies deep inspiration but not auditory stimuli. Case 5. From left to right: responses to a deep inspiration. Ice applied to face during signal and a further deep inspiration. The finger constricts poorly to both toe and deep inspiration while the toe responds only to deep inspiration. Symbols as in Fig. 1. From R.W.Gilliatt, L.Guttmann and D.Whitteridge. 1947. Inspiratory vaso-constriction after spinal injuries. (*J. Physiol.*, **107**, 67).

In co-operation with Gilliatt and Whitteridge (Gilliatt *et al.*, 1948) we studied further reflex activities of the isolated cord which may play a part in the vasomotor readjustment mechanism. It has been established from the results of earlier workers that a single deep inspiration causes vasoconstriction and a decrease in electrical response of the skin (Stürup *et al.*, 1935). Table 12 and Figs. 122a–c demonstrate our findings on inspiratory vasoconstriction from which it is clear that, in high complete cord lesions above the sympathetic outflow to the hands, deep inspiration still elicits vasoconstriction in the fingers, which can prevent or at least delay fainting due to postural hypotension in these patients. From these observations, it can be assumed that inspiratory vasoconstriction is purely a spinal reflex taking place in the thoracic region of the isolated cord. The afferent fibres concerned in this reflex enter the spinal cord mainly in the upper thoracic region, but the possibility that the limits of entry are somewhat wider than this cannot be excluded. In this connection, it may be mentioned that a deep breath may cause dilatation of the pupils (Somogy 1913). Recently, Silver (1971) has shown that this inspiratory vasoconstrictor reflex can be elicited in complete cervical lesion even during the stage of spinal shock at a vital capacity of the lung of 400–900 ml.

As a result of these and other observations, it has been possible to restore the redistribution of blood flow from the viscera by this vasoconstrictor reflex and other factors. The application of an abdominal binder or cuffs around the calves and the prescription of 20–25 mg of ephedrine before raising the patient from the horizontal to the vertical position and, in particular, resistance exercises producing the squeezing effect of muscular contraction on the vascular system have proved invaluable in overcoming circulatory maladaptation to posture in these high cord lesions. They prevent the dangerous pooling of blood in the paralysed parts of the body and promote the circulatory adjustments necessary to meet the metabolic requirements not only for restoring the upright position of the tetraplegic when sitting in a wheelchair and also standing in parallel bars (with the help of a physiotherapist) but even for athletic performances. These patients are, for instance, able to participate in archery and table tennis, with the bow or bat fixed to the hand. The pull of the bow is accomplished by a hook fixed on the other hand, as the fingers are paralysed (see Chapter on Sport).

Cardio-vascular changes during halothane anaesthesia

Spinal paraplegics, in particular, those above T5/6, need careful attention when undergoing general anaesthesia. This applies to the possible development of hypotension as well as autonomic hyperreflexia during operative procedures, such as transurethral resection or external sphincterotomy. Recently, extensive studies have been reported on the cardio-vascular problems connected with general anaesthesia (Troll & Dohrmann, 1975; Welphy *et al.*, 1975; Anderson & Thomas, 1975).

Effects of the renin–angiotensin system on blood pressure

It is well known that the enzyme renin releases angiotension I and II which in turn releases aldesterone from the adrenal cortex and acts as vasoconstrictor on blood vessels (see also chapter on Renal Deficiency). Johnson, Park & Frankel (1971) have been engaged in research on the effect of the renin–angiotensin system on postural hypotension in cervical lesions. These authors investigated the action of angiotensin following intravenous infusion in patients with cervical cord transection and found that the fall of blood pressure was abolished when raising the patient from the horizontal to 45° head up position. This is an important contribution to the problem of postural hypotension in cord transection above T5, where the splanchnic control is crippled, and further investigations will establish how far the use of angiotensin injection can be utilized in the prevention and treatment of postural hypotension in these patients.

CUTANEOUS VASCULAR RESPONSES TO MECHANICAL AND CHEMICAL STIMULATION (TRIPLE RESPONSE, REFLEX ERYTHEMA, DERMOGRAPHISM)

The term triple response (Lewis), which is now generally used for reflex erythema and dermographism, is characterized
a. by an initial, sharply defined vasodilatation of all skin vessels restricted to the line of stroke evoked by the end of the reflex hammer or by a dragging needle;
b. a flare with irregular margins spreading for variable distances outside the region of the stroke and caused by dilatation of the arterioles of the surrounding area of the skin;
c. local oedema (weal) of variable intensity over the line of stroke.

The neurogenic mechanism of the various components of the triple response has been investigated by various authors (Breslauer, 1919, L.R.Müller, 1931, and in particular by Lewis & Grant, 1925), and this reflex phenomenon is considered as an axon reflex resulting in vasodilatation of the skin arterioles due to direct mechanical stimulation of peripheral vaso-motor nerves or as a result of chemical stimulation by a histamine-like substance (H-substance of Lewis), liberated by cells of the skin along the path traced by the stimulation.

My own observations on this cutaneous reflex response in complete transverse lesions of the spinal cord can be summarized as follows:

In the initial stages following cord transection, mechanical stimuli by stroking with blunt or sharp instruments elicit no significant difference in the extent of the spreading flare between the normal and paralysed area of the skin but the flush may last longer in the dermatomes below the transection. This is understandable if one remembers that, in the initial stages following transection, the paralysis of the vasoconstrictors may be very conspicuous. However, once the reflex function of the isolated cord is developed and with the recovery and, indeed, increase of the vasoconstrictor tone, the effect in the paralysed area to cutaneous stimulation is vasoconstriction—i.e. the line made by the stroke is of white colour (dermatographia alba). This is in distinct contrast to the spreading flush above the level of the lesion, which is particularly obvious in the segment or segments just above the level of the lesion (dermatographia rubra). Thus, in complete transection of the thoracic cord, the level of the lesion is clearly defined by the increased cutaneous vasodilatation and sometimes weal formation in the border zone above the transection. Chemical stimulation by intracutaneous histamine injection confirmed these findings obtained by mechanical stimulation—i.e. decrease of spreading flush in the paralysed area and increase and longer lasting spreading flush in the border zone above the level of the lesion. This is in accordance with Cooper's (1950) findings. These investigations have clarified the neurogenic mechanism of the triple response. While it is accepted that the triple response is primarily an axon reflex, this reflex is modified by the reflex action of the spinal cord.

DISTURBANCES OF THERMOREGULATION

Changes of blood flow and temperature regulation, as a result of the large scale redistribution of blood which follows the vasoconstriction in the paralysed part of the body caused by bladder distensions, have been described in this book (page 327ff).

This chapter is concerned with the disturbances of blood flow and temperature regulation in paraplegics and tetraplegics due to environmental influences.

The maintenance of body temperature (homeothermia) depends on the nervous integration and co-ordinated reflex function of three systems:

(a) Surface receptor system consisting of cold and warm receptors in skin and certain mucous membranes. There are two main groups of temperature receptors associated with the sensation of cold and heat respectively, those which react with a maximum discharge at temperatures around 30°C and those with a maximum discharge around 40°C. 'Cold spots' have been found associated with Krause's end bulbs which are distributed in the skin (Weddell, 1941), while the corpuscles of Ruffini are associated with spots sensitive to warmth. Hensel & Zotterman (1951) found that there are not only separate types of receptors for warmth and cold but that the afferent fibres of the warmth receptors are of larger caliper than those of cold receptors. Both have a steady discharge rate at temperatures between 20° and 40°C. However, there is still some discrepancy of opinion as to whether there are, in fact, separate receptors for warmth and cold or whether the free endings which are concerned with pain sensation are also concerned with temperature (Weddell et al., 1955; Oppenheimer et al., 1958).

(b) Afferent transmitter system which conveys impulses from the surface receptors to the thermoreceptive and integrative structures in the anterior and posterior part of the hypothalamus via peripheral nerves, sympathetic and spinal cord. It was found by Ranson and his co-workers (1937, 1939) in long-term experiments on cats and monkeys that small lesions in the anterior hypothalamus diminish or abolish the response to body warming (heat loss mechanism), while lesions of the posterior hypothalamus also abolish the response to body warming (heat production mechanism). These experimental findings in animals have been confirmed by clinical observations in man that anterior hypothalamic lesions result in hypothermia. Widespread hypothalamic destruction tends to result in poikilothermia (Erickson, 1938; Ranson 1940; Burgi, 1953; Haymaker & Anderson, 1955).

(c) Efferent transmitter system which mediates impulses from the cerebral stations to all peripheral organs subserving regulation of body temperature through descending

pathways which traverse the postero-lateral hypothalamus, tegmentum of the mid-brain
and pons, reticular formation of the oblongata, lateral columns of the spinal cord to the
anterior roots and sympathetic nerves.

It has been established from studies of earlier workers that animal and man with
transection of the cord at higher level at air temperature of 26·6°C are essentially poikilotherm (Pflüger, 1878; Pembrey, 1897; Gardiner & Pembrey, 1912; Freund & Strassmann,
1912; Holmes, 1915; Sherrington, 1924; Foerster, 1936) but if they are kept at 20·2°C
they may regain some degree of temperature control against cold (Thauer, 1931; Clark,
1940).

The inability of tetraplegic patients to control their body temperature is particularly
apparent in the immediate stages following cervical cord transection, where these patients
behave as poikilotherms, and the mechanisms of heat production and heat loss are out of
control. In hot climates, environmental hyperthermia may have serious metabolic
effects, and, therefore, the nursing of these patients in an air-conditioned ward has been
found effectual in preventing hyperthermia (Cheshire & Coats, 1966). According to
Benedict & Lee (1938), the value of hypothermia lies in a reduction of the oxygen requirement of living tissues as their temperature falls, and, according to Bigelow *et al.* (1950)
and Horvath *et al.* (1953), oxygen requirements at 34°C are approximately 20½ less than
at 37°C. The lowest temperature in acute tetraplegics recorded at the Stoke Mandeville
Spinal Centre was 29°C and the highest 40–40·6°C. However, two of our patients—one

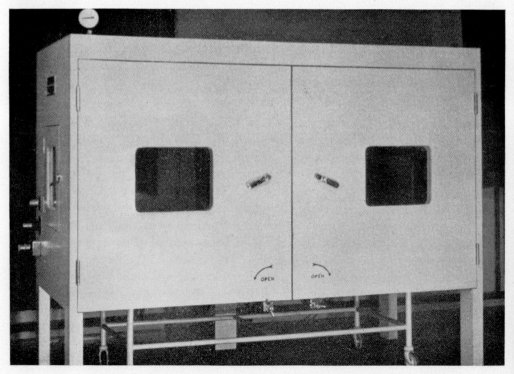

FIG. 123a. From Guttmann (1947) *The Post Graduate Medical Journal*, **231**, 337.

with a severe though incomplete lesion below C4, the other with an incomplete below C6, who developed, after cervical cord injury, a brain-stem complication with unconsciousness for several days—developed hyperthermia of 42°C and 41°C respectively. Both, however, recovered following largactyl injections, intravenous drips of ice-cold saline,

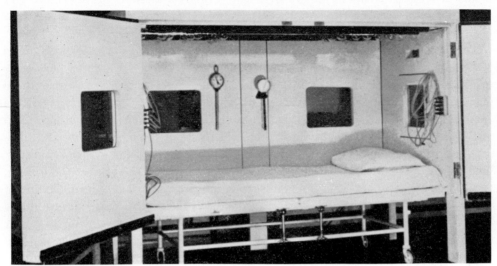

FIG. 123b. From Guttmann (1947) *The Post Graduate Medical Journal*, **231**, 337.

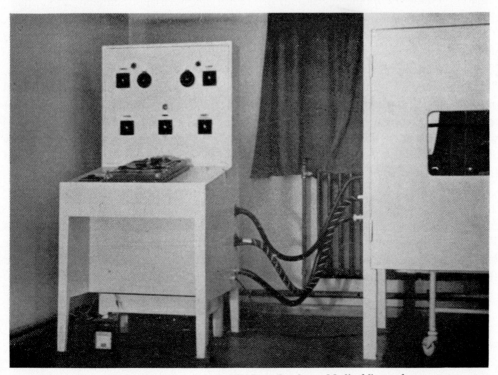

FIG. 123c. From Guttmann (1947) *The Post Graduate Medical Journal*, **231**, 337.

and kept in a cool room covered with sheets only. Both are still alive, with their incomplete tetraplegia of spastic type and speech disturbances of brain-stem type (slow, hesitant and slurred speech which is particularly pronounced in the case with the C4 lesion).

Detailed experimental studies on temperature control in late stages of tetraplegia and paraplegia were carried out by me in 1958 in co-operation with Silver and Wyndham on 4 cervical patients (one incomplete with touch sensation present to L1–L3 on right side only), two thoracic lesions (T4 and T8) and a normal control.

The same experimental procedure was adopted in each study. The subjects, all in good health condition, were stripped and rested nude for 1 hr on hospital beds at an environmental temperature of 27°C. Thereafter, they were transferred either to an environmental temperature of 18–20° or 35–37° for $1\frac{1}{2}$–2 hr. The cold temperature conditions were obtained in a room open to the outside air but shielded from direct and most reflected radiation from the sun on the colder days of summers of 1954 and 1956. Air in the room was circulated slowly by means of a small electric fan to avoid gradients. The study at 35–37°C was made in a specially constructed heat chamber (Guttmann, 1947) (Fig. 123). The heat source was a series of infra-red electric heaters in the roof of the 'hot box', but the patient was shielded from direct radiation. The air heated in this way was circulated slowly. Humidity in the 'hot box' was constant between 40–50 per cent during the exposure of the cervical subjects, but tended to rise to 60–70 per cent when the other subjects, who sweated, were studied. The temperatures given of all the environmental conditions were globe thermometer readings, as they take account of radiation. Globe thermometer readings in the hot box were approximately 20°C higher than the air temperature but were within 1°C in the neutral and cold temperatures. The sweat glands function was detected by the Quinizarin (Chinizarin) Dye Method which has been shown to be very sensitive (Guttmann, 1937, 1947).

Rectal temperature was measured every 15 min with a clinical rectal thermometer. Skin temperature was measured by means of a copper–constantan thermocouple stretched over a Y-shaped applicator; the e.m.f. was recorded on a Cambridge Instrument galvanometer specially constructed for skin temperature measurements. Skin temperatures (Ts) were measured at the forehead, chest, side, fingers, toes and anterior surface of the body above and below the level of the cord lesion. Average skin temperatures were calculated from the formula:

$$Ts = 0.7T \text{ of trunk} + 0.1T \text{ of foot} + 0.1T \text{ of finger} + 0.1T \text{ of forehead.}$$

Metabolism was measured twice in each air temperature condition by means of a Benedict–Roth type of apparatus and was determined over 5-min intervals. K int, the heat conductance of the tissues, and K air, the conductance of the air, were determined from the equation due to Hardy & Soderstrom (1938):

$$K \text{ int} = \frac{M \pm S}{Tr - Ts}$$

and similarly,

$$K \text{ air} = \frac{M \pm S}{Ts - Tr}$$

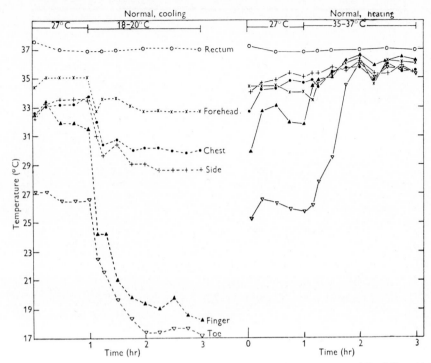

FIG. 124a. Temperatures of normal man during 1 hr of rest at 27°C, followed by 1–2 hr of exposure at 18–20°C and 35–37°C.

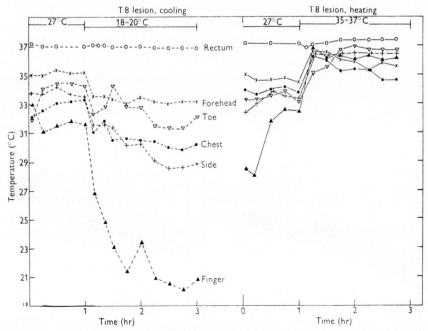

FIG. 124b. Temperatures of patient case 1, with lesion below T8. Guttmann, Silver and Wyndham: Thermoregulation in the Spinal Man. *Brit. Journ. Physiol.* (1958), **142**, 406.

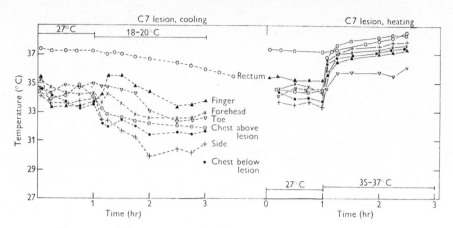

FIG. 124c. Temperatures of patient case 4, with lesion below C7.

where M = rate of metabolic heat production (cal/m² hr)

S = rate of heat storage (cal/m² hr)

Tr = rectal temperature (°C) and Ts skin temperature (°C).

Our studies have shown that tetraplegics with transverse lesions below C6 and T4 at a neutral air temperature of 27°C, maintain constant rectal temperature at approximately 37°C, as do paraplegics below T8. However, in cool air at 18–20°C, there were definite differences between tetraplegics and the normal control as well as with the paraplegic below T8. These two controls maintained constant rectal temperature by cooling of the extremities, initial fall of body heat and rise in metabolism by shivering (Figs. 124a and b). Our tetraplegics, exposed nakedly, like the controls, to 18–20°C air temperature, cooled rapidly and as shown in Fig. 124c the rectal temperature fell to 35·5°C

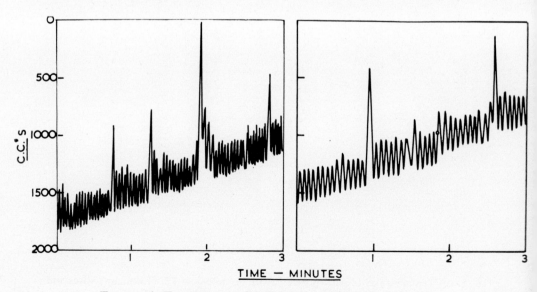

FIG. 124d. Temperatures of patient case 2, with lesion below T4.

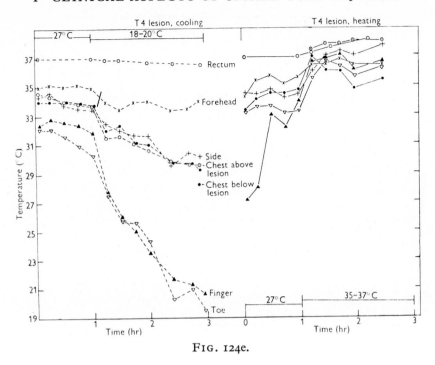

FIG. 124e.

in 2 hr due to lack of shivering, which occurred only in the few remaining muscles above the level of the lesion, thus raising the metabolism by only 50 per cent. Johnson & Spalding (1964, 1966) confirmed these observations but their cervical patients did not respond to cooling to such extent as was found in our experiments on rapid cooling. It may be remembered in this connection that Sherrington (1924) cooled the hind limbs of animals with complete transection of the cord and shivering occurred only in muscle groups innervated above the level of the transection.

In hot air at 35–37°C, the two control subjects maintained a constant body temperature, due mainly to evaporation of sweat. Tetraplegics, who do not sweat over the body or, if so, only minimal, showed rapid rise of rectal temperature to 38·5C in 1½ hr, when panting and distress became apparent. Fig. 124d is a spirometer tracing of a complete tetraplegic below C7 in the neutral environment and at 35–37°C and demonstrates the increased rate and smaller tidal volume in heat.

The patient with a transverse lesion below T4, although complete below that level as far as motor and sensory functions were concerned, showed a marked fall of both toe and finger temperatures which contrasted with those of the cervicals; he also showed some sweating below the level of the lesion, indicating that the lesion had not interrupted completely the sympathetic control to the lower limbs (Fig. 124e).

While our studies clearly show that the patients with complete transverse lesions of mid-cervical cord, when exposed naked to low or high temperatures cannot regulate temperature at will, as do paraplegics below T5, we did not exclude the possibility that cervical-lesion patients when conditioned to lower or higher temperatures would show better regulatory adjustment. Indeed, further experience has shown that this is the case.

TABLE 13

Subject	Level	Time injury (years)	Temperature (°C)		Foot blood flow (ml/100 ml foot/min)		
			Last before heating	Increase	Last 10 min before heating	10th–20th min during heating	Increase
G.P.	C5	0·7	36·15	0·10	5·8	5·4	−0·4
A.W.	C6/C7	0·8	35·45	0·20	0·5	0·3	−0·2
E.F.	C6/C7	1·0	36·50	1·60	3·7	1·9	−1·8
J.V.	T1	—	36·05	0·25	0·5	0·7	0·2
		0·9	36·85	1·00	4·7	5·6	0·9
D.H.	T1	1·0	35·75	1·10	5·0	5·3	0·3
	C6/T3	8·7	37·05	1·30	9·2	9·3	0·1
R.B.			37·60	0·45	9·4	9·5	0·1
I.H.	T4	—	36·55	1·10	7·6	6·7	−0·9
S.M.	T5/T6	0·7	36·30	1·65	2·9	3·5	0·6
P.W.	T7/T6	1·3	36·50	0·85	3·7	3·4	−0·3
A.H.	T8	1·1	35·75	1·75	3·3	3·1	−0·2
A.H.	T10/T9	0·4	36·75	1·30	1·6	1·7	0·1
	T10/T11	9·0	36·90	0·60	1·5	1·6	0·1
D.C.			37·30	0·55	1·5	2·0	0·5
A.H.	T10/T11	0·8	36·35	1·10	5·3	4·7	−0·6
J.G.	T11	6·2	37·30	1·20	1·9	2·0	0·1
A.S.	T11	—	36·95	0·50	5·0	5·4	0·4
	T11/T12	1·8	36·95	0·60	1·7	2·6	0·9
C.N.			37·15	0·40	3·7	4·0	0·3
G.Y.	L1	0·8	37·10	0·45	2·7	4·9	2·2
G.T.	L2	—	36·95	0·35	3·8	7·6	3·8
W.M.	L2	2·3	36·65	0·60	2·3	7·1	4·8
G.W.	L4	—	37·20	0·35	8·6	10·4	1·8
J.C.	L3/L5	1·1	36·70	1·25	2·6	7·1	4·8
P.C.	S	—	36·75	0·60	1·5	6·8	5·3
F.B.	None	—	36·60	0·60	4·1	8·4	4·3
	None	—	37·00	0·70	1·8	4·4	2·6

From Cooper, Ferres and Guttmann: Vasomotor response in the foot to raising temperature in the paraplegic patient (1957), J. Physiol. 136, 547.

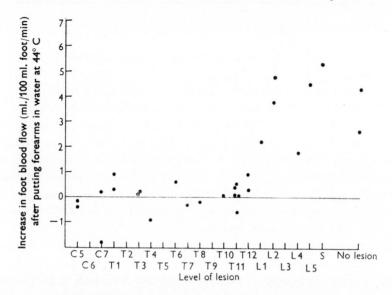

FIG. 125. Foot blood flow changes following body warming plotted against the level of the spinal cord tension. The flow changes are calculated as described in the text for preparation of Table 12. From Cooper, Ferres, Guttmann (1957) Vasomotor response in the foot for raising body temperature in the paraplegic patient. *J. Physiol.*, **136**, 555.

In this connection, it may be noted that in Clark's (1940) experiments, cervical spinal cats which had been kept for some time at 27–30°C were more easily chilled than were the same cats when previously accustomed to environmental temperature at 21° C.

In connection with temperature regulation in the spinal man, foot bloodflow in response to raising body temperature by heating of both arms immersed in water of 40–44° for 30–40 min was studied in 1957, in co-operation with Cooper and Ferres, in 21 subjects with complete lesions ranging from C5 to L5 levels and normal controls.

Oral temperatures were taken at intervals with a clinical thermometer which was left in the mouth for a minimum of 3 min. In two experiments, the skin temperatures of the great toe was measured by means of thermocouple which was strapped to the toe with adhesive tape. The foot blood flow was measured in the sitting as well as supine lying position in the same subject.

There was no increase in foot bloodflow in patients with transverse lesions between C5 and T10, although the oral temperature showed a marked rise, while patients with lesions below L1 and normal controls produced marked vasodilatation in the foot following arm warming. Table 12 and Fig. 125 demonstrate our results.

From these observations, it was concluded that the upper level of vasomotor outflow from the spinal cord to the foot, occurs at L1 and may also include T11–T12. This appears to be higher than the level for sudomotor function to the foot found by electrical stimulation of the preganglion trunks (Randall *et al.*, 1955), but is more in accordance with histological studies (Sheehan, 1941).

Responses of the pilomotor system

The pilomotor system plays a particularly essential part in the heat regulation in furred animals. Although its function is rudimentary in man, compared with that in furred animals, it is associated with shivering, vasoconstriction, increase of heart rate, elevation of metabolic activity, etc., in the production and maintenance of body heat in man.

Accompanying the vasomotor fibres to the skin are sympathetic postganglionic fibres, which on excitation elicit contractions of the smooth muscles, bringing the papillae into prominence and producing erection of the hairs (cutis anserina, gooseflesh). The erection of the hairs reduces radiation of body heat. Diencephalic impulses regulating body temperature descend the antero-lateral tracts of the spinal cord to the grey substance of the intermedio-lateral horns from where the peripheral innervation through post-ganglionic fibres and anterior roots commences.

Reflex disturbances of the pilomotor system following spinal cord lesions have been subject of research in the past, and reference is made especially to André-Thomas' monograph *Le Reflèxe Pilomoteur* (1921) in which he described, in particular, a great variety of pilomotor reflex disturbances in syringomyelia due either to increase or lack of diencephalic excitability caused by complete or partial interruption of the diencephalic-spinal pilomotor fibres or due to destruction or irritation of the lateral horn chain. Thomas found no pilomotor disturbances in polio as in his view the infectious process is confined to the anterior horns only. This is not in accordance with my own observations as far as the function of the sweat glands is concerned. During the polio epidemic in 1932 in Silesia, I found amongst 223 patients several cases where, in addition to the destruction of the anterior horns, the intermedio-lateral horns were also affected resulting in disturbances of sudomotor function. In some patients, these disturbances—either hyper- or hypohidrosis—were confined to the paralysed limbs, in others there were considerable dissociations between the motor paralysis and the disturbances of sweating (Fig. 128). One patient—a 23 year old woman with pregnancy of 8 months—with ascending motor paralysis died from respiratory paralysis. The histological examination of the spinal cord showed not only most severe destruction of the anterior horns throughout the whole length of the cord but the lateral horns were also affected by the inflammatory process (Guttmann, 1933).

In complete transverse lesions of the spinal cord, the paralysis below the level of the lesion also involves the pilomotor system. In cervical and T1/T2 transections, the pilomotor paralysis affects the whole body, including both upper limbs. In lesions below T5, pilomotor function in the upper limbs and chest is preserved, and the lower the thoracic lesion the more the areas of the trunk showing pilomotor response to cooling and other stimulation above the cord lesion. In fact, in complete lesions with segmental supralesionary hyperreflexia, increased pilomotor response may be part of the autonomic hyperactivity in the affected segmental dermatomes. In complete lesions below L2, there is no paralysis of the pilomotor function.

Once the stage of spinal shock has subsided and the exaggerated reflex function of the isolated cord has developed, the spinal pilomotor reflex is one of the components of the mass reflex and can be elicited in the skin areas below the level of the lesion either alone or in combination with flexion contractions of the spastic legs, detrusor contraction of the bladder or other visceral activity in the paralysed part of the body.

Sudomotor function

Sweat glands activity, apart from the vasomotor control, represents the most important mechanism for maintaining homeothermia in man by regulating heat loss. This function of the sweat glands depends on the integrative control of the various afferent and efferent components of the peripheral and central nervous system, amongst which the spinal cord, anterior and posterior roots and the pre- and post-ganglionic innervation play their part. Thermoregulatory as well as reflex disturbances of the sudomotor system can be readily demonstrated in man by applying dye methods amongst which the Starch–Iodine Method (Minor, 1927) and the Quinizarin (Chinizarin) Compound (Guttmann, 1937) have proved the most satisfactory.

CORTICAL CONTROL

Certain cortical areas, especially the sensory-motor cortex but also the precentral area (field 6), exert some regulatory influence on the sudomotor function. This was concluded from observations in unilateral cerebral paralysis, Jacksonian epilepsy (Toporkoff, 1925; Guttmann & List, 1928; Guttmann, 1931) as well as from results of electrical stimulation of cortical centres and from cortical excisions within the sensory-motor region (Guttmann, 1931). In this connection, the case of one of my patients described in my monograph on X-ray diagnosis by contrast methods, published in Vol. VII, 2, of the *Handbuch der Neurologie* of Bumke and Foerster (Guttmann, 1936) may be mentioned, who, apart from a spastic paresis of the left hand and arm, was suffering from Jacksonian epilepsy, starting in the extensors of the left hand and fingers and progressing into the whole left arm. There was distinct sweating of the left hand and forearm during and after the seizures. The underlying cause of these seizures was found to be a large frontal para-saggital meningeoma of the right side, which I removed. The tumour reached distally just into the hand and finger areas of the motor cortex. Following operation the patient had at first a complete left hemiplegia from which, however, in due course he made a full recovery, including return of the isolated finger movements of his left hand. For several days, the hemiplegia was accompanied by outbursts of profuse sweating over practically the whole left side of the body, and from time to time one could see large beads of sweat appearing over the left forearm. Toporkoff (1925) described in a patient an outburst of sweating over the right hand extending to the elbow as aura before an epileptic attack. Moreover, sweating over that area also occurred as equivalent of seizures lasting for 1 hour. Fig. 126 shows one of my patients suffering from Jacksonian epileptic fits which always started in the hypothenar muscles of the left hand. Thermoregulatory sweat test showed start of sweating in the left hypothenar, and during the further stages this man showed a relative hyperhidrosis over the left arm and trunk. Other cases of this kind have been described previously (Guttmann & List, 1928).

During electrical stimulation of the left sensory cortex by Foerster, in a case of focal epilepsy manifesting itself by paraesthesia and clonic contractions of the right foot and leg, I observed during continued stimulation of the left cortical focus for the abdominal muscles, a clear outburst of sweating confined to the right abdominal region. The sweat secretion continued for some time after the electrical stimulation had ceased. Following the excision of the foci for foot, leg and abdomen of the sensory-motor cortex by Professor Foerster, resulting in spastic paralysis of the right leg associated with sensory disturbances up to an area just above the umbilicus, the thermoregulatory sweat test, using

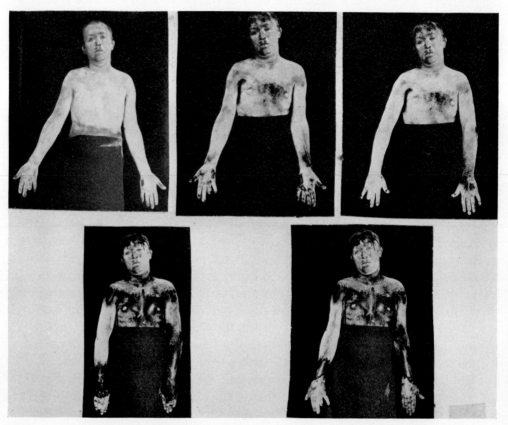

FIG. 126.

Minor's starch–iodine technique showed earlier onset of sweating followed by hyperhidrosis in the affected areas. In another patient I excised the left frontal oculo-motor field (area 8), because of focal epilepsy originating from that area. Following the operation and also three days later there was distinct though only temporary hyperhidrosis over the left side of the face. These observations reveal a somatotopic division of the thermoregulatory centres of the cortex. Penfield & Boldrey (1937) reported that 'perspiration seems to have occurred once as a result of low precentral stimulation'.

In this connection, experimental studies of Langworthy & Richter (1930), Wang & Lu

(1930) and Schwartz (1937) on skin resistance ('psychogalvanic reflex') are of import-ance. These authors found that stimulation of the cat's motor cortex gave rise to a distinct drop in skin resistance mainly on the contralateral side of the body, and it is well known that the galvanic skin response depends mainly on the activity of the sweat glands.

While some of these observations demonstrate some excitatory effect of the cortical centres on sweat gland activity, their major function seems to be an inhibitory one. For, it is a well-known fact and confirmed by the cases mentioned above that destruction of the cortical areas 4, 6, and 8 results also in hyperhidrosis of the opposite side of the body. This may be explained as a release phenomenon on subcortical mechanisms sub-serving thermoregulation, which in these circumstances act unrestrained from cortical inhibition. These observations in man and animals also show a considerable overlapping between representation of autonomic mechanisms subserving thermoregulation, such as sweating and somatic motor representation in the cortex, which explains the correlative reaction of these two systems. However, there is no clear correlation between the intensity of sudomotor changes and the degree of motor paralysis.

Hypothalamus

The experimental research work of Karplus & Kreidl on the function of the hypothalamic area, published in a series of papers between 1909 and 1937, has been fundamental in clarifying a great deal of the confusion and mysteries attached to the function of this vital part of the brain. They demonstrated in the cat and monkey, by their results obtained from stimulation of the hypothalamic region, especially its anterior part, and following destruction of this area, the importance of the hypothalamus as the regulatory centre for the activity of the various autonomic mechanisms, including sweating. The sudomotor function, the most effective mechanisms of lowering the temperature in man, was already noticed by Karplus & Kreidl (1910) in response to hypothalamic stimulation, and this mechanism was later studied in detail by Hasama (1940).

From all the evidence which is available from the numerous experimental and clinical data, it would appear that the anterior part of the hypothalamus (preoptic and supraoptic region) is primarily concerned with the regulation of heat loss (Keller & Hare, 1932; Keller, 1938; Teague & Ranson, 1936; Ingram, 1940), and only by major destruc-tion affecting also the lateral area of the hypothalamus are heat production, heat main-tenance and heat loss out of control.

The supranuclear sudomotor fibres descend from the diencephalon through pons and oblongata, where a partial crossing of the fibres takes place so that each half of the spinal cord contains sudomotor fibres for both halves of the body. Therefore, unilateral cordo-tomy produces only hypohidrosis below the level of the lesion. In the oblongata, most sweat fibres travel through an area occupied by the lateral reticulo-spinal tract.

Spinal cord

Within the spinal cord the supranuclear sudomotor fibres pass through the posterior aspect of the antero-lateral tract very close to the lateral pyramidal tract and the border zone of the intermedio-lateral horns, where the segmental synapse with the ganglion

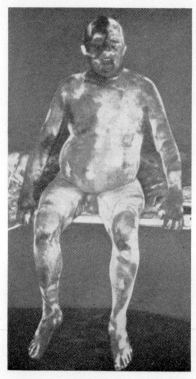

FIG. 127.

cells of the grey matter takes place. Unilateral cordotomy of the antero-lateral tract only results in ipsilateral hypohidrosis below the level of the lesion if the dorso-medial part of the antero-lateral tract is severed. Experience has shown that cordotomies at the level of C2–C3 may spare sudomotor fibres, with the result that only those fibres are interrupted which innervate distinct areas only, such as trunk and leg dermatomes, as shown in Fig. 127 of a patient who had a cordotomy carried out by Foerster on the left side below C2 because of intractable hyperpathic pain, following neuroma formation in his right hand resulting from an ulnar nerve injury. The thermoregulatory sweat test showed hypohidrosis over the left side of the face, trunk and leg, while the sudomotor function of the left shoulder and left arm was spared (Guttmann & List, 1928). This finding indicates that in the cervical cord there is a somatotopic arrangement within the supranuclear sudomotor tract, which as is known, also exists for the various modalities of sensation in both spino-thalamic and posterior column tracts. The fibres for the upper limb lie in the most medial part of the lateral and adjacent anterior horns, while those for the lower limb lie more laterally along the rostral border of the lateral pyramidal tract. This also explains the segmental or regional type of disturbance of sweating in incomplete lesions or recovering, initially complete lesions of the spinal cord, especially in the cervical cord.

In the chapter on pilomotor function, attention was drawn to disturbances of temperature regulation, as revealed by sudomotor deficit resulting from destructive processes affecting the intermedio-lateral horns themselves, such as polio or syringomyelia. Fig. 128 demonstrates a man with severe residual paralysis from poliomyelitis (see atrophy of left shoulder and arm), where the thermoregulatory sweat test revealed profound hypohidrosis over the left side of the trunk and arm, contrasting with a compensatory hyperhidrosis of the homologous parts of the body on the right side of the body in addition to the left side of the face. This phenomenon, which I termed peri- and supralesionary reflex sweating, was described in detail previously in connection with peripheral and central lesions of the nervous system in a paper on motor and autonomic border zone reflexes (Guttmann, 1933). Fig. 129 shows the perilesionary hyperhidrosis

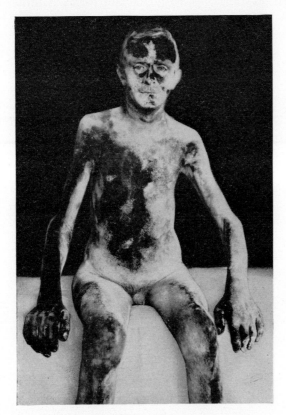

FIG. 128.

in a man in whom the cervical sympathetic ganglia had been removed. It shows most strikingly the readjustment forces innate in the nervous system to compensate for any sudomotor deficit by evolving this reflex response to restore and maintain homeothermia. Fig. 130 shows the result of a thermoregulatory sweat test of a man who complained of increased sweating on the left side of the trunk and right axilla. The sweat test revealed this disturbance as compensatory hyperhidrosis for a segmental anhidrosis on the right chest and upper abdomen. An- or hypohidrosis involving one or several segments is not infrequently found in syringomyelia (Guttmann & List, 1928).

Spinal roots

It is a well-established fact that the preganglionic sudomotor fibres leave the intermedio-lateral horns via the anterior roots and connect with the ganglia of the sympathetic chain through the rami communicantes albi and that each anterior root has its connection with several sympathetic ganglia. Thomas, Head and Foerster have tabulated the segmental sudomotor centres in the medio-lateral horns in relation to the sympathetic ganglia via anterior roots. Their findings correspond fairly closely with each other. There is no doubt that nociceptive responses arising from visceral irritations—for instance as a result of afflictions of the gall-bladder, may reflexly lead to segmental hyper- or hypohidrosis, as mentioned before as Viscero-Sudomotor Reflex (Guttmann, 1938).

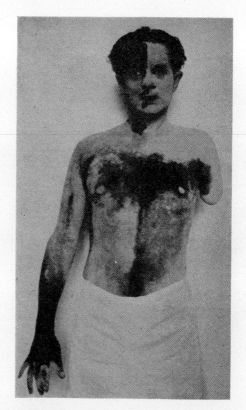

FIG. 129. From *Journal Anatomy*, London, 74 (1940) 538. Disturbance of sweat secretion after extirpation of certain cervical sympathetic ganglia.

In analysing the relationship of anterior and posterior roots to sudomotor function it has been proved by Foerster (1936) that electrical stimulation of the peripheral end of a divided anterior root always elicits marked sweating over a greater or lesser number of dermatomes. However, when the corresponding peripheral end of the divided posterior root was stimulated prior to the stimulation of the anterior root, vasodilatation occurred in the cutaneous distribution of the posterior root but there was anhidrosis in that area. This was confirmed by the starch–iodine technique in a patient suffering from intractable pain due to cancer metastases in the pelvis where, before a bilateral cordotomy was performed (Professor Foerster), the electrical stimulation of the peripheral end of the divided 5th thoracic posterior root resulted in vasodilatation of the cutaneous distribution of this root. Electrical stimulation of the divided 5th anterior root elicited marked sweating, which started in T6 dermatome and extended distally to T10. Moreover, the outburst of sweat also spread in cephalad direction involving T3/4 dermatomes. However, there was anhidrosis in the cutaneous area corresponding, though slightly larger, to the vasodilator area obtained previously by the electrical stimulation of the 5th posterior root thus demonstrating inhibition of sudomotor function (Guttmann & List, 1928).

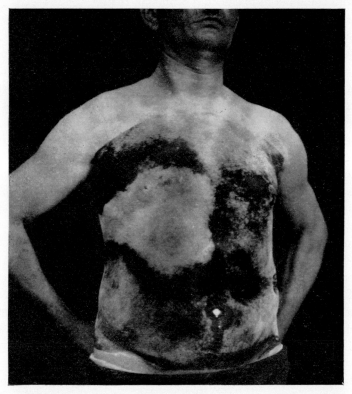

FIG. 130.

Although these effects of electrical stimulation of the distal part of the divided posterior roots is undeniable, there still persists discrepancy of opinion amongst workers in this field as to whether the posterior roots conduct true efferent nerve fibres, which on stimulation evoke segmental vasodilatation and sudomotor inhibition. It was Stricker (1876) who first demonstrated the vasodilatator effect following stimulation of posterior roots in animal experiments, and his findings were confirmed by Werziloff (1896), Bayliss (1901) and Dieden (1915) in animals and by Foerster (1924, 1927) in man following electrical stimulation of a great number of the peripheral end of divided cervical, thoracic, lumbar and sacral posterior roots. It was also found that the resection of cervical, upper thoracic and lumbo-sacral posterior roots resulted in temporary hypothermia of the arm and leg respectively. However, this disturbance soon disappeared and local cutaneous thermal and mechanical stimuli elicited undisturbed vasodilatation. As far as the sudomotor function was concerned, only temporary hyperhidrosis followed the resection of several adjacent posterior roots. In fact, in one case following the resection of the posterior roots of L5–S5 on the right side by Foerster, the thermoregulatory sweat test which I carried out several weeks later revealed an hypohidrosis over the whole posterior aspect of the right leg. Although no definite conclusion could be made from this single case, the possibility that this hypohidrosis was the result of transneural degeneration of ganglion cells in the corresponding intermedio-lateral autonomic centres of the spinal cord could not be excluded (Guttmann, 1930).

In connection with the vasodilator and inhibitory sudomotor effects following electrical stimulation of posterior roots, which suggest efferent function of fibres within these roots, the anatomical studies of Ken Kuré and his co-workers in animals (1930) and Gagel (1930) in man may be mentioned. These authors described intact myelinated nerve fibres of thin calibre in the central part of the divided roots and, moreover, Gagel found degeneration of these fibres in the peripheral part of these roots at later stages. From these findings, he thought to prove the existence of efferent nerve fibres in the posterior roots originating from the intermedial cells of the lateral horns. Foerster accepted this view with regard to the vasodilator effect and I came to the same conclusion with regard to sudomotor inhibition. However, this concept is not in accordance with Bayliss' views. This author, while confirming the vasodilator effect of posterior root stimulation as found by Stricker (1876), denied the existence of true efferent fibres and advanced the theory of 'antidromic' conduction through the posterior roots. Lewis (1928), agreeing with Bayliss' theory, postulated that the antidromic conduction liberates histamine (H-Substance) which is responsible for the vasodilator effect. In this connection, it may be noted that in man there is always a long latent period following faradic stimulation of the peripheral part of a divided posterior root, until vasodilatation appears in the cutaneous distribution of that root, which is in contrast to the immediate effect of faradic stimulation of anterior root fibres on the muscular system as well as sudomotor function. If Lewis' concept of the release of the H-Substance evoked by antidromic conduction is correct, this would also explain the inhibition of sweating, since Hara (1932) described an inhibitory action of histamine on sweating. As far as the anatomical proof of the existence of efferent inhibitory nerve fibres in the posterior root is concerned, Ken Kuré's and Gagel's conclusions were not accepted by other workers in this field (Barron & Mathews, 1935; Hinsey, 1934; Okelberry, 1935; Sheehan, 1935; Story, Corbin & Hinsey, 1936; Toennies, 1938), and from all evidence available so far no definite conclusion can be drawn in this rather complex problem.

Effects of complete and incomplete transverse lesions of the spinal cord on sudomotor function

Complete interruption of the sudomotor pathways between the hypothalamic region and the sympathetic outflow abolishes the thermoregulatory function of the sweat glands, resulting in anhidrosis. Since Riddoch's & Head and Riddoch's classical studies (1917) during the First World War on soldiers with spinal cord transection, details of the disturbances of sweating in complete and incomplete lesions of the spinal cord have been repeatedly reported (Guttmann & List, 1928; Guttmann, 1931, 1953, 1954, 1969; Guttmann & Whitteridge, 1947; List & Peet, 1938–39).

The extent of thermoregulatory loss of sweat gland activity following complete lesion depends on the level of the lesion and the time which has elapsed after injury. In the early stage following cord transection, the sudomotor deficit is more extensive and corresponds more closely to the level of sensory loss than in later stages, when the last normal segment above the level of the transection through its anterior root connection with its corresponding sympathetic ganglia has developed its maximal function overlapping into several dermatomes below the level of the sensory loss. In complete lesions of the cervical cord, including C8 and T1, the thermoregulatory sweat test shows anhidrosis over the whole body, apart from a few pin-points of sweat over face and neck if some sudomotor fibres of the cervico-thoracic junction have escaped damage. Such patients cannot stand heat well and on increasing heat stimulation in the sweat cabinet feel uncomfortable and soon mobilize auxiliary heat regulatory mechanisms, such as increased rate of respiration (panting), mottled cutaneous vasodilatation over the body and increased renal function. However, in later stages of complete tetraplegia, the patient acquires a better tolerance to heat. The thermal readjustment is due to the improved vasomotor control and the increased function of those sudomotor fibres which initially escaped permanent damage at the time of injury.

The question arises whether and to what extent the isolated cord itself can take part in this process of thermoregulatory readjustment, similar to its co-ordinated reflex function in restoring posture. Randall & Seckendorf (1961) described sweating, though considerably reduced below the level of the lesion, in 5 patients with complete transection of the cord at various levels (verified by laminectomy) 1 to 11 years after injury. These findings were contrary to Benzinger's conclusions (1959, 1960) that cutaneous thermo-receptive impulses play no part in the production of sweat. This problem has been re-examined by me in co-operation with Randall and Silver on patients with clinically complete lesions of the cervical and upper thoracic cord, using both the Quinizarin dye (Guttmann, 1937, 1947) and starch–iodine techniques (Randall, 1946). It was found that in some of these patients, when subjected to high degrees of heat in the sweat cabinet (Fig. 123) for longer periods, sweating did occur in the form of patches of minute pin-points of sweat scattered irregularly over some areas below the level of the lesion, including the feet. As reflex sweating (see later) due to visceral activity—i.e. detrusor contraction of the bladder—could be excluded, these findings could indicate thermo-regulatory sudomotor responses of the isolated cord to intense heat stimulation. However, as in our cases no laminectomy had been carried out to verify anatomical transection of the cord, no definite conclusion can be drawn from these cases. Moreover, it cannot be excluded that the positive response of the scattered patches of sweat glands below the level of a transection of the cord are due to local axon reflexes resulting from direct heat stimulation of the skin. In this connection, it may be noted that Bickford (1939) produced sweating by direct faradic cutaneous stimulation which occurred in a very circumscribed

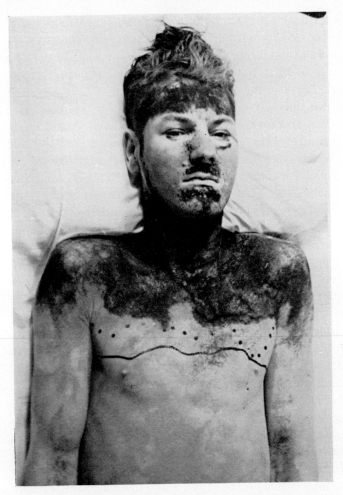

FIG. 131a. ...... pain sensibility; ———— touch sensibility. Early stage of thermoregulatory sweating in relation to pain and touch sensibility in complete T4 lesion.

area around the electrodes. His results were in accordance to those obtained by Lewis & Marvin (1927) for pilomotor function (goose skin).

The thermoregulatory disturbances of sweating occurring in the early and late stages of the test in a complete lesion below T3/4 is demonstrated in Fig. 131a. While in the early stage of the sweat test, using the Quinizarin dye method, there was rapid and profuse sweating over face, neck, shoulders, upper limbs and upper chest (supra-lesionary hyperhidrosis), there was anhidrosis below that level which corresponded closely to the level of the sensory loss. However, in the final stage of increased heat stimulation, sweating occurred well below the sensory level tapering down and gradually diminishing in intensity to T10 dermatome. The particularly profuse sweating over the areas of compensatory hyperhidrosis mentioned during the initial stage is still visible (Fig. 131b). While complete lesions below T5 and T6 show almost identical anhidrosis below the umbilicus and marked dissociation between the loss of sensibility and loss of sweating (Fig. 131c) complete lesions between T7, T8 and T9 show anhidrosis only below the 12th dermatome, and in those below T9/10 some diminished sweating may also extend to the proximal area of the legs. The sweat glands for the lower limbs are innervated by the segments of the thoraco-lumbar junction (T10–L2/3). Complete lesions at and below T12 show more or less marked sweating over the legs but sweating may be diminished over the feet and back of the legs. On the other hand in complete spastic lesions at that level there may be outbursts of spontaneous hyperhidrosis which may be very troublesome to the patient (see chapter on Spasticity).

Autonomic borderzone reactions

Mention has already been made of hyperhidrosis developing above the level of complete cord lesions. The exaggerated activity of sweat glands is particularly conspicuous in the segments nearest the lesion and reveals itself by early onset of sweating and a band-like form of hyperhidrosis. The hyperhidrosis may be associated with increased muscular vasomotor and pilomotor responses, and these reflex responses are elicited by afferent excitation as revealed clinically by a borderzone-hyperpathia.

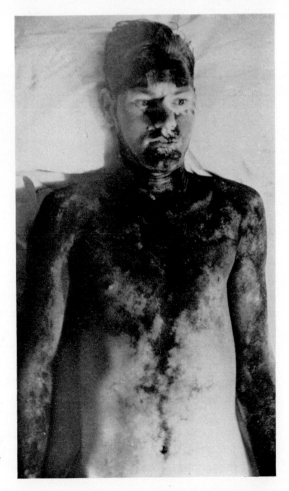

FIG. 131b. Final stage of thermoregulatory sweat test in T4 transection of the cord.

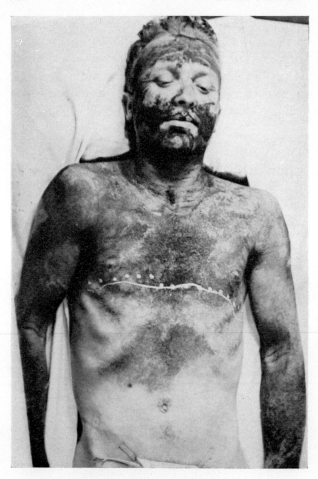

FIG. 131C. ...... pain sensibility;
——— touch sensibility. Marked
dissociation between loss of sensibility and loss of sweating in
complete T5 lesion.

Incomplete cord lesions

The somatotopic arrangements of the sudomotor tract within the spinal cord explains
the segmental or regional type of thermal sweat disturbance in initially incomplete lesions
of the spinal cord. This is shown in a case of incomplete lesion of the mid-cervical cord
which demonstrates the thermoregulatory sudomotor disturbances over the right side
of the forearms, trunk and leg and also shows the dissociation to the disturbances of
sensibility (Fig. 132).

The somatotopic arrangements of the sudomotor tract also explain the scattered
segmental recovery of initially complete transverse lesions which, in incomplete cervical
lesions, might for instance, start first in the abdominal area on one side, before sudomotor
recovery takes place in other parts. This is shown in the case of a young man who had a
neuro-fibroma at the level of C5/6, which was removed by Professor Cairns in Oxford.
Before the operation there was a complete transverse spinal syndrome below C5 with a
lower motor neurone paralysis of the left deltoid and incomplete paralysis of the left
biceps in addition to complete sensory loss below C4 and loss of control of the bladder.

The thermoregulatory sweat test (Quinizarin technique) before the operation showed only hypohidrosis in the face especially on the left side, and also some pin-points of sweat over the upper chest and right arm; otherwise there was complete anhidrosis. The patient made an excellent recovery, including the left deltoid and biceps, and when he left hospital he was able to walk without support, and bladder and bowel function had returned. Fig. 133 shows the scattered segmental recovery of sudomotor function two months after the operation.

Incomplete lesions involving the posterior columns only or in combination with the pyramidal tracts but sparing the spino-thalamic tracts do not show disturbances of sweating.

Conus–cauda equina lesions do not show signs of anhidrosis; in fact, in some patients

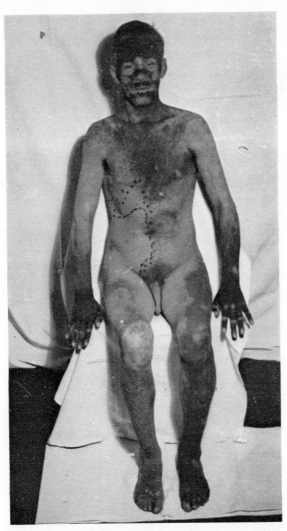

FIG. 132. – – – pain, ×·×·× temperature. Dissociated disturbance of sweating in recovering cervical lesion

with cauda equina lesions, spontaneous outbursts of sweating occur in the paralysed lower limbs. However, if the conus–cauda equina lesion is complicated by overlaid peripheral lesions such as sympathetic ganglia, plexus or peripheral nerves these can be easily demonstrated in the thermoregulatory sweat test by anhidrosis in the distribution of these injured peripheral sections of the nervous system. Fig. 134 demonstrates the complete loss of thermoregulatory sweating in a case of lumbar sympathectomy. Fig. 135 shows a case of pressure lesion at the capitulum fibulae resulting in a pressure sore in a case of conus–cauda equina lesion below L2 (loss of pain sensibility marked by dots) which revealed anhidrosis over the distribution of the lateral popliteal nerve and also within the scar of the healed sore over the capitulum fibulae.

Reflex sweating

The sweat gland activity in spinal paraplegics is not only of interest from a thermo-regulatory point of view, but it also represents an outstanding component of widespread reflex responses of the skeletal muscles and autonomic mechanisms (mass response), once the uninhibited reflex activity of the isolated cord has developed (List & Pimenta, 1944; Guttmann, 1953). Reflex sweating is elicited by many extrinsic and intrinsic stimuli in the paralysed part of the body, and this has been described in the chapter on the bladder.

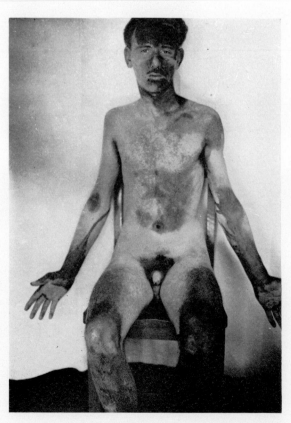

FIG. 133.

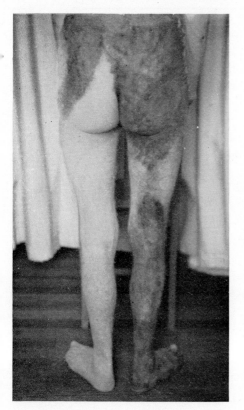
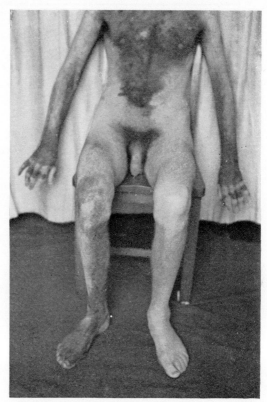

FIG. 134. Only partial sympathectomy on the right lumbar region.

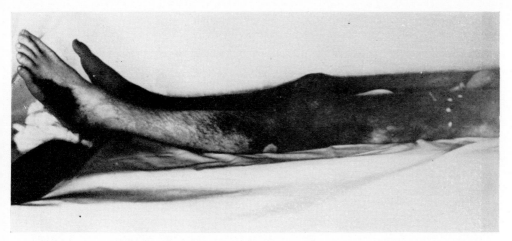

FIG. 135. . . . . . . level of sensory loss. Superimposed paralysis of the left external popliteal nerve as a result of a pressure of the capitulum fibulae in a case of conus-cauda equina lesion below L1.

Head & Riddoch (1917), in their classical paper on reflex changes following transection of the spinal cord, summarized the following circumstances which were found to precipitate reflex sweating below the lesion on the 259th day following transection of the cord in an officer who was struck by shrapnel in the mid-thoracic region:

1   spasms of the legs, especially repeatedly induced flexion reflexes;
2   an enema;
3   catheterization;
4   change of temperature—e.g. when being lifted out of his bath sweating appeared over his whole body, especially his lower extremities, but there was no change of pulse or pupils during such hyperhidrosis.

From my own experience I can confirm this observation but further factors evoking reflex sweating should be mentioned:

1   Change of posture, in particular in cervical lesions. In some patients, reflex sweating may occur when a patient is placed in the prone position, in others when placed on one side. Lately it was found in a tetraplegic when raised from the horizontal to the upright position, in particular when standing in the parallel bars.
2   Any acute infection of the bladder or an acute pressure sore or following infection from ingrowing toe-nails.

Details of reflex sweating elicited by bladder distension and hyperactivity are given in section on bladder disturbances.

CHAPTER 27

DISTURBANCES OF THE BLADDER AND
UPPER URINARY TRACT

Terminology and definition

The term 'neurogenic bladder' (McLellan, 1939) is used generally as a collective term primarily for dysfunctions of the urinary bladder resulting from lesions of the peripheral or central parts of the nervous system. Moreover, in recent years the term 'neurogenic bladder' has often been specifically associated with injuries of the spinal cord or cauda equina. Yet, this term is really a misnomer, as the function of the normal bladder is in itself neurogenic. The neurogenic dysfunctions of the bladder may be due to brain lesions (cortex, hypothalamus, midbrain, pons or oblongata), or affliction of the spinal cord at, above or below the spinal micturition centre in the lumbosacral cord. Furthermore, they may result from lesions of the sympathetic innervation or from spinal roots and their peripheral ramification or from abnormalities of the autonomous intramural innervation of the bladder wall. Therefore, in future, more accurate definition for neurological disorders of the bladder will be necessary, such as 'neurogenic vesical or bladder dysfunction' due to cortical, or subcortical or spinal cord etc., lesions, which will facilitate generally acceptable nomenclature.

Any consideration of vesical disorders resulting from affliction of the nervous system must always include recognition and evaluation of the anatomical structures and their abnormalities—either congenital or acquired—which have existed previous to the neurological lesions, as they may greatly influence the abnormal function resulting from the neurological deficit. In this connection, special attention must be paid to the pre-existing habits of micturition.

Some anatomical aspects

Certain relevant anatomical data are reviewed here which are fundamental for the understanding of the physiology and pathophysiology of the bladder and ureter in their relationship to renal function and pathology. In particular, the close anatomical connections of the bladder–ureter complex explains the direct route taken by ascending infection.

The human bladder is a multi-layered, muscular, membraneous hollow organ, varying in shape and capacity, which serves as a fluid reservoir. In the new-born, the bladder is of ovoid shape and lies chiefly in the abdomen adjacent to the ventral abdominal wall. From the apex of the bladder the medial umbilical ligament, a residual of the obliterated urachus, extends to the umbilicus, as also do the two lateral umbilical ligaments which are residua of the obliterated umbilical arteries. The knowledge of these anatomical connections are of importance as they may give rise later to abnormalities, as will be seen later. In the adult, when emptied, the bladder lies totally within the pelvis and has the form of a tetrahedron, but when filled it assumes an oval, pear shaped or circular form. This fluid reservoir is provided with emptying and closing mechanisms consisting of smooth and striated muscles.

The muscles of the forces of the emptying mechanism consist of: (a) Three, though not distinctly separate, smooth layers of detrusor muscle originating embryologically, with the exception of the trigone, from the allantois. The trigone (Trigonum vesicae Lieutaudy) originates embryologically from those parts of the cloacal wall from which the Wolff's ducts run out. The mucosa of the trigonal area is smooth and differs distinctly from the other parts of the bladder wall which has a reticular contour formed by the detrusor bundles. The detrusor represents the main expulsive force. (b) Striated muscle groups consisting of diaphragm and abdominal muscles.

The forces of the closing or fluid retention mechanism consist of: (a) striated external urethral sphincter and the striated muscles of the pelvic floor (perineal muscles, bulbo— and ischiocavernosus and levator ani), originating embryologically from the cloacal muscles. (b) Smooth muscle bundles of the bladder neck which, however, are intermingled with striated muscle bundles originating from the external urethral sphincter (Wesson, 1920; McCrea, 1926). Thus, the detailed muscular arrangement of the bladder is rather complicated and somewhat confusing. Outer and inner dorsal and ventral longitudinal muscle bundles are intertwined with transverse and circular muscle bundles, and at the vesical neck there exists interlacing of smooth and striated muscle fibres. Taking part in the formation of the vesical neck, which extends from the internal urethral meatus to the circular part of the external urethral sphincter, including the prostatic

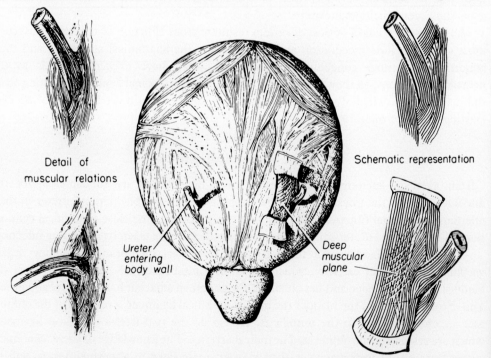

Detail of
muscular relations

Schematic representation

Ureter
entering
body wall

Deep
muscular
plane

FIG. 136. Ureterovesical junction. R. T. Woodburne in *The Neurogenic Bladder* (Ed. S. Boyarski) Publ. Williams & Wilkins, Baltimore, 1967.

part of the urethra, are the outer and inner longitudinal fibres and transverse bundles of the bladder base and also elastic tissues. (c) Circular bundles surrounding the internal urethral orifice from the trigonal muscle. The vesical neck also contains striated muscle fibres deriving from the external urethral sphincter. Bors *et al.* (1954) found striated muscle fibres at the bladder neck in 19 out of 20 resections of the bladder neck but only at the anterior commissure (12 o'clock).

The closing or fluid retention mechanism has been the subject of controversy for some time. The traditional concept of the existence of a true annular internal vesical sphincter (Uhlenhut *et al.*, 1953) has been denied in recent years in particular by Woodburne (1960, 1967) on account of his studies on macerated preparations after stripping the bladder from its adventitia. Fig. 136 demonstrates Woodburne's findings. He confirmed the views of previous authors (Le Gros Clark, 1883; Griffith, 1895) that there is no specific smooth muscle sphincter at the vesical neck. On the contrary, there is a continuity of bladder and urethra and the arrangement of the detrusor fibres are such as to open mechanically the proximal part of the vesical neck. However, recently Ichim & Burghele (1970), who studied the fibres of the detrusor by a 'transparency method' on human bladders 24 hours after death, came to the conclusion that there exists a smooth internal sphincter. In these experiments the upper pole of the bladder was opened, a cold light cystoscope introduced and the bladder was filled with saline. Through the transparence of the illuminated bladder, the course of the detrusor fibres as well as the anatomical structures of the trigone and the bladder floor, with its 'trigonal mouthpiece' forming a morphological unit with a rich vascular supply, can be studied from the outside. These authors found of special interest the annular formation of the bladder orifice which plays the role of a smooth sphincter merging posteriorly with the trigone. Moreover, one can see with this method the elastic connective tissue which serves as a support and insertion point of the smooth muscle fibres and completes the muscular–connective tissue ring of the bladder floor. This ring has the function of a smooth sphincter. In the area of the ring the mucosa is fixed to the deep layers.

THE LYMPHATIC SYSTEM OF THE BLADDER

Since Masgagni (1787) and Cruikshank (1790) described the lymphatic vessels in the bladder, the problem of localization and distribution of the lymph vessels in the bladder has been the subject of repeated discussion in the literature. Although the views expressed are controversial, the majority of histologists agree that neither the urothelium nor the submucosa contain lymph vessels and that the lymphatic system is localized in the muscle layers (Renyi-Vamos, 1960). Lymph vessels from the upper vesical wall cross the arteria obturatoria and its accompanying veins and join lymph glands which are situated along the arteria hypogastrica and arteria iliaca externa. The lymph vessels originating from the bladder neck join together with those from the prostate and seminal vesicles, the lower lumbar lymph glands. Knowledge of this anatomical distribution of the lymph gland system helps to understand the course of infection within the bladder and urogenital tracts.

Anatomical relationship between bladder and ureter

Detailed reviews on the anatomy and physiology of the ureter and its relationship to the vesico-ureteric and pelvi-ureteric junctions have been published in recent years which have revealed certain controversial views on this subject (Narath, 1951; Frey & Quénu, 1965; Woodburne, 1967; Bors & Comarr, 1971). Since Waldeyer's description of the 'uretersheath' in 1891 particular attention has been paid by numerous workers to the anatomical arrangements of the vesico-ureteric junction (McMahon, 1938; Pieper, 1951; Correy & West, 1953; Uhlenhut et al., 1953; Woodburne, 1960; Hutch, 1962; Tanago & Pugh, 1963). Their and other investigators' findings have clarified the intrinsic muscular and elastic fibre connections which exist between the intravesical part of the ureter and the bladder wall, especially the trigone. These intricate connections form the anatomical basis of an efficient function of the ureteric orifices in preventing vesico-ureteric reflux and also mutual contamination of urine with seminal fluid excretion, the latter being prevented by a proper reciprocal function of the close muscular connection between the ureteric orifices and ejaculatory ducts. On the other hand, it is obvious that neurogenic dysfunctions of bladder and urethra may adversely affect this intricate system of tissue connections at the vesico-ureteric junction and thus the function of the ureteric orifices. Moreover, these close tissue connections also explain the direct route of ascending infection from the bladder into the ureters and kidneys. Talbot (1958, 1968) has drawn attention to the continuation of the subepithelial tissue of the bladder with that of the ureter, renal pelvis and interstitial tissue of the kidney and thus establishing a direct pathway of bacterial invasion. How far Waldeyer's 'sheath', which according to Woodburne (1967) is not a connective tissue substratum but a space between detrusor fascicles and terminal ureter, plays an essential role in the accumulation of infective material producing early ascending infection, remains to be seen. Having attended a great number of necropsies of paraplegics who died from ascending infection and pyelo-nephritis, I was always impressed by the continuous and uniform fibrous mass extending from the bladder and involving the whole upper urinary tract and kidneys which could represent the final outcome of direct ascending infection. This does not exclude, of course, other pathways of bacterial spread through lymphogenic and vascular channels, such as haematogenic origin of renal cortical abscesses, but the direct route of ascending infection seems to be the most common.

The innervation of the ureter is still a controversial subject, especially concerning motor function. The ureter receives its innervation from the renal plexus, the upper and lower end of the intermesenteric plexuses (L2–L5) and from the superior hypogastric plexus and hypogastric ganglia (Mitchell, 1935, 1950). Lermonth (1931) found that electrical stimulation of the peripheral end of the presacral nerve produces contraction of the ureteric orifices in man. Lutzeier (1963) reported a decrease of the tone of the ureter following sympathectomy which is in accordance with Langworthy's & Murphy's observation (1939) who found ureteric dilatation following sympathectomy in the cat. There is difference of opinion amongst authors as to whether spinal anaesthesia had any influence on tone and contractility of the ureter (Lapides, 1948; Rutishauser, 1962; Skalol & Morales, 1966). Drugs are known to affect ureteric activity and alpha and beta adrenergic receptors have been demonstrated in the ureter (Boyarski et al., 1966, 1971; Rosset et al., 1967). The difficulty in assessing the action of motor nerve innervation of the ureter lies in the well-known fact that the ureter, completely deprived of its nerve supply, still contracts to stimulation. Bors & Comarr (1952, 1971) mention amongst other points, as indirect evidence of the nervous influences on ureteral motor activity, a different incidence of reflux occurring in upper as compared with lower motor lesions of the spinal cord. This is not in accordance with my own observations on the relationship between ureteric reflux and level of cord lesions. However, there is also some disagreement regarding the sensory innervation of the ureter. Head (1893) mapped out cutaneous areas of referred ureteric pain over the L1–L2 segments. According to Foerster (1936) the radicular sensory innervation of the ureter includes T9–L2. White & Garrey (1942) have shown that division of the posterior spinal roots T12–L2 abolished pain resulting from distension of the renal pelvis.

CONGENITAL STRUCTURAL ANOMALIES

Before considering details of the vesical neuro-physiology and pathophysiology, certain congenital structural anomalies may be mentioned briefly which may prevent, a priori, a co-ordinated reciprocal function of the vesical closing and emptying mechanisms. They may involve the bladder itself and may lead to intravesical obstruction. The more common are the congenital bladder diverticulum, the extrophy (i.e. eversion of the dorsal bladder wall which may be associated with absence of the ventral bladder and lower abdominal walls), reduplication of the bladder which may be complete or incomplete or trigonal folds which may result in obstruction of the vesical outlet. On the other hand, urethral anomalies such as congenital urethral stricture resulting in stenosis of the external meatus, hypospadias or congenital diverticulum may be the primary cause of vesical dysfunction. Of special interest are urechal cysts. They develop as a result of persistence of the lumen of the allantoic stalk which may result in a small cavity with epithelial lining becoming filled with fluid and developing later into a larger cyst surrounded by a thick wall of connective tissue (Kuntz, 1965). There may be no connection of such a cyst with the bladder or external opening at the umbilicus; on the other hand such a persistent allantois lumen, called a patent urachus, may connect with the bladder and develop into an umbilico-urinary fistula. Recently I saw a young man with a complete traumatic tetraplegia below C5/6 and chronic urinary infection, who developed, at the end of 1969, 3 years after his injury, a swelling and inflammation around the umbilicus with high temperature. Aspiration of this swelling by the family doctor revealed a large amount of pus from a infected urechal cyst beneath the umbilicus. Following opening of the cavity there was a temporary urine discharge through the umbilicus indicating connection of the urechal cyst with the bladder. A contrast filling of the cyst carried out on 18 December 1969 through the sinus of the umbilicus showed a cavity lying anteriorally above the bladder. At that time, no communication with the bladder was found (Fig. 137a), neither did a cystography of the bladder show any communication of the

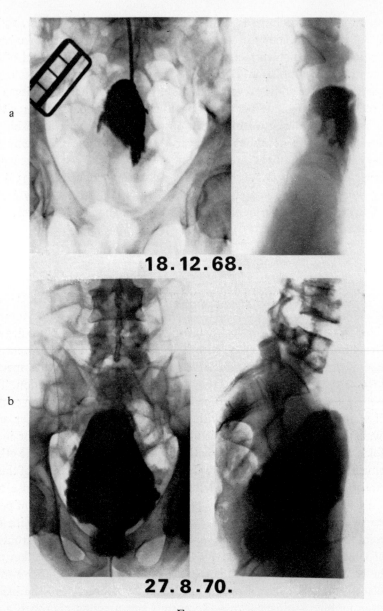

FIG. 137.

urechal cyst with the umbilicus (Fig. 137b) although the lateral X-ray of the bladder showed some structural abnormality of the apex of the bladder.

PHYSIOLOGICAL AND PATHOPHYSIOLOGICAL ASPECTS

Since Mosso & Pellacini's cystometric studies in 1882, anatomists, neurologists, physiologists and urologists have been engaged in a great variety of studies on the complex act of micturition and its relationship to the peripheral and central parts of the nervous system in normal and pathological conditions. The history of this research over the last 60 years contains a considerable number of contributions which have been fundamental in furthering the understanding of the innervation of the intricate process of storage and emptying of the urinary bladder (Elliot, 1907; Barrington, 1914–41; Head & Riddoch, 1917; L.R.Müller, 1918–31; Denning, 1924; Weston, 1920; McCrae, 1926; Hovelacque, 1927; Stöhr, 1928; Learmonth, 1931; Langworthy and his associates, 1933–40; Denny-Brown & Robertson, 1933; Evans, 1936; Munro, 1936–52; Talaat, 1937; McLellan, 1939; and others). The congregation of most patients with spinal cord injuries in Spinal Units during the Second World War has been a new and acute incentive to research on the pathophysiology of the human bladder and a vast literature on this subject has accumulated. This has resulted in a greater awareness of the complexity of the vesical dysfunction following complete and incomplete lesions of the spinal cord and its effects on the function of the upper urinary tract as well as on the cardiovascular system and other autonomic mechanisms. Yet, in spite of the advances made in the last 25 years in the development of sophisticated techniques of investigation of the urinary tract, there still exist gaps in our knowledge. Controversial concepts have arisen regarding both physiological aspects and the management of the abnormal vesical function.

The act of micturition

The act of micturition in physiological conditions with intact nervous control can be defined as a co-ordinated powerful reflex response at spinal segmental level to stretch of the bladder wall when the volume pressure reaches its physiological threshold and provokes the desire to void and thus initiates micturition. The ways in which the expulsive and closing forces perform their functions in the act of micturition have been the subject of intensive studies. Barrington (1921), on account of animal experiments, postulated six reflexes at hind-brain and spinal level involved in the act of micturition. Van Duzen's (1935) concept based on Young et al. observations (1921, 1926) and his own studies distinguishes three phases in the act of micturition:

1 Contraction of the trigone depressing the posterior portion of the internal vesical orifice which is then opened.

2 A wave of detrusor contraction originating in the area of the internal vesical orifice, extending towards the dome of the bladder and exerting a lateral pull on the internal orifice which opens it further. (The effacement of the internal neck as a result of the detrusor contraction due to its insertion into the area of the vesical neck has also been confirmed by Lapides et al., 1960.)

3 Contraction of the abdominal muscles increasing the intra-abdominal pressure and thus the expulsive power of the detrusor contraction. (Mullner (1951) found in fluoroscopic studies that volitional voiding starts with increased abdominal pressure accompanied by reciprocal relaxation of the pelvic floor.) This elicits a powerful pull on the vesical neck initiating contraction of the bladder base spreading upwards and involving the whole bladder musculature. Conversely, volitional interruption of micturition begins with contraction of the pelvic floor muscles, resulting in elevation of the whole base of the

bladder and abrupt closing of the vesical neck. Burgheli & Ichim (1970) stimulated electrically the motor nerves of the bladder, following introduction of a cold-light cystoscope through an opening above the posterior border of the trigone and filling the bladder with saline. From that position, the function of the bladder could be observed and registered by endovesical cinematography. Following stimulation of the nervi pelvici through double electrodes the pressure produced by detrusor contractions overcomes the resistance of the tone of the sphincter system and voiding occurs. However, 10–15 seconds later the stimulating effect on the sympathetic fibres in the plexus pelvicus, where both parasympathetic and sympathetic fibres are mixed, evokes contraction of the smooth sphincter and the bladder emptying is stopped. This is accomplished by the longer latent period of sympathetic stimulation. From these observations, the authors assume, as already mentioned above, the existence of a smooth internal sphincter which plays a part in the closing mechanism of the bladder.

Although modern anatomical research (Krantz, 1951; Woodburne, 1960, 1967) is in accordance with the views of previous authors (Le Gros Clark, 1883; Griffiths, 1895) that anatomically there is a continuation of bladder and urethra and that the detrusor muscle fibres open mechanically the proximal part of the vesical neck, there is no doubt about the reciprocity between the expulsive action of the detrusor and the inhibitory action of the vesical neck. The response of the vesical neck (internal sphincter complex) is like that of the external urethral sphincter opposite to that of the detrusor muscle. Denny-Brown & Robertson (1933), recording simultaneously vesical, urethral, rectal, perineal and abdominal wall pressure, found reflex relaxation of the detrusor when the sphincters contracted and vice versa. However, in normal conditions, the inhibitory function of the vesical neck complex is less essential during micturition than during sexual function, where contraction of the smooth muscle bundles of the vesical neck is important and acts like a trap-door in preventing regurgitation of the ejaculate into the bladder during orgasm. It is well known that, following prostatectomy, this trap-door action is abolished and regurgitation of the ejaculate into the bladder during orgasm occurs as a result of the destruction of the prostatic and membranous structures of the urethra. The disturbed balanced reciprocity between the forces of expulsion and the inhibitory function of the vesical neck complex is the primary cause of bladder dysfunction in lesions of the central nervous system. This will be discussed later.

Desire to micturate is precipitated primarily by increased bladder volume initiating reflex detrusor contraction followed by relaxation of the sphincter complex. The relationship between bladder volume and the first desire to void varies individually. Best & Taylor (1935) found first desire to void at about half the volume of the bladder content required to cause irresistible urgency of micturition. During sleep in the adult, when conscious awareness of bladder distension is eliminated, afferent impulses emanating from the distended viscus may be strong enough to interrupt the sleep, thus restoring desire to void and promoting volitional voiding. In very young children who have not full control, these afferent impulses may initiate voiding without arousing consciousness and bed wetting is the result.

The reflex action of the bladder is also subject to volitional and emotional impulses which in certain extrinsic (for instance cold) or intrinsic conditions may facilitate micturition before the bladder is sufficiently distended to act reflexly. Conversely, these influences may inhibit vesical emptying in spite of desire or stop the flow of urine abruptly once it has started. Prostatectomy may not necessarily prevent the ability to stop the urine flow at will. The effect of stressful psychiatric interview on raising intravesical pressure has been demonstrated by Straub *et al.* (1950). The emotional incontinence in subjects with cerebral atherosclerosis or brain tumours is well known. On the other hand, normal subjects may, through embarrassment, have difficulty in overcoming their inhibition to micturate at will or on desire in the presence of a doctor or nurse. In others the visual or auditory stimulus of running water may be necessary to facilitate volitional voiding. This practice is sometimes adopted in training children.

Posture also has an influence on the ability to micturate, and certain normal subjects are unable to pass urine in supine position even by using strong abdominal pressure. Others are able to pass only small quantities of urine in that position and moreover, the rate of urine flow is diminished, and greater or lesser quantities of residual urine result.

While the active contraction of the abdominal muscles during the act of defaecation is essential, their degree of action in the act of micturition varies considerably from individual to individual of both sexes according to circumstances. Certain individuals use abdominal pressure only at the end of micturition. Denny-Brown & Robertson (1933) found that abdominal wall contractions were not necessary to initiate and sustain micturition. They also observed 'after contractions' at the end of voiding which were associated with an increase in intrarectal pressure and contraction of the abdominal muscles. These after contractions which were particularly pronounced when the urine volume was small, were not considered to be the result of rise in abdominal pressure. Electro-myographic studies have confirmed the variability of muscular activity of the abdominals in micturition on desire or volition (Bors, 1963). However, the flow rate of urine depends, apart from the volume, on the action of the abdominals and diaphragm in raising intra-abdominal pressure.

Wilful suppression of desire to micturate leads to temporary inhibition and relaxation of the detrusor muscle, in the same way as volitional suppression influences the function of colon and rectum, which clearly indicates control of central stations of the nervous system on the function of smooth muscles. Protracted suppression of releasing the distended bladder normally sets up a feeling of considerable discomfort leading eventually to irresistible urge to micturate accompanied by more or less pronounced cardiovascular and other responses of autonomic mechanisms such as shivering, piloerection and sweating. Habitual restraining of micturition in spite of large fluid intake, as is the case in excessive beer or tea drinkers, results in increasing bladder capacity and may lead eventually to chronic over-stretching of the detrusor muscle and reduction of its expulsive power. These pre-paraplegic, individually varying habits of micturition, should always be taken into consideration when dealing with patients suffering from bladder dysfunction due to affliction of the nervous system, in particular in spinal paraplegics and tetraplegics.

The question of sequence and latency in the reciprocal action between the detrusor muscle and the internal and external sphincter complex and muscles of the pelvic floor is still a matter of controversy (Denny-Brown & Robertson, 1933; Hinman *et al.*,

1954; Mullner, 1958; Murphy & Schoenberg, 1960; Petersen *et al.*, 1962; Abramson *et al.*, 1962; Glahn, 1970, 1974).

Abramson and his associates combining electromyography of the pelvic floor muscles with suprapubic cystometry, found a variable delay of detrusor contraction following relaxation of the pelvic floor. The electrical silence of the striated muscles of the pelvic floor preceded the detrusor contraction by 2–20 seconds. Bors (1963) came to the conclusion that 'pelvic floor relaxation seems to precede or coincide with the detrusor action more often than following it, depending on individual variations'. Hinman *et al.* (1954) found during cineradiography the following sequence of events in nulliparous women:

1 Isometric detrusor contractions and opening of the internal sphincter.
2 Relaxation of the perineal muscles.
3 Emptying contractions of the detrusor.
4 Closure of the external sphincter.
5 Contraction of the perineal muscles and elevation of the bladder base.
6 Closure of the internal sphincter with relaxation of the detrusor.

HIGHER CONTROL OF MICTURITION BY CORTICAL AND SUBCORTICAL STATIONS

From all that has been said, it is obvious that supraspinal stations—i.e. cortical and subcortical structures—exert, under normal and pathological conditions, a considerable influence on the complex act of micturition as they do on other autonomic mechanisms such as gastro-intestinal function, vasomotor control, temperature regulation, sweating, etc.

Cortical influences

Cortical centres situated in areas 4 and 6 are supposed to exert some degree of inhibitory control of the reflex function of the bladder (Lewis, Langworthy & Dees, 1935). Kleist (1934) and Foerster (1936) localized the cortical representation of bladder and rectum in the lobulus paracentralis just above the fissura calloso-marginalis. Adler's hypothesis (1920) of two cortical vesical centres, one for the detrusor, situated in the lobulus paracentralis, and the other for the vesical sphincter mechanism situated in the convexity of the brain between the cortical representation of leg and arm, was not substantiated by other authors (Kleist, 1934; Foerster, 1936). However, recently Gjone *et al.* (1963) found in the chloralized cat that stimulation of the sensori-motor cortex elicited intermixed facilitatory and inhibitory responses on the micturition reflex. Actually, the absence of inhibitory cortical control in the young infant is correlated to the late development of cortical centres.

The representation of vesical function in the cortex is bilateral, and it is well known that unilateral cortical and subcortical lesions have no or only very transient effect on sphincter control, as has been confirmed in recent years by Rothfield & Rabiner (1954).

On the other hand, bilateral cortical affliction in the adult, in particular those affecting the frontal lobe and parasagittal areas (gunshot injuries, parasagittal meningioma), may produce, even in the absence of raised intra-cranial pressure, bladder dysfunctions which are similar or identical to that of a young infant. Foerster (1936) found, following bilateral destruction of the vesical cortical fields, firstly retention of micturition necessitating catheterization, followed later by reflex micturition and incontinence which could last for a considerable time. In patients with gunshot injuries of both paracentral lobes during the First World War, he found that the bladder paralysis was combined with isolated paralysis of both feet and toes. Fig. 138 shows the X-rays of one of my own patients from the Second World War who sustained a brain injury of the upper parietal region, resulting in a spastic paresis without sensory disturbances of the right arm and particularly the right leg with paralysis of most of the dorsi- and plantarflexors of the right foot and toes and, in addition, a marked spastic paresis of the dorsi- and plantar-flexors of the left foot and toes. There was, therefore, no doubt that he had a bilateral lesion of the paracentral lobe, more on the right than on the left. He was suffering from extreme urgency and precipitous incontinence. Moreover, after micturition, urgency returned after a few minutes and he passed again several ounces of urine. He died in 1965 from metastases of a carcinoma of the sigmoid colon. Recently, Andrew & Nathan (1964) found that frontal lobe lesions caused frequency and extreme urgency of micturition

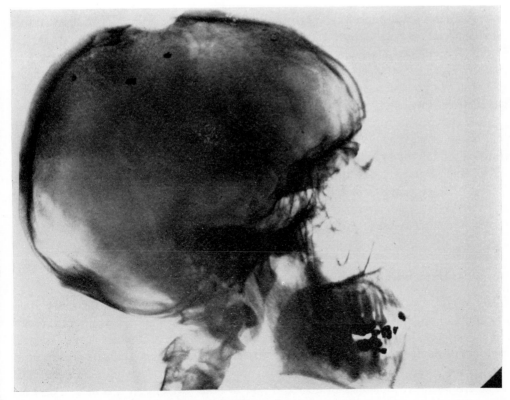

FIG. 138.

when the patient was awake and there was incontinence during sleep. Olivecrona (1935) described bladder dysfunctions in patients with parasagittal and frontal tumours. Foerster (1936) described a case of metastatic hypernephroma of the gyrus fornicatus of the left side reaching into the lobulus paracentralis who suffered for 8 years from focal epileptic fits, which started as a rule in the right big toe but repeatedly also with sudden involuntary micturition. On the other hand, a unilateral meningioma of the lobulus para-centralis, causing focal epileptic fits starting in the contralateral big toe and foot, may not necessarily elicit vesical dysfunction, as described in another of Foerster's patients. During my visiting professorship at Duke University, Durham, U.S.A., in 1969, I saw several patients from the Vietnam War with parasagittal injuries of the cortex who were suffering from disturbances of micturition (frequency, urgency and incontinence). Some of them had initially urine retention for varying periods.

Subcortical influences

In recent years the work of Tang & Ruch (1955, 1956, 1967) has revealed more details of the subcortical control of the brain which has amplified and clarified the findings of previous workers in this field (Barrington, 1921, 1925; Kabat et al., 1936; Langworthy et al., 1940). Following transhypothalamic, intercollicular, supra- and infracollicular decerebration in the normal cat, they found a number of descending pathways exerting both facilitatory and inhibitory influences on the micturition reflex. From their studies they concluded: (a) Oblongata and posterior pons have no micturition centres but are merely 'way stations' of descending inhibitory and facilitatory pathways of higher cerebral centres. This is contrary to Kuru & Koyama's (1961) views, who considered oblongata and posterior pons as seats of actual micturition centres. (b) However, the anterior pons has a strong facilitatory influence on the spinal segmental micturition reflex. (c) This pontine centre is in turn restrained by cerebral areas above the intercollicular level. In transection of the mid-brain (intercollicular decerebration) the pontine centre is released from central inhibitory influences, resulting in lowering of the threshold of the micturition reflex. Ruch & Tang found the volume of fluid necessary to elicit the micturition reflex to be as low as 4 and 8 ccs as compared with the normal threshold for micturition of 40/80 ccs in correlation with the size of the cat. Transection below the pontine centre results in complete loss of micturition reflex.

Descending and ascending pathways within the spinal cord

There is still discrepancy of opinion with regard to the localization of the descending cerebral pathways within the spinal cord (Budge, 1864; Foerster & Gagel, 1932; Hun-sicker & Spiegel, 1933; Wrack, 1943). According to Rothfeld & Rabiner (1954), cortical impulses to the sacral spinal micturition centre are mediated through fibres arising from the cerebral cortex and they transverse the cortico-spinal tracts. From my own experience on antero-lateral cordotomies in man and that of other workers in this field (Foerster, 1936; Kahn & Rand, 1952), it can be concluded that bilateral cordotomy of the spino-thalamic tract results in immediate disorganization of the micturition reflex. However, as to whether the fibres descending from the facilitatory cerebral centres transverse into lateral columns and those of the inhibitory areas run into the ventral columns still needs clarification. Kuru *et al.* (1960) studying the connections of the pontine area with the Marchi degeneration technique found descending fibres running down into the lateral reticulo-spinal tract decussating at the midlumbar level of the spinal cord and terminating in the intermedio-lateral cell column of the sacral cord. They also found afferent connections to the thalamus. Nathan & Smith (1958) concluded from their studies following cordotomy in man that the pathways for voluntary control of micturition lay in a transverse equatorial plane passing through the ependymal canal. Efferent and afferent fibres running more medially. However, their evidence given by their anatomical sections of the cord following cordotomy does not appear to be conclusive.

Spinal segmental and peripheral control of micturition

The synaptic connections of ascending and descending nervous pathways subserving micturition take place in the lumbo-sacral segments of the spinal cord which represent the spinal micturition reflex centre. Destruction of this centre, in particular of its sacral part, results in depriving the bladder of its reflex function and it has to rely on its intramural autonomous nerve supply only. From the spinal vesical centre originates the peripheral control and integration of vesical reflex function. The efferent and afferent components involved in the peripheral innervation of the forces of expulsion and retention are:

A. EFFERENT INNERVATION

1. *The sympathetic innervation* derives from L2, L3 and L4 segments. Their pre-ganglionic fibres pass to the inferior mesenteric ganglion and their post-ganglionic fibres traverse through the hypo-gastric nerves to the bladder wall and urethra. The participation of the sympathetic innervation in the act of micturition has been the subject of controversies for some time. In particular, the effects of stimulation of the sympathetic nerves on micturition are not unequivocal. The old concept (Elliott, 1907) that the hypo-gastric nerves constrict the sphincter and inhibit the tone of the detrusor muscle has been rejected by Van Duzen (1932) and Evans (1936), who found no convincing evidence that the sympathetic system plays any part in the act of micturition, especially with regard to the internal sphincter complex. Other investigators supported the view that sympathetic stimulation results in contraction of the internal sphincter orifice and the detrusor, followed immediately by the latter's relaxation (Learmonth, 1931; Langworthy, Kolb & Lewis, 1950; Kuntz & Saccomano, 1944; Ingersoll, Jones & Hegre, 1954). See also Burgheli's and Ichim's observations reported above. Langworthy and his colleagues held the view that sympathetic stimulation is mainly concerned with the mechanism of ejaculation, and Learmonth found discharge of seminal fluid in man following stimulation

of the superior hypogastric plexus. Conversely, following resection of the plexus or the upper lumbar ganglia, the power of ejaculation is abolished or at least greatly impaired, while bladder function remains unimpaired.

2. *The parasympathetic innervation* originates in S2, 3 and 4 segments and reaches the bladder and urethra through the pelvic autonomic rami (nervi erigentes). It represents the chief efferent mechanism in the act of micturition. Stimulation of the pelvic nerves always results in vigorous contraction of the detrusor muscle. Unilateral stimulation of the pelvic nerve elicits strong contraction of the ipsilateral side of the detrusor but also, although diminished, contraction of the opposite detrusor. Stimulation of the central end of a severed pelvic nerve, while that of the opposite side remains intact, causes contraction of the whole bladder after a latent period of a few seconds (Ingersoll *et al.*, 1955). Conversely, resection of the pelvic nerves results in flaccid paralysis of the bladder.

3. *Somatic volitional innervation* originates in S1 and S2 segments and reaches the striated musculature of the urethra and pelvic floor through the pudendal nerves. Stimulation of the pudendal nerves elicits elevation and closure of the vesical neck (Ardran *et al.*, 1956; Noix, 1960). Pudendal anaesthesia (Lapides *et al.*, 1955) or pudendal neurotomy does not result in incontinence (Wertheimer & Michon, 1928).

B. AFFERENT INNERVATION

Afferent impulses mediating sensation of bladder distension and pain is conveyed by the pelvic and pubic nerves but also by the sympathetic innervation. Afferent impulses arising from the bladder are conducted through the pelvic nerves, while those arising from the external sphincter and partly also from the vesical neck travel through the pudendal nerves. However, Bors (1952) concluded from his experience with transurethral resection of the bladder neck that pain can still be experienced in spite of complete anaesthesia resulting from pudendal nerve block. According to Learmonth (1931), pain and touch sensations are conveyed by parasympathetic and sympathetic fibres. In Denning's (1924) animal experiments with bladder distension, the uneasiness of the animal caused by bladder distension was not relieved by pudendal neurectomy but was greatly diminished following resection of the pelvic and hypogastric nerves.

Although the parasympathetic afferents mediate sensation of bladder distension and pain, sympathetic afferents also convey these sensations in complete spinal cord lesions above the level of the transection (Guttmann & Whitteridge, 1947). The findings of Langworthy *et al.* (1940) that the bladder is sensitive to thermal stimuli are not in accordance with the results of other authors (Waltz, 1922; Nathan, 1952), and it is suggested that the disagreement regarding thermal sensibility of the bladder is due to associated thermal stimulation of the urethra which is actually sensitive to thermal stimulation.

C. AXONAL INNERVATION

Modern studies using electron microscope and microelectrode have furnished details of the intricate axon innervation of individual muscle cells of the detrusor (Caesar et al., 1957). It was found that one axon innervates a number of smooth muscle cells, and one muscle cell may be in contact with several axons. Stretch receptors in the bladder have been described (Iggo, 1955), and it was found that stretch increases excitability by depolarizing the muscle cell (Ursillo, 1961).

GENERAL DOCUMENTATION
AND CLASSIFICATION

For a comprehensive classification and documentation of vesical disorders sequential to lesions of any parts of the nervous system and their effects on other organs of the organism especially the upper urinary tract, the evaluation of a considerable number of data arising from clinical and experimental investigations is indispensable. In modification with those outlined recently by Bors (1967), Bradley (1967), Markland et al. (1967), the following investigations have to be considered:

1. *Full neurological examination* to determine onset, site, type, completeness and duration of the neurological affliction. In addition to defining the deficit of motor, sensory and autonomous functions, attention should be paid to investigations of the state of reflexes in the lower limbs and, especially, to the bulbo-cavernosus, anal and cremasteric reflexes during the stage of spinal shock as well as during the various phases of reflex return.

2. *Clinical evaluation of bladder function.* This includes examination of micturition at will, on desire, preparaplegic habits of micturition, flow rate, ability to stop flow, participation of the abdominal muscles in the act of micturition, onset of retention, urgency, and frequency as well as types of incontinence. In lesions of central stations of the nervous system, in particular complete lesions of the spinal cord above the level of the thoraco-lumbar junction, the essential points to be considered are: duration of spinal shock, onset or permanent absence of reflex micturition, date of onset and cessation of catheterization, degree of residual urine, infection, symptoms of bladder distension and automatic detrusor activity resulting in local sensation with or without associated cardio-vascular and other autonomic responses, facilitation of voiding by various types of trigger mechanisms, last but by no means least the patient's ability to adjust himself to his bladder dysfunction.

3. *Diagnostic and experimental tests of bladder and renal function*

a Residual urine tests (in lying and vertical positions).
b Detailed laboratory urine analysis including specific gravity test, cells, protein

electrolytes, culture (type of infection) and renal function tests (blood urea, creatinine clearance, B_2-microglobuline osmolality).

c   Straight X-ray of urinary tract (demonstration of stones and/or chronic constipation).

d   Cystometry combined, if indicated, with sphincterometry (determination of tone and changes of bladder function).

e   Intravenous pyelogram (renal and ureteric changes, early pyelitis).

f   Cysto-urethrogram by fractionized slow filling of bladder and delayed X-ray. (Demonstration of shape and capacity of bladder, diverticulosis of urethra and bladder, types of reflux, ureter kinking and blockage.)

g   Voiding cysto-urethrogram with fluoroscopy combined, if indicated, with cineradiography.

h   Cystoscopy, if indicated, for retrograde pyelography or to determine hypertrophy of bladder neck, blockage at external urethral sphincter, internal bladder orifice, or ureteric level and other structural pathology.

i   Diagnostic anaesthesias (mucosal, pudendal, epidural, subarachnoid block, all of which are rarely indicated).

j   Radio-isotope test for renal function, if indicated.

k   Electro-myography and electrical stimulation test, if indicated.

l   Dip slides urine test (Dennis Guttmann and S. R. Naylor, 1967) for out-patients to minimize in-patient check ups of paraplegics in employment.

DYSFUNCTIONS OF THE BLADDER IN SPINAL CORD AND CAUDA EQUINA LESIONS (CLASSIFICATION AND TREATMENT)

Amongst the afflictions of the various stations of the nervous system, those of the spinal cord and cauda equina, in particular, have been the subject of intensive investigation and research after the Second World War, with regard to vesical disorders, and they can be more readily classified than can afflictions of other parts of the nervous system, such as cortical and subcortical lesions. How far future documentation and patient planning with the aid of a computer will be possible, remains to be seen (Carter & Jackson, 1971).

I. Stage of spinal shock (vesical hypo- or areflexia) retention and overflow incontinence (ischuria paradoxa)

In the initial stage of an acute transverse spinal cord lesion, regardless of level and whether the lesion remains complete or in due course becomes incomplete, all connections between the spinal vesical reflex centre and its facilitatory and inhibitory cerebral centres are interrupted. In this stage, termed by Marshall Hall (1841) 'spinal shock', there is a depression and imbalance of the reflex activity of the isolated cord for all efferent and afferent stimuli. As a result, any volitional or reflex function of the bladder is abolished. There is no desire to urinate, and the bladder no longer responds to an appropriate degree of distension by efficient reflex contraction. Commensurate with the flaccid paralysis of the skeletal muscles, there is at first a flaccid paralysis of the detrusor muscle as well as the striated bladder muscles. Although the bladder wall, thanks to its autonomous intramural innervation and its inherent elasticity, is not completely atonic, no effective detrusor contractions are elicitable to overcome the passive blockage of the vesical orifice. Therefore, retention of urine occurs. Voiding through overflow will take place only when the maximum of expansibility of the bladder wall is reached and the passive blockage of the bladder exit and that of the paralysed external urethral sphincter are overcome by excessive intravesical pressure (ischuria paradoxa, overflow incontinence). If over-distension of the bladder is allowed to continue, long standing atonicity of the bladder wall is inevitable, resulting in adverse effects on detrusor function once the period of spinal shock has subsided.

The duration of the initial stages of bladder paralysis varies from 8 days to 6–8 weeks. In complete lesions above the thoraco-lumbar junction, the duration of this stage depends on various factors:

1 Hypotonicity of the bladder wall due to chronic habitual over-distension developed previous to the spinal cord lesion.

2 Delayed development of reflex automatism of the isolated cord in upper thoracic and cervical lesions not infrequently as a result of the degree of longitudinal damage of the cord associated with its transverse lesion. In such cases the knee and ankle jerks may also be diminished for longer periods than usual.

3 Age of the patient (in young individuals reflex micturition may occur within a few days following complete transection of the cord).

4 Efficiency of the initial management of the bladder, in particular whether or not over-distension during the stage of spinal shock and severe infection was avoided or whether the initial treatment was carried out by intermittent catheterization or by permanent drainage with an indwelling catheter.

II. Stage of automatic or autonomous micturition

Once the stage of spinal shock has subsided, level and type of the cord or conus–cauda equina lesion, whether complete or incomplete, are determining factors in the pathophysiology of the bladder. A distinction has to be made between transverse lesions above the thoraco-lumbar junction without damage to the spinal vesical centre and those where this centre or its afferent and efferent nerve roots are involved either by direct destruction (conus–cauda equina lesion) or by longitudinal damage associated with the transverse lesion at higher level. These facts explain the great varieties of bladder dysfunction occurring in spinal cord lesions. The following types of spinal cord bladder can be distinguished:

A. THE AUTOMATIC REFLEX BLADDER (SUPRA-NUCLEAR, ALSO CALLED UPPER MOTOR NEURON TYPE)

EARLY AND INTERMEDIATE STAGES OF VESICAL REFLEX ACTIVITY

In complete transverse lesions above the lumbar–sacral segments, provided the reflex arc has remained intact, reflex micturition develops as soon as the stage of spinal shock has subsided and the isolated cord develops its automatic reflex function, unrestrained from cerebral influences. Once a sufficient degree of distension of the bladder wall is reached, sensory receptors in its wall evoke, through their afferents, reflex contraction of the detrusor muscle, resulting in opening of the bladder exit, and promote reciprocal relaxation of the external urethral sphincters and the muscles of the pelvic floor. Reflex automatism of the bladder may occur earlier than that of the skeletal muscles of legs, especially the knee and ankle jerks, while bulbo-cavernosus, anal reflex and plantar response, as a rule, appear earlier than reflex activity of the bladder. Details of this have been published elsewhere (Guttmann, 1953).

In the early phase of bladder reflex automatism, tone and function of the detrusor are still greatly diminished; therefore, its expulsive force is less effective and larger amounts of residual urine will result. The duration of this phase of reflex activity of the bladder varies from case to case, and intermittent catheterization will still be necessary for some time to avoid larger amounts of residual urine until the tonicity of the detrusor and its expulsive force are strong enough, in due course, to ensure micturition without or with the least amount of residual urine (intermediate stage).

As a rule, 5–10 per cent residual urine of the full capacity of the bladder is acceptable, provided stagnation of the urine is prevented by large fluid intake. Hyporeflexia of the bladder may persist for longer periods in those transverse lesions where the initial management of the bladder has been inefficient, especially when over-distension and severe

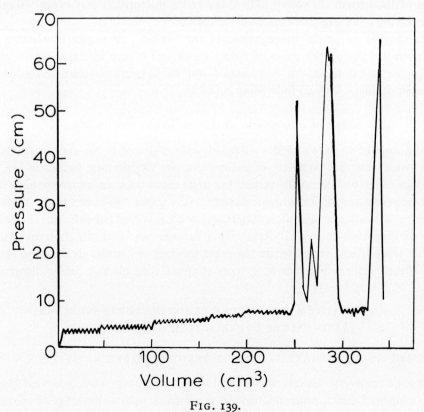

FIG. 139.

infection of the bladder has been allowed to develop or pre-paraplegic bladder abnormalities were present.

III. Final Stages

(a) CO-ORDINATED VESICAL REFLEX FUNCTION

Once full reflex automatism has developed, various types of automatic bladder may emerge. In the ideal form, especially in incomplete transverse lesions, the detrusor will react with one strong contraction, as occurs in normal individuals, once the critical point of bladder distension is reached, and the bladder will be almost completely emptied. This reflex micturition may occur, according to the bladder capacity, every 2–4 hours, and amounts of 250–350 ccs of urine may be expelled. This is the ideal type of co-ordinated automatic reflex bladder. However, in the majority of complete cord lesions with otherwise co-ordinated vesical reflex function, several detrusor contractions may occur in response to bladder distension to ensure complete emptying (Fig. 139).

(b) DISCO-ORDINATED VESICAL REFLEX FUNCTION

The relation between distension of the bladder and the reflex responses of opening and closing mechanisms is often disturbed at one stage or another. The resulting disturbances of reflex micturition in both complete and incomplete lesions have to be analysed individually by special investigations, as mentioned previously. The causes of these

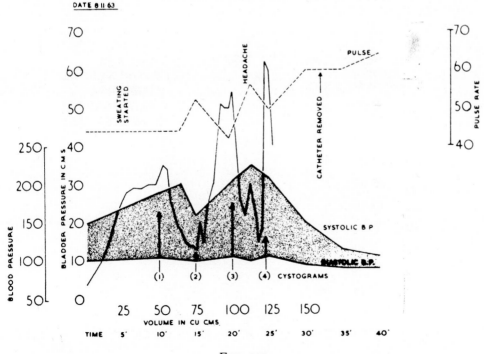

FIG. 140.

disturbances may lie primarily in dysfunction of the afferent or efferent components of the vesical reflex arc and its synaptic connections, resulting in hypo- or hyperreflexia of the bladder. Furthermore, flexor or extensor spasms of skeletal muscles resulting from the heightened reflex activity of the isolated cord itself may also influence the reflex activity of the bladder. For instance, flexor spasms of the legs may interrupt reflex micturition in progress. Moreover, any irritative process elsewhere in the organism, such as an ingrowing toe nail, may greatly increase the spasticity. On the other hand, structural changes in the various compartments of the urinary tract itself, such as diverticulosis, hypertrophy of the bladder neck, changes of the external urethral sphincter, and above all, those produced by active infection, may be responsible for increased vesical dysfunction. All these abnormalities influencing each other, may eventually affect capacity and shape of the bladder.

The most serious and troublesome type of disco-ordinated automatic bladder is the uninhibited-hypertonic cord bladder, whereby even small amounts of urine evoke very frequent detrusor contractions of varying intensity, producing almost constant voiding of smaller or greater quantities of urine (reflex incontinence). It is obvious that the smaller the capacity of the bladder, such as is the case in fibrous contracture of the bladder as a result of prolonged suprapubic or urethral catheter drainage by indwelling catheter, the more frequently these emptying contractions occur. The following cystometrograms are examples of uninhibited vesical hyperreflexia in complete lesions below C7 and T2 respectively (Figs. 140 and 141) which in the case of C7 already caused hypertension at filling of 50 ccs and in the case of T2 at 150 ccs bladder volume.

In incomplete transverse cord lesions, where the afferent and efferent connections between the spinal cord and the cerebral regulatory centres are not completely inter-

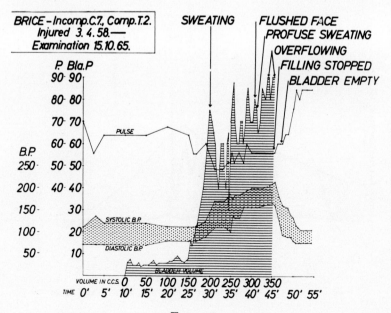

FIG. 141.

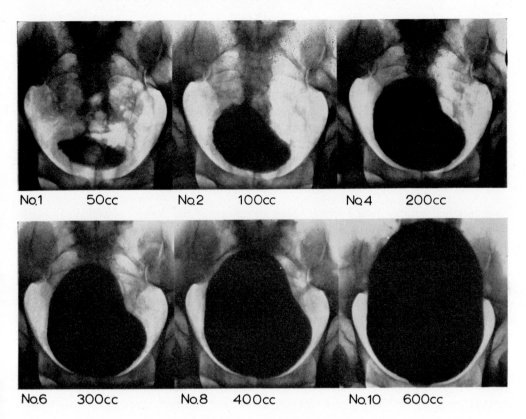

No.1   50cc   No.2   100cc   No.4   200cc

No.6   300cc   No.8   400cc   No.10   600cc

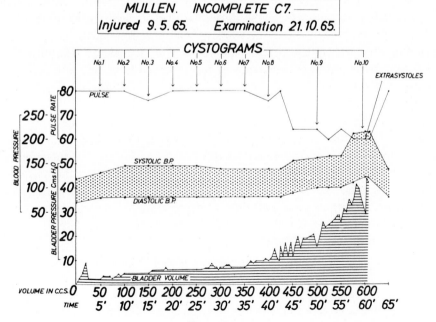

FIG. 142.

rupted, the facilitatory central impulses may outweigh the inhibitory ones and cause urgency of micturition with varying degrees of incontinence. As in complete lesions the symptoms of autonomic hyperreflexia, especially those of the cardio-vascular system, can be elicited in relationship to the size and expansibility of the bladder. Fig. 142 demonstrates the relationship of cystometrogram to cystography in a case of incomplete lesion of C7 where the increase of bladder pressure only started at 450 ccs eliciting bradycardia and hypertension reaching its maximum at bladder volume of 600 ccs.

Effects of bladder distension and vesical hyperactivity on somatic and autonomic systems

As mentioned before, during spinal shock all reflexes of the skeletal as well as autonomic systems are either abolished or diminished. Nevertheless, considerable distension of the bladder in cervical and upper thoracic lesions may produce cardiovascular and other autonomic reflex responses. Silver (1971) reported on cardiovascular reflexes during spinal shock. It was found that during the period of spinal shock inspiratory vasoconstriction and autonomic hyperreflexia resulted in response to distension of the bladder. Tulloch & Rossier (1975) in an experimental study on the autonomic nervous system and the bladder during spinal shock, found that the urethral muscle responded to drugs earlier than the detrusor muscle. Stimulation with parasympathicomimetic drugs caused some rise in intravesical pressure but much greater rise of intraurethral pressure. During spinal shock bladder evacuation was accomplished with the Credé manoeuvre combined with alpha adrenergic blockage and beta adrenergic stimulation.

The heightened reflex activity of the automatic bladder has its repercussions on both somatic and autonomic mechanisms both below and above the transverse lesions. The volleys of afferent impulses from the distended bladder wall and contracting detrusor may radiate unrestrainedly along the whole reflexogenic zone of the isolated cord. This in turn may elicit widespread reflex responses of skeletal muscles, resulting in flexor or extensor spasms of the legs, involving in higher thoracic lesions also the abdominal, intercostal and trunk muscles and in cervical lesions even muscles of the upper limbs (see Fig. 106).

Of special interest are the widespread reflex responses of autonomic mechanisms set up by distension of the bladder and vesical hyperactivity in the spinal man. It was shown by Carmichael, Doupe & McSwiney (1939) that distension of the duodenum in non-paraplegic healthy men produced vasoconstriction, more marked in the toes than in the fingers, and the same was found by Stürup (1940) following distension of the oesophagus. Circumscribed disturbances of sweating, corresponding to the segmented distribution of the gall-bladder, have been described as due to a viscero-sudoral reflex (Guttmann, 1938). In one of the cases published a change of functional state of sweat glands activity was studied in relation to a severe gall-bladder attack. While the sweat test carried out immediately following the attack showed an almost complete anhidrosis in the distribution of the 7th and 8th thoracic dermatomes on the right side, a relative hyperhidrosis was found in the same area as compared with the left side in tests before and three days after the attack when the patient had only little discomfort.

Sherrington (1899) described a sharp rise of blood pressure following distension of the gall-bladder in a spinal cat and Watkins (1938) and Talaat (1938) reported a rise of blood pressure in animal experiments when the bladder pressure was raised. Head & Riddoch (1917), in their classical paper on reflex responses in traumatic paraplegic soldiers of the First World War, described the effects of bladder activity on sweating, which was also previously described by Bowley (1890) in a case of traumatic tetraplegia. André-Thomas (1921) published his studies on pilo-erection responses made during the

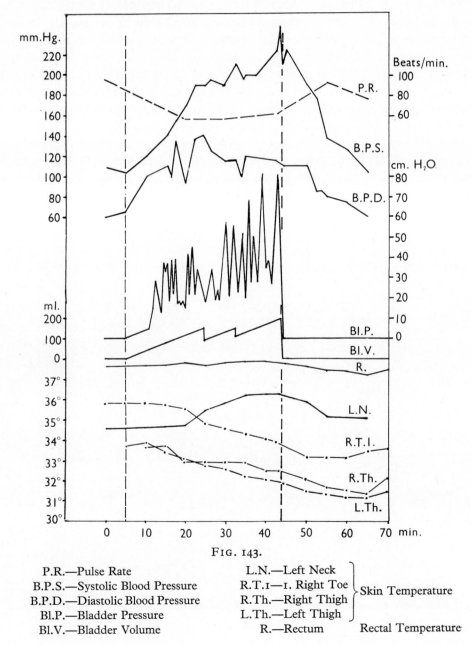

FIG. 143.

P.R.—Pulse Rate
B.P.S.—Systolic Blood Pressure
B.P.D.—Diastolic Blood Pressure
Bl.P.—Bladder Pressure
Bl.V.—Bladder Volume

L.N.—Left Neck
R.T.1—1. Right Toe
R.Th.—Right Thigh
L.Th.—Left Thigh
R.—Rectum

Skin Temperature

Rectal Temperature

First World War on paraplegic soldiers and demonstrated that distinct reflex responses could be elicited by stimulation above and below the lesion of the spinal cord (see chapter on the Pilomotor system).

In 1944, during my early cystometrographic studies on traumatic paraplegics of the Second World War, I observed distinct responses of the cardiovascular system during bladder distension, especially marked in complete transverse lesions above T5—i.e. above the splanchnic outflow—which called for more detailed investigation. With my colleagues of the Department of Physiology, Oxford University, Whitteridge, Gilliatt, Cunningham, Phillips and Wyndham and members of my medical staff, the cardiovascular changes as well as the responses of the sudo- and pilomotor systems were systematically studied. Every member of the team had one specific task, such as filling the bladder and registering bladder volume and bladder pressure, measuring blood pressure, pulse, respiration, sweating, pilo-erection, vasomotor and temperature changes. All these various recordings had to be carried out simultaneously and timed at regular intervals. The results obtained were reported in various publications (Guttmann & Whitteridge, 1947; Gilliatt, Guttmann & Whitteridge, 1947; Guttmann, 1963, 1954, 1968; Cunningham, Guttmann, Whitteridge & Whyndham, 1953). In due course our findings were confirmed in various countries by many other workers in this field (Thompson & Witham, 1948; Robertson & Wolff, 1950; Bors & French, 1952; Kurnick, 1956; Hodgson & Wood, 1958; Martens, Harms & Jungmann, 1960; Rousseau, Freedman, Boyarsky & Abramson, 1962; Garnier & Gertsch, 1963–64; Corbett, Frankel & Harris, 1971; and others), some of them using

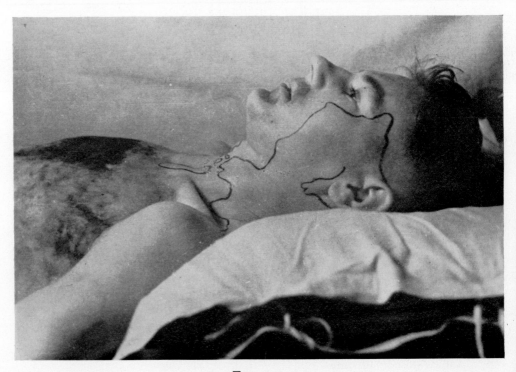

FIG. 144.

modern sophisticated monitoring techniques which allowed the study of the various parameters mentioned above to be carried out by only one or two workers.

The symptomatology of the autonomic hyperreflexia as a result of bladder distension is demonstrated by the results obtained in one of my first patients with a complete lesion at T4 (Fig. 143). As can be seen, during the experiment of bladder filling, marked by the two vertical lines, the increasing bladder volume elicited detrusor contractions which became increasingly powerful. There was a sharp rise in both systolic and diastolic blood pressure with values up to 240/135. This was associated with a marked bradycardia. Distinct changes of body temperature also developed. While the skin temperature below the level of the lesion, as measured in the thigh and toes, fell markedly, the temperature above the level of the lesion, as measured in the neck, rose. The temperature in the rectum increased only slightly, if at all. Patches of vasodilatation appeared above the

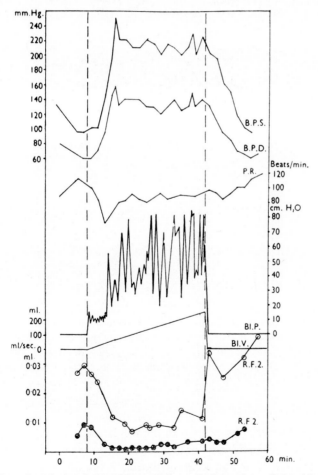

FIG. 145. Complete lesion below T2–3. Effect of distension of the bladder on the blood flow through a finger in a patient with a high lesion. B.P.S., systolic blood-pressure; B.P.D., diastolic blood-pressure; P.R., pulse rate; Bl.P., bladder pressure; Bl.V., bladder volume; R.F.2, —·— pulse volume in right index finger. (From L.Guttmann and D.Whitteridge (1947), *Brain*, **70**, 361.)

level of the lesion, especially engorgement of the veins in the neck and temporal area, indicating increased venous pressure and were associated with blockage of the nasal air passages. In Fig. 144 the areas of vasodilatation in face and neck are marked by the black lines. The reflex sweating in this case is shown in Fig. 153. Fig. 145 demonstrates the effect of distension of the bladder on blood flow through the right index finger in a complete lesion below T2/3, resulting in vasoconstriction. This was also found in other high lesions in both fingers and toes, in particular in complete lesions of the cervical cord below C6. It may be noted that it was sometimes impossible to take blood samples from the foot veins during the stage of vasoconstriction, indicating their participation in the

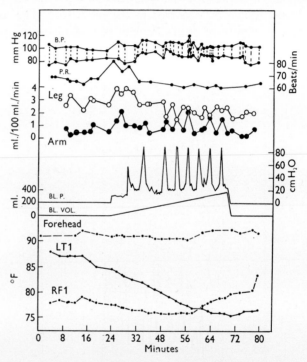

FIG. 146. Bladder distension in patient (4). Lesion below T6 on left, T7 on right. From above downwards, at the beginning of observations, blood pressure systolic and diastolic, pulse rate, blood flow in calf, ○——○, blood flow in forearm, ●——●, bladder pressure, bladder volume, skin temperatures from forehead, left hallux (L.T.1) and right thumb (R.F.1). From Cunningham, Guttmann, Whitteridge and Wyndham (1953) *J. Physiol.*, **121**, 581.

powerful active vasoconstriction present in the whole vascular bed of the paralysed area. Donegan (1921) produced evidence for such venous constriction in animals. Yet, even in these high lesions, face, neck and forearm showed a vasodilatation.

In special experiments in co-operation with Cunningham, Whitteridge & Wyndham (1953) we studied heart output, venous pressure and muscle bloodflow. Records taken at the height of a detrusor contraction of the bladder in a case below T6 showed a fall in bloodflow in the calf and a rise in bloodflow in the forearm. In a patient with a lesion below

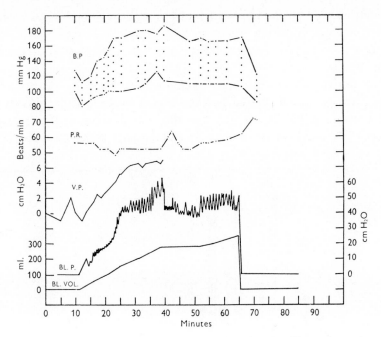

FIG. 147. Bladder distension in patient (1). Lesion below C7. From above downwards, blood pressure systolic and diastolic, pulse rate, venous pressure, bladder pressure, bladder volume.

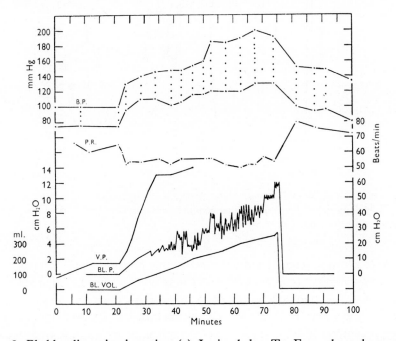

FIG. 148. Bladder distension in patient (2). Lesion below T1. From above downwards, blood pressure systolic and diastolic, pulse rate, venous pressure, bladder pressure, bladder volume.

T6 on the left and T7 on the right, the blood flow through both forearm and calf was found to fluctuate widely during distension of the bladder; the greater changes coincided exactly with the peaks of the detrusor contraction with a rapid return towards normal as soon as the detrusor contraction was over. If, however, observations were not made at the height of the detrusor action, changes were found to be small (Fig. 146).

Venous pressure was measured by means of a saline manometer connected to a wide bore transfusion needle inserted into the anticubital vein. The patients lay flat with the foot of the bed raised by foot blocks and the arms abducted at the shoulder. The

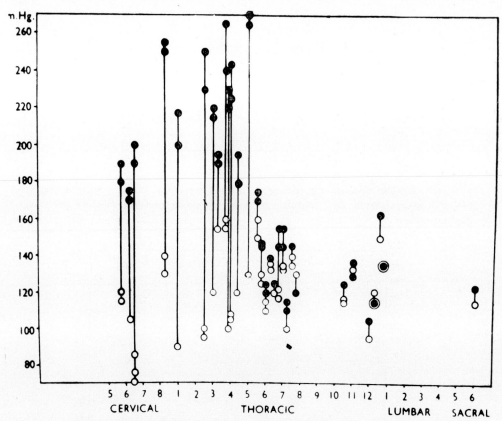

FIG. 149. The relation between blood-pressure changes and the level of the lesion. —◯— systolic blood-pressure before distension of the bladder. —●— systolic blood-pressure during distension of the bladder.

patients were allowed to reach a steady state in this position before venous pressure was recorded, and the measurements were made in relation to the sternal angle. As shown in Figs. 147 and 148 in complete lesions below C7 and T1 there was a sharp rise of venous pressure to 7 and 14 cm H_2O respectively during bladder distension and detrusor action. This was in contrast to only slight rise of venous pressure and insignificant changes in blood pressure and pulse, in spite of vigorous detrusor contractions raising the bladder pressure to over 60 cm H_2O, in all lesions below T6, as in the low lesions the vascular bed above the cord transection is large enough for compensatory distribution of blood through vasodilatation. Fig. 149 demonstrates the relation between blood pressure changes and the level of lesion and shows the great rise of systolic blood pressure in complete lesions above T5/6 during distension and hyperactivity of the bladder as compared with lesions below that level.

Cardiac output during distension of the bladder, as determined by Grollman's acetylene rebreathing method (Douglas & Priestley, 1948), was found not to change

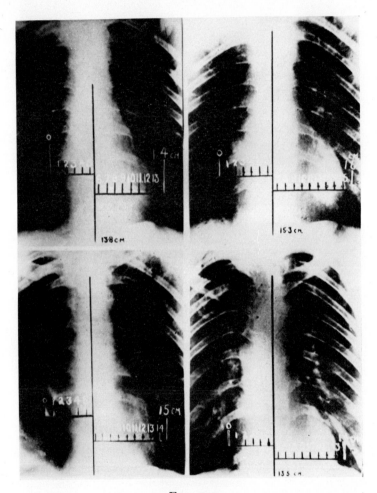

FIG. 150.

significantly. In a special study carried out in co-operation with our radiologist, Dr H.Jones, it was found that, in lesions above T5, the diameter of the heart may increase by as much as 1·5 cm at the height of the considerable redistribution of the blood following the increased bladder pressure and blood pressure (Guttmann, 1954) (Fig. 150). The electro-cardiogram revealed considerable arrhythmias in high transverse lesions (Fig. 151) which did not occur in complete lesions below T5/6. These are discussed in more detail in the chapter on pregnancy and labour, for the autonomic hyperreflexia found in the spinal man is by no means confined to hyperactivity of the bladder.

Outbursts of sweating and pilo-erection are also regular components of the autonomic hyperreflexia due to bladder distension. In cervical and upper thoracic lesions sweating

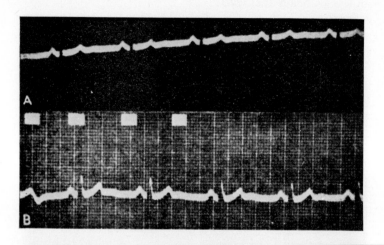

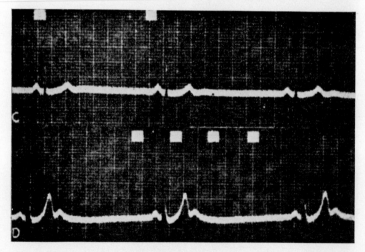

FIG. 151. Complete lesion below T3. Electrocardiograms before (A and B) and during (C and D) distension of the bladder, in a patient with a high lesion. A and C lead II, B and D lead IVR. Notice the slowing of the heart rate and the increase in size of the U wave especially in lead IVR. (From L.Guttmann and D.Whitteridge (1947), *Brain*, **70**, 361.)

usually started over the forehead and face (upper lip) either bilaterally or unilaterally, spreading later to both arms and chest, tapering off to T7/8 but rarely progressing beyond T10 dermatome. Fig. 152 demonstrates the profuse reflex sweating at the height of bladder distension in a man with a transection of the cord below C8/T1 due to gunshot injury. In the case of T3/4 lesion, shown in Fig. 144, reflex sweating started at the level of the lesion spreading to both axillae and tapering off to T8 (Fig. 153). Fig. 154 shows the final stage of reflex sweating in a complete lesion below T5 involving the trunk down to T11 but also partly the legs and proximally the medial parts of the arms including the hands. (Note that sweating is less pronounced on the left arm where the sphygmomanometer cuff compressed the blood circulation.) In lesions of T7–8 reflex sweating was not found to be a regular component of the autonomic response as compared with high cord

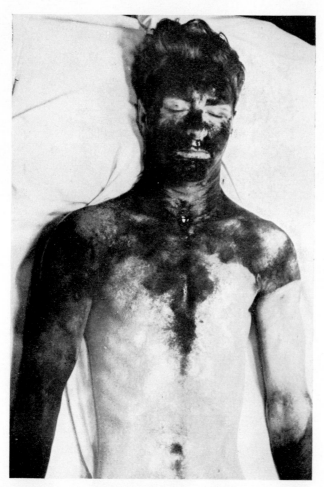

FIG. 152. The white area on the upper left arm is caused by a sphygmomanometer.

lesions, especially when the transverse lesion was associated with a longitudinal lesion. If present in these cases, it involved the distal part of the trunk and the lower limbs. In some subjects the part of the spinal sudomotor centres at the cervico-thoracic and thoraco-lumbar junctions respectively may show a specially marked degree of hyperactivity resulting in a rapid and exaggerated sudomotor response to bladder distension or any other intrinsic or extrinsic stimulus. This explains the band-like area of hyperhidrosis found in certain dermatomes, as shown in Fig. 155 of a complete lesion below T7 following

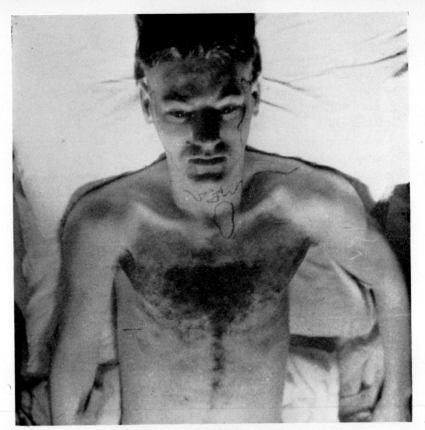

FIG. 153.

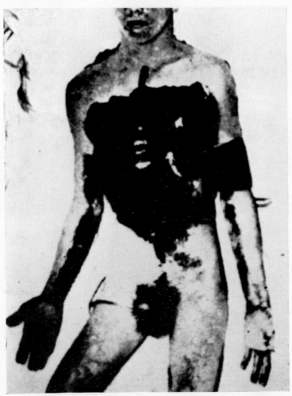

FIG. 154. The dark area above the left elbow is caused by a sphygmomanometer cuff depressing reflex sweating in left forearm and hand.

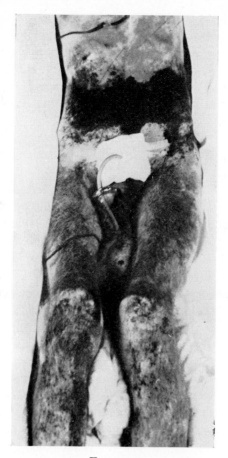

FIG. 155.

gunshot injury, where such profuse band-like hyperhidrosis occurred between T8 and T10 indicating the state of distinct hyperactivity of these segments of the cord situated just below the level of the cord transection. Further details of sudomotor and pilomotor response in the spinal man are discussed in the respective section on sudo- and pilomotor disturbances.

Subjective symptoms

The large scale redistribution of blood resulting from the vasoconstriction in the paralysed areas following distension and hyperactivity of the bladder is associated with certain subjective symptoms. Patients with complete transverse lesions may complain about discomfort in the abdominal and particular the suprapubic region or in the penis, followed by an undefined ascending sensation in the midline of the body; furthermore they may experience a feeling of oppression in the chest associated with difficulty in breathing, shivering sensation or feeling hot, and pounding headache, in particular in the back of the head or between the eyes. An officer remarked: 'I always know when my bladder is full because my heart starts to pound and to beat very slowly against resistance'. Other patients experienced hot ears when their bladders were distended or when passing urine automatically. Some patients with complete lesions below T7 or T10 with hyperpathic zones at the level of the cord transection may complain about increased pain at that level when the bladder is distended. However, all these subjective and objective manifestations described promptly disappear when the bladder (or any other viscera) distension and hyperactivity is released, as demonstrated in all Figs. at the end of the experiment.

Mechanism

In analysing the complex mechanism involved in the hyperactivity and dysfunction of the autonomic system, it can be stated that the primary reflex response to vesical reflex hyperactivity is vasoconstriction, as evidenced by the sharp decrease of blood flow, blood volume and skin temperature. This leads to a large scale compensatory redistribution of blood within the vascular bed in areas above the level of the spinal cord transection shown by vasodilatation in fingers and face including the nasal mucosa. Thus hemostasis is safeguarded in all patients of middle and, in particular, lower thoracic lesions, and blood pressure within narrow limits is maintained. However, in high thoracic and cervical lesions the finger vessels are also involved, as shown by their intense vasoconstriction, and therefore the remaining compensatory vasodilator response is unable to prevent the sharp rise of blood pressure. It is known that in man the fingers receive their vasomotor innervation from the 3rd to the 7th or 8th thoracic roots and the splanchnic nerves take their origin from the 5th to 11th thoracic roots. It was clearly shown that distension and hyperactivity of the bladder sets up intense arterial and venous vasoconstriction in the vessels of the finger, and the strong constrictor impulses from the isolated cord are able to overpower any vasodilatation which may be induced by the action of higher centres on the vasomotor fibres of T3 and T4 innervating the fingers. However, while in these high lesions the fingers show vasoconstriction, vasodilatation in arms, neck and head was still found in mid-cervical lesions. This will be discussed later.

There is no evidence that the changes in heart output are responsible for the blood pressure changes but changes in the peripheral vascular resistance play a very important, if not the most important, part. The increase of blood pressure is most likely to be responsible for the observed bradycardia—sometimes with a pulse rate of 48 p.m.—as part of a depressor reflex elicited by the intact aortic and carotid sinus nerves. The question arises whether the catecholamines, adrenaline and noradrenaline, are liberated and to what extent they are responsible for the raised blood pressure.

Special studies were therefore undertaken to examine the effect of excessive bladder activity on plasma catecholamine levels in patients with complete lesions at various levels to determine whether the liberation of adrenaline and/or noradrenaline may be responsible for the raised blood pressure. Although in a complete T5 and C6 lesion adrenaline, and to a lesser degree noradrenaline, greatly increased just before bladder and blood pressure reached their maximum and fell once the bladder pressure was released, as shown in Figs. 156 and 157, this problem needs further investigation and the same applies to the relation between renin and excessive bladder activity.

The mechanism of the vasodilator effect found in cervical lesion is of special interest. The vasodilatation involves the shoulder, upper chest, neck, ears and face and is of patchy type, associated with congestion of the naso-pharyngeal mucosa resulting in blockage of the nasal air passage. It is well known that vasodilatation in the face combined with nasal congestion is the regular and immediate effect of paralysis of the vasoconstrictor fibres following cervical sympathectomy or transection of the cervical cord. However, there is no evidence that in high cord lesions the vasodilatation in these areas resulting

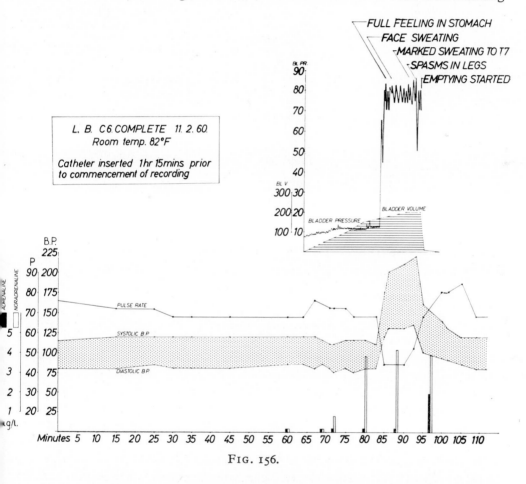

FIG. 156.

from excessive bladder activity is due to 'paralytic' vasodilatation as there is every sign of increased sympathetic activity. On the other hand, if, in high cord lesions, the vessels of face, neck and upper arms are controlled by the isolated cord, then one would expect that they would constrict as do the vessels of the fingers. However, they behave as if the vasoconstrictor influence of the isolated cord were overpowered by an active vasodilator mechanism excited by the intact carotid sinus nerves or entirely under the control of higher centres. While the vessels of the hand and fingers are controlled by the isolated cord and are constricting to a degree that the blood flow drops to zero, as shown in the pletysmogram, face, neck and upper arms show marked vasodilatation, which has all the appearance of being a readaptive mechanism. In this connection, it may be remembered that vasodilatation in the tongue was found following stimulation of the chorda tympany (Machol & Schilf, 1928), moreover, the Vidian nerve is thought to mediate vasodilator fibres for the nasal mucosa (Schilf, 1937). Another possibility for this striking vasodilator responses may be the release of a powerful vasodilator substance similar to the effect of the stimulation of posterior spinal roots. Vasodilatation seems to be a predominant function of the vasomotor systems in face, neck and upper chest in man, and

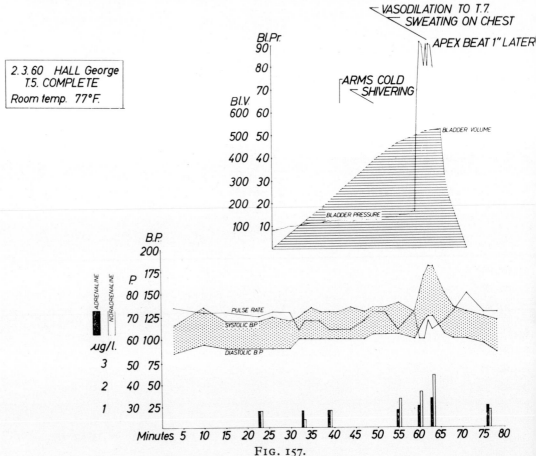

FIG. 157.

the patchy type of vasodilatation observed during bladder distension in patients with high cord lesions resembles very much the flushing elicited almost regularly by emotions in many normal subjects, especially women.

The sudden rise in blood pressure no doubt leads, as shown by the visible engorgement of the temporal and supraclavicular vessels, to a sudden increase in intracranial blood flow and, mechanically, to passive vasodilatation, experienced by the patients as pounding headache and head-fullness. Therefore, passive vasodilatation may also play a part in the vasodilator response of the cutaneous circulation in face, neck, upper chest and upper arms, as well as in the naso-pharyngeal mucosal circulation leading to stoppage of the air passage (called by some authors Guttmann sign).

The clinical significance of the autonomic hyperreflexia

Knowledge and recognition by the medical and nursing attendants of the various components of the reflex responses of autonomic mechanisms, especially the cardio-vascular phenomena, is most essential for an appropriate management of paraplegics and tetraplegics. It must be realized that these reflex responses represent stress or alarm signals of excessive activity of a viscus in the anaesthetic area of the body and they may be the only indicator of impending abdominal catastrophy. Complaints of headaches by patients with high cord lesions, in particular, have to be taken seriously and not be treated casually by aspirin or other drugs as they may be caused, for instance, by bladder distension due to acute blockage of an indwelling catheter or large residual urine due to obstruction at the external or internal sphincter complex or by a stone at any level of the urinary tract which needs appropriate measures. Obstruction in the intestinal tract by constipation may be another cause of these autonomous reflex responses. Neglect of these manifestations of stress in the organism may sometimes elicit epileptic fits and, if not counteracted early, may cause cerebral haemorrhage (see chapter on Pregnancy and Labour). On the other hand, the awareness of some of these phenomena by the patient, such as flushing, feeling of heat, sweating, etc., can be utilized for the patient's training to employ adequate stimuli for emptying the bladder at regular intervals in accordance with fluid intake.

B. THE AUTONOMOUS CONUS–CAUDA EQUINA BLADDER (NUCLEAR–RADICULAR OR LOWER MOTOR NEURON TYPE)

Destruction of the ganglion cells and their synapses within the spinal bladder centre itself or its nerve roots, in complete lesions of the conus–cauda equina, results in inter-ruption of the connections between bladder and spinal vesical centre. The bladder has become autonomous. Effective detrusor contractions do not occur and voiding depends on the usually ineffective control of the autonomous intramural innervation of the bladder wall which is incapable of provoking appropriate powerful emptying contrac-tions to bladder distension. Therefore, micturition is activated by abdominal pressure and depends on the efficiency and power of the abdominal muscles. Cystometry shows either a flat curve with feeble and irregular contractions or, in patients where the bladder wall has become rigid, a greater or lesser steep slope of its tonus limb. There is dribbling or stress incontinence, if the external urethral sphincter and the muscles of the pelvic floor are de-efferentated, but the bladder can be emptied more or less satisfactorily by manual pressure, assisted by abdominal pressure at regular intervals. There are exceptions to this rule. One of our patients was admitted several months after cordectomy because of an intramedullary tumour. The whole spinal cord with its roots below T9 had been removed, yet cystometry revealed some moderate though irregular detrusor contractions with considerable voiding effect. In this case, the autonomous intravesical innervations had undoubtedly reached an unusual degree of compensatory function.

C. MIXED FORMS OF VESICAL DYSFUNCTION

In some cases of conus–cauda equina lesion or longitudinal lesions at higher level, the destruction of the spinal bladder centre or its roots is only partial and there may be various forms of dissociation in the paralysis of detrusor, external urethral sphincter and pelvic floor muscles. This results in mixed forms of autonomous and automatic bladder function. Provided the sacral arc has escaped total damage, greater or lesser co-ordinated detrusor contractions may develop once the acute phase of bladder atonicity has passed. On the other hand, paralysis of striated muscles of the closing mechanism of micturition, the remaining or re-established detrusor function may cause dribbling incontinence.

D. VESICAL DYSFUNCTION FOLLOWING POSTERIOR ROOT DEGENERATION

Special mention may be made of the dysfunction of the bladder following destruction or degeneration of all sacral posterior roots. This is seldom found in traumatic lesions in its classical form but is often associated with tabes dorsalis and diabetic neuropathy. The loss of sensibility results in loss of desire to urinate and consequently the bladder becomes increasingly distended and atonic. Voiding occurs in the form of continuous dribbling incontinence. The cystometric curve is flat with a shift to the right.

MANAGEMENT AND RECONDITIONING OF BLADDER DYSFUNCTION

GENERAL CONSIDERATIONS

This represents a complex process of re-adjustment of the bladder function to the neurological deficit. In this process, urinary retention as well as urinary incontinence has to be considered. The sooner and the more in detail the patient is made aware of his individual type of bladder dysfunction, the sooner he may become conscious of his own responsibility and active co-operation in overcoming his vesical disability, especially in later stages when he has regained his upright position and is up and about in his wheel-chair or when his walking capability is restored.

The aims of the management in any stage of bladder paralysis are as follows:

1 Prevention of infection.
2 Prevention of overdistension of the bladder.
3 Prevention of local damage to urethra and bladder by manual expression, instrumentation, irrigations with irritant chemical solutions and artificial drainage.
4 Maintenance or restoration of a satisfactory bladder capacity.
5 To make the patient catheter-free as soon as possible by restoring in incomplete cord lesions efficient volitional or, in complete lesions, reflex micturition per urethram with no or the least possible degree of residual urine or incontinence. In conus–cauda equina lesions, efficient micturition should be accomplished by training and development of strong power of the abdominal muscles.

These aims reveal at once the multiple tasks and profound responsibility which confronts every physician or surgeon who is dealing with spinal paraplegic and tetraplegic patients both in acute and later stages of bladder paralysis. Today, these unfortunate people have the right to expect the best and not the second best treatment—i.e. the employment of those methods of management which from all experience have proved the most efficient to accomplish the desired aims, in particular the prevention of infection.

Methods and techniques of management

We have to consider the following procedures used so far:

1 Permanent non-interference with urinary retention resulting in overflow incontinence.
2 Manual expression.
3 Urethral drainage by (a) intermittent catheterization, (b) continuous drainage through indwelling catheter with or without tidal drainage or other forms of irrigation.
4 Suprapubic drainage (a) by aspiration, (b) suprapubic cystostomy and catheter drainage, (c) cutaneous vesicostomy.
5 Urethrostomy.
6 Conservative and surgical methods of reconditioning in later stages.

A. INITIAL MANAGEMENT

There is general agreement that from the efficiency of the initial treatment of the paralysed bladder the whole prognosis of spinal cord sufferers depends not only for their early return to a useful life but indeed for their life expectancy. It must be remembered that, even today, in spite of all advances made in the treatment of these patients during the last 25 years, ascending infection of the urinary tract resulting in renal deficiency is still the main killer. However, there is still discrepancy of opinion amongst workers in this field regarding the most effective method of preventing over-distension, local damage and infection of the bladder in the crucial initial and early stages of bladder paralysis in spinal cord lesions. In the following, the various methods used in the initial and early stages of bladder paralysis will be discussed and evaluated.

Non-interference

As a rule, the paralysed bladder is never sufficiently distended after an acute spinal cord injury as to warrant immediate drainage by any method. In fact, voiding may occur immediately as a result of the acute impact of the trauma, and patients have been admitted to accident departments with wet underwear. Moreover, in many cases of spinal injury the rate of renal secretion is retarded due to traumatic shock, especially in those associated with injuries to other parts of the body (crush syndrome). Fluid intake should be restricted during this period. This is particularly important in tetraplegics because of the disturbed water metabolism as a result of the loss of the vasomotor control which follows the interruption of the vasoconstrictor fibres in the cord. The belief that increased fluid intake will establish at this stage micturition by reflex detrusor action is erroneous. Moreover, as already pointed out, larger fluid intake in these high lesions carries the danger of developing pulmonary oedema. Therefore, the bladder can be left alone for 12–24 hours until percussion of the suprapubic region reveals increasing distension of the bladder or, in *a priori* incomplete lesions, distension provokes discomfort or distress due to reflex responses of autonomic mechanisms. During the period of non-interference by instrumentation, repeated attempts by *gentle* manual pressure and massage upon the lower abdomen or combined with digital massage per rectum may be carried out to elicit voiding.

Retention and overflow incontinence. However, it cannot be overstressed that permanent non-interference with urinary retention allowing maximal distension of the bladder resulting in overflow incontinence has proved a most unsatisfactory method resulting in chronic over-distension, hydronephrosis through back pressure and detrusor damage, and must be condemned, the more so as it does not prevent bladder infection.

Continuous manual expression. Vellacott & Webb Johnson (1919) described seven cases of spinal cord injuries in which manual expression only was carried out and an automatic bladder developed after three weeks. Four of these patients had sterile urine but three developed infection of the bladder. This method, although abandoned in due course because of its hazards, such as inability to prevent ascending infection of the urinary tract and the danger of rupture of the bladder as already reported in one of Vellacott's & Webb Johnson's cases, has been recently revived by Golding (1968) who claimed satisfactory results in twenty-five patients. He found that by this method an automatic bladder developed in 7 to 30 days and the residual urine slowly decreased; moreover all patients showed a normal intravenous pyelogram. However, Cook & Smith (1971) who tried this method on six patients who had not been catheterized previously and had a normal intravenous pyelogram on admission, found that all patients developed urinary infection and hydronephrosis; three of them developed deep vein thrombosis. In view of these disastrous results these authors rightly discontinued further trials with this method. Golding's results should, therefore, be considered as an exception rather than a rule.

Urethral drainage. While, during the Second World War, urologists and other surgeons following Thomson-Walker's views condemned urethral catheterization and advocated suprapubic cystotomy as the method of choice for the initial treatment of the paralysed bladder, which was then widely accepted, further experience during and after the war has revealed the hazards and disadvantage of this method. Today, this method is rarely used by spinal cord specialists unless there is a strict indication (see later). It is now generally agreed that the method of choice for the immediate and early management of the paralysed bladder is urethral catheterization. However, authors still differ whether at this stage urethral drainage should be done by continuous drainage with an indwelling catheter, with or without a closed receptacle system and with or without irrigation or tidal drainage, or by intermittent catheterization.

THE NON-TOUCH TECHNIQUE OF INTERMITTENT CATHETERIZATION

In 1947 following experiences with paraplegics who were admitted to the Stoke Mandeville Centre immediately after injury, I advocated the non-touch technique of intermittent catheterization as the method of choice for the treatment of the paralysed bladder during the spinal shock and the early stages of paraplegia. In due course this method has been further developed and its standard improved (Guttmann, 1949–63; Guttmann & Frankel, 1966). Details of the method and its evaluation are described hereunder:

Intermittent catheterization is instituted if after 12–24 hours voluntary or reflex function of the bladder has not developed and gentle manual pressure upon the bladder region or digital massage per rectum has proved unsuccessful, and the bladder has become distended.

The reason why intermittent catheterization in the immediate and early stages of paraplegia is infinitely preferable to immediate continuous drainage by an indwelling catheter, can be summarized as follows:

1 Immediate and early drainage of the paralysed bladder by indwelling catheter of any type, including Gibbon's catheter, leads invariably to early bladder infection which in a great number of cases occurs within 2–4 days if not within 24 hours. Therefore, in this respect there is really no difference between indwelling urethral catheter and drainage by suprapubic cystostomy whether with or without tube insertions.

2 An important reason for first using intermittent catheterization and not an indwelling catheter is to allow the urethral mucosa to become accustomed gradually to the foreign body. It must be remembered that in the state of spinal shock and flaccidity, the tone of all tissues including that of the urethral and bladder mucosa is greatly diminished, and as a result the threshold to pressure is lowered and injury to the mucosa facilitated. Consequently, an indwelling catheter, especially one of larger size, kept *in situ* without being changed for several days or even weeks, tends to produce ischaemia of the tissue by constant pressure especially on the peno-scrotal angle of the urethra resulting in a pressure sore leading to abscess and eventually to that most dreaded complication, peno-scrotal fistula. Kyle (1968) stressed the obstructive effect of the catheter on the ducts of the many glands which open in the urethra and considered this as the cause of the persisting foci of infection 'which remained after the offending instrument has been abandoned'.

3 In incomplete cord lesions and those complete ones, especially in young people, where early return of voluntary or reflex function can be expected, provided no bladder infection has occurred, intermittent catheterization encourages the physiological stimulus for micturition, namely some bladder distension by setting up the appropriate impulses to the spinal reflex bladder centre and thus promoting early return of detrusor activity in these cases. Using this regime of bladder management, we found, particularly in young patients with complete lesions above T10, the appearance of automatic reflex-micturition as early as 8–10 or 14 days after injury. Therefore, the old teachings of physiologists and neurologists that automatic reflex-micturition after complete lesions occurs only after 6–8 weeks can no longer be accepted dogmatically.

The view held by urologists and other surgeons for so many years that, with inter-mittent catheterization, the paralysed bladder cannot be kept sterile longer than 2 days is absolutely unfounded, provided proper aseptic precautions are taken. That the old prejudice against intermittent catheterization has not been overcome, is shown by the astonishing statement made as late as 1959 by Prather in the U.S.A.: 'It is generally agreed that in the management of spinal cord injuries intermittent catheterization drainage is the worst form of treatment which can be used'.

I have always considered intermittent catheterization in the acute stages of paraplegia and tetraplegia as a major medical and not a nursing procedure. It should, therefore, be carried out exclusively both in men and women by a medical officer familiar with the non-touch technique and not left to the nursing staff, let alone to orderlies or 'tech-nicians'. Over the years, this concept has been consistently adhered to, and intermittent catherization has continued to be the method of choice in the management of the paralysed bladder during the caute stages of paraplegia and tetraplegia. It has been found, that by using this regime the paralysed bladder can be kept sterile in the great majority of patients not only for many weeks but indeed often throughout the whole period that catheterization has been needed. I am, of course, aware that other workers in this field, even some in spinal units, would argue that they have not sufficient staff or time to carry out intermittent catheterization and revert to the immediate method of urethral drainage by an indwelling catheter. However, I cannot accept such arguments as valid in this field of medicine since they are not acceptable in any other field by our profession. It must be stressed that the time taken in carrying out the technique of intermittent catheterization with all its meticulous care, is well spent in preventing the disastrous complications associated with ascending infection of the urinary tract resulting in chronic invalidism and early death of these unfortunate people. This is particularly vital in those patients who, in addition to the spinal injury, have associated injuries to the chest and other parts of the body, where the organism has to deal with all the potential complications of these injuries and, no doubt, it can do so more readily, if it is not interfered with by an additional infection of the urinary tract.

Immediate indwelling catheterization may be indicated for the determination of osmolal output in acute renal failure following acute traumatic paraplegia. This is now very rare.

Technique and procedure

Figs. 158a–d demonstrate the instrumentation and technique. The instruments arrive in an autoclaved sealed catheterization pack and after opening the photograph demon-strates the contents. The penis, the foreskin retracted, after preliminary cleaning with Savlon 1 per cent solution, is put through a small hole in the sterile paper towel and held with a piece of sterile gauze. The doctor, with sterile gown, mask and sterile gloves, then cleans the glans penis, especially the meatus, again with 1 per cent Savlon solution. The catheter is contained in a 1-inch nylon envelope open at one end which contains the lubricant (0·05 per cent Hibitane); the catheter is pulled out of this envelope with a sterile forceps and is ready for use without further lubrication. The doctor gently introduces

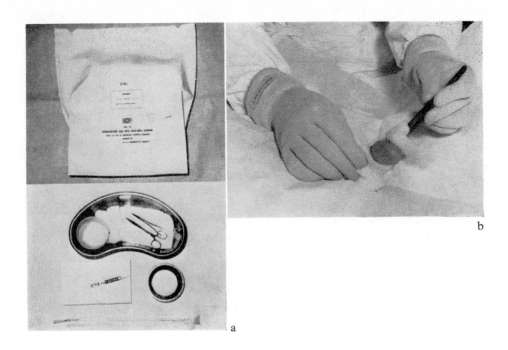

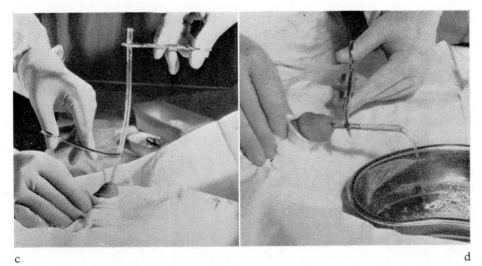

FIG. 158a. Autoclaved catheterization pack. The upper half of the photograph shows the sealed paper bag and the lower half shows the contents. b. Catheterization: the penis has been put through the small hole in the sterile paper towel, the foreskin has been retracted and the penis is held with a piece of sterile gauze; the doctor is cleaning the glans with 1 per cent Savlon solution. c. The doctor is gently introducing the already lubricated catheter, the blunt end of the catheter is supported with forceps held by an assistant. d. The catheter is in the bladder, it is removed as soon as the bladder has been completely emptied. From Guttmann and Frankel (1966) *Paraplegia*, **4**, 63.

the catheter, the blunt end of the catheter is supported with forceps held by an assistant. The catheter used for this procedure is a plastic Jacques catheter, size 8 or 10 E.G. Since plastic catheters have been introduced, urethritis is now rare. The catheter is immediately removed once the bladder has been completely emptied.

Early circumcision, especially in patients with long and narrow foreskin, is highly advisable to prevent infection of meatus and urethra and paraphymosis. In patients who are admitted in the first few days after injury with an indwelling catheter already *in situ*, it is advisable to take a swab for culture from the meatus and urethra as well as a urine specimen before intermittent catheterization is started to ascertain whether or not infection had already occurred. In such a case it is safer to start antibiotic treatment, even if there is only bacteriuria without increase of white cells and protein.

Cervical patients have, not infrequently, an initial period of water retention with oliguria during the first few days after injury and during this time need only, as a rule, twice daily catheterization. At about the 3rd–6th day or soon after, often a profound diuresis occurs, and 3 or 4 litres of urine may be secreted in 24 hours. During such diuresis, the fluid intake should be temporarily reduced, and the patient be catheterized four or more times a day. If the period of diuresis is overlooked by the medical and nursing staff, over-distension may occur in this acute stage resulting in discomfort and exaggerated reflex responses of autonomic mechanisms, especially increase of blood pressure. After the diuresis is over, fluid intake should be adjusted so that each catheterization at approximately 9 a.m., 2.30 p.m. and 10 p.m. yields between 500 and 700 ml in adults, and every care must be taken to see that the bladder never becomes over-distended. This in itself shows the great responsibility of the staff concerned with the management of paralysed patients in the acute stage. On three times daily catheterization in patients who are unable to pass any urine, the fluid output in correlation with fluid intake should average 2 to 3 litres in 24 hours.

Care must also be taken to empty the bladder completely, as it is known that in the recumbent patients, in particular those with flaccid lesions, the lowest point of the bladder is not necessarily drained by the catheter (Doggart, Guttmann & Silver, 1966). Therefore, change of position and abdominal pressure is used at the end of the catheterization to obtain any residual urine and thus prevent stagnation in the bladder. The importance of regular turning of the patient in the acute and early stage and the early restoration of his upright position to avoid stagnation in the urinary tract cannot be overstressed. When, in adults, the residual urine becomes less than 500 ml, catheterization can be reduced to twice daily, and when less than 250 ml to once daily, and when less than 100 ml catheterization can be stopped provided an efficient automatic reflex bladder, in lesions above the thoracolumbar junction, or an autonomous bladder in conus-cauda equina lesions, emptied by powerful abdominal pressure has developed. However, the residual urine has to be checked once or twice a week for several more weeks.

Before 1954, it was our practice to give prophylactic penicillin or sulphonamides or alternatively Aureomycin or later Tetracyclin during the first week or two of catheterization. However, since antibiotics are not given routinely as urinary prophylactics, the patients with associated injuries should be treated with intramuscular penicillin or other antibiotics for the first week or two for the prevention or treatment of chest or other infections. This applies, of course, also to patients who have been admitted with infected urine as a result of an indwelling catheter.

In recent years, I introduced a combination of hexamine-mandelate (250 mg) and methionine (250 mg) manufactured in one tablet as an acidifying agent and called G.500 (this drug is manufactured by Harker, Stagg Ltd, Emmott Street, London E.1). This combination obviates the dispensation of the many tablets necessary if these three drugs are taken separately to establish a satisfactory acidity of the urine with a pH of 5 and under. This combination is, therefore, much less troublesome for the patient. The initial dosage of 16 tablets a day can be gradually reduced to find a proper maintenance dose in the individual cases. It must be noted, however, that G.500 was found ineffective in preventing alkaninity of the urine during proteus infection (Fig. 159).

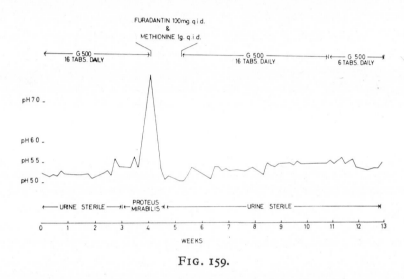

FIG. 159.

ASSESSMENT OF STERILITY

Urine is sent for bacteriological examination very frequently during intermittent catheterization, at least three times a week, and if infection occurs as judged by the appearance of the urine to the naked eye and confirmed by microscopic examination a systemic antibiotic course is started at once while awaiting results of culture and number of white cells.

The commonest organisms found in the infected patients, especially those who were admitted with an indwelling catheter, were *K. aerogenes*, mixed growth, *Ps. pyocyanea*, *Proteus mirabilis*, *B. coli*, Providence, *Strep. faecalis* and *Serratia*. *Strep. faecalis*, which previously was considered to be non-pathogenic, has been shown to be a precursor of infection with other organisms by a few days, and as pure *Strep. faecalis* infection was often associated with pyuria this is included in the list of pathogens.

Results on admission and during early stages of paraplegia are based on catheter specimens, results on discharge on carefully taken mid-stream specimens (except in those patients who were discharged with a permanent indwelling catheter). If the Path. Lab.

reports large bacterial growth without increase of white cells and protein in the urine and in the absence of clinical signs of infection another specimen should be sent at once to find out whether the bacteriuria found was due to contamination.

Urine was regarded as sterile if, in the absence of anti-bacterial drugs, it contained less than 4 white cells per mm^3 and gave no growth on culture. In doubtful cases, the examination was repeated. The bacteriological methods used in our material have been described by Milner (1963).

It is of utmost importance that specimens are examined immediately or within half an hour of collection, as when the urine is left standing bacteria multiplies. If the examination cannot be carried out immediately, the urine specimens should be refrigerated. We were fortunate in having excellent co-operation from our Pathology Department and this should be the aim in all Spinal Centres. Dennis Guttmann and G.Naylor (1967) introduced the dip-slide method for bacterial examination of urine which has been developed further by Dennis Guttmann (1970). This method which has been proved particularly useful for out-patients check ups, can be easily modified for clinical use for hospital in-patients.

RESULTS

It is of interest to survey the results achieved with intermittent catheterization. A statistic over a period of 6 years on 313 patients (Guttmann, 1963) showed that 39 per cent were admitted with sterile urine following initial treatment with intermittent catheterization while on discharge 61 per cent were sterile and catheter free. In 1966 a more comprehensive report was published on the management of the paralysed bladder in the acute and early stages during an 11 year period on 476 traumatic paraplegics and tetra-plegics —409 males and 67 females, admitted to Stoke Mandeville Spinal Centre within the first 14 days, most of them within the first 48 hours after injury (Guttmann & Frankel, 1966). The patients were followed up after discharge from the Centre at least yearly but often more frequently, especially those who were infected and had developed complications. Check-ups included urine culture, cell and protein counts, blood chemistry and intravenous pyelogram. In some cases, cystograms and clearance tests were also included. At the time of the publication of the report 298 males and 46 females had had check-ups.

Table 14 demonstrates the state of the urine on arrival at the Centre in relation to treatment before arrival. As can be seen, the results where no catheterization or only intermittent catheterization had been employed by the referring hospital are infinitely superior to those where a Gibbon catheter was used and even more so to those where a Foley catheter was employed. Already at this stage a greater percentage of females were infected.

Table 15 demonstrates the state of urine on admission and discharge, the males catheterized exclusively by the doctor in charge of the case showed 64·8 per cent sterile urine, the females only 49·3 per cent. In analysing these figures, however, only the male patients are considered, as the number of female patients is too small to be assessed in percentage. It was found that of the 92 male patients who were not catheterized before admission to the Centre 63 (68·5 per cent) were sterile on discharge. Of the 157 who had

TABLE 14

Treatment before arrival	State of urine on arrival	
MALES 409		
	Sterile	Infected
No catheterization	92	0
Intermittent catheterization	157	7
Foley catheter	45	61
Gibbon catheter	36	9
Suprapubic	0	2
	330 (80·7%)	79
FEMALES 67		
	Sterile	Infected
No catheterization	12	0
Intermittent catheterization	17	7
Foley catheter	7	20
Gibbon catheter	4	0
	40 (59·7%)	27

TABLE 15. Patients admitted within 14 days of injury between 1.1.54 and 31.12.64

MALES		409	FEMALES		67
On admission			*On admission*		
Sterile	330	(80·7%)	Sterile	40	(59·7%)
Infected	79		Infected	27	
On discharge			*On discharge*		
Sterile	263	(64·3%)	Sterile	33	(49·3%)
Infected	146		Infected	34	

TOTAL MALE AND FEMALE ON DISCHARGE

Sterile	296	(62·2%)
Infected	180	

intermittent catheterization before admission, 109 (69·4 per cent) were sterile on discharge, while of the 45 treated with Foley catheters before admission 27 (60 per cent) were sterile on discharge and of the 36 treated with Gibbon's catheter before admission 23 (63·9 per cent) were sterile on discharge. Of the 7 infected cases who had intermittent catheterization before admission, 4 were sterile and 3 remained infected on discharge; of 61 infected patients who were treated with an indwelling Foley catheter, 31 (50·8 per cent) were sterile on discharge and 30 remained infected; of 9 infected patients treated by Gibbon catheter on admission, 5 were sterile on discharge and 4 remained infected. Of the 2 patients infected by suprapubic cystostomy on admission, one became sterile following closure of the suprapubic drainage and one remained infected.

This analysis clearly demonstrates the high efficiency of intermittent catheterization

TABLE 16. Neurological lesions and sterility on discharge (males and females)

	Total	Sterile on discharge	Infected on discharge
Cervical:			
Complete	79	44 (55·7%)	35
Incomplete	102	65 (63·7%)	37
T1–T5:			
Complete	37	22 (59·3%)	15
Incomplete	6	4	2
T6–T12:			
Complete spastic	72	41 (56·9%)	31
Complete flaccid	45	22 (48·8%)	23
Incomplete spastic	23	18 (78·3%)	5
Incomplete flaccid	13	10 (76·9%)	3
Below T12:			
Complete spastic	6	4	2
Complete flaccid	51	32 (62·7%)	19
Incomplete spastic	12	9 (75%)	3
Incomplete flaccid	30	25 (83·3%)	5
Total	476	296 (62·2%)	180

in the prevention and overcoming of infection of the paralysed bladder in the initial and early stages of traumatic paraplegia. Table 16 demonstrates the neurological lesions and sterility of the bladder on discharge in males and females, and Tables 17a and b show the length and results of follow-ups in males and females.

The reasons may be discussed why our results in female patients have been less favourable than in the male. There are several possible explanations for the higher incidence of infection in females:

1 Anatomically, the development of ascending urethral infection is easier in the female than in the male. Moreover, some may have been infected before injury. As an example, a female patient with non-traumatic paraplegia was admitted a short time after the onset of paraplegia, and the cystogram showed a grossly crenated bladder obviously resulting from long standing chronic infection before her paraplegia.

2 The preparation for catheterization in the female is more difficult, again on account of the female anatomy.

3 As pointed out before, in all male paraplegics intermittent catheterization was universally performed by the medical officers, while, in the female, catheterization was allowed to be carried out by the nursing staff. It has since been decided that the medical officer should also perform the intermittent catheterization in the early stages in female paraplegics and results have improved (Walsh, 1968).

4 In some female cases, intermittent catheterization was abandoned in favour of a temporary indwelling catheter when an automatic bladder developed before the patient was able to get up and the bed was wetted between catheterizations. Even then, indwelling catheters were used in such patients only when the urine was infected, but the presence

TABLE 17a. Length and result of follow-up (males)

Years after injury	Number of last check-ups	Sterile on first discharge	Infected on first discharge	Sterile at check-up	Infected at check-up	Originally infected sterile now	Originally sterile infected now
1	84	53 (63·1%)	31	44 (52·4%)	40	2	11
2	42	25 (59·5%)	17	19 (45·2%)	23	3	9
3	53	38 (71·4%)	15	36 (67·9%)	17	6	8
4	37	25 (67·6%)	12	21 (56·8%)	16	2	6
5	26	11 (42·3%)	15	6 (23·1%)	20	1	6
6	21	13 (61·9%)	8	9 (42·9%)	12	3	7
7	15	6	9	10	5	4	0
8	5	0	5	3	2	3	0
9	5	2	3	4	1	2	0
10	20	5	5	5	5	1	1
Total	298	178 (59·7%)	120	157 (52·7%)	141	27	48

TABLE 17b. Length and result of follow-up (females)

Years after injury	Number of last check-ups	Sterile on first discharge	Infected on first discharge	Sterile at check-up	Infected at check-up	Originally infected now sterile	Originally sterile now infected
1	11	6	5	5	6	0	1
2	7	3	4	3	4	1	1
3	9	5	4	4	5	2	3
4	5	2	3	3	2	1	0
5	3	1	2	1	2	0	0
6	3	0	3	1	2	1	0
7	4	1	3	2	2	1	0
8	2	2	0	2	0	0	0
9	1	0	1	1	0	1	0
10	1	0	1	0	1	0	0
Total	46	20 (43·5%)	26	22 (47·8%)	24	7	5

of the catheter prevented rapid and complete eradication of the infection. On the other hand, although the number of female paraplegics was too small at the time of the stastics to assess whether a higher rate of infection would be reflected in later complications, it is interesting to note from our results that more women became sterile during follow-up than became infected.

Recently Frankel (1969) reported an improvement of sterile urine in women since their intermittent catheterization has been carried out by a medical officer. Although the figures at the time of the report were small (15), there had been a considerable improvement in the state of the women, as 10 out of 15 (67 per cent as compared with under 50 per cent reported in 1966) had sterile urine.

The effects of intermittent catheterization on complications

Hydronephrosis

Thirty-five patients (7·4 per cent) developed hydronephrosis of varying degrees; of these 14 were unilateral and 21 bilateral. Neurological lesions of these patients is shown in Table 18 and the time lapse between injury and diagnosis of hydronephrosis is demonstrated in Table 19. Thirteen of these 35 patients had only dilated renal pelves but normal calyces and of these 6 had sterile urine, which confirms the well known fact that sterile urine as such does not necessarily prevent hydronephrosis if dysfunction of the opening or closing mechanism of the spinal cord bladder develops at a later date, although this occurs much less often than in patients who developed early infection of the urinary tract. Twenty-two patients had frank hydronephrosis but, of these, only 3 had sterile

TABLE 18. Hydronephrosis and reflux related to neurological lesions

	Hydronephrosis	Reflux
Cervical:		
Complete	4	5
Incomplete	5	2
T1–T5:		
Complete	4	3
Incomplete	0	0
T6–T12:		
Complete spastic	5	4
Complete flaccid	8	4
Incomplete spastic	0	1
Incomplete flaccid	1	0
Below T12:		
Complete spastic	0	0
Complete flaccid	4	0
Incomplete spastic	1	0
Incomplete flaccid	3	2
Total	35	21

TABLE 19. Time between injury and first diagnosis of complications

Time after injury	Hydronephrosis	Reflux	Stones
Less than 3 months	0	2	0
3 to 6 months	6	8	0
Over 6 to 12 months	11	5	2 (1 bladder)
Over 1 to 2 years	6	3	3
Over 2 to 3 years	6	1	3 (1 bladder)
Over 3 to 4 years	3	0	
Over 4 to 5 years	2	1	
Over 5 to 6 years	1	1	2
Over 6 to 7 years			1 (1 bladder)
Total	35	21	11 (3 bladder)

urine. Three of the 22 had gross hydronephrosis, all were infected. Of the 9 cases with hydronephrosis with sterile urine, 5 showed spontaneous improvement, 3 were unchanged and one deteriorated. This man, a traumatic tetraplegic since 10 November 1961, whose bladder was always sterile, developed a mild unilateral hydronephrosis about three years after injury, as the result of a large residual urine. A bladder neck resection was carried out (Dr Walsh) to relieve the back pressure. This operation, while eliminating the residual urine, proved otherwise unsuccessful, as it resulted in ascending infection of the urinary tract and further increase of hydronephrosis.

In 6 other patients with hydronephrosis, the hydronephrosis developed as a result of infection and high residual urine. They all also had ureteric reflux. Four were treated with antibiotics and indwelling catheter and of these two improved and two remained unchanged. Three of the patients with hydronephrosis were found to have ureteric strictures one, three and five years after injury. They were treated by ureterolysis with considerable improvement, but a certain degree of hydronephrosis persisted in all three.

VESICAL URETERIC REFLUX

Twenty-one patients (4·4 per cent) including 2 females had ureteric reflux, 15 unilateral and 6 bilateral. Their neurological lesions are also shown in Tables 18 and 19. All these patients had been infected before cystogram, at which reflux was demonstrated. Six patients with reflux leading to hydronephrosis have been described in the preceding section, of the remaining 15 patients 4 were treated successfully with antibiotics and had normal cystogram and I.V.P. later. One patient was treated with temporary Foley catheter while 10 had to have a permanent indwelling catheter; of these 5 subsequently had cystograms without reflux but the indwelling catheter was retained because of chronic infection which did not subside with antibiotic treatment.

DIVERTICULA OF BLADDER

The majority of patients did not have cystograms but of those who did 12 (2 sterile) showed the appearance of diverticulosis or trabeculation and a further 80 (6 sterile) showed only slightly irregular bladder outlines.

RENAL STONES

Eight patients (1·7 per cent) including 2 females developed renal stones, three bilateral, five unilateral. The time lapse between injury and diagnosis of the stones is shown in Table 19. All these patients had had severe urinary infection before these stones were diagnosed, and in all 8 patients, stones were removed surgically (Dr Walsh). In 3 patients there has been no recurrence, in 5 the stones recurred and further removal was attempted in 3. In 2 of these the stones have recurred. Two of these patients died.

BLADDER STONES

Three patients (0·6 per cent) 2 male, 1 female, developed bladder stones, 2 while being treated with Foley catheters. The stones were removed by cystoscopy in 2 cases and in 1 by open surgery. This outstandingly low instance of calculosis in bladder and kidneys compares most favourably with 22·5 per cent of calculosis amongst 351 patients of the Second World War reported previously (Guttmann, 1953) and other authors with even higher percentage of calculosis (see later).

URETHRAL FISTULAE

In spite of the many thousands of intermittent catheterizations performed in this large number of patients during the many years of study, there has been not a single case of urethral, peno-scrotal or vesico-vaginal fistula. This is now confirmed by other workers in this field and Jacobson & Bors (1970), in their report on spinal cord injury in Viet-namese Combat pointed out that none of their patients treated with intermittent cathe-terization developed peno-scrotal pathology. For the sake of the paralysed patients, this achievement alone, apart from the other satisfactory results obtained, more than justifies the amount of effort expended on this form of management of the spinal bladder in the early stages following spinal cord injury. Moreover, the amount of money spent on equip-ment and personnel for intermittent catheterization at these early stages of bladder paralysis is more than compensated by the avoidance of prolonged and even permanent hospitalization later for costly treatment of complications developing as a result of inadequate management of the bladder in the early stages. Thus, by proper initial treat-ment of the paralysed bladder much misery and chronic invalidism and indeed early death of these patients can be greatly minimized or altogether prevented.

In recent years more and more workers in the field of traumatic paraplegia in this and other countries confirmed most encouraging results with intermittent catheterization as the method of choice in the immediate and early management of the paralysed bladder. Walsh (1968) published a report of 97 patients (92 male and 5 female) treated at Stoke Mandeville since the publication of 1966 mentioned above, the majority of whom (60) were admitted within 48 hours of injury. Of the 92 early cases studied, 85 (92·4 per cent) were admitted with sterile urine and 76 (82·6 per cent) were discharged with sterile urine. Only one case was found to have a stone in the left renal calculus and showed a bilateral vesical ureteric reflux. The stone was removed surgically and the patient discharged with sterile urine and mild degree of hydronephrosis on the left side. Dollfus & Molé (1969) published their experience on intermittent catheterization covering a period of 3 years and 4 months after injury. Eighty-two per cent of urines were sterile in men and 67 per cent in women. Fourteen patients were followed up after discharge up to 2 years and their urine was found sterile in 92 per cent. Other authors who reported encouraging results are Brussatis (1953); Rossier & Brumer (1964); Ehalt (1965); Bors (1967); Comarr (1968); Hardy (1968); Key (1968); Cibeira (1968); Adler (1969); Talbot (1970); Gibbon et al. (1969); Jacobson & Bors (1970); Pearman (1971). Hardy's state-ment (1968) that the incidence of calculus formation has quite considerably dropped since his use of intermittent catheterization in selected cases represents an interesting confir-mation of our experience. At the second meeting of the Group of Neuro-Urological Research of the Faculty of Medicine of the University of Saar (Homburg) in Mulhouse, France (November, 1970), Legner, an experienced urologist, declared that intermittent catheterization by the method described here was the only right method also for the urologist.

Recently Stickler *et al.* (1971) studied the mode of development of urinary infection in 9 male paraplegics who were treated by intermittent catheterization during the early stage of paraplegia. In 4 of the 9 cases the organisms eventually responsible for the bladder infection could be isolated from the urethra or from its external meatus before they invaded the urine. They found variation in the rate at which different organisms established themselves in the urinary tract and reached a level of 10^5 organisms/ml in the urine. In 5 of these 9 patients the invading bacteria were present at 10^5 organisms/ml of urine prior to the production of a pyogenic infection. From these few observations, the authors came to the conclusion that the penile cleansing performed before the insertion of the catheter rarely sterilized the external meatus of the urethra. To conclude that 4 sterile cases out of 9 constitutes a rare incidence is in itself open to question. Although this should not lead to generalization, in view of the vast number of sterile bladders achieved by the non-touch technique of countless intermittent catheterizations described above and by other authors, it demonstrates the importance of meticulous cleansing of the meatus before inserting the catheter and the education of the medical staff in this respect. As already mentioned, in this connection, early circumcision in paraplegics is highly recommended in particular in patients with long foreskin, to diminish the danger of transferring infection from the meatus and urethra.

Continuous drainage by indwelling catheter

In the foregoing section some reasons have been given why continuous indwelling catheter drainage of the paralysed bladder is an unsuitable method for the immediate and early treatment, the most important being that it leads invariably to early infection. This seems to be now the general view of all experienced workers in the field of spinal cord injuries. Hardy (1968), in his comprehensive analysis of 400 cases treated in a 10 year period between 1956 and 1965 by indwelling catheter drainage, states 'all but a very small number of the 400 cases had some infection at some time during the catheter period' and 'that infections make up the most significant part of the complications of the indwelling urethral catheter and that cases with infection of the epididymis were the most troublesome'. Of special interest is the high incidence of calculi formation in Hardy's cases following indwelling catheter drainage, namely 49 out of 400 (12·25 per cent). These unsatisfactory results were obtained in spite of the fact that Hardy employed a meticulous technique of catheterization, including apparatus which had been pre-packed and autoclaved, and there was a separate pack for each procedure in each case. Chlorhexidine solution was used for cleaning the meatus and foreskin and 1 per cent Chlorhexidine cream was instilled into the urethra before the passage of the catheter, which was changed only once a week and was connected with a closed drainage system comprising a polythene tube and drainage system. The catheter mainly used was a self-retaining Foley type catheter 16 to 22 French gauge with a 5 cc balloon. The defects of this type of catheter described by Hardy are:

1   insidious deflation of the balloon,
2   occlusion of the lumen of the catheter by pressure within the balloon,
3   occlusion of the lumen of the catheter by distortion of the balloon inflated eccentrically,
4   failure of the balloon to deflate when required.

These observations are in accordance with our own with this type of catheter. The failure of the balloon to deflate when required necessitated either bursting the balloon by overdistension, which is a bad method, as fragments of the rubber give rise to calculus formation later, or dissolving the latex of the balloon by ether or chloroform, which unless sterile paraffin was introduced into the bladder gave rise to irritation of the mucosa. Before puncturing the balloon by surgical procedure, it is worthwhile trying to pull the inflated balloon slowly and gently through the urethra. As Dr Melzak at Stoke Mandeville repeatedly found, this gradually dilates the urethra to some extent and changes the balloon's shape into a sausage-like elongation due to the elasticity of its wall. In recent years rubber catheters have been replaced more and more by plastic catheters which cause far less allergic reaction than occurs with rubber catheters in certain hypersensitive patients.

A more serious though rare complication of prolonged indwelling catheter drainage is the pressure of the balloon within the bladder against the symphysis in women who spent the whole day sitting in their wheelchair. The combined prolonged pressure from

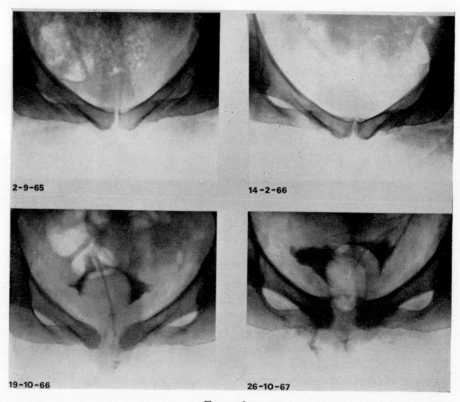

FIG. 160.

the pelvic floor on the one hand the pressure from the balloon within the bladder on the other may lead to a destruction of the symphysis resulting in separation of the ossa pubis as shown in Fig. 160 of one of our former, rather obese, female paraplegic patients, who was treated with an indwelling Foley catheter because of severe incontinence.

Gibbon et al. (1969) consider, as the main hazard of continuous catheterization by indwelling catheter, blockage of the system by mucus or phosphatic debris which, in the presence of bladder infection, may lead to acute pyelonephritis. The special small calibre plastic catheter of 1·5 or 2 mm overall diameter devised by Gibbon (1956, 1958) has been used as indwelling catheter in 100 patients who had been admitted to the Southport Spinal Centre within 14 days of their injury. Neither routine use of anti-bacterial or penile dressings were used. In all, the urine became infected 'sooner or later' and in spite of closed drainage the urine remained sterile only 'for a week or more'. This is in accordance with our own experience at Stoke Mandeville with this type of catheter. Kyle (1968), the urologist at the Perth Spinal Unit in Australia, admits that with small calibre catheters, particularly Gibbon's catheter, one sees fewer strictures; however, he found these very small catheters only efficient in clear urine. They are easily blocked, as we also found, and thus render the control of infection more difficult. For this reason he found that they caused more nursing problems, and, therefore, interference. This does not prove the views expressed by Cosbie Ross in 1960 that 'it is not necessary to change the catheter and drainage continues for many weeks with little interference. Cross infection is eliminated and nursing time saved'. From his experiences Kyle came to the conclusion that 'the best prophylaxis is not to use indwelling catheters unless essential' and in the Perth Spinal Centre intermittent catheterization is used whenever possible.

Jacobson & Bors (1970) published a survey of 114 actual combat injuries of the Vietnam War, 79 complete and 35 incomplete lesions of various levels, the majority being low thoracic and lumbo-sacral injuries; 77 (67 per cent) of the spinal injuries had major associated injuries to other parts of the body. Almost all had urinary infection from catheter, and the genito-urinary complications were numerous such as epididymitis 14 (12·8 per cent), renal stones 14 (13 per cent), bladder stones 56 (49·1 per cent), hydronephrosis 20 (11·4 per cent), peno-scrotal complications with abscess, diverticulum or fistula 8·8 per cent. Of special interest is the fact that 5 patients developed pseudo-papillomata and 2 squamous carcinoma, grade 1 and grade 2 respectively, of the urethra. Such most unsatisfactory results could be at least minimized and great misery later prevented even in war time if the responsible Government Department, in particular, the military medical authorities, would issue strict instructions that the medical staff in base hospitals, where the wounded in many instances can be admitted in the shortest possible time by field ambulance or helicopter, are properly trained in the initial treatment of the paralysed bladder. Autoclaved catheterization packs, as described on page 373 (Fig. 158a) can now be manufactured from disposable material and should be part of the equipment of first aid stations and base hospitals. It should be possible for a medical officer to carry out proper cleansing of the penis, in particular the meatus with Savlon etc. before inserting the catheter into the bladder even under war-time conditions, as one expects him to carry out aseptic operations under these conditions. The most important initial management of these severely wounded soldiers is their evacuation by air to their home country with highest priority. Moreover, after arrival their *immediate* transfer to *Spinal Injuries Centres* should be organized and they should not be kept in General Military or Veteran Hospitals where, as a rule, the staff is not acquainted with the comprehensive management of spinal injured patients. From all my experiences during and after the Second World War in this and other countries, I am convinced that as a result of the inadequate management in General Hospitals, these unfortunate victims of war developed all the complications under the sun, so well described by Jacobson & Bors on spinal cord casualties of the Vietnam War, before they were admitted to specialized Spinal Unit for, what is called, 'rehabilitation'. All too often 'lack of staff' is given as argument or excuse for immediate permanent drainage of the acutely paralysed bladder by an indwelling catheter. Hence the high percentage of bladderstone. Glane (1974) reported removal of vesical stones in no less than 40 per cent.

Tidal drainage

Although tidal drainage was introduced by Lawer (1917) in this country, no great interest was taken in this method until it was developed by Munro in the U.S.A. (1935) for both the immediate and long-term treatment of the paralysed bladder, and during the Second World War it was widely used. He himself has improved his original tidal drainage apparatus by two later models (1952). We have found Riches' design at Stoke Mandeville very satisfactory, which, being fitted with a manometer, can also be used for cystemetrography.

The principle of tidal drainage is based on siphonage with the help of irrigating fluid which is elicited whenever a predetermined intravesical pressure has been reached, thus the bladder is alternately filled and emptied automatically. However, in practice, it works satisfactorily only if its management is fully understood and continuously controlled by the medical and nursing staff day *and* night and also by the patient. Munro (1952) himself has tabulated causes of functional failure, such as air leaks, using a wrong type of Murphy dropper, formation of a trap in the long catheter connections, kinks in the connections, leakage of urine around the catheter, if the apparatus is not properly adjusted, and mistakes in the adjustment of height of the siphon curve. According to Munro the proper height of the siphon curve should be set at 1 or 2 cm above the bladder level during the stage of spinal shock when the bladder is atonic; once the bladder becomes automatic, at 10 to 13 cm for the reflex bladder and at 15 to 18 cm for the hypertonic bladder. During and immediately after the Second World War we have used tidal drainage extensively but later it has only been used in selected cases in later stages in patients with infected bladders to clear the bladder from debris, mucus and small stones. It has not been used in the immediate and early stages of spinal injuries as it does not prevent early infection.

Suprapubic cystostomy

In my Monograph in Volume Surgery of the History of the Second World War (1953), I reported that 300 out of 351 traumatic paraplegics of the Second World War had supra-

pubic cystostomy carried out for bladder drainage before admission to the Stoke Mandeville Spinal Centre. In the majority of them (210) this was done within 3 days after
injury. Every case admitted with suprapubic drainage, whether with or without urethral
catheterization prior to the cystostomy, showed signs of infection of the urinary tract,
and in a considerable number of cases the infection was of an ascending type, including
pyrexial attacks, stone formation in bladder, ureter and kidneys, leading to pyo- or
hydronephrosis. It may be stressed that epididymo-orchitis was not prevented by suprapubic drainage. These findings did not prove the opinion held by urologists in that time
that suprapubic cystostomy 'if done early will prevent serious infection' (Riches, 1943),
nor has it been proved that urinary infection could be avoided if suprapubic cystostomy
was of high type (Donovan, 1947). As one would expect, the infection was introduced
and maintained by the suprapubic tube, whether it was of retaining type such as Pezzer,
Malecot, Foley or any other type of catheter, especially if the catheter was left in the
bladder for longer periods. In numerous cases, it was difficult to withdraw the suprapubic
catheter on admission as it was encrusted with phosphates. In lesions of any level where
the suprapubic drainage was continued for some time, the bladder was repeatedly found

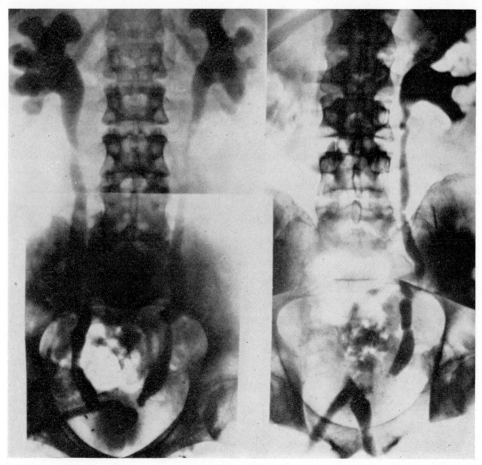

FIG. 161

to be extremely contracted. In several cases with contracted bladders, various degrees of hydroureter and hydronephrosis were found, as shown in Fig. 161, in spite of the fact that cystoscopy did not reveal blockage of the ureteric orifices. This observation is at variance with the opinion held generally at that time that the main factor in the development of hydroureter and hydronephrosis was back pressure from the dilated bladder.

Experience has shown that there is no evidence that the neurological level of a spinal cord lesion as such is responsible for the vesico-ureteric reflux, but that the chronic inflammatory changes of the ureters themselves producing ureteritis and periureteritis are the decisive factors. On the one hand, these changes lead to impairment of the elasticity and destruction of the valve-like action of the ureteric orifices, resulting in vesico-ureteric reflux as already suggested by previous observations (Hagner, 1912; Kretschner & Greer, 1914; Prather, 1944; Talbot, 1949; and others); on the other hand the ureteritis leads to impairment of elasticity and contractility of the ureter itself. Adhesions between ureter and surrounding tissues caused by peri-ureteritis are responsible for the increased tortuosity and kinking of the ureter which gives rise to mechanical obstruction.

In my Monograph of 1953 evidence has been given of the bacteria, such as Staph. pyogenes, Str. haemolyticus, coli, proteus, which were obtained from cultures taken from the bladder end of the catheter and which were different from the urine cultures.

Suprapubic cystostomy does not prevent the development of an automatic bladder though, as a rule, the recovery of the detrusor action was found greatly delayed as compared with that following intermittent catheterization. It is, therefore, understandable, why suprapubic drainage does not prevent development of epididymo-orchitis, once the infected urine is expressed by the reflex detrusor action through the posterior urethra. The reflex detrusor action becomes, naturally, the more frequent the smaller the capacity of the bladder as the result of contracture.

All these facts have endorsed my conclusion drawn from the war experience (Guttmann, 1947) that there is no reason whatsoever to consider suprapubic drainage as a satisfactory, let alone, as the method of choice in the immediate and long term treatment of the paralysed bladder. In fact, my and other authors' experience definitely contra-

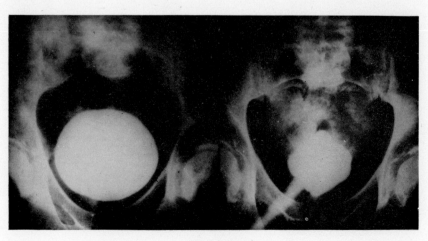

FIG. 162.

indicates its indiscriminate use and routine performance as immediate and early treatment of the paralysed bladder in both war-time and peace-time injuries of the spinal cord and cauda equina (Munro, 1935, 1945; Talbot, 1946; Donovan, 1947; Martin & Davis, 1948; Freeman, 1949; Cosbie Ross, 1960; and others). Suprapubic cystostomy as a temporary measure is indicated only if a spinal cord injury is associated with direct injury to the urethra or if the first urethral catheterization reveals a marked urethral stricture which cannot easily be overcome. In later stages, suprapubic cystostomy may be indicated in a case of urinary fistula which cannot be healed by conservative or surgical treatment. The sooner suprapubic drainage is discontinued the better the prospect of checking urinary infection and restoring a good capacity and satisfactory control of the bladder. While we succeeded after the war, in a case of incomplete transverse lesion below T10 with suprapubic cystostomy of 5 years and 4 months standing (Fig. 162), in establishing a satisfactory bladder function with good capacity as shown in Fig. 162, this represents an exception. In the great majority, we were able to discontinue suprapubic drainage within a year. While we did not experience major complications following spontaneous closure of the suprapubic sinus, apart from repeated break down, serious complications due to intraperitoneal extravasation including fatal peritonitis have been reported (Pate & Bunts, 1948; Reite & Comarr, 1954; Bunts, 1958).

In cases in which suprapubic drainage has been continued for long periods, healing of the suprapubic wound is always delayed, and even if the tract has been excised surgically it still has a tendency to break down, even, as we found, after many years. Based on personal experimental studies on catgut as an undesirable suture material for nerve sutures (Guttmann, 1943), better healing results after excision of the suprapubic track were obtained by using stainless steel wire, a procedure which has also been adopted for surgical closure of urethral fistulas.

In conclusion, the view expressed by Ogier Ward & Riches (1944) that, in cases of complete transverse lesion of the spinal cord, a properly conducted cystostomy opening is infinitely preferable to an automatic bladder, and their strong recommendation that suprapubic drainage should continue in such cases, has not been confirmed by the experience gained in this Centre and by other workers in this field. Actually, the view held that suprapubic cystostomy as an immediate or early treatment of the paralysed bladder is only indicated in very exceptional cases, as mentioned above, is now generally accepted in this country and abroad.

Cutaneous vesicostomy

In recent years, suprapubic drainage as early urological management of paraplegic patients has been revived in the form of the tubeless or what is called, cutaneous vesicostomy in the U.S.A. by Blocksom (1957), Lapides et al. (1960, 1962, 1964), Arduino & Miller (1960), Felton & Read (1960), Leal, Scributis & Lloyd (1963), Bernstein-Hahn (1965), Rosenthal et al. (1967) and others. However, strong criticisms have been made by American and other physicians and surgeons, in particular those with extensive experience in paraplegia (Bors, Comarr, Ebel, Habib, Susset, Talbot, 1963; Guttmann & Frankel, 1966; Gibbon et al., 1969; Cibeira, 1970; Bors & Comarr, 1971). Comarr, in particular, has dissociated himself immediately from Lapides' statement that 'if the bladder does not come around within 2 weeks after injury this is the indication to do it'. It may be noted that Lloyd, who himself was in favour of cutaneous vesicostomy instead of the use of a permanent suprapubic mushroom catheter in the *occasional* case only when such form of bladder drainage becomes necessary, made his view abundantly clear: 'to do frequent and routine cutaneous vesicostomy early in the course of paraplegia is inexcusable'. Kyle (1968) calls cutaneous vesicostomy 'an unreasonably traumatic procedure, hard to manage and necessitating the wearing of complex and expensive apparatus'. Krahn *et al.* (1964) stated that all their 7 patients undergoing the Lapides' vesicostomy were failures and required intubated drainage later. Laskowski & Brantley Scott (1965) performed the Lapides' vesicostomy in 45 patients, 44 of them with spinal cord lesions, who (1) were unable to empty the bladder effectively, (2) required prolonged tube drainage and (3) had a poor prognosis for neurological recovery (no detailed information was given about the meaning of this point). Although there were no deaths, wound infection was the most common early postoperative complication (8 cases), the others being necrosis of the distal part of the bladder flap (5), prolonged urinary leakage (2), atelactasis (1), paralytic ileus (1). The most common late complications were: technical difficulty with the collecting device (8 cases) encrustations of skin flap due to growing hair (4), bladder calculi (4), tight stoma (3) renal calculi (2) and vesical eversion (1). Moreover, squamous metaplasia was found in all 13 cases where biopsies were performed and cystitis glandularis occurred in 2 patients. These tissue changes may, as is known, lead later to carcinomatous development. Yet, incredible as it may seem, in spite of all these results the authors consider the incidence of postoperative complications as acceptable. Karafin & Kendall (1966) reported one death. These experiences clearly contra-indicate Lapides' view (1964) to employ cutaneous vesicostomy as a 'standard treatment in paraplegics within a week or two after injury'. This concept ignores so profoundly the natural forces of physiological adjustment in the spinal cord including the return of bladder function. This procedure represents a grave mistake and is a serious retrograde step in the early management of paraplegics and tetraplegics as it adds a considerable local damage to the bladder wall in addition to its neurogenic lesion. It would result in most, if not all, of the unhappy consequences of tubed suprapubic cystostomy of 30 years ago and would create a very serious situation, especially if this surgical procedure were followed up by workers with little experience with the complex problem of paraplegia and tetraplegia. In this connection, the quoted reports published by Krahn *et al.* and Laskowski & Brantley Scott are highly significant. It is therefore, gratifying that this method is rejected by urologists and other workers concerned with the treatment and rehabilitation of paraplegics and tetraplegics, including those who unfortunately still adhere to the method of urethral drainage by indwelling catheter as initial and early treatment of these patients because of lack of staff or other reasons, to carry out intermittent catheterization.

Closed methods of suprapubic catheterization

The old technique using a trocar and canula for the introduction of a self-retaining catheter of a larger size, has been generally abandoned, and during the Second World War it was replaced by Riches' method of suprapubic catheterization (Riches, 1943), employing a very small catheter (16F) fixed to a trocar. Whatever closed technique is used, care has to be taken that the trocar is inserted well above the pubis in the midline and, in particular, that the bladder is maximally distended and the patient lies in head down position. These precautions may diminish the risk of injury to the peritoneum, as during bladder distension the peritoneum is raised, and thus an uncovered area of the bladder is exposed through which the trocar can be pushed into the bladder. However, it must be remembered that the peritoneum down to the pubis forms a pouch in front of the distended bladder which may even contain small gut (MacAlpine, 1948). In such cases, the danger of causing peritonitis with any closed method is great, especially if the distended paralysed bladder is already infected whether spontaneously or by previous urethral catheterization, and extravasation of urine occurs. Moreover, the catheter, although firmly fixed to the trocar, may break lose either on entering the abdominal fascia or, in particular, before entering the bladder, by the resistance of the muscular bladder wall. This may result in peritonitis, as happened to one of my own patients during the war, which induced me to give up suprapubic catheterization by any closed technique. Furthermore, once the catheter is inserted and suprapubic drainage is established, great care has to be taken by the nursing staff not to pull out the catheter after this procedure on turning the paralysed patient, especially if a small catheter has been used, for it may be difficult or even impossible to insert a new catheter through the very small opening. Actually, if the small catheter is pulled out during the night and this is not realized immediately and rectified by the nursing staff or by the patient, the small fistula may close within hours.

Because of the potential hazards of infection, encrustations and stone formation following urethral catheterization, Smith, Cook & Robertson (1969) revived suprapubic catheterization by using a 6 in. or 8 in. plastic canula with a hollow bevelled trocar which, after insertion through a mid-line stab over the upper part of the anterior wall of the distended bladder may remain in position for several weeks. The authors themselves frankly admit the disadvantage of this method which they discovered in their 12 male patients treated with that technique. Although 6 of the 18 cannulae inserted kinked within as early as 2 days, each cannula lasted at an average of 13 days (0 to 45). Moreover, 7 of the 12 patients eventually had a urethral catheter because a member of staff was uncertain of the technique for re-insertion of the cannula after it had blocked due to a kink. Deposits within the cannula were not avoided although the authors did not consider them as significant.

In a paper on problems in the early management of bladder paralysis, Cook & Smith (1970) reported about a modification of their technique by using an infant peritoneal dialysis catheter in 4 patients, but again it was not possible to control infection satisfactorily (2 patients had an indwelling catheter before suprapubic catheterization).

From all the data given so far by these authors, it cannot be said that their technique and its modification (1970) represent an improvement on any other form of suprapubic catheterization including Riches' method. On the contrary, the not infrequent kinking of their cannula (6 out of 18), the lasting of each cannula at an average of only 13 days and, in particular, the fact that 7 out of their 12 patients eventually had an urethral catheter because a member of staff was uncertain of the technique for re-insertion of the cannula after it had blocked due to a kink, are additional risks to the other hazard of suprapubic drainage described previously. They should be a warning to anybody with less expertise than Mr Smith against employing this technique of suprapubic catheterization in the immediate and early management of paraplegics and tetraplegics. Moreover, the statement and conclusion made in their latest publication—an account of only 4 patients (1970)—'in the knowledge that even in the best hands intermittent catheterization produces nearly 40 per cent of infected urine on discharge from hospital it has been decided to continue with fine suprapubic catheters' are as surprizing as they are misleading. As their results were based on studies in male patients, comparison should of course, have been made with the results reported on male patients treated with intermittent catheterization, of which the authors must have been fully aware, namely 69·4 per cent out of 157 patients sterile on discharge from hospital (Guttmann & Frankel, 1966), 82·6 per cent out of 92 patients on discharge (Walsh, 1968), 82·3 per cent on 17 patients on discharge and 92 per cent on 14 patients on follow up 2 years and longer (Dollfus & Molé, 1969). Intermittent catheterization has been accepted by many workers in this field as the method of choice in the initial and early treatment of the paralysed bladder in spinal cord injuries. It is the safest method in the immediate and early management of the paralysed bladder and every traumatic paraplegic and tetraplegic really deserve to be given the benefit of this method.

Perineal urethrostomy

There is general agreement that this method suggested by Lewis (1945) is the worst possible method in the management of bladder paralysis, whether in the acute, early or late stages, and it is only mentioned here to be condemned. Performed through the bulbus urethra, it results in scrotal and prostatic sepsis. Moreover, it prevents the patient from sitting in a wheelchair as the pressure of the catheter against the perineal structure inevitably produces pressure sores which may be of disastrous type, as was found in the case of a boy with spina bifida who was transferred to Stoke Mandeville (Fig. 168).

CONCLUSIONS

From all the experiences gained so far, it can now be concluded that the non-touch technique of intermittent catheterization has proved to be highly effective and superior to any other form of initial and early management of the paralysed bladder following complete and incomplete cord and cauda equina lesions, in preventing infection and fistulae and minimizing stone formation, hydronephrosis and other serious complications of the uro-genital system.

The non-touch method of intermittent catheterization is considered as a medical and not a paramedical procedure and, therefore, should be carried out in the initial and early stages of paraplegia and tetraplegia in both male and female patients by a medical officer familiar with the details of this method as long as voluntary or reflex function of the bladder has not fully returned. The custom so long accepted, even in some Spinal Injuries Centres, to delegate, because of shortage of medical staff, this delicate, and for the patient so vital, initial treatment to nurses and other paramedical staff is to be deprecated. For, it is as much the responsibility of the administrative authorities, as it is of the physicians and surgeons in hospitals and, in particular, Spinal Injuries Centres, concerned with the initial and early treatment of spinal cord injuries, to ensure that sufficient staff is available to carry out this important part of the comprehensive management of these seriously ill patients in the early stages of paraplegia.

Generally speaking, a newly paralysed patient needs 150–200 intermittent catheterizations before the return of automatic or autonomous bladder function, in young patients and incomplete lesions naturally less. If one balances the time taken by the medical officer to carry out proper intermittent catheterization, which preserves a sterile bladder for many weeks or throughout and avoids early complications, against time-consuming and costly treatment of later complications arising from continuous drainage by indwelling urethral catheter or suprapubic drainage, including repeated surgical procedures with all the paraphernalia involved, one can be in no doubt that in the patient's interest the employment of sufficient medical staff is more than justified.

B. MANAGEMENT IN THE INTERMEDIATE AND LATE STAGES

The aims of management in the intermediate and late stages are to make the patient catheter-free as soon as possible and to adjust him to his ultimate bladder dysfunction. Hand in hand with these aims goes the control of bladder infection by mechanical procedures, chemotherapy and antibiotics to prevent ascending infection and safeguard the kidneys from destruction. Although the treatment is divided into conservative and surgical procedures, in practice both are interrelated in many cases.

The objects to be pursued can be summarized as follows:

1 Control of residual urine and retention in the early intermediate stage.
2 Control of incontinence.
3 Reconditioning of the patient to his micturitional dysfunction.
4 Continuous drainage by indwelling catheter in later stages.
5 Control of infection by mechanical procedures, acidifiers, chemotherapy and antibiotics.
6 Management of late complication.

1. Control of residual urine and retention in the early intermediate stage

In the early intermediate stage of bladder dysfunction, following the stage of spinal shock in complete lesions above the lumbo-sacral cord, the reciprocal reflex mechanism between the expulsion forces of the detrusor contractions and the relaxation of the sphincter complex and the muscles of the pelvic floor are imperfect for some time in ensuring complete evacuation of urine, and persistent residual urine results. This occurs in cases following discontinuation of indwelling catheter drainage who are infected as well as in cases treated by intermittent catheterization who have sterile urine. Therefore, intermittent catheterization must be continued at gradually increasing intervals and residual urine tests must be carried out systematically to ascertain the amount of residual urine, which may vary within wide limits. If it is small in amount (under 1–2 oz) with a bladder capacity of at least 10 oz there is no harm, as long as stagnation of urine, which represents an ideal medium for bacteriological growth, is avoided by a high fluid intake.

Cystometric studies should be carried out in that stage to ascertain the development of the reflex activity of the detrusor and its expulsive power. Parasympathetico-mimetic drugs such as Carbamylcholine chloride (Carbachol, Doryl), the urethane of choline, in doses of 1–5 mg by mouth 2–4 times daily or 0·00025–0·0005 g intramuscularly have proved useful in improving reflex micturition by increasing the expulsive power of the detrusor and promoting voluntary micturition in incomplete lesions. Another very effective cholinergic agent in hypotonic bladder is Urecholine (Beta-Methylcholine urethane) recommended by Lee (1950) in doses of 5 mg subcutaneously or 5–50 mg orally 3–4 times daily. Side effects of these cholinergic drugs are gastro-intestinal disturbances, sweating and lacrimation and they should be avoided in patients with a history of gastro-duodenal ulcers and asthma. Moreover, we found that the beneficial effect of these drugs is by no means uniform in neurologically comparable lesions of the same level; in fact in some cases the degree of urinary retention increased, presumably, these drugs stimulate the sphincter complex as much as the detrusor.

Treatment of retention in later stages

Conservative

In later stages, when the reflex activity of the isolated or diseased spinal cord is increased, larger amounts of residual urine may be due to the increased reflex activity of the internal and external sphincter complex. There are no specific drugs available to relax solely the heightened reflex function of the sphincter mechanism. Moreover, in this stage the reflex activity of the detrusor itself is increased resulting in frequent but ineffective micturition with greater or lesser amounts of residual urine. One has, therefore, to rely on drugs which have a generally depressant effect on spasticity, which are discussed in the section on spasticity. However, temporary local suppression of the heightened reflex activity of the sphincter complex including the pelvic floor muscles by local anaesthesia of urethra and bladder outlet through instillation of anaesthetics such as 60 ml of 0·1–0·25 per cent solution of Pantocaine can be achieved, thus diminishing the resistance of the sphincters and increasing the expulsive power of the detrusor. The increase of detrusor capacity by topical anaesthesia was described by Bors & Comarr (1970), who in addition found that suppression of the mucosal impulses also results in the reduction of the skeletal spasticity in some patients. Whether it is necessary to achieve relaxation of the pelvic floor by simultaneous anaesthesia of the external anal sphincter by instillation of 5–10 ml of Nupercainal ointment into the rectum will have to be decided from case to case. Relaxation of the external anal sphincter was demonstrated electro-myelographically (Bors & Blinn, 1957; Rossier & Bors, 1962). One can fully agree with these authors that this simple procedure can be carried out with impunity several times weekly or even daily before more drastic procedures (see later) are contemplated to eliminate or greatly reduce residual urine by increasing the expulsive force of the detrusor. In some cases, the temporary reduction of urethral resistance of the urinary outflow by repeated urethral dilatation using increasing calibre of catheters may facilitate the development of co-ordination between bladder and sphincter function. It must also be remembered that while reflex—or, in incomplete lesions, voluntary-micturition is in progress—the force of the urinary stream can be increased by raising the intravesical pressure by contractions of the abdominal muscles, or in the case of paralysis in higher lesions above T5, manually.

A powerful function of the abdominal muscles is of particular importance in overcoming residual urine in lower motor neuron lesions affecting the spinal micturition centre itself or its spinal roots in cauda equina lesions resulting in an autonomous bladder. Emmett (1954) found that contraction of the intact abdominal muscles, as is the case in lesions below T12, raises the intravesical pressure to 50–70 cm water, which we confirmed in our cystometric studies and which is sufficient to evacuate the bladder, provided there is no obstruction at the bladder or urethral outlet by hypertrophy of the bladder neck, external sphincter or increased spasticity. Therefore early physiotherapy to the abdominal muscles while the patient is confined to bed, and restoring his upright posture as early as possible have proved essential in the management of residual urine. Moreover, the full co-operation of the patient, who must be made aware of his bladder dysfunction, is indispensable. This will be discussed in the section on reconditioning.

Surgical

In the vast majority of complete paraplegics and tetraplegics satisfactory reflex—or in incomplete lesions, voluntary micturition can be established. There remains, however, a group who in later stages develop structural changes at the urethra and/or vesico-urethral levels causing disturbances of the hydrodynamics resulting in retention of urine and larger amounts of permanent residual urine necessitating surgical treatment.

In general, surgical procedures designed to overcome urinary retention can be divided (a) into those to overcome the structural resistance of the peripheral sections of the urinary tract mentioned above, (b) into those to reduce or abolish the action of certain components of the vesical and/or urethral nerve supply. Under certain circumstances a combination of both procedures may be necessary.

(a) 1: Transurethral resection of the external sphincter

In recent years the importance of the obstruction of the external urethral sphincter as the cause of urinary retention has become more and more apparent. It was in particular, Cosbie Ross and his colleagues (1958, 1960, 1963, 1966) who developed the resection of the external urethral sphincter as a useful method to eliminate its resistance. The indication for this operation is made by thorough observation with the aid of a vesico-urethrogram and urethroscopy. The operation was carried out by Ross initially with the cold punch technique, several strips being resected from the posterolateral aspect of the external sphincter. Although this technique was successful, the postoperative complication was severe and dangerous venous bleeding. Since Ross improved his technique by coagulating first the two posterolateral areas to be cut with diathermy current, the danger of massive postoperative bleeding has been greatly reduced, and the functional results regarding the elimination of the obstruction have been very satisfactory.

The good result of transurethral sphinterotomy, as a reliable procedure for alleviating chronic retention due to detrusor-sphincter dysfunction, has been confirmed in recent years by many workers in this field. This operation has been advocated even in early stages of retention both in upper and lower motor neurone lesions, if, by accurate diagnosis, the external urethral sphincter is found to be the site of obstruction (Leriche et al., 1974). However, it should be done in selected cases only and not become a routine operation in early stages of urinary retention. This applies, in particular, to incomplete cord lesions, and I agree with Perkash (1975) that in these patients this operation should be deferred for at least 2 years and that medication (Dantrolene and others) in combination with systematic training of the patient may eventually overcome the retention. Moreover, one has to consider the loss of penile erection which may follow transurethral sphincterotomy, which, obviously in incomplete cord or conus-cauda equina lesions but also in complete lesions, must be considered as a serious complication. Recent publications have drawn attention to this problem (Thomas, 1974; Dollfus et al., 1974; Hachen, 1974; Walsh, 1974).

The initially excellent results of transurethral resection of the external urethral sphincter may not be permanent and infection and fibrous-sclerosis of the sphincter may necessitate re-operation. How far the recently advocated modified technique of sphincterotomy (O'Flynn, 1973; Perkash, 1974; Madersbacher, 1974) of making 4 cuts each 5–6 mm in the 12 o'clock region, instead of or in combination with the generally accepted resection at 3 and 9 o'clock, will improve the permanent results remains to be seen. This technique is based on the anatomical findings of an aggregation of striated fibres at 12 o'clock in the anterior commissure (Bors et al., 1954; Oelrich, 1964; Sant, 1972), and this may account for the successful results achieved by Madersbacher and Perkash.

(a) 2: Open operations

Surgical procedures by open operation to eliminate or reduce urethral resistance are Young's (1953) Y–V plasty of the vesical neck which is mainly used in children, or the perineal membranous urethroplasty introduced by Semans (1949, 1960). This latter operation consists in freeing and transecting the membranous urethra and re-uniting the prostatic apex with the pelvic diaphragm. However, any operation within the perineal region of paraplegics and tetraplegics may facilitate the development of pressure sores later and this method is not practised in this country as the method of choice in eliminating urethral resistance in spinal paraplegics and tetraplegics. Although Bunts (1961) considered membranous urethroplasty in 3 of 12 operated cases as a necessary adjunct to trans-urethral resection, and in 5 cases a feasible alternative to transurethral resection, in 4 patients transurethral resection became necessary afterwards. Moreover, urinary infection remained in all patients.

(a) 3: Transurethral resection of the bladder neck

This operation, first introduced by Emmett (1945), has proved from all experiences to be the most important surgical method in the treatment of urinary retention due to obstruction at the vesico-urethral junction be it caused by hypertrophy of the bladder neck or spasticity. At Stoke Mandeville this operation has been carried out successfully for many years, and our results are in accordance with the experiences of many other surgeons in both upper and lower motor lesions. Fig. 163 shows the result of TUR in a case of complete lesion below T5 who, about 5 years after injury, developed a profound bladder distension due to hypertrophy of the bladder neck. However, authors still differ as to

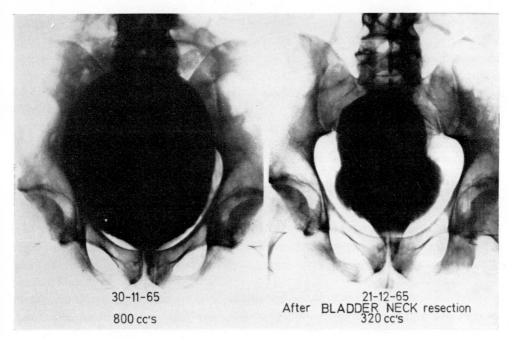

30-11-65

800 cc's

21-12-65
After BLADDER NECK resection
320 cc's

FIG. 163.

whether the resection should be done round the clock (Emmett, 1959) or not. Bors (1957); Cosbie Ross (1960), Gibbon *et al.* (1965) favour limited resection, a view shared by Walsh. Bors & Comarr (1971) resect the vesical neck in areas where tissue is prominent, usually the posterior lip and the lateral folds. This means a resection from 3 through 9 o'clock. Only if this fails is the resection of the anterior lip included. While the amount of resected tissue has varied widely throughout the years, there has been a trend in recent years not to resect more than 2–4 g. Baker *et al.* (1950) and Burns & Kettridge (1958) extended the resection to the proximal margin of the external sphincter. The instrumental technique of TUR varies. While Gibbon *et al.* (1965) employ the cold punch, probably the majority of surgeons are using diathermy.

With regard to the time when TUR is indicated, there is also difference of opinion amongst workers in this field. There is, however, now the tendency to perform TUR at an earlier date than was the rule previously, although as early as 1947 Bumpus *et al.* advocated TUR in upper motor neuron lesions 2–6 weeks after return of reflex activity of the spinal cord had occurred. Bors & Comarr (1971) are now inclined to perform TUR after three months—when intermittent catheterization fails to establish satisfactory micturition in paralysed patients with lower motor neurone lesions. While I agree that TUR should not be delayed for long, I am not in favour of any dogmatism regarding the time for TUR performance. Having regard to the great variability of bladder dysfunction in paraplegics and tetraplegics and the varying speed of the patient's adjustment to his bladder dysfunction, every case should be considered individually. Moreover, it must be remembered that only repeated observations will show whether the site of obstruction is really the vesico-urethral junction only or whether the external urethral sphincter is the major obstruction. In certain cases Walsh combines TUR with urethral sphincter resection, using the diathermy technique. This is also preferred by Bors & Comarr (1971) who are using the Bugbee electrode instead of the Collins knife as used by other surgeons. Caldwell (1970), however, considers damaging the mucosal surface in sphincterotomy as unphysiological. He has, therefore, been using, in cases of retention in women, the retropubic approach, dividing the sphincter at 3 and 9 o'clock, which leaves the lining of the urinary tract undamaged while dividing the sphincter muscle. However, no follow-up details of this operation were given.

(a) 4: Operations for electric detrusor stimulation

Operations designed to implant electrodes for direct electric stimulation of the destrusor muscle have been performed in spinal cord patients in recent years by various authors (Bradley *et al.*, 1963; Bunts, 1964; Scott, 1965; Susset, 1966, 1968; Hagman *et al.*, 1966 and others) to overcome retention of urine. A review of the literature shows that so far about 80–90 patients were subjected to this operation. However, so many methodical and technical imperfections have been described that this operation cannot be considered so far of practical use in spinal cord lesions. The implantation of detrusor stimulators demands a large uncovering of the bladder because of the impossibility of assessing the full detrusor contraction from one optimal single point. Failures in the implanted receiver have occurred, and the receiver had to be removed and replaced by another in a second operation. Furthermore, rupture of the electrodes, infection and necrosis of the tissues, surrounding the implanted apparatus or spreading of the electric current, causing pain and contractions of the muscles of the pelvic floor and adjacent skeletal muscles were other undesirable side-effects of this method. Above all the therapeutic results of this procedure, in particular, their permanence, are unsatisfactory so far. It is obvious that this surgical procedure is contra-indicated in the immediate and early stages of paraplegia and tetraplegia and, if at all contemplated in future, should be the last resort, provided its failure can be avoided by further research. At a Symposium held in March 1976 in Frankfurt on Electrical Stimulation of the Neurogenic Bladder, Ichim (Rumania) reported about 10 patients in whom electrodes were implanted for direct detrusor stimulation even during spinal shock. This approach completely neglects the achievements made in the recovery of bladder function and it is utterly contrary to the principles of treatment and rehabilitation of paraplegics and tetraplegics and should be rejected. It may be noted that at that Symposium several speakers with experience on this subject, with the exception of one (Merrill, USA) reported about failure of this method.

(a) 5: Muscle transplantation to increase detrusor function

Transplantations of the rectus abdominis (Boshamer, 1951, 1960) or of the gracilis (Ingelman-Sundberg, 1957) into the bladder wall have been used in some cases of lower motor neuron lesions to increase voiding pressure and to overcome urinary retention. Although the authors claim satisfactory results, reports of long-term detailed follow up of the patients are not available. The value of this surgical approach in the treatment of retention seems very doubtful and was never used at Stoke Mandeville.

(a) 6: Urinary diversion

While suprapubic cystostomy, as mentioned before, has very rare indications and, as a rule, as a temporary measure only in cases with local uncontrollable damage of the urethra by strictures or fistulae, it has no place in the treatment of persistent vesical urinary retention in view of the better understanding of the vesical pathophysiology and the advances made in the more adequate methods of treatment of this condition in spinal cord lesions, such as TUR and resection of the external urethral sphincter. However, from all experiences gained, cutaneous vesicostomy and urethrostomy are contra-indicated in the treatment of paraplegics and tetraplegics in both early and late stages of spinal paraplegia and tetraplegia.

Supravesical diversions by ileal or colonic conduits are also deprecated in the treatment of vesical urinary retention. Their indication in urinary incontinence, ureteric reflux and hydronephrosis with renal deficiency will be discussed in the following chapters.

(b) Neurosurgical procedures on components of the vesical and urethral nerve supply

It can be said that most of the neurosurgical procedures advocated in the past for the relief of the external sphincter and vesico-urethral obstruction have been practically abandoned in favour of transurethral external sphincterotomy and transurethral resection of the bladder neck.

(b) 1: Pudendal neurectomy—pelvic neurectomy

This operation was strongly advocated by Cosbie, Ross & Damanski (1953). However, in practice this proved to be a rather tedious operation, and unless it is done bilaterally and all branches of the nerve are excised the results are either only temporary or unsuccessful. Moreover, bilateral pudendal neurectomy inevitably leads to loss of penile erection and impotence.

(b) 2: Pelvic neurectomy (resection of the parasympathetic outflow)

This operation, which is now hardly ever carried out for denervation of the external sphincter and bladder neck, also leads inevitably to impotence.

(b) 3: Sacral rhizotomy

Anterior and posterior rhizotomy was advocated by Meirowski *et al.* (1952) and Brendler *et al.* (1953). This operation, if carried out bilaterally from S1–S5, will certainly denervate the external sphincter and relieve blockage of the urinary outflow but will at the same time denervate all muscles of the pelvic floor and destroy the power of erection. The result of partial or selective resection of anterior and/or posterior roots is uncertain.

(b) 4: Intrathecal alcohol block

The elimination of the sacral root supply of the external sphincter and muscles of the pelvic floor can be much more easily accomplished by chemical destruction through an intrathecal alcohol block (Guttmann, 1946, 1953, 1973), as compared with the tedious operation of sacral rhizotomy. However, this procedure should be reserved for selected cases only—i.e. those complete upper motor neurone lesions with intractable spasticity of the lower limbs and trunk in addition to deformity and contracture of the uninhibited bladder, resulting in spastic obstruction at the vesico-urethral junction and external urethral sphincter. With regard to technique, indications and results see chapter on Spasticity, pages 402–550.

2. Control of incontinence

(a) Passive overflow or passive incontinence is the result of overdistension of the paralysed hypotonic bladder in both upper and lower motor neuron lesions, if no drainage was established at the proper time. Rapid evacuation of an overdistended bladder by catheter drainage should be avoided in order to give the bladder wall the chance to adjust itself to a small volume, as otherwise haemorrhage may occur within the bladder.

Passive incontinence may also develop in tabes and diabetic neuropathy due to degeneration of the afferent pathways when, as a result of the loss of sensibility, there is no desire to urinate, and the bladder becomes atonic and dribbling incontinence ensues. In progressed cases, wearing of a urinal will be indispensable in addition to intermittent catheter drainage. In less progressed cases the treatment consists, apart from controlling infection, in teaching the patient to adjust the frequency of micturition, using abdominal pressure, in relation to the amount of fluid intake. Moreover, fluid intake should be restricted from 7 p.m. and/or the patient should interrupt his sleep once or twice at night to avoid nocturnal incontinence.

Patients with lower motor neuron lesions as a result of traumatic lesions or myelodysplasia, associated with spina bifida resulting in autonomous bladder, often suffer from passive incontinence to various degrees, especially if the sensory elements are affected more severely than the motor, and the urethral resistance is low as a result of the paralysis of the urethral spincter and the bulbo-cavernosus muscles, and the anal reflexes are absent. Such patients will need urinals or, in certain cases, surgical urinary diversion, especially in cases of spina bifida, if hydronephrosis, hydroureter or other anomalies of the upper urinary tract exist, representing co-existent anomalies to the lower motor neuron lesions. Nash (1967) reported on urinary diversion in congenital paraplegia in 473 children, in 448 (about 95 per cent) of whom the causative lesion was spina bifida or dysplasia. Seventy female children have been subjected to ileal loop diversion at various ages and various stages of their pathology. Children below the age of 5 were excluded from this operation. The post-operative mortality was nil, 50 girls operated on between 1955–63 were followed up. There was a late mortality due to renal failure of 7 (14 per cent), 3 in the first 4 months, one in the 3rd year, 2 in the 4th year and one in the 10th year. Nash considered ileal loop as the most satisfactory method in dealing with incontinence arising from congenital paraplegia in the female. However, in incomplete lower motor neuron lesions, whether traumatic or non-traumatic, the passive incontinence can be reduced to manageable proportions by training the patient to habits of self-management. This can even be achieved, as I found, in spina bifida children, provided the mother is instructed to correlate the amount of fluid intake and the time of expressing the child's bladder to avoid dribbling incontinence.

(b) Stress. A special form of passive incontinence in lower motor neuron lesion is the stress incontinence due to weakness of the external urethral sphincter and the muscles of the pelvic floor. Loss of urine will occur during various types of stresses such as coughing, laughing, brisk movements, jumping or lifting of objects, even in patients who otherwise have learned to control their incontinence. Such patients may, therefore, prefer to wear a urinal.

Vincent (1959–68) studying the effect of perineal elevation found that, when the ischiorectal region and perineum is elevated beyond a certain point by mechanical means, the flow of urine is stopped or prevented from starting. He used this procedure in female patients with stress incontinence to show that with applied mechanical pressure urine did not leak on coughing. For patients with only weak pelvic floor muscles, Vincent recommends simple exercises consisting of tightening the anus and buttocks as powerfully as possible, sometimes with the aid of electrical treatment of the perineal region. In other patients, the control is achieved by using an appliance 'in the form of a wide belt which holds a saddle piece, with a balloon on its upper surface, tightly pressed against the anus and perineum'. However, in complete lesions with the great amount of elevation necessary to keep the bladder outlet closed, the author himself stressed the danger of developing pressure sores (Vincent, 1968).

(c) Active. Active incontinence develops due to reflex activity of the automatic bladder in upper motor neuron lesions. It occurs when the critical point of bladder distension is reached and the emptying reflex is elicited. It is obvious that the smaller the capacity of the bladder the more frequently are the detrusor contractions evoked. The most troublesome reflex incontinence is the result of the uninhibited function of the dysco-ordinated contracted automatic bladder, and it is particularly distressing in the female paraplegic, as, for anatomical reasons, they cannot be fitted with a urine-tight urinal. They have to

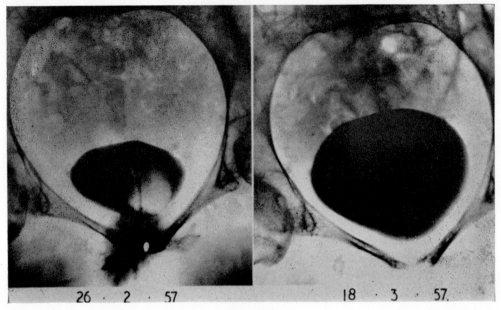

FIG. 164.

rely on absorbent pads, fixed by plastic pants which have to be changed frequently. The aim of management of this type of incontinence is to reduce the spasticity by relaxing drugs such as Pro-Banthine (Probantheline Bromide) in doses of 10–30 mg which is supposed to be more effective and with less severe side-effects (postural hypotension, dizziness, dryness etc.) than Methanteline Bromide (Banthine) which is used in the U.S.A. Etamon (Tetrethylammonium) which has an anticholinergic effect was found to eliminate uninhibited detrusor contractions (Nesbit *et al.*, 1947; Jönsson & Zederfeldt, 1957). Bors & Comarr (1970) found a potentiating effect of Banthine plus Atropin in reducing detrusor hyperactivity in order to prevent structural contracture. However, in cases with intractable spasticity, resulting in bladder contracture, transformation of the uninhibited bladder into an autonomous one by selective anterior rhizotomy or by intrathecal alcohol or phenol injections will be necessary if the conservative treatment fails to improve that condition which can make the patient's life most miserable by adding to the incontinence hyperreflexia of autonomic mechanisms. Fig. 164 shows the excellent result of an intrathecal alcohol block in a girl of 24 with a complete thoracic cord lesion and a disco-ordinated spastic bladder with almost continuous reflex-incontinence which made her life utterly miserable and prevented her from returning to a useful life. Since alcohol block she is continent, expressing her bladder at regular intervals, and is for many years employed as an art teacher. In very selected cases of women who have developed a dilatation of the urethra by the use of ever-increasing sizes of indwelling catheters and are continuously incontinent, urinary diversion by ileal conduit can be justified.

(d) Precipitous. Precipitous micturition is a form of incontinence which is found in both traumatic and non-traumatic incomplete lesions of the spinal cord as well as in other afflictions of the central nervous system, such as multiple sclerosis, where frequency and urgency may represent one of the early symptoms of the disease. Precipitous micturition also occurs in brain lesions. Drugs such as Atropine or Probanthine may have some transitory beneficial effect on reducing the hyperexcitability of the detrusor mechanism but the best result can be achieved by systematic training of the patient to correlate the amount of fluid intake with emptying the bladder at regular intervals which depend on the degree of precipitancy. Change of temperature, in particular cold weather, may have an adverse effect on precipitancy and increase incontinence. The wearing of a urinal may be necessary in numerous cases of non-progressive incomplete cord lesions, at least temporarily, to avoid anxiety and embarrassment until better control is achieved. However, a greater number of patients with complete lesions will have to depend on wearing a urinal permanently.

Electrical treatment of incontinence

This is still a very debatable problem. In Great Britain Caldwell (1963, 1967) was pioneering in the field of electrical control using an implantable device, designed by the Medical Research Connal's Sphincter Research Unit in Exeter. Alexander & Rowan (1968) introduced an external electrode system for use in female patients, in which a standard vaginal pessary served as a standard electrode carrier. Similar devices have been reported by de Soldenhoff & McDonnell (1968) and Edwards (1971). Hopkinson (1971), using intra-anal plug electrodes, reported his results of five years' experience on various types of incontinence and claimed 53 per cent cures. However, others report control only by continued use of the prescribed apparatus. In analysing critically all these reports, it can be concluded that electrical control of urinary incontinence is still uncertain and depends very much on the proper selection of cases. However, if satisfactory results in incomplete lesions of the spinal cord could be achieved even only in 30–40 per cent by the intra-anal plug electrode, it would be worthwhile trying before contemplating major surgical procedures.

URINALS

There are various designs of urinals for male paraplegics on the market, of which the most suitable are those which are the least likely to cause injury to the anaesthetic skin and deeper tissues, in particular the penis, and which can be properly cleansed. One-piece urinals, in which the sheath, top and reservoir bag cannot be detached from each other, are, as a rule, not suitable for paraplegics, as in some the rubber top is too hard. The Stoke Mandeville type of urinal is shown in Fig. 165. It has the advantage over other designs that the various parts of the urinal can be easily disconnected, which facilitates cleansing. It consists of a double bag with a one-way valve between and on top of that a second one-way valve. The urinal's top which is either straight or of swan-neck type, is provided with a detachable sheath which is replaceable at low cost. There are several sizes of the sheath varying from $\frac{1}{2}$ in to $1\frac{1}{2}$ in in diameter to ensure an accurate fit to the penis. The one-way valve between the urinal top and upper reservoir bag has an internal diameter of $\frac{3}{8}$ in to prevent back pressure in patients resulting from strong detrusor activity.

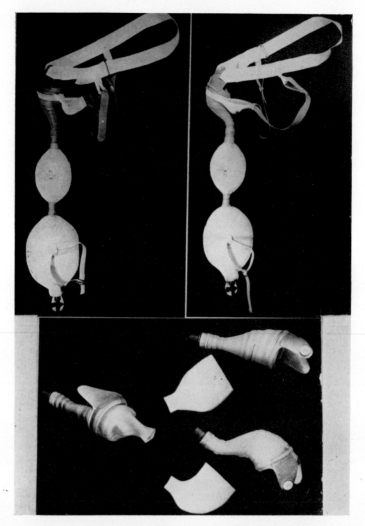

FIG. 165.

The top piece of the urinal and each bag reservoir can be disconnected for cleaning purposes. New sheaths are needed from time to time but, in contrast, to one-piece urinals, the main parts of the Stoke Mandeville type may last for 1 year to 18 months. (Manufacturers Down Bros., Mayer and Phelps, 32 New Cavendish Street, London W1). This urinal, as most of the other types, is supplied with a canvas belt and suspensory straps to the front and back of the urinal top where they are fixed by buttons. It is obvious that in cervical lesions with loss of finger movements the urinal has to be applied to the patient by his attendant. In Great Britain, paraplegics and tetraplegics are supplied with two urinals by the Health Service on doctor's prescription.

An alternative type of urinal which has become very popular in this and other countries, is the condom type of urinal. It was first used in U.S.A. The great advantages of this urinal are (a) that there is no hard material in contact with the genital region,

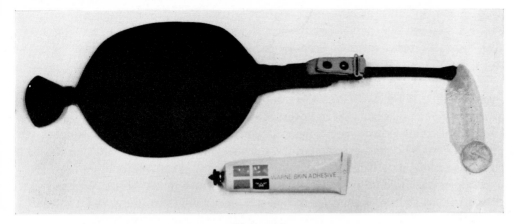

FIG. 166.

especially no constricting pressure exerted on the penis, (b) it can be easily applied and removed. However, in cervical lesions with paralysis or great weakness of the finger muscles this urinal as any other type has to be applied by the patient's attendant, (c) it can be used by patients with very short and retractable penis and even for small children. Its disadvantage is the increased cost (one condom for 23–24 hours plus Latex adhesive solution). Furthermore some patients become allergic to Latex and develop a rash on penis and groin. The least irritating Latex at present is that manufactured by the American firm Dow-Corning but it is more expensive. In some patients allergic reactions can be prevented by first spraying the proximal part of the penis where the condom is fixed with Nobecutane (New Skin) before applying the Latex solution. Fig. 166 shows the details of the condom urinal which is connected by a plastic connector with a rubber tube which in turn is connected with a supra-pubic type of container bag. To apply the condom the penis, proximal to the glans up to the symphysis pubis, is coated with Latex solution, then the condom is rolled over on to the penis, leaving about one inch of the sheath distal to the penis, and gently pressed around the penis until the adhesive is dry. The distal opening of the condom should be at least $\frac{1}{4}$ in to avoid back flow of urine during micturition. For a small child the condom can be substituted by a plastic finger stall. The adhesive can be removed with ether or surgical alcohol and the condom should never be removed without first removing the adhesive as otherwise this will be harmful to the skin of the penis. The condom urinal can also be prescribed in Great Britain under the Health Service regulations.

From the beginning, the patient has to be made aware by the medical and nursing staff about the vital importance of his personal hygiene, and the sooner he is trained the better for his health and future independence. Careful washing and drying the genital area should be a daily routine to avoid offensive urinary odour which would make the paraplegic socially unacceptable. Of special importance is the proper use and cleaning of whatever type of urinal. When applying the urinal, it is essential to ensure that no or minimal pressure is exerted on the posterior surface of the penis or on the scrotum and groins and that the penile skin is not twisted under the sheath. Careless handling of the urinal may result in a pressure sore, especially over the posterior aspect of the penis, which in one of our patients, admitted from home, resulted in a urethral fistula. Therefore, the penis must be inspected carefully on removing the urinal every day and if a skin lesion is found the urinal should not be worn until the lesion is healed.

Furthermore, the urinal should be arranged in such a way that free urine flow is ensured and reflux of urine into the trousers is prevented, which may occur when the patient is seated in his chair on an unsuitable rubber cushion. Some years ago, I designed a horse-shoe shaped sorbo rubber cushion which slopes towards the front and facilitates the urine flow. The rubber reservoir of the urinal is fixed to the leg and care should be taken that the holding band is not too tightly fixed.

Paraplegics should be provided with two urinals which should be used alternatively to ensure regular proper cleaning and drying. For cleaning, the urinal is first soaked in Steroxol solution (Chlorine and Detergent) and then thoroughly rinsed with plain water. Thereafter it is soaked for 1–2 hours in 10 per cent Milton solution (Sodium hydrochloride 1 per cent sodium chloride 16·8 per cent, chlorate sulphate, carbonate and calcium chlorate) or 15 per cent Dakins solution (Chlorinated lime, sodium carbonate and boric). For drying, the urinal should be hung up away from direct heat. At least once a week the various sections of the urinal should be taken apart and the junction points cleaned separately. After cleaning the catheter, the patient should wash his hands thoroughly with soap and running water. His finger nails should be cut short.

For the night, urinals other than the condom type should be discontinued and replaced by a suitable container. Glass or metal bottles with hard unprotected top rings should be avoided and replaced by containers of light plastic material to prevent pressure sores.

DRAINAGE BAG

All that has been said about the care of the urinal also applies to the drainage bag connected with the indwelling catheter. The urinal commonly used for this purpose was the G.U. supra-pubic bag but in recent years more and more plastic bags either disposable or supplied with a tap which can be opened to drain the urinal are used, which have the advantage that one can see the condition of the urine especially the degree of sediment and mucus, and as this bag is marked one can measure the amount of urine drained at different times. Whether this equipment or other types of containers are used, a closed drainage system between the catheter and the drainage bag has to be established, both during the day and the night, by attaching the catheter to the nozzle of the rubber urinal or plastic container or by means of sterile glass and tube connections with a Winchester which does not represent a closed drainage system and following sterilization should contain some antiseptic fluid. If the male paraplegic with an indwelling catheter is lying in bed and the catheter is connected with the urinal or Winchester the connecting tube should never be placed back between the legs to drain behind the patient because of the danger of producing damage to the urethra, but the catheter should be placed forward and upwards from the end of the penis.

As pointed out earlier, no satisfactory urinals for female paraplegics have yet been found, and it is even more important to restore bladder continence in these patients by early training. It is our experience that this has proved more satisfactory than in the male. Those females who, because of their particular bladder dysfunction (dys-co-ordinated spastic automatic bladder), cannot achieve this have to be satisfied with regular changing of soft absorbant pads unless trials with Vincent's technique are made first (see p. 401) which, as pointed out, has the risk of developing pressure sores in complete lesions. Keane of the Spinal Unit in Dublin developed a suction device, called Urovac, which prevents continuous incontinence in bed-ridden female patients with progressed multiple sclerosis by electrically controlled suction. This apparatus can be fixed to several patients in the ward and through a common tube the urine is sucked out into a large container outside the ward to prevent offensive odour. However, for female paraplegics who are able to move about in their wheelchairs this device has so far not proved successful.

3. Reconditioning of bladder function by training—self-care

The paralysed patient should be made fully aware and in detail of his bladder dysfunction by the medical and nursing staff, and this should start as early as possible during the intermediate stages to ensure his full co-operation and develop his own responsibility for the control of his bladder dysfunction. As soon as he is catheter-free he must learn to correlate the fluid intake with emptying the bladder at regular intervals according to bladder capacity and presence or absence of infection. The amount of fluid intake varies between 3–6 pints within 24 hours, and in the presence of bacteriuria—i.e. non-active urinary infection—he will have to drink 5–6 pints of fluid to flush the kidneys and ureters and prevent stagnation in the urinary tract by more frequent micturition. Moreover, the pH should be tested and the urine should be kept acid by taking acidifyers regularly. The times at which fluid is taken has to be arranged in accordance with daily life activities and the bladder emptying routine. Paraplegics who are at work, sports meetings, or travelling abroad should take a bottle of fluid (water, fruit drinks, tea) with them to continue their routine. During pyelitic attacks, in addition to a course of antibiotic treatment the fluid intake has to be increased, if necessary by intravenous drip. In complete, upper motor neuron lesions, especially above T5, the patient must learn to appreciate the importance of certain sensations as indication of bladder distension, such as tightness at the level of the lesion, vague ascending sensation, hot flushes in face and/or upper chest, head fullness, headaches, sweating or goose skin. Therefore, he has also to be acquainted with certain 'trigger' mechanisms such as coughing, straining deep breath and rhythmic tapping of the suprapubic area, rubbing the inner side of the thighs or the glans penis or peri-or intra-anal digital stimulation to set reflexly into action the emptying mechanism of the bladder. Egede Blahn (1970) compared suprapubic rhythmic manual pressure (SRMP), carried out by optimum technique, i.e. using pointed pressure with the apex of the fingers instead of flatly applied pressure with the palm or volar plan of the fingers and other 'trigger' mechanisms. Measuring intravesical and abdominal pressure electromanometrically he found that SRMP setting up a stretch reflex of the bladder evoked reflex micturition more effectively than other trigger mechanisms. The efficiency increases with the duration and speed of SRMP.

In lower lesions of the spinal cord and cauda equina the strengthening of the abdominal muscles by systematic exercises, starting while the patient is still confined to bed, are essential for developing to a maximum the power of abdominal pressure to ensure satisfactory micturition with the least amount of residual urine. All this can also be achieved in children with both upper and lower motor neuron lesions, if the training of the child is started early, and the adopted habit of micturition is continued at home under the supervision of the parents, especially the mother.

Jousse *et al.* (1964) also stressed the importance of training female paraplegics to control their bladder dysfunctions and outlined a programme of training. Fifty per cent of 80 cases with complete lesions and 80 per cent of 103 incomplete lesions regained mastery of useful bladder control.

4. Continuous drainage by indwelling catheter in later stages

The number of paraplegics and tetraplegics who need permanent continuous drainage by indwelling catheter has certainly decreased in recent years as a result of the advances made in the initial management of the paralysed bladder. However, there are still those who, because of a particular dysfunction of their urinary tracts, need this form of urinary drainage either permanently or temporarily for varying periods during the intermediate and late stages following cord and cauda equina lesions. Therefore, it is essential to instruct the patient as well as his attendant at home, before his discharge from hospital, in the basic principles and techniques of bladder care with an indwelling catheter.

The most popular type of indwelling catheter today is the Foley type for urethral and also for suprapubic drainage in those few patients, where, from rare reasons mentioned earlier, the latter form of bladder drainage is indicated. A good deal of research has been carried out both by medical staff and manufacturers to improve the original rubber type of Foley catheter, and in recent years it has been replaced by plastic material which is infinitely less harmful to the urethra than that made from rubber. In particular, urethritis and allergic reactions are less seen with the plastic material. However, faults still occur with the balloon as described earlier in the book and the ideal indwelling catheter for long-term drainage is not yet developed. The small side-tube for distending the balloon with sterile water or saline is occluded either with a special spiggot, with the fluid injected under pressure by an adaptor fitted to the syringe, or by a rubber stopper already fixed to the tube. In the latter case, the fluid to distend the balloon has to be introduced through a small needle which perforates the rubber stopper. Catheters are used in various sizes but, as a rule, no larger sizes than 14 or 16 F gauge should be used in the male. In the female with wide urethra, it is sometimes necessary to use a larger size. The balloon should not be larger than 5 cm^3 but again in women a larger size may be necessary. For suprapubic drainage, the balloon should not be distended more than with 3 cm^3.

The frequency of changing the indwelling catheter is of great importance. The custom, unfortunately still widely used, to leave the catheter in for 1–2 weeks or even longer as a routine is deprecated as this inevitably leads to complications, in particular collection of mucus, stone formation and damage to the mucosa of bladder and urethra. It is our practice to change the catheter at first every other day and later 2–3 times a week, and this has proved very beneficial to the patient. The exception, leaving the catheter connected with a closed drainage system longer than 3 days, will be discussed later.

Catheterization at home, self-catheterization

Once the patient is at home, he can be provided with a sterilization set, rubber gloves and catheters from his District Medical Officer of Health, and his catheter is usually changed by the District Nurse unless he is able to carry out the catheterization himself with scrupulously aseptic precautions, helped by a member of his family. At Stoke Mandeville, we have trained certain paraplegics, being discharged with an indwelling catheter, in self-catheterization. He (and his attendant at home) are specially trained in the principle and technique of changing the catheter, and from all our experience gained it can be concluded that this has proved more satisfactory than the catheterization carried out by a medical practitioner or district nurse who are not familiar with this type of patient or are too busy to carry this out regularly. Even women can carry out self-catheterization efficiently, and I have watched one of my female patients performing this procedure who sustained a complete transverse lesion below T6 in 1943. She has done this for many years most skilfully, using a mirror placed in front of her legs which are spread apart. Autoclaved disposable catheterization sets including disposable catheters of the kind as shown in Fig. 158 have recently been manufactured, and although this has increased the cost, it greatly facilitates self-catheterization and is undoubtedly more safe and less time-consuming.

CATHETER BLOCKAGE

Patients with indwelling catheter must also be made aware of the symptoms resulting from bladder distension (see p. 336) following blockage of their catheter due to kinking, mucus, stones or due to failure to empty the bag or Winchester. Immediate steps must be taken to relieve the blockage, which is of particular importance in cases with reflux into the upper urinary tract or in high cord lesions.

5. Measures of controlling infection

(a) Mechanical procedures

BLADDER WASHOUTS

In cases with indwelling urethral or suprapubic catheters, irrigation of the bladder should be carried out at least once a day, especially in the morning. Bladder washouts should be done with a syringe rather than with a funnel as the pressure used by the syringe facilitates the cleaning of the bottom of the bladder, in particular in crenated bladders with diverticulosis. However, care must be taken not to distend the bladder in order to avoid autonomic hyperreflexia. In this connection, it may be noted that Riddoch (1917) mentioned in his classical paper, that one of his patients complained about 'head fullness' during bladder washout, which was the instigation to my own research on the effects of bladder distension on the cardio-vascular system. It is also useful to turn the patient during the washout from the supine into semi-lateral position, which will facilitate the removal of mucus and sediment. The fluid used for bladder washouts should be tepid (85–90°F). The solutions recommended for irrigating bladder with alkaline urine are 0·5 per cent acetic acid, 4 per cent boric acid, Zephiron 1 : 1000 or flavozole 1 : 2000. When the urine is acid, normal saline or potassium permanganate 1 : 2000 is recommended. If pyocyanea infection of the urine is prevalent, washouts with phenoxetol sol. 2·4 per cent, followed by saline, used for 2–3 days, proved effective. In cases with phosphatic deposits, we have used Suby's solutions G and M (Suby, Suby & Albright, 1942) which like Renacidin sol. 10 per cent (as recommended by Mulvaney et al., 1960 and Bors & Comarr, 1971) has proved useful in dissolving gravel and bladder stones of small size. However, caution is suggested with the use of renacidin for bladder irrigation in the presence of reflux, as acute damage to the kidney may occur. The efficiency of these irrigations is increased by frequent changes in the solutions employed with a view to producing changes in the pH of the urine.

Tidal drainage has also been used for bladder irrigation in later stages of paraplegia, but it is of use only if it is understood by all concerned including the patient. We have used it in suitable cases only during the day under proper control and found it in such cases very useful in cleansing the bladder from sediment, mucus and even small stones. Other authors who also still use tidal drainage in selected cases, are Talbot (1963) and Ascoli (1968). The reason why this method has been given up by many workers, is the difficulty in assessing accurately the height of the tidal drainage loop in accordance with bladder dysfunction. Also the drip rate of the fluid has to be controlled.

In all patients with continuous catheter drainage, fluid intake or large quantities (3–6 pints) is even more important than in catheter-free patients to avoid stagnation in the upper urinary tract.

There is no doubt that, in the majority of paraplegics and tetraplegics who, because of their particular bladder dysfunction in later stages, need long-term continuous drainage by indwelling catheter, this regime of mechanical procedures has proved beneficial in keeping the bladder and upper urinary tract infection at a low grade. Moreover, in catheter-free patients who, due to infection or, in the case of a sterile bladder, as a result of changes in the co-ordination of the emptying and closing reflex mechanisms, develop complications of the upper urinary tract, temporary indwelling catheter drainage in combination with bladder washouts and increased fluid intake, can prevent further deterioration of the bladder dysfunction and preserve the integrity and function of the renal parenchyma. The efficiency of these procedures can be greatly increased by the employment of acidifyers, chemical drugs and antibiotics.

(b) Antibacterial agents (acidifyers, chemotherapeutics, antibiotics)

Before the introduction of the sulphonamides and antibiotics, acidifyers such as hexamine, mandelic acid, acid sodium phosphate, ammonium benzoate and ammonium chlorate were the favourite drugs to combat infection of the urinary tract. Of these, hexamine (10 g three times daily) certainly has an inhibitory effect on bacterial growth by liberating formaldehyde in acid urine with a pH of 4–5. In pyelitic attacks, I found previously intravenous injections of 5 cm³ cylotropin (hexamine, sodium salicylate and caffeine) once or twice daily effective. However, prolonged treatment had the disadvantage, like Urotropine (the trade-mark of hexamine) by mouth, in causing haematuria. Ammonium benzoate and, in particular, ammonium chlorate are now seldom used because of their adverse gastro-intestinal effects. Ascorbic acid (1 g 3–4 times daily), introduced by Donald & Murphy (1959) without the combination of chemotherapeutic drugs, has not proved effective. In series of cases, throughout the years, we tried various combinations of acidifying agents, amongst them a combination of hexamine and hippuric acid to potentiate the acidifying effect, but this combination did not prove successful. However, the combination of methionine (Kass & Sossen, 1959) and hexamine-mandelate, manufactured as G500 (see p. 349), has proved an effective acidifyer of urine, but it cannot prevent alkalinity in severe infection with B. proteus because of its hydrolysing effect of urea into ammonia. Moreover, some patients are hypersensitive to the unpleasant taste and smell of methionine on prolonged treatment.

Of all the chemotherapeutic antibacterial agents, Furadantin (nitrofurantoin) has proved very effective against Gram-positive and Gram-negative organisms, and it acts well with acidification by G500. The doses prescribed are: 50–75 mg for adults and 5–10 mg for children four times a day during or immediately after meals, and this is given for eight to ten days or even longer in special cases, but should not be continued for more than 19 days. In cases where a course of antibiotics does not clear the urine, it is very worth while to start a short course of Furadantin and the urine may become crystal clear. During my weekly consultant visits to the Duchess of Gloucester House, the hostel for paraplegics, who are employed in the surrounding industries, I always inspect the urines of the residents and on occasions a short Furadantin course of 6–8 days is prescribed, if a urine is found to be cloudy and containing mucus and sediment in a resident, who is known to have recurrent though sub-clinical urinary infections, and within a few days the urine becomes crystal clear. Side effects of Furadantin are, as a rule, insignificant and consist mainly of a sickly feeling. A few patients who are allergic to the drug may develop raised temperature with lung involvement. Moreover, polyneuropathy was observed in patients who had been treated with doses of 200–400 mg daily for longer periods (Spencer, 1962; Rubinstein, 1962).

With the discoveries of Sulphanilamide and its many derivatives and, in particular, the antibiotics, a new era in the treatment of the infection of the urinary tract began and our facilities for a more specific treatment of the various types of micro-organisms have vastly increased. Of the sulphonamides, sulphadiazine and sulphamezathine proved in pyelitis more suitable than the less soluble sulphathiazole. A well tolerated and readily soluble sulphonamide is gantrisin (sulphonamide-isoxasole, Hoffmann-La Roche) which neither crystallizes nor has harmful effects on the renale tubules. Whereas the sulphonamides were used in the treatment of both Gram-positive and Gram-negative organisms, with the introduction of penicillin for wider clinical use during the war, attempts were made to treat urinary infections with penicillin. Since 1944, I treated acute urinary infections with three hourly intramuscular injections of 30–50,000 units of penicillin up to a total of 3,000,000 units and found it effective not only against Gram-positive organisms but also against atypical coli of the paracolon group. With the discovery of streptomycin and broad spectrum antibiotics as well as nitrofurantoin (furadantin), penicillin became somewhat forgotten in the treatment of urinary infections. However, in the late 1950s resistance of Gram-negative organisms became more and more apparent at Stoke Mandeville. Milner (1963) of the Pathology Department, in identifying separately members of the Paracolon group, showed that most of the organisms previously called Paracolon bacilli were Providence and most of the strains of Providence were resistant to the antibiotics available at that time. My colleagues Colley & Frankel (1964) carried out systematic studies on 32 paraplegic patients with Providence urinary infections. Of the 30 strains of Providence, the majority (23) were isolated as biotype 21 and 7 were of biotype 27. The sensitivity of these Providence strains was determined against the following antibiotics: pencillin (Penicillin G), ampicillin (Penbritin), methicillin (Celbenin), cloxacillin (Orbenin), phenothicillin (Broxil), propicillin (Brocillin), tetracycline, streptomycin, nitrofurantoin, colymycin, trimethoprim and kanamycin. Nearly all strains were sensitive to penicillin and ampicillin, all strains were sensitive to kanamycin and trimethroprim but only few were sensitive to the other antibiotics. Pencillin G was found very effective in the treatment of Providence urinary infection. Of the 32 patients treated with Penicillin G 1,000,000 units 6 hourly for 6 to 10 days, Providence was eliminated in 30 patients but it recurred in 5 patients after 4 weeks. Two of these patients were treated again and in one the Providence was eliminated and the urine remained sterile for $2\frac{1}{2}$ years, in the other patient the Providence infection recurred three times after penicillin treatment. Although further experiences at Stoke Mandeville have shown that Providence strains as any other strains may become resistant against any antibiotic including Penicillin G, these studies on the beneficial effect of Penicillin G in the treatment of certain acute and subacute urinary infections are worthwhile remembering. Colley & Frankel also refer to one patient who had been unsuccessfully treated with Furadantin, tetracycline and streptomycin for a chronic Providence infection and who was cured of this infection while having treatment with Penicillin for a superficial boil. His urine remained sterile for three years. It may also be mentioned that Penicillin was also successfully used in the treatment of Proteus septicaemia (Hutchinson & Randall, 1947; Holloway & Scott, 1956). Bors & Comarr (1971) in assessing the frequency of micro-organisms encountered in 489 urine cultures on 33 spinal cord injury patients, found the following to be the most frequent: *Proteus mirabilis* (21·8 per cent), *Proteus Rettgeri* 17·2 per cent, *Pseudomonas* 14·7 per cent, *Aerobacter aerogenes* 13·2 per cent and *Escherichia coli* 11·8 per cent and Paracolon-Providence 6·5 per cent. This would correspond more or less—allowing variations in frequency within these groups—to the experience of most workers in this field.

The many brands of new antibiotics developed in the last 10–15 years have given the clinicians a great choice in the treatment of urinary infection, although none has proved a universal remedy for the various groups of Gram-negative organisms. One of the most popular antibiotics used is still the tetracycline group (Terramycine) which, however, as any other antibiotic, should not be used routinely but should be reserved for active bladder infection as evidenced by a bacterial count of more than 100,000 ml and increased number of white or red cells, and especially in pyelitic attacks. There is no doubt that pyuria is clinically more significant and therefore more indicative for immediate action than bacteriuria.

When streptomycin became available, we carried out systematic studies on the effect of this antibiotic on mono- and pluribacterial urinary infections in paraplegics with various types of bladder paralysis (Guttmann, 1953). In accordance with previous investigators (Petroff & Fricas, 1946; Pulaski, 1946) we found streptomycin effective, especially in those cases who were catheter-free or did not require regular catheterization. Administrations of streptomycin in pyelitic attacks, both in catheter-free patients and those still under suprapubic or urethral drainage, resulted in dramatic clinical improvement, with prompt disappearance of septic effects, decrease of leucocytosis and improvement of renal function. The antibacterial effect of streptomycin was also seen in cases with very long standing urinary infection, as found in the few survivors (mainly incomplete lesions) from the 1914–18 World War.

The routine course of streptomycin treatment, as used at Stoke Mandeville in an acute infection of pyelo-nephritic type, was as follows: Intramuscular injections were at first given at three-hourly intervals, the first three doses being 0·8 g each, followed by three doses of 0·5 and this was followed by doses of 0·2 g, to a total amount of 8 g, in special cases up to 10 g. No adverse toxic effects of any significance were observed in the great majority of patients during and after the treatment described. Some patients would only complain of paraesthesia in fingers and a sensation of tightness in the face, especially around the mouth, lasting one or two days. In a few cases, slight dizziness for a day or two was observed, especially when the patient changed his position. Some patients with raised blood urea felt very sleepy during the first day which induced us to reduce the amount of the first high doses. Two tetraplegics who had previously had a course of streptomycin without any adverse reactions developed allergic attacks to local streptomycin application to their pressure sores. One patient developed some deafness.

With this regime applied to the first 100 patients with closed bladders, immediate sterility of urine was achieved in over 50 per cent. However, only 16 per cent remained sterile after four up to seventeen months. In certain cases with pluri-bacterial infections or those who became re-infected, a second or third course carried out at various periods succeeded in eliminating these organisms. In one case, the urine was infected with proteus Morgagni and staphylococcus pyogenes. The first course of streptomycin (7·9 g) eliminated the proteus but not the staphylococcus, although the latter was found to be sensitive to streptomycin but resistant to penicillin. Nevertheless, it was eliminated by a course of 10 million units of penicillin. The urine became re-infected with B. coli but became sterile after a second course of streptomycin (10 g) and it was found to be still sterile after 6 months.

Although dissociations were repeatedly found between the therapeutic effect and the sensitivity of organisms to streptomycin, the therapeutic effect of this antibiotic on the patient's clinical condition is unquestionable. A frequent voluntary statement of patients as a result of the streptomycin treatment was 'I feel much better in myself, less tired, not so hazy, more energetic'—in other words they were less toxic. The antibacterial effect of streptomycin increases as the alkaline reaction of the urine becomes stronger (Abraham & Duthie, 1946), and, therefore, we have used Potass. citr. in doses of 30 to 60 g three times daily during the treatment to ensure a pH of 7 or more in cases without raised blood urea.

Unfavourable conditions for the elimination of infection by any antibiotic treatment are marked trabeculation and diverticula formation of the bladder, continuous urethral or suprapubic drainage, obstruction of the upper urinary tract by calculosis and undrained abscesses. The two latter complications, naturally, have to be dealt with first surgically, but a course with antibiotics may at least prevent general septicaemia.

In spite of the ever increasing number of new antibiotics we still use streptomycin as a most valuable agent against urinary tract infections, the more so as its price has considerably decreased in view of the many rival products.

COMPLICATIONS OF THE URINARY TRACT AND THEIR MANAGEMENT

A. FISTULAE AND DIVERTICULA

(1) Suprapubic fistulae

Breakdown of a suprapubic scar resulting in a urinary fistula was found to be not an infrequent occurrence in our war-time patients (Guttmann, 1953). This complication occurred particularly in patients with long-standing suprapubic drainage, in whom the suprapubic tract was allowed to close spontaneously but it also followed surgical closure. Actually break-down of the suprapubic tract may occur many years after spontaneous or surgical closure. We found not infrequently that a breakdown of the scar and the development of an abscess followed by a fistula could be avoided if, as soon as the patient noticed the slightest sign of a swelling or inflammation of the scar, diversion of the urinary stream by a temporary indwelling urethral catheter was introduced immediately and combined with bladder washouts and treatment with sulphonamides and antibiotics. If this procedure proved unsuccessful, excision of the whole fibrous track and resuture became necessary using either fine steel wire or braided nylon rather than catgut as suture material, as being less likely to cause reactions. However, the best prevention of this complication is discontinuation of suprapubic drainage at the earliest possible date, and our best results were achieved in those paraplegics in whom this was possible after controlling the bladder infection.

(2) Urethral fistulae and diverticula

The most frequent site of urethral fistulae is undoubtedly the peno-scrotal junction produced by an indwelling catheter, especially if it is of larger size and left *in situ* for 7 days or longer, as shown in Fig. 167. This results in a pressure lesion of the posterior urethra followed by a peri-urethral abscess which eventually breaks through the scrotal skin or urethra at the peno-scrotal junction, as shown in Fig. 167. Griffiths & Walsh (1961) reported 31 urethral fistulae found in 2,060 (1·5 per cent) male paraplegic patients

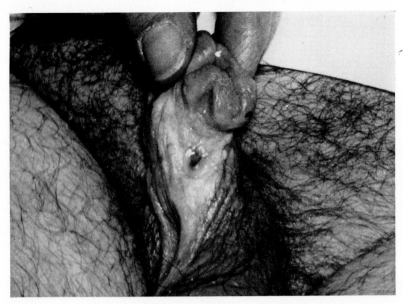

FIG. 167.

admitted to Stoke Mandeville over a period of 16 years, 16 of which were caused by long-standing indwelling Foley catheters. During that period only 2 patients developed urethral fistulae whilst at Stoke Mandeville, although the majority of the 2,060 at some time had been treated by an indwelling catheter which, however, was invariably changed three times a week by a skilled medical officer. Moreover, in this connection, it may be again referred to our report (Guttmann & Frankel, 1966) on 476 acute traumatic para-plegics and tetraplegics who were treated over an eleven-year period by intermittent catheterization using the non-touch technique. Not a single urethral, peno-scrotal or vesico-vaginal fistula occurred in spite of the many thousand intermittent catheterizations which were carried out during that long period.

The incidence of peno-scrotal fistulae has been frequently reported in the literature of other authors. Comarr & Bors (1951) found 43 (7 per cent) fistulae among 619 patients and recently (1971) 445 (21 per cent) peno-scrotal lesions among 2,074 patients, Bunts (1958) found 10·6 per cent fistulae in 1,000 patients. One of the reasons for the high percentage of peno-scrotal fistulae found in certain Spinal Units is most probably the fact that they receive their spinal cord injuries mainly, if not entirely, at later stages follow-ing injury after inadequate management elsewhere, where catheterization in the acute and early stages had been left to unskilled medical and, in particular, paramedical staff.

In one patient a vesico-urethral fistula occurred following extensive transurethral resection which healed by urinary diversion through an indwelling urethral catheter.

Fistulae may also occur due to external causes. They may develop in the perineal area or in the urethra, either at or distally from the peno-scrotal junction. Perineal fistula which invariably follows urethrostomy may, as mentioned earlier, lead to disastrous consequences, especially if associated with pressure sores, as shown in the case of a boy with a spina bifida, as shown in Fig. 168, and this method is now generally condemned.

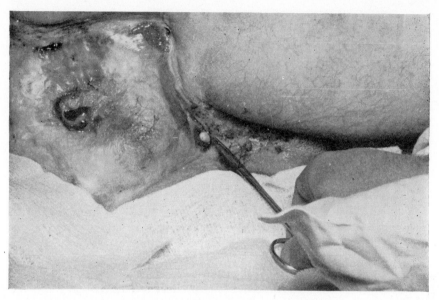

F IG. 168.

External urethral fistulae also develop as a result of pressure from rubber glass urinals, condoms, penis clamps, the latter used by some surgeons for preventing incontinence, and by faulty position of the patient in bed. In patients with pressure sores over the sacrum who have to be nursed in prone position, great care has to be taken to ensure that the penoscrotal area is free from pressure by being positioned in the gap between the adjacent pillow—or sorbo rubber packs.

One patient admitted during the war to the Centre, with extensive pressure sores and suprapubic drainage, had a vesico-rectal fistula which healed spontaneously, and in 2 patients vesico-rectal fistulae developed as a result of penetrating cancer of the bladder. Both died. One female patient developed a vesico-vaginal fistula which healed spontaneously.

Treatment

The treatment of urethral fistulae consists in combined conservative and surgical procedures. Actually fistulae, especially those in the bulbous urethrae, may heal spontaneously.

Success of the surgical treatment depends largely on the condition of the fistula, i.e. whether the fistula is associated with a stricture or not. Griffiths & Walsh (1961) described eleven cases of urethral fistulae without an associated stricture, and all healed eventually although two and even three surgical closures were necessary. However, in eight of these patients excision of the fistulous track resulted in development of a diverticulum. Various surgical techniques have been described in the literature for the closure of fistulae associated with strictures but not a single one has proved to be reliable for all cases. In one of the patients, described by Griffiths & Walsh, Donovan, urologist in Birmingham, successfully closed the fistula and at the same time opened the large urethral stricture with bougies and carried out a split-skin inlay. The fistula recurred a year later and eventually healed after 4 surgical attempts. In a case operated in two stages by Griffiths, using the Denis Browne technique, the fistula closed but reopened later, and in due course a moderate-sized diverticulum developed. Of 4 other cases of fistula and stricture at the peno-scrotal junction who were operated upon, 2 were failures due to recurrence of the urethral stricture. These difficulties with the surgical repair of fistulae associated with urethral stricture were also encountered by other workers in this field. Diversion of the urinary flow by suprapubic drainage in these cases does not, as a rule, guarantee a successful primary closure of a fistula as this diversional procedure does not prevent detrusor action and thus voiding through the urethra occurs, and in the experience of Griffiths & Walsh, Comarr (1959), Bors & Comarr (1971) and others, repeated trials were necessary to close the fistula. Therefore this diversionary procedure, let alone that by perineal urethrostomy, has been abandoned.

The key to the solution of this difficult problem is prevention and there cannot be any doubt that with the adoption of a meticulous technique of urethral catheterization as proved by the non-touch technique, the incidence of urethral fistulae will profoundly decline.

(3) Urethral diverticula

Urethral diverticula which are of different shape and size are not infrequent results of long-standing indwelling catheter drainage, especially with larger size of catheters (Fig. 169), but may also develop as a result of a stone lodged in the urethra (Fig. 170). Diverticula can be easily demonstrated by urethrography. The incidence of this complication varies with different authors. Comarr & Bors (1951) reported 61 (50 per cent)

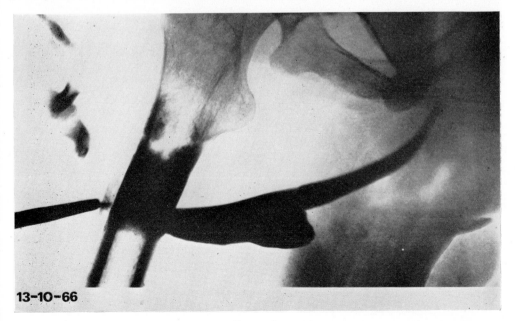

13-10-66

FIG. 169.

diverticula amongst 122 patients, Bunts (1958) found 4·6 per cent in 1,000 patients and Griffiths & Walsh (1961) found 19 (9·5 per cent) diverticula in routine urethrograms on 200 patients.

Treatment

With regard to treatment of urethral diverticula it was always our practice to leave a small diverticulum untreated unless it increases in size, accumulating infected urine and debris and thus becoming a permanent source of maintaining infection. Griffiths & Walsh considered the inversion or invagination of the sac into the urethra, as recommended in the American literature, as undesirable, as this procedure results in urethral obstruction with all its complications. Before contemplating excision of a diverticulum of larger size the patient is instructed how to evacuate the sac by digital compression after micturition, to prevent stagnation of urine, and this can be associated with urethral washouts. Large, especially multiloculated urethral diverticula and those resulting in a fistula, naturally need surgical treatment.

Bors & Comarr (1955–58) reported perineal urethral diverticula as a result of complete ischiectomies including the pubic ramus and damage to the urogenital ramus, an operation carried out for repair of pressure sores. We have not seen that serious complication in our material, as we consider such radical procedure unnecessary.

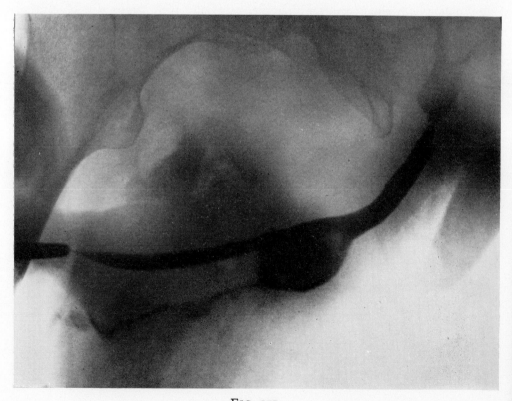

FIG. 170.

(4) Stone-formation

There are two main factors causing formation and growth of stones in the upper urinary tract following spinal cord injuries:

a   Infection, especially with urea splitting organisms producing alkaline urine, which favours precipitation of calcium phosphate, ammonium magnesium phosphate and calcium carbonate, and

b   Hypercalciuria resulting from decalcification of bones, caused by enforced bedrest and recumbency leading to stagnation of the urine flow. The nucleus of a stone may be formed primarily within the renal tissue or the so-called Randall's plaque (Randall, 1937), in the basement membrane of a tubule or beneath the epithelium of the renal papilla, and from there it finds its way into a renal calyx. On the other hand, a stone may develop in the urinary passages as a result of precipitation of salts or as a result of infection resulting in tiny semi-solid lumps of coagulated fluid or dead epithelium. Nordin et al. (1967) distinguish between two main types of renal stones according to whether, (1) in addition to calcium phosphate, they contain either calcium oxalate, associated with increased excretion of calcium or oxalate or both, and (2) magnesium ammonium phosphate (MAP) which is associated with chronic infection of the urinary tract. There is no doubt that in our material stones removed from paraplegics are of MAP type.

In the development of bladder stones, foreign bodies, in particular fragments of the tip of catheter or the burst balloon of a Foley catheter, hair, wire or thread suture following closure of a suprapubic fistula, may be contributory factors. Moreover, small renal stones transferred through the ureter into the bladder or posterior urethra can grow considerably in size through phosphatic sediment if not removed in time. In my monograph (1953), the X-rays of a case of traumatic paraplegia below T11/12 with suprapubic drainage were described showing two stones in the bladder and one in the posterior urethra. A urethrogram following the removal of the stones demonstrated a large diverticulum resulting from the stone at the peno-scrotal junction. Fig. 171 shows a collection of the various types and sizes of stones encountered throughout the years at Stoke Mandeville. Special attention is drawn to the two large bladder stones, one lying on top of the other like millstones, found in a paraplegic woman and successfully removed by Dr Walsh. It is interesting to note that these overriding stones caused grinding noises in the patient's lower abdominal region, but when the patient reported hearing these noises, she was promptly treated with tranquillizers! (This case who later became pregnant has been described on page 192.)

Stones in paraplegic patients consist of phosphates and carbonates of calcium, magnesium and ammonium. Their chemical properties have been studied in detail, in particular by Mulvaney (1964) and recently by Burr (1972), the biochemist of Stoke Mandeville Spinal Centre. He employed for the analysis of stones the electron microprobe method used by geologists to examine rock samples, and Figs. 172, 173 show a section of a ureteric stone and the tracings obtained by this section for calcium, magnesium and phosphorus. Of particular interest is the part marked with an arrow in the tracings at which the calcium concentration falls almost to zero but the magnesium concentration is so high that the tracing is off the scale, while there is no apparent change in the phos-

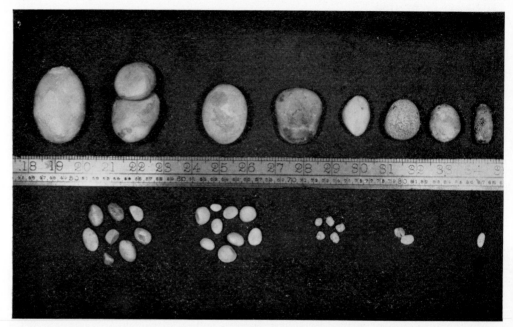

Fig. 171.

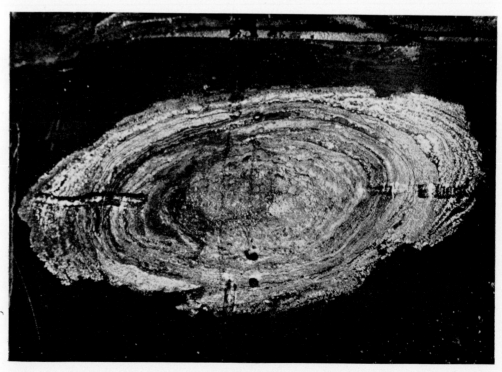

Fig. 172.

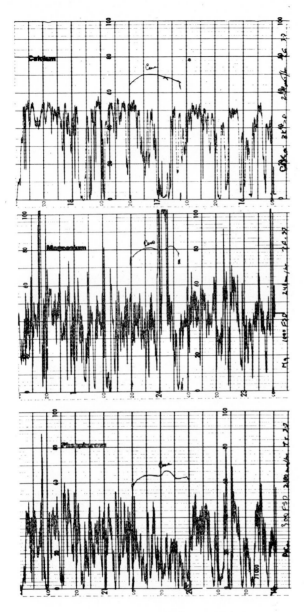

FIG. 173.

phorus concentration. Although the original stone nucleus in a few paraplegic patients may be urate, oxalate and even cystine, the secondary stone consists of calcium phosphate in the great majority of cases. Amongst our paraplegics, there was one patient who, before his paraplegia, had an oxalate stone, and when he developed a larger stone following his spinal injury the stone nucleus was oxalate.

The incidence of calculosis following spinal cord injuries has been repeatedly reported in the literature, and from the statistics published in this country, Canada and U.S.A.

TABLE 20

Author	No. patients	Percentage
Comarr (1955)	1,104	6·8
Damanski & Gibbon (1956)	116	14·7
Bunts (1959)	1,000	5·7
Comarr *et al.* (1962)	1,507	8·2
Guttmann & Frankel (1966)	476 (treated with intermittent catheterization) (Admitted within 14 days of injury most of them within 48 hr)	0·43 ⎰ 1·7 (renal) ⎱ 0·6 (bladder)
Bors & Comarr (1968)	2,322	10·9

during and in the early years after the Second World War, which were compiled in my monograph of 1953, the incidence of calculosis varied between 20–68·7 per cent. My own statistic of 351 traumatic paraplegics from the Second World War revealed a calculosis of 22·5 per cent. In the great majority of these patients, the initial treatment had been suprapubic cystostomy. The considerable improvement made ever since in the management of paraplegics and tetraplegics resulting in prevention of calculosis, is best shown in statistics published on a larger number of patients during the last 15 years or so, as shown in Table 20.

Comarr (1955) and Damanski (1962) found renal calculi to be more frequent in patients with lower motor neuron lesions and also they form more frequently in patients with complete than with incomplete transverse lesions (Prather, 1947; Bunts, 1959). Age and long bone fractures are also factors in raising the incidence of calculosis (Rossier & Bors, 1965). Moreover, according to Bors (1951) and Comarr *et al.* (1962), renal stones are more prevalent on the right than on the left side in both traumatic paraplegia and polyomyelitis.

Treatment

In discussing the treatment of calculosis, preventive measures should be mentioned first. The most important of all these measures in spinal cord injuries is, of course, the prevention of infection. As shown, this is best achieved by intermittent catheterization as described earlier in this book, and by transfer of these patients to a Spinal Injuries Centre immediately or within the first few days after injury. At least as important is the prevention of stasis of the urine flow due to enforced bed rest and recumbency. The prevention of crystallization of calcium salts in the kidneys during the stage of hypercalciuria in the early weeks after paraplegia by a large fluid intake in correlation to the number of catheterizations and keeping the urine acid, is also essential. The regular turning of the patient from the start day *and* night is as essential for the prevention of stone formation as it is for the prevention of bed sores. When lying in supine position, the patient, unless he has fractures of the ribs or a haemothorax, should be encouraged to carry out exercises with a chest expander which increases the blood flow and facilitates the blood circulation also in the paralysed part of the body. Needless to say, the sooner the paraplegic and tetraplegic can be raised from the horizontal to the upright position and be transferred to a wheelchair the better.

Once stones are formed, even small ones, they have little tendency to disappear when the patient is able to get up, nor can they be dissolved quickly by agents such as solution G or M (Suby, Suby & Albright, 1942) or Renacedin. If patients are admitted in later stages with bladder or renal stones of larger size, surgical removal as early as possible is indicated, as without their removal there is no hope of controlling the infection of the urinary tract.

Vesical calculi of small or medium size should be crushed under direct vision whenever possible, and many stones can then be washed out by irrigation. Greatest care and gentleness should be exercised in carrying out this operation. Violent suction of the debris following litholapaxy must be avoided at all cost, as this could result in greater damage, including rupturing, the already damaged bladder wall or, especially in lesions above T5, in profound autonomic hyperreflexia, in particular of the cardio-vascular system. Large bladder stones are best removed suprapubically.

Ureteral stones should be reduced by solutions G or M or in certain instances by Renacidin so that their extraction by manipulation of the ureteral cather or by a loop becomes possible. If the ureter stone has caused blockage of urine flow and an acute hydro- or pyonephrosis has developed, attempts may be successful to push the stone up into the pelvis and release first the pressure from the kidney which is followed by washouts of pelvis and calyces through the ureteral catheter, which could then be left *in situ* for 24 hours for drainage and for further irrigation. This procedure has proved most effective in bringing down the raised temperature (as a rule of swinging type), which the patient may have had for several days before admission. If a pyelitic attack does not respond to an appropriate course of antibiotic treatment with temperature returning to normal within three or four days, or a rise of temperature recurs after a few days, blockage in the upper urinary tract by a stone or other cause may be suspected and the patient should be re-admitted to a spinal unit without delay, which might be a life saving measure. Blockage of a ureter or pelvis by a stone will produce not only a pyonephrosis but generalized septicaemia if immediate surgical relief is not carried out. Silver & Martindale (1970) described a case of septicaemia as a result of a calculus in the left proximal ureter producing blockage and hydronephrosis of the left kidney. Blood cultures grew the same organisms, proteus and B aerogenes, as found in the urine.

The management of renal stones is in the great majority of patients surgical. While small quiescent stones in the upper or lower calyces may be left alone and watched for some time, pelvic stones should be removed at an early date by pyelostomy. There is now general agreement amongst urologists and spinal specialists that nephrectomy for calculosis should be avoided in paraplegics and tetraplegics as long as possible, and that renal stones of large size including stag-horn type can be removed by nephrostomy.

It may not always be possible, for one reason or another, to remove completely multiple or stag-horn type renal stones, and the instillation of dissolving solution through nephrostomy, pyelostomy or ureterostomy tubes may be necessary, unless, as in the case of a residual stone or stones in the lower calyces, an amputation of the lower renal pole is preferred at a later date. However, great care has to be taken regarding the time of onset, the number of drops employed and the duration of these dissolving solutions. At Stoke Mandeville, we have given preference to Suby's solution G and M but have also used Renacidin, first used by Mulvaney (1959–64). It may be noted that several fatalities were reported in the literature following the use of Renacidin (Auerbach *et al.*, 1963; Fostvedt & Barnes, 1963), and as a result the manufacturers of Renacidin withdrew the drug from the market. In one of our patients—a complete paraplegia below T5 who was suffering from hydronephrosis and calculosis in the left kidney—a nephrostomy was carried out and 12 days after the operation a Renacidin instillation through the nephrostomy tube was started. However, one day after this treatment the patient developed haemorrhagic urine and an acute renal failure. He was immediately transferred to the renal unit of Princess Mary's R.A.F. Hospital, Halton, for haemodialysis, where he gradually recovered after some stormy weeks. Two months after the onset of the acute renal failure, he was discharged from the Spinal Injuries Centre and returned to his job three months later. However, in due course he died on account of progressive renal deficiency from which he was already suffering before the operation. Scibutis *et al.* (1962) also reported bleeding and raised temperature during irrigation by Renacidin and also found it disappointing in its use for bladder stones. It does not replace clean surgery but may be indicated for patients who previously had operations and for whom additional surgery of the kidneys would be hazardous. Bors & Comarr (1971), who considered the 5 fatalities reported following Renacidin treatment to be a result of faulty technique rather than the drug itself, are still in favour of this therapy for dissolving renal stones and during 1965 and 1967 succeeded in achieving complete dissolution in 30 out of 47 patients; in 11 patients the size of the stone was either reduced or further growth arrested, 3 patients did not tolerate the treatment and 3 patients had stag-horn stones too old and too large for Renacidin therapy. These authors have taken special precautions, such as restricted flow rate, never exceeding 20 drops per minute, restricted flow duration of Renacidin of 1 hour alternating with saline 3, 2 or 1 hour respectively depending on the patient's tolerance, furthermore by using a Fr.N 4 or 5 urethral catheter as inflow channel and as outflow channel a plastic catheter of minimum Fr.N 6. Moreover, if the patient shows malaise, nausea or bloodstained fluid with either Renacidin or saline instillation, this is at once stopped but is resumed after at least 24 hours of freedom from symptoms. In spite of these precautions, I feel one should be very circumspect in the use of Renacidin in patients with raised blood urea and other signs of renal deficiency combined with calculosis.

(5) Vesico-ureteric reflux

Changes of the hydrodynamics in bladder and ureter leading to vesico-ureteric reflux have been of increasing interest during the last 15 years to nephrologists, spinal specialists and urologists alike. Kjellberg *et al.* (1957) reported 37 per cent of reflux in a large series of non-paraplegic children with urinary tract infection without demonstrable obstructive lesion. Rosenheim (1963) and his team of co-workers found reflux in 76 per cent out of 55 non-paraplegic patients with radiological evidence of chronic pyelonephritis, and over a period of 4 years 23 (64 per cent) out of 36 of his patients with apparent primary chronic pyelonephritis had vesico-ureteric reflux.

The main cause of reflux in spinal cord lesions is the disorganization of the reciprocal vesico-ureteric function as a result of ascending infection. It is generally agreed that the lower portion of the ureter is particularly vulnerable to ascending infection from the bladder and also to increased vesical pressure. As the intravesical section of the ureter with its longitudinal muscle fibres plays an essential part in the prevention of back flow of urine from the bladder, bacterial invasion of this region may easily lead to impairment of the elasticity of the valve-like action of the ureteric orifice and disrupt the reciprocal vesico-ureteric function and its hydrodynamics. Alterations in the juxta-ureteric bladder wall was previously considered by Hutch (1958) as the cause of the development of reflux whether congenital or acquired. Dilatation of the lower segment of the ureter has been described by Talbot & Bunts (1949) as the first sign of a vesico-ureteric reflux, which we confirmed in our own paraplegic patients.

Vesico-ureteric reflux may be transient or permanent. It occurs unilaterally and bilaterally although more often unilaterally, and it may change from one side to another in the course of alterations of the vesical dysfunction (Fig. 174).

The standard method of demonstrating reflux has been cystography which in recent

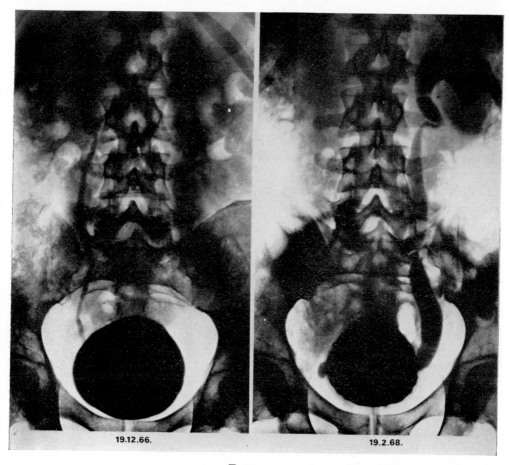

19.12.66.   19.2.68.

FIG. 174.

years has been supplemented or replaced by cinefluoroscopic or radioisotopic techniques (Bitker & Pagnot, 1964). However, from all our experience, cystography still represents an efficient standard method. Smith (1966) compared both methods in 145 children and came to the conclusion that the ciné method yielded only slightly better results than cystography in detecting reflux. The advantage of cinéradiology in the evaluation of reflux is the demonstration of the flow rate and antiperistaltic waves which may affect either part or the whole length of the ureter up to the renal pelvis and calyces. Moreover, this method can be combined with recordings of volume and intravesical pressure. Intravenous pyelography, revealing certain hydrodynamic changes in the urinary tract, not infrequently make detailed cystographic studies necessary. They may show dilated parts of the ureter, saccule formation or constriction in the lower end of the ureter (Cosbie Ross, 1960), either unilaterally or bilaterally, furthermore, tortuosity and kink formation of the middle and upper sections of the ureter.

In 1963, I reported 343 patients with complete or incomplete lesions of the spinal cord in whom 512 cystographic studies had been carried out. Over 300 patients were examined during 1961–63, amongst them 122 in the early stages following injury or disease. In numerous cases cystography was repeated several times.

The standard technique adopted was to have the first X-ray film taken after filling the bladder slowly when the patient was relaxed (resting film). In some cases, a second resting film was taken after 5–10 minutes to ascertain whether reflux had then occurred. This was followed by a film taken during bladder pressure raised by straining either voluntarily or passively, or by provoking reflex detrusor function (micturating film).

Reflux was found in 75 out of the 343 cases (22 per cent). Of these, 221 had upper motor neuron lesions with more or less marked spasticity, and the incidence of reflux was 43 (19 per cent), while 122 cases had lower motor neuron lesions with flaccidity, and amongst these 32 (26 per cent) had reflux. These findings confirmed previous views (Guttmann, 1953) that there was no evidence to assume a particular neurogenic lesion of the ureter as a direct aetiological factor of reflux, as far as type, degree and level of the cord lesion was concerned. This was not in accordance with the view expressed by Bors & Comarr (1955) and Damanski & Gibbon (1960), who considered reflux occurring more frequently in upper motor neuron lesions than in lower motor neuron lesions. Bors suggested as explanation, that the preservation of the sympathetic innervation of the trigone in low-cord lesions may have some protective effect upon the ureteric orifice which accounts for the low incidence of reflux in lower motor neuron lesions. However, there is no proof that cord lesions at and above T5, including cervical lesions, where the whole splanchnic control is crippled, show a higher incidence of reflux than cord lesions below that level. The arbitrary classification of cord lesions described by Damanski & Gibbon, dividing their cases into those above T9, T9–T11 and T11, is not acceptable as a proof of their theory from a neuro-physiological point of view that reflux is prevalent in upper motor neuron lesions. Actually, Bors & Comarr (1971) in a recent statistic of Long Beach V.A. Hospital on 866 patients, in contrast to their data given in 1955, also found, in confirmation of my own observations, a higher percentage of reflux in lower motor neuron lesions (38·6 per cent) than in upper motor neuron lesions (27 per cent). The concept that the cord lesion itself has a direct effect on the incidence of reflux

TABLE 21. Time between injury and first diagnosis of reflux

Time after injury	Reflux
Less than 3 months	2
3 to 6 months	8
Over 6 to 12 months	5
Over 1 to 2 years	3
Over 2 to 3 years	1
Over 3 to 4 years	0
Over 4 to 5 years	1
Over 5 to 6 years	1
Total	21

has led workers in this field to carry out neurosurgical procedures, such as pudental neurectomy, sacral neurectomy, anterior or posterior rhizotomy, or intrathecal alcohol block. However, from the results described it cannot be concluded that these operations had any therapeutic effect on the reflux.

It is worthwhile mentioning that of my 122 patients who had a cystogram within the first 12 months following paraplegia and tetraplegia 34 had a sterile urine and there was no reflux. Of the 85 patients with infected urine only two had reflux. Moreover, it may be remembered (see page 381) that the incidence of vesico-ureteric reflux of the 476 patients admitted to Stoke Mandeville immediately or within the early days after injury and treated with intermittent catheterization was only 4·4 per cent (21 patients), 15 had unilateral and 6 bilateral reflux (Guttmann & Frankel, 1966). All these patients had been infected before the cystogram at which reflux was demonstrated, and in 6 of them the reflux was associated with hydronephrosis. Table 21 demonstrates the lapse of time between cord injury and first diagnosis of the reflux.

These findings show contrary to my previous observations described in 1963, that reflux can, in fact, develop already in the early months in the presence of bladder dysfunction as a result of ascending infection of the vesico-ureteric junction and the ureter itself, associated with alterations of shape and size of the bladder. Although reflux may occur in bladders of any shape or capacity, this was found particularly as a result of long standing suprapubic or urethral drainage, leading to fibrous contracture of the bladder (Fig. 161).

Treatment

The treatment of vesico-ureteric reflux is still a matter of discussion. It can be divided into conservative and surgical procedures. From all the experiences gained it can be concluded that there is no procedure employed for the treatment of this complication which has proved consistently or permanently successful. This applies in particular to the various anti-reflux surgical procedures advocated, be they corrective procedures at the vesico-ureteric junction such as introduced by Hutch (1952, 1963), Politano & Leadbetter (1958), Bischoff (1962), Winter (1966), or neurosurgical procedures such as posterior or anterior rhizotomies (Brendler *et al.*, 1953), sacral nerves neurectomy

(Scheibert, 1954), resection of the nerves at the vesico-ureteric junction (Bors, 1955; Ivatsu, 1961), intrathecal alcohol block or urinary diversions such as cutaneous ureterostomy, ileal conduit (Bricker, 1950) or colonic loop. Recently Cashion & Moeller (1975) made a study of sacral rhizotomies carried out over 20 years to reduce ureteral reflux and came to the conclusion that this procedure is not indicated. Walsh (1967) reported about our experience in 10 patients with ileal conduits most of them done elsewhere. None was free of troubles, the commonest one being skin trouble. One patient who had an ileal conduit done at Stoke Mandeville Centre died afterwards from ileus and peritonitis, another with an ileal conduit done elsewhere, a man of 67, had to be operated upon be-

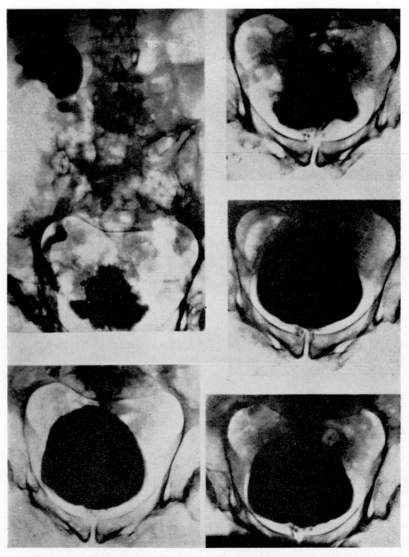

FIG. 175. From 21st Congress of German Society of Urology (1965, Springer, Berlin) page 112.

cause of bowel obstruction due to adhesions around the operated site. There is by no means general agreement amongst urologists themselves as to the most suitable method of urinary diversion. Cosbie Ross (1967) considered diversion of urine by ileal loop to be indicated only in stage III of ureteric reflux with progressive renal deterioration. Alternatively, he recommended a segregated colonic loop, especially when only the left kidney was functioning. In favour of this operation he considered the fact that a prolonged dissection of the mesocolon was unnecessary, furthermore the anastomosis between the iliac colon and upper rectum gave less rise to the development of postoperative ileus than following ileal loop diversion. However, he condemned uretereo-colonic anastomosis in the presence of associated defects in the control of defaecation. Retief & Key (1967) in accordance with observations of Cibert *et al.* (1958), Pelot & Voestlin (1961), Pelot (1963), Vernet *et al.* (1960) and Truc *et al.* (1962), preferred in their few cases of urinary diversion (6 out of 210 cases) a colonic conduit because of its better tone as compared with the ileal loop.

Since 1944 we have pursued a conservative approach to the management of vesico-ureteric reflux, in particular in grades I and II—i.e. light and moderate degrees of reflux without or with light or moderate dilatation of the upper urinary tract. For, reflux may disappear by proper bladder training—i.e. correlation of fluid intake and voiding at regular intervals and combating infection. Hardy (1963) described patients who had reflux for many years, amongst them one patient with reflux of 17 years duration, without harmful effects. He has also seen bilateral reflux occurring and recurring and resolving itself. What can be achieved by conservative treatment, even in cases with highly contracted, deformed and trabeculated bladder following long-standing urethral drainage with dilatation of the kidney and tortuous ureter, is demonstrated in one of our patients followed up for several years. Fig. 175 shows the disappearance of the reflux and remarkable improvement of the bladder almost to its normal size and shape. If reflux is the result of obstruction at the bladder neck TUR is the treatment of choice.

In cases with reflux of grade III—i.e. gross dilatation of the ureter with kink formation at any level leading to blockage of urine flow and resulting in hydronephrosis and renal deficiency, ureterolysis was found to be beneficial in restoring or improving the hydrodynamics of the urinary tract (Guttmann, 1953).

Urinary diversions have been carried out in the form of cutaneous ureterostomy, nephrostomy and ileal loop operation in only a few and very selected cases suffering from progressive reflux, frequent pyelonephritic attacks and renal deterioration. The advantage of cutaneous ureterostomy is the avoidance of the potential complications of laparatomy. In particular, it allows renal catheterization and the urine is free of mucus.

Our conservative approach is in accordance with that of other specialists in this field, such as Hardy (1963), Bors & Comarr (1967, 1971), Talbot (1967), Tarabulcy, Morales & Sullivan (1967) and others. Tarabulcy, Morales & Sullivan (1967) reviewed the successes and failures of various forms of management of reflux in a group with acquired and another with congenital reflux. The follow up of patients in both groups was between two and five years. The methods of treatment evaluated were:

1 scheduled voiding 2–3 hourly,
2 continuous bladder drainage,

3 TUR of vesical neck,
4 anti-reflux procedures,
5 ileal conduit.

Of all these procedures the most satisfactory results were achieved by scheduled voiding and urethral catheter drainage.

Amongst the neuro-surgical procedures intrathecal alcohol block was recommended for ameliorating certain types of reflux (Maury *et al.*, 1963). My own experience in this respect since 1946 is, that, while it is true that in some cases of contracted and disco-ordinated automatic bladders reflux may disappear following alcohol block, in others it appeared after the block. This procedure is not indicated for the treatment of reflux *per se* but to transform complete transverse lesions with intractable spasticity of skeletal muscles, including uninhibited detrusor dysfunction into lower motor neuron lesions.

Results on pudendal nerve anaesthesia and resection to eliminate obstruction due to spasticity of external urethral sphincter have been reported by Bors *et al.* (1950, 1954) and Cosbie Ross & Damanski (1953). While the effect of anaesthesia after novocaine or xylocaine is uncertain and in any case only temporary, bilateral resection of pudendal nerve will result not only in relaxation of the external sphincter but also paralysis of the pelvic floor muscles, elimination of the bulbo-cavernosus and anal reflexes. It also abolishes erection and emission. Therefore, one will have to think twice whether this procedure is justified to eliminate spasticity of the external urethral sphincter in view of the more suitable method of removing the obstruction by resection of the external sphincter. Moreover, the scars as a result of the operation in the ischial area may facilitate the development of pressure sores.

(6) Hydronephrosis—pyonephrosis—retroperitoneal fibrosis

Non-obstructive hydronephrosis following spinal cord injuries above the thoraco-lumbar junction may be caused by neurogenic spasms of muscle fibres of the pelvi-ureteric junction or calyces. Just as early infection of the bladder may elicit detrusor spasms once the heightened reflex-activity of the isolated cord has developed, so may spasms of the pelvi-ureteric junction and/or calyces be caused by early ascending infection, resulting in alteration of the normal rhythm of relaxation and contraction between the calyces system and pelvi-ureteric junction. Under normal circumstances, the calyces eject their contents into the renal pelvis which in turn empties itself into the ureter. Disturbances of the emptying mechanism at the pelvi-ureteric junction, due to obstruction, will result in stagnation of urine in the pelvis resulting in, what is called, pelviectasis or pelvic type of hydronephrosis. In these cases, the I.V.P. will show dilatation of the renal pelvis, while the calyces may be of normal shape and size.

However, if the pelvis is intrarenal, its capacity for enlargement is limited and a calyceal type of hydronephrosis will predominate. In the majority of our cases, the hydronephrosis commenced in the calyces system, as revealed by dilatation of individual or all calyces varying in size from clubbing to 'cannon-ball' deformity. In the great majority, hydronephrosis following spinal cord lesions, except where caused by congenital defects and abnormalities, is the result of obstruction which may occur within any section

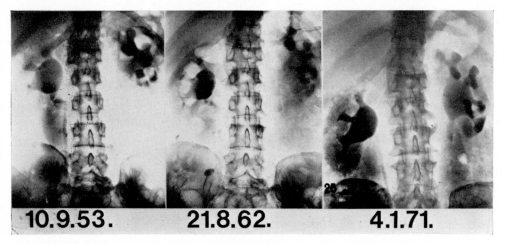

FIG. 176.

of the urinary tract. Hydrodynamic dysfunction resulting from structural alteration in urethra, bladder or ureter, may develop without infection of the urinary tract. However, the main cause of hydronephrosis is ascending infection from the bladder which could be prevented by proper management from the start as reported earlier.

Attention has been drawn in my monograph of 1953 to the development of hydronephrosis caused by periureteritis and panureteritis setting up inflammatory adhesions between the various segments of the ureter—mainly the lower and upper ones—and the surrounding tissues, resulting in ureter-kinking in coronal and sagittal directions and in certain cases producing strictures of the ureter. While there is no doubt that the primary cause of retroperitoneal fibrosis in spinal paraplegics is the ascending infection of the urinary tract, it would be of interest to examine whether in these patients abuse of analgesic drugs such as phenacetin, codein-phosphate and paractanol play an additional cause, as postulated recently by Lewis *et al.* (1975) in non-paraplegic patients. Patients, admitted with long-standing infection, have shown grotesque forms of hydroureter and hydronephrosis, and one wondered, sometimes, how it was possible not only to survive but even lead an active and useful life with such renal pathology for so many years. In this connection, the following case is indeed an instructive example:

On 25 August 1953 a man, aged 38 years, was admitted, who on 27 October 1943 had sustained a fracture-dislocation of T12/L1, resulting in an incomplete transverse spinal cord syndrome below T11 with only partial motor paralysis of the distal muscles of the left foot and analgesia from T11–L3 on the left and S4/5 on the right, dribbling incontinence and a residual urine of 8 oz but being able to pass 20 oz of urine by expression. The urine was infected with *B. proteus*, and an I.V.P. revealed a bilateral hydronephrosis with a very large dilatation of the right pelvis and a kink of the right ureter at the ureteropelvic junction (Fig. 176). Unfortunately, there was no record of any I.V.P. done elsewhere. He was treated with antibiotics and courses of Pituitrin, without effect on the hydronephrosis by the latter (from the natural history of this patient it would appear that, at the age of 4, he had had some kidney trouble which was called a chill). During regular check-ups in the following years, the urine was found to be sterile, B.P. and blood urea were always normal, but there was no change in the bilateral hydronephrosis. When, in 1962, there was some deterioration in his condition and he was absent from work (employed as a civil servant) for the first time in 10 years, the blood urea was found to be raised (51 mg per cent) and he showed a residual urine of 7 oz with a bladder capacity of 16 oz, and cystography showed some diverticulosis of the bladder. On 8 June 1962, a TUR round the clock was carried out (Dr Walsh) which reduced the residual urine to 1·5 oz; in due course, the blood urea became normal again (24–32 mg per cent), and the urine became temporarily sterile, but he needed courses of antibiotics from time to time followed by G500 to acidify the urine. I.V.P. two months after bladder neck resection showed only slight improvement of the hydronephrosis (Fig. 176), but subsequent I.V.P.s did not show any change in the large hydronephrosis, as shown by the I.V.P. of 4 January 1971 (Fig. 176). Blood urea 35 mg per cent, sugar and electrolytes normal, urine sterile, BP 135/90, the pulse 54, blood count normal. He is now working full time at Headquarters of the Department of Social Security.

This case shows how a large hydronephrotic kidney can adjust itself for many years to the metabolic needs of the organism and maintain its metabolic homeothesis.

Treatment

Bloch, in 1923, recommended ureterolysis as treatment for hydronephrosis, resulting from panureteric fibrotic adhesions for non-paraplegic patients. I advocated this procedure for our paralysed patients in the early years of our work, and it has been carried out successfully by Mr Griffiths and Dr Walsh ever since. It was found possible to free the kinked ureter from its dense adhesions and to straighten it out by combining in certain cases the ureterolysis with a nephropaxy. In the case of a very elongated ureter as a result of kink formations, it may be necessary to alter the course of the ureter by fixing it to the psoas fascia outside the peritoneum.

In cases with non-obstructive type of hydronephrosis, Yates-Bell (1949, 1953) recommended a course of fresh Pituitrin consisting of 0·5 cm³ intramuscularly every day for 2 weeks, 0·5 cm³ on alternative days for 2 weeks and a maintenance dose of 0·5 cm³ once a week for 6 weeks. This treatment is based on the stimulating effect of Pituitrin on the ureter eliciting rhythmic contractions, as described by Tona (1928, 1936). We have confirmed the beneficial effect of this treatment in a few selected cases of unilateral hydronephrosis with normal blood urea (Guttmann, 1949). Fig. 177 shows the cystograms of a traumatic paraplegic below T4 before and after Pituitrin treatment. After daily intramuscular injections of 0·5 cm³ of Pituitrin for 18 days there was a marked improvement of the gross hydroureter and hydronephrosis, and 42 days after completion of Pituitrin treatment the cystogram and I.V.P. showed practically normal ureter and kidney. In another case (cauda equina L4), in which Pituitrin also had profound beneficial effect on the hydronephrosis, there was a recurrence when the treatment was discontinued. However, a further course of treatment had again a prompt effect which was maintained with a dosage of 1 cm³ Pituitrin every three days. Some patients were hypersensitive to 1 cm³ Pituitrin and developed diarrhoea—therefore it is safer to use o·5 cm³. Bell rightly pointed out, that there will be no benefit from this treatment in cases with large residual urine, long standing fibrotic hydroureter and obstruction at the uretero-pelvic junction, which is in accordance with our experience.

If hydronephrosis, especially a bilateral one, progresses, causing symptoms of renal deficiency, further steps have to be taken to eliminate obstruction and ensure free urine flow and at the same time combat infection, as outlined earlier in this book by the various methods of diversion.

It has been pointed out earlier (page 399) that any urinary diversion procedure in spinal cord sufferers is rarely indicated and should be reserved for highly selected cases. In this connection, Susset's paper (1966) on 'Hydronephrosis and Hydroureter in Ileal Conduit Urinary Diversion' may be quoted. This paper is of importance and should be

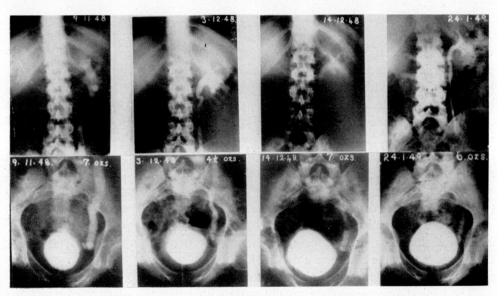

FIG. 177.

quoted in some detail, as the author adopted a rather 'dynamic' surgical approach and his indications for this operation are open to criticism. During the years between 1957–64, 138 patients were subjected to cutaneous uretero-ileostomy. Of these patients, only 78 (representing 155 ureters), who had had preoperative and postoperative pyelograms were included in his report. Forty-one patients had a meningomyelocele and 29 were 'various paraplegics', amongst them 18 adults. It was unfortunate that the author in his statistics did not specify the results obtained in the meningocele and 'various paraplegics' groups. The dilatation of ureters and kidneys were classified as follows:

I   ureters mildly dilated in lower portion mainly without obvious hydronephrosis;
II   mild hydronephrosis with early blunting of calyces;
III marked hydronephrosis with calyceal dilatation;
IV   very large dilatation affecting pelves and calyces with obvious parenchymal atrophy;
V   very large, bag-like hydronephrosis with little parenchyma left, and very poor concentration of opaque media.

From his results, Susset himself came to the conclusion that the ileal urinary diversion cannot be considered as a procedure of choice when the upper urinary tract is normal, actually 42 per cent of normal ureters showed some degree of dilatation following operation. The same consideration also applies to patients with mild dilatation (29 per cent were made worse). On the other hand, he considered this operation as the procedure of choice when the ureter was decidedly dilated, although there was an improvement in severe dilatation in only 44 per cent (no details given regarding degree and duration of the improvement) and 32 per cent remained unchanged. One can hardly imagine that any spinal specialist could ever agree with the views expressed in this paper, as far as patients with spinal cord lesions are concerned. Actually in the discussion following this paper, Dr Bors and Dr Comarr expressed their criticism.

Pyonephrosis

Unilateral or bilateral pyonephrosis developing in the terminal stages of chronic pyelone-phritis, particularly if associated with amyloidosis, is not an unusual *post-mortem* finding. However, the incidence of acute pyonephrosis due to obstruction of the ureter or pelvis by stones or panureteric stricture has greatly declined during the last 20 years, as a result of the advances made in the treatment of spinal cord injuries. In our series, reported earlier of 476 paraplegics and tetraplegics treated by intermittent catheterization in the initial and early stages of bladder paralysis, there was not a single case of this most serious complication. Walsh (1970) reported an incidence of pyonephrosis in 39 out of 3,458 patients (1·13 per cent), admitted to Stoke Mandeville over a period of 17 years (1950–67), and since that statistic only 2 further cases have been seen in the last 4 years.

In 23 out of 32 patients operated upon by Walsh himself, stones were found to be the cause of obstruction; in 12 of these, they were associated with stricture or periureteric fibrosis; in 7 cases the cause was a ureteric kink due to intramural as well as periureteric fibrosis; in 2 cases the cause of obstruction was not confirmed.

The clinical symptomatology usually starts with a pyrexial attack from which the patient does not recover promptly in spite of antibiotic treatment; although the initially high temperature may subside and may even be subnormal, the patient remains listless, loses appetite, feels 'liverish' and appears ill. There may or may not be increased leuco-cytosis, depending on the effectiveness of antibiotic treatment, but persistent leucocytosis over 10,000–12,000 may be important for the diagnosis. Blood urea may not be greatly increased. Lowering of haemoglobin under 70–65 per cent and red cells under $3\frac{1}{2}$ millions may be an important sign of general toxaemia in cases with long-standing obstruction. An immediate straight X-ray may be of great diagnostic value in detecting stones as the cause of obstruction, and in cases without greatly increased blood urea an I.V.P. may clarify the site of the ureteric obstruction.

The first case of obstructive pyonephrosis due to ureteric stones, admitted to the Centre in 1944 within the first 3 weeks after its opening, was a soldier who was blown up by a mine on 4 May 1943 and sustained a complete conus–cauda equina lesion below L2/3. This case may be recorded in some detail, as it led to our very selective approach to nephrectomy, which hitherto had been the conventional treatment of pyonephrosis.

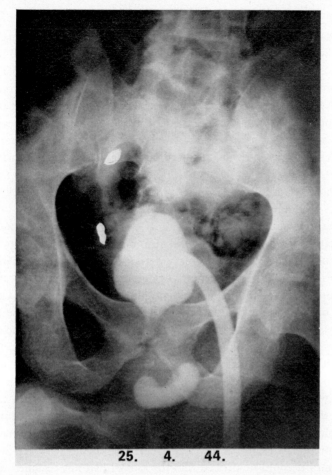

25. 4. 44.

FIG. 178a.

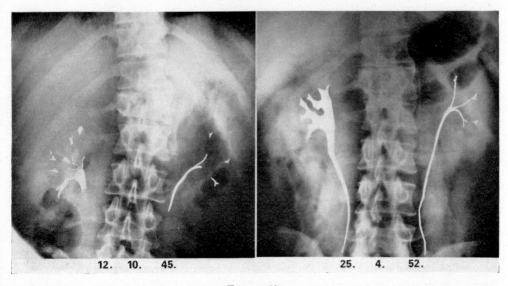

12. 10. 45.   25. 4. 52.

FIG. 178b.

This man had had a suprapubic drainage since the day of injury, and he developed several pyelitic attacks with high temperatures before admission. He was nursed for 6 months on plaster beds elsewhere, and, apart from ascending infection of the urinary tract, he also developed pressure sores. The bacteriological examination of the urine showed only *Esch. coli*, but swabs taken from the catheter end (Malecot) within the bladder showed heavy growth of *proteus, Staph. pyogenes* and *B. haemolytic* streptococci. The bladder was treated by tidal drainage through the suprapubic catheter, and at first great amounts of mucus and debris were removed. The plaster bed was, of course, discarded immediately after admission.

Two months after admission, he developed another pyelitic attack with rigor and vomiting, which did not respond to treatment. There was pain in the right upper abdominal region spreading to the back associated with tenderness. Hgb. 93 per cent, leucocytosis of 22,000, temperature 101° rising to 104° but subsiding within the next 3 days. An X-ray showed two stones in the right ureter (Fig. 178a). A cystoscopy performed by Mr Riches (later Sir Eric Riches), the first urological consultant to the Centre, revealed, in addition to a great amount of dirty granulations hanging like grapes around the catheter beneath the suprapubic opening in the bladder, a complete obstruction of the right ureter at 10 cm (upper calculus), and thick pus came from the ureteric catheter. On immediate exploration, the right ureter was found to be grossly thickened and intensely hyperaemic, and the right kidney was extremely congested and greatly enlarged. The ureter above the upper stone near the pelvis was incised, the stone removed and the distal stone milked up and removed through the same opening. A catheter passed up to the kidney drained copious thick pus, and the kidney was thoroughly washed out with saline. Although this was a classical example of a pyonephrotic kidney, which at that time would have been a clear indication for immediate nephrectomy, Mr Riches agreed, albeit reluctantly, to postpone the operation until it could be proved that the kidney had not regained its function and remained the main source of infection. It may be noted that the renal pus showed some of the bacteria, especially *B. haemolytic* streptococci, as found previously in the suprapubic catheter specimen. The decision to refrain from nephrectomy in this paraplegic was guided by the consideration that, in all probability, the left upper urinary tract was also infected.

Actually, this man's condition improved dramatically after the operation. The right kidney regained its function, and subsequent I.V.P.s showed practically normal outlines and good secretion of both kidneys (Fig. 178b). The suprapubic drainage was discontinued in October 1945 ($2\frac{1}{2}$ years after injury) after he had developed good detrusor action and the bladder had become automatic, and, in due course, the urine became sterile. He made an excellent rehabilitation and became a member of the first wheelchair polo and basketball teams, and while still an in-patient started work in a factory in Aylesbury with 6 other paraplegics. After his discharge from hospital he was employed full time for many years in open industry, living as a resident at our Hostel for employable paraplegics, the Duchess of Gloucester House in Isleworth, London. In 1954, he developed vascular hypertension, resulting, in due course, in considerable cardiac and aortic changes, including a temporary left cerebral thrombosis and some sclerotic retinal changes, which forced him in 1959–60 to give up full-time employment. Until that time, regular check-ups showed sterile urine and blood urea varying between 23 and 38 mg per cent. With increase of the hypertensive disease, he developed nephrosclerosis and eventually renal failure and died on 21 August 1961 at the age of 50, 18 years after injury.

Of the 32 patients reported by Walsh (1970), one died 5 weeks after operation due to perforation and haemorrhage of an acute gastric ulcer, probably the result of steroid treatment. In 3 cases, nephrectomy was carried out at a later date, following the initial operation (nephrostomy or T-tube in the ureter), when it was proved that the kidney had not regained function and remained highly infected. One of these, a woman, had apparently been obstructed for several months and, when first drained, the pus was sterile. The second case had a perinephric abscess involving the bowel and he had been obstructed for 28 days. The third case had a periureteric abscess and had been obstructed for 21 days. In all the remaining 28 cases, the affected kidney resumed excretion of urine within 24 hours and some within 3 hours. The degree of function varied according to the degree of impaired renal function before the pyonephrosis. In 21 cases, I.V.P.s before and after the operation were available; of these, 7 cases showed normal findings before and after; in 7 cases the previous impairment remained unchanged, and in 7 there was deterioration of renal function—i.e. increased hydronephrosis or impaired dye concentration. The period between operation and last I.V.P. varied from 2 months to 15 years. Ten of the 21 cases showed satisfactory renal function more than 5 years later.

From all these observations, it can be concluded that immediate nephrectomy in paraplegics and tetraplegics is very rarely, if ever, justified.

(7) Diagnosis and management of acute and chronic renal failure

Reference has been made earlier in this book to the serum protein changes following the acute and later stages of spinal cord injuries. The clinical symptoms of renal deficiency are oliguria, anaemia, derangement in the ratio between blood and urine osmolality and disturbances in the urine sodium and potassium concentrations. Tubular damage leading to irreversible tubular necrosis is the detrimental result, if proper management is not applied as early as possible. Therefore, in view of the therapeutic advances made in recent years, early diagnosis of renal deficiency is vital, and the determination of tubular concentration in the presence of oliguria as well as regular blood pressure readings and, above all, careful and detailed examination of the urinary sediment are of utmost importance. Unfortunately, in spinal cord injuries, the bacterial examination of the urine, important as it is, has become so routine that sometimes the proper evaluation of the urinary sediment is neglected. As is well known, the presence of red cells, particularly red cell casts, is indicative of glomerular damage; granular casts indicate parenchymal renal damage, and the presence of a necrosed papilla may indicate necrotizing papillitis. As pointed out earlier (page 346), increase of protein, white cells and epithelial cells indicates acute inflammation of bladder or ureter, even in the absence of bacteriuria, or may be the precursor of bacterial infection.

Stott *et al.* (1972) have listed the following criteria of established acute renal failure:

Increasing uraemia with a blood urea greater than 150 mg/100 ml

Low urinary urea concentration

Urinary sodium concentration greater than 20 mEq/l

Urine osmolality less than $1\cdot1 \times$ the plasma osmolality

Failure to respond to mannitol in a dose of 300 ml of 20 per cent solution given intravenously.

A high dose intravenous urogram may be helpful, as described by Brown *et al.* (1970), especially where obstructive uropathy is suspected.

Comparative studies on the endogenous creatinine and urea clearances were undertaken at various stages following spinal cord injuries (Doggart, Guttmann & Silver, 1966). Special attention was paid to renal function in the immediate and very early stages of complete traumatic lesions. The creatinine clearance test was found superior to the urea clearance test as a measure of glomerular filtration rate. In the immediate stages, glomerular filtration rate, as indicated by the creatinine clearance test, was found remarkably normal. In contrast, the blood urea level was profoundly raised as a reflection of tissue breakdown. Only in one case (T10 complete), associated with disruption of the pelvis and bilateral haematoma of the groin, was the serum creatinine found to be raised on the first day following injury (2·7 mg per cent); clearance was 73 ml/min, blood urea 83 mg per cent. There was oliguria which, however, improved, and on the second day serum creatinine was 0·9 mg per cent and blood urea 44 mg per cent. The level of the complete lesion was found to have no significant influence on renal function.

Although creatinine clearance is generally considered as the most reliable method of detecting renal damage, it may not be possible to detect very early deterioration of renal function with this method owing to the ability of the kidney to compensate. In recent years, Bernier *et al.* (1968) and Harrison *et al.* (1968) found that B_2-microglobulin—a low molecular globulin fraction, described by Berggård and Bern (1968)—is increased in patients with renal disease proportional to the degree of renal dysfunction. This low molecular weight protein is produced in the body by lymphocytes and its urinary excretion is markedly increased in patients with dysfunction of the renal tubuli which normally catabolize B_2-microglobulin. Therefore, in normal circumstances, B_2-microglobulin is present in only trace amounts in human serum and urine. Recently, Lindan *et al.* (1972) confirmed increased high serum levels and increased urinary excretion and clearance of B_2-microglobulin in 17 out of 25 paraplegics and tetraplegics. From these findings, it would appear that the B_2-microglobulin test is more sensitive as compared with standard renal function tests such as creatinine clearance, X-ray and protein.

Acute renal failure following traumatic shock (crush syndrome)

In acute traumatic paraplegia, acute renal failure can be produced by either severe renal ischaemia (Brun, 1954) or by nephrotoxic substances released from damaged haemoglobin (Shen *et al.*, 1943) and myoglobin (Bywaters, 1944). Oliguria may also result from dehydration due to inadequate fluid replacement, especially after abdominal surgery and in patients suffering from paralytic ileus. The estimation of the urine specific gravity, or, if possible, the urine and plasma osmolality, may be invaluable in the differential diagnosis of oliguria in these circumstances. In the case of dehydration, the urine specific gravity will be above 1020 and the urine osmolality generally above 500 mOsmols/kg and considerably above the plasma osmolality (normally 275–285 mOsmols/kg), whereas in acute tubular necrosis the specific gravity of the urine is 1010 or less and the osmolality not greater than the plasma osmolality. In these patients, hourly urine output to assess the volume and concentration of urine and detect the presence of haem components in addition to blood urea determination is essential. In such a case the insertion of an indwelling catheter, under scrupulous aseptic precautions by a medical officer, is preferable to intermittent catheterization. The determination of the specific gravity of the urine may be misleading if large molecules such as glucose, protein or dextron are present in the urine.

If oliguria is found to be due to dehydration, rapid fluid replacement with dextrose saline is given. A litre or more may be infused in 1 to 2 hours. Measurement of the central venous pressure is helpful in judging the rate of fluid replacement and to prevent circulatory overload, particularly in patients with cardiac embarrassment.

The immediate and early admission of spinal cord injuries to the Spinal Centre in acute renal failure, as a result of general traumatic shock following haemorrhages due to multiple injuries associated with the cord lesion (crush syndrome), has greatly declined in recent years, thanks to a better understanding of the mechanism of this condition in accident and surgical departments, and, particularly, as a result of improved therapeutic facilities provided in the intensive care units of general hospitals. Our routine treatment of traumatic shock, throughout the years, consisted of blood transfusions followed by selective hydration with dextrose–saline to combat ischaemia, hypoxia and haemorrhages associated with the spinal cord injury, and to restore blood volume. With these conservative procedures, supplemented in recent years, if necessary, by mannitol, which has proved renoprotective, renal perfusion and function have improved, thus preventing tubular obstruction by casts. Barry *et al.* (1967) made the following recommendation for mannitol treatment of oliguria:

'1   When detected, oliguria should be treated promptly by immediate infusion of 20 g of hypertonic mannitol during a 5–10 minutes' interval.

'2   If urine flow increases to 40 ml/hr or more during the two hours following mannitol infusion, sustained hydration should be established and intermittent 20 g infusion of mannitol used only as needed to maintain urine flow at 100 ml/hr. Mannitol usually must be considered a temporary measure to protect the kidneys while the basic cause of depressed renal function (e.g. dehydration, hypotension) is being corrected.

'3   If urine flow increases, but to less than 40 ml/hr, the patient should be re-evaluated and, if practical, an acute 500 ml infusion of isotonic saline or dextrose should be administered, followed by a second dose of mannitol.'

These authors wisely suggest some precautions. All oliguric patients should receive the initial trial dose, as there is no way to predict response, but this dose is considered as harmless. However, unless urine volume exceeds 100 ml/hr, under no circumstances should more than 100 g of mannitol be given in 24 hours.

Frusemide may also be used in the diagnosis of acute renal failure. When oliguria is observed, 40 mg frusemide is given intravenously. If in the next hour less than 40 ml of urine is produced, 250 mg frusemide is given. If despite this a diuresis of 60 ml of urine or more is not established in the next two hours, treatment for acute renal failure is instituted.

In the stage of oliguria during traumatic shock, attempts to 'flush out the kidneys' by excessive fluid administration have proved to be wrong, as this may easily lead to circulatory overloading and precipitate pulmonary oedema, especially in upper thoracic and cervical lesions. Since protein catabolism liberates potassium in the body, the amount of dietary protein and electrolytes should be restricted and a carbohydrate diet of 1,000–1,500 calories be given during the stage of oliguria. Gastric suction, which may be necessary in acute dilatation of the stomach and vomiting should be used with care as severe alkalosis may develop. Cantarovich *et al.* (1973) have described the use of high dose frusemide administration in acute renal failure. They recommend giving 2,000 mg in divided doses daily during the oliguric phase, and have shown accelerated recovery of renal function with reduction of the period of oliguria by using this method. If these conservative measures fail and anuria and uraemic symptoms develop, the patient should be immediately transferred to a hospital where haemodialysis or peritoneal dialysis are available, which may constitute a life-saving measure. This happened just recently in one of our traumatic paraplegics, a man aged 23 who, having fallen from a scaffolding (40 ft), sustained in addition to a fracture dislocation of L2 resulting in an initially complete paraplegia below T12/L1, a right Colles fracture, a fracture of right scaphoid, dislocation of right elbow, fracture of right pubic ramus, butterfly haematoma at the perineal region and haematoma of right hip. He was transferred to Stoke Mandeville one day after injury (1 December 1970) severely shocked but conscious (BP 110/80, temp. 97°F). Blood urea rose from 108 to 125 mg per cent, potassium 7·3 mEq/l (he had vomited 200 ml blood-stained fluid, while in the ambulance, and 10 ml blood-stained fluid were aspirated on admission). As intravenous mannitol treatment (20 g in 250 ml saline) did not result in any improvement of the severe oliguria, he was immediately transferred to the Dialysis Unit at the nearby R.A.F. Hospital, Halton, where the blood urea rose on the same day to 145 mg per cent, white cells 15,900. He received altogether 17 dialyses, the last on 11 December 1970. Diuresis started on 11 December 1970, reaching 1L by the 16th and 4L by the 22nd. He was readmitted to Stoke Mandeville on 29 December 1970 with a blood urea of 104 mg per cent which by 18 January 1971 had decreased to 42 mg per cent; potassium and chlorides normal. The patient has made some motor recovery, especially in the right leg and also some sensory recovery.

Mitchell (1965) of the Dialysis Unit at Halton described 5 cases who were previously transferred from our Spinal Centre. Three of them had acute renal failure following traumatic shock and 2 were in acute failure of chronic renal deficiency. Two of the cases with acute renal failure resulting from post-traumatic shock due to multiple injuries may be quoted here from Mitchell's paper.

'Thirty-four year old male (G.S.) was admitted to hospital on 29 July 1962 following an accident in which a tractor toppled over on him. He sustained a fracture of the 11th thoracic vertebra and fractures of the right 12th rib, the transverse processes of the 2nd, 3rd and 4th lumbar vertebrae and the right ulnar styloid process. He had burns of the fingers and right palm. He was transferred to the National Spinal Injuries Centre the

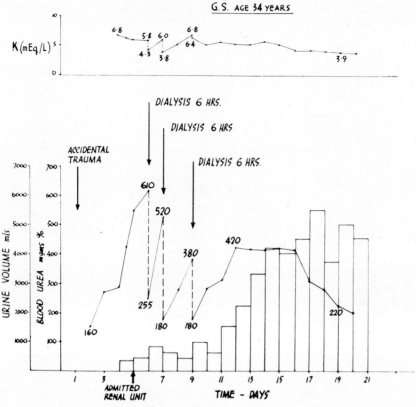

FIG. 179. Chart showing plasma ureas, plasma potassiums and urine volumes of patient G.S. during period of acute renal failure. From Mitchell (1965) *Paraplegia*, **2**, 254.

following day, during which he developed a left hemiplegia. Parietal burr holes showed bruising of the brain but no collection of blood.

'Oliguria had been present since the accident and on 2 August he was admitted to the Renal Unit with a plasma urea of 550 mg per cent and a plasma potassium 6·0 mEq/l. At the beginning of dialysis later the same day the plasma urea was 610 mg per cent and plasma potassium 5·8 mEq/l. Six hours dialysis continuing into the early hours of the morning lowered the plasma urea to 255 mg per cent and the plasma potassium to 4·3 mEq/l. The plasma urea and potassium and the urine volume is illustrated in Fig. 179. Three dialyses with one- and two-day intervals respectively were required to control the biochemical disturbances. Diuresis began on the 11th day and thereafter the blood urea rose more slowly, levelled out then fell spontaneously. He returned to Stoke Mandeville in the diuretic phase on the 20th day of his illness with a plasma urea of 200 per cent.

'The paraplegia remained but after a course of rehabilitation he became independent and was discharged home on 2 June 1963. By November 1963 he was generally well, and noted to have a normal urea clearance and creatinine clearance of 102 ml/min. Persistent urinary infection was a residual problem.'

'A 36 year old male (W.P.) was admitted to hospital on 4 September 1963 following an accident in a mine; a rock fell on to his back. He was severely shocked, had multiple.

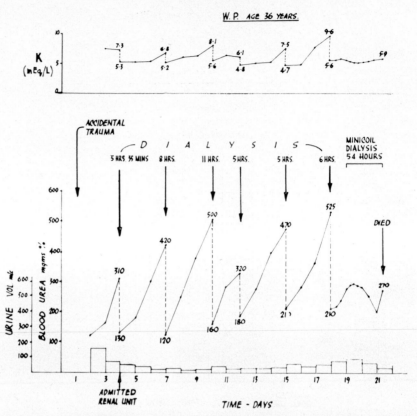

FIG. 180. Chart showing plasma ureas, plasma potassiums and urine volumes of patient W.P. during period of acute renal failure. From Mitchell (1965) *Paraplegia* **2**, 254.

fractures of the ribs and pelvis and a fracture dislocation of the third lumbar vertebra. Because of a T10 paraplegia he was transferred to Stoke Mandeville the next day. He was discovered to have acute renal failure with a rapidly rising blood urea and was admitted to the Renal Unit on 7 September with a plasma urea of 300 mg per cent and potassium of 7·2 mEq/l. Fig. 180 illustrates the progress of the plasma urea and potassium and of the urine output. In spite of five dialyses in 11 days, he developed uraemic changes in his gastrointestinal tract, first manifested by the onset of haematemesis on 19 September. A subsequent dialysis on the Kolff twin-coil artificial kidney was carried out using regional heparinization, but in spite of maintaining the patient's clotting time at normal levels and improving the biochemical changes of uraemia the gastrointestinal bleeding continued. An attempt was made to maintain the biochemical improvement by continuous haemodialysis using a 'Minicoil' (Lawson *et al.*, 1962) and to keep pace with the blood loss by transfusion until it became obvious that the condition was irremediable. The patient died 24 September. Fig. 180 shows plasma ureas, plasma potassiums and urine volumes during dialyses. *Postmortem* examination showed fracture dislocation of the body of the third lumbar vertebra, fractures of the pelvis and of the 8th to 11th ribs and lateral processes of the 2nd and 3rd lumbar vertebrae, extensive haemorrhage into the para-spinous and psoas muscles, diffuse gastroenteritis, pre-pyloric peptic ulcer, bilateral renal tubular necrosis with focal renal cortical necrosis, and necrosis of the lower lumbar cord.'

These observations indicate the great value of dialysis as an early renoprotective and life-saving therapeutic procedure in the immediate stage of spinal cord injuries associated with multiple injuries of the body. Dialysis should be considered if oliguria does not improve within a few hours following blood transfusions and mannitol infusion, and the blood urea shows a tendency to rise. In order to prevent early irreversible damage of renal tissues, it is safer to transfer the patient to the nearest Dialysis Unit before the blood urea has reached the 150–200 mark.

Acute renal failure in chronic renal insufficiency

There is general agreement amongst all workers in the field of spinal cord afflictions that, in spite of the advances made in the treatment of these patients during the last 25 years or so, the prevention or early management of chronic renal deficiency resulting from ascending infection of the urinary tract still leaves much to be desired. Although it is recognized that certain chronic renal diseases carry a worse prognosis than others, ascending infection of the urinary tract, including pyelonephritis, should be considered as one of the potentially reversible causes of renal insufficiency. Long experience in this field has shown, without any doubt, that paraplegics as well as tetraplegics, in spite of chronic infection leading to renal deficiency, not only can remain alive, but indeed lead a life worthwhile living for many years, which only 25 years ago would have seemed impossible.

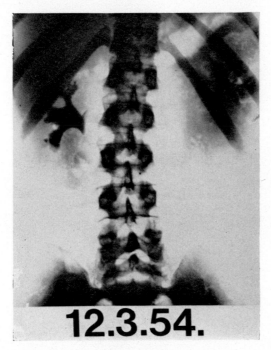

FIG. 181.

Therefore their expectancy for an active and useful life could still be vastly prolonged, if all the modern therapeutic facilities of recent years including dialysis treatment could be employed for them in good time. There is still reluctance amongst some nephrologists in charge of Dialysis Units to give paraplegics suffering from chronic renal deficiency, including those employed, an equal chance for dialysis treatment, including home dialysis, with non-paraplegics suffering from this calamity, on the grounds that it is a hopeless task—a defeatist attitude which prevailed 25 years ago towards the treatment of paraplegics generally. Therefore, consideration should be given to the inclusion of dialysis facilities in the larger Spinal Centres, if there is not a Dialysis Unit in the immediate neighbourhood.

An example of what can be done even in a case of very advanced renal deficiency is shown by the following case:

T.N., now 35 years of age, sustained a fracture dislocation of C5 on 25 June 1953 resulting in an incomplete tetraplegia. He was admitted to Stoke Mandeville from Belfast on 16 February 1954 with marked urinary infection, a stag-horn calculus in the right kidney (Fig. 181) and multiple healed pressure sores. He had a nephrolithotomy in 1954 and made an excellent rehabilitation, and at the time of discharge in December 1954 he was able to walk with the aid of sticks, and took up employment with the British Railway immediately, where he has worked ever since. He married and became the father of two children. In due course he had a recurrence of stones in the right kidney, and an I.V.P. on 1 June 1960 showed an hydronephrosis of the right kidney, while the left had remained normal (Fig. 182a). He had another nephrolithotomy in 1960 but in August 1966, when he

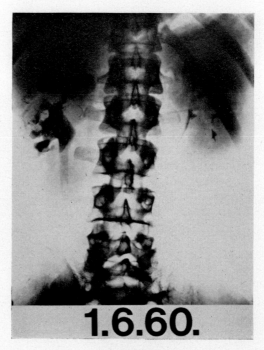

FIG. 182a.

developed a perinephritic abscess and the kidney was found not to be functioning, it was removed by Dr Walsh. The left kidney was functioning well and only showed mild enlargement of calyces, as shown in Fig. 182b. The histological examination of the kidney revealed, apart from multiple abscesses, amyloidosis. Nevertheless he greatly improved, blood urea was within normal limits and the urine became sterile and remained so, apart from one recurrence. In the following years blood urea gradually increased (55 mg per cent in 1969) and he developed in 1969 a nephrotic syndrome with hypertension. During a check up on 13 February 1970, BP was 175/120 but fell later to 140/90. In March 1970 he was admitted as an emergency because of worsening of his nephrotic syndrome. He had rapidly gained over two stones in weight and developed extensive peripheral oedema. Renal function was deteriorating; urinary protein excretion varied between 500 to 2,000 mg per cent, there were some hyaline and granular casts, 10–30 white cells, urine sterile, blood urea 89 mg per cent, sodium 135, potassium 5·3, increasing to 6·6 mEq/l, Hgb. 72 per cent, marked hypoproteinaemia (Alb. 1·1, Glob. 2·6). He was transfused with 2 pints of whole blood on 19 March 1970 and was given Resonium and sodium bicarbonate, and carbohydrate diet was instituted. Rectal biopsy on 16 March 1970 did not show evidence of amyloidosis. On 23 March 1970 he developed a hypertensive attack (BP 230/150), pulse 52 due to autonomic hyperreflexia, which was treated with Ansolysen and temporary indwelling catheter to prevent bladder distension. When, during the following days, the blood urea rose to 129 mg per cent, the anaemia increased (Hgb. 63 per cent) and the oliguria worsened, he was transferred in April to the Dialysis Unit at Halton, where following peritoneal dialysis and removal of oedema fluid his condition

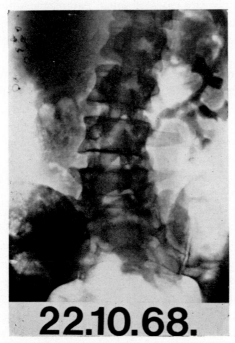

22.10.68.

FIG. 182b.

much improved. As his domicile was in London, he was transferred on 16 May 1970 to
the Dialysis Unit of St Thomas' Hospital under the care of Dr Norman Jones, F.R.C.P.,
where he was accepted following initial peritoneal dialysis for a chronic haemodialysis
programme in view of his excellent adaptation to his illness and his stable and supporting
family background, and home dialysis was arranged. From Dr Jones's report on 6
January 1972 it would appear that the patient carried out his own dialysis well at home.
As he was very eager to have a renal transplant this was carried out in the beginning of
January 1972—the first time in a traumatic tetraplegic—when a good match donor
kidney became available. The operation was successful, and he was discharged home on
11 February 1972. He kept well for several months. However, in early April he started
complaining of backache, and eventually it was found that he had developed abscesses
involving his spine and caused by aspergillosis. It was this disease with its complications
which eventually led to his death on 11 June 1972. The day before he died the blood urea
level was 52 mg per cent and the plasma creatinine 2·1 mg per cent and the kidney
transplant was functioning well right up to the time of death. It is really a tragedy having
regard to the good function of the transplanted kidney that he had to die from aspergillosis. It is hoped that in future paraplegics who need kidney transplantation for renal
deficiency as a result of pyelonephritis will not be excluded from this new treatment.

Renal transplantation has made considerable progress during the last 5 years.
Amongst the criteria quoted for selection of recipients of renal allotransplantation
such as age, failure to respond to good conservative management etc., absence of active
systemic infection is mentioned, and Nolan (1972) postulates that every possible attempt
must be made to suppress infection of the urinary tract before transplantation. Therefore, it is obvious that only rare cases of spinal paraplegia suffering from renal failure
may be eligible for renal transplantation. The selection should be made in the first
place by the medical staff of the Spinal Injuries Centres during the regular check ups
of their patients.

Urine analysis and urine culture as well as detailed blood analysis and diastolic blood
pressure are the key to the diagnosis of early and progressive renal deficiency. Moreover,
positive results of rectal biopsies will ascertain whether chronic renal deficiency is
associated with amyloidosis, although negative rectal biopsies do not exclude renal
amyloidosis, as shown by the histological findings in this case following nephrectomy of the
right kidney.

Multiple factors are often operative in causing deterioration of renal function, and
amongst them occult sepsis from chronic tonsillitis and tooth decay or osteomyelitis
resulting from pressure sores may be mentioned. The importance of proper dental
hygiene and care cannot be overstressed, and patients with early renal deficiency should
have regular dental check-ups and septic teeth should be removed immediately. Toxic
agents are also instrumental in causing acceleration of renal deficiency and indeed acute
renal failure. The case of chronic renal deficiency, who developed acute renal failure,
following Renacidin treatment, mentioned earlier (page 423) is a striking example in this
respect, and the constant use of pain-killing drugs, especially those containing Phenacetin
should also be mentioned in this connection. Products of protein catabolism also have
toxic effects and, therefore, protein intake should be reduced in acute exacerbation of

chronic renal failure, associated with oliguria or anuria, and replaced by carbohydrate diet. The special protein and mineral free diet consisting of glucose, peanut or olive oil and vitamins, introduced by Bull *et al.* (1949, 1953), which we used to prescribe for these patients in previous years, has been abandoned because it was too nauseating even when given by stomach tube.

Mineral metabolism. Particular attention has been paid in recent years to potassium hemostasis and its disturbances in chronic renal failure, whereby protein catabolism and metabolic acidosis play an essential part. Paeslack (1965) found hyperkalaemia in 5 cases and hypokalaemia in 2 cases with progressed renal deficiency amongst 36 paraplegics, in whom detailed investigations of the mineral metabolism had been carried out. Hypokalaemia may result from increased loss of potassium due to diarrhoea, vomiting, anorexia and diuretics, and this may cause adverse cardiac effects (Tucker *et al.*, 1963). In some cases, especially where renal failure is due to chronic pyelonephritis, hypokalaemia may result from failure of renal conservation of potassium and the excretion of large amounts of this ion in the urine. On the other hand, metabolic acidosis may cause hyperkalaemia in oliguric patients with acute renal failure (see page 445).

Treatment consists of control of acidosis by sodium bicarbonate and adequate glucose intake, and in cases of persistent vomiting and diarrhoea, a slow intravenous infusion of dextrose–saline should be given. Resonium-A (Sodium Polystyrene Sulphonate) is indicated in hyperkalaemia associated with severe oliguria or anuria and 15 g should be given 3–4 times daily by mouth in a little water. Resonium should be discontinued as soon as the serum potassium level falls to 5 mEq/l to avoid potassium depletion. Therefore, biochemical control is necessary during treatment.

Anaemia. Anaemia, associated with more or less profound albuminuria, as found in the case described earlier, is one of the classical symptoms of progressive renal deficiency. Anaemia may be obscured in certain cases by haemoconcentration as a result of vomiting, diarrhoea and excessive use of diuretics. Its main causes are: blood loss, particularly due to gastrointestinal haemorrhages, haemolysis associated with severe abnormalities of red blood cells, associated with thrombocytopaenia (haemolytic-uraemic syndrome) and deficiency of the bone marrow, which according to Moor (1957) and Erslev (1967) does not respond with compensatory erythroid hyperplasia in the presence of anaemia. The important researches of Jacobson *et al.* (1957), Erslev (1960, 1967), Naets (1960), Reissmann *et al.* (1960) have shown that hypoxia caused by anaemia will result in stimulating activity of erythropoitin, an erythropoitic hormone in the plasma, which promotes differentiation of bone marrow stem cells to early red cell precursors (Erslev, 1960). These findings have confirmed my views about the importance of the oxygen carrying erythrocytes in preventing tissue hypoxia and, therefore, the need of blood transfusions in paraplegics suffering from pressure sores and osteomyelitis associated with pyelonephritis and renal deficiency (Guttmann, 1946, 1949, 1953). In a time, when, during the Second World War, plasma transfusions were generally used to combat nutritional deficiency, we found blood transfusions, particularly of fresh blood, as the quickest and most effective therapeutic agent in restoring and maintaining a satisfactory nutritional condition in paraplegics. In certain stages of renal deterioration with anaemia, blood transfusions were found to have a distinct beneficial effect in raising the haemoglobin value and diminishing albuminuria and blood urea. Undesirable effects of repeated transfusions of full blood can be obviated by transfusions of packed red cells. Additional treatment with vitamins and iron following blood transfusion is also desirable. However, once renal deficiency has become greatly advanced, blood transfusions were found of very limited or of no value at all. No time should be wasted in continuing the conventional conservative treatment, and dialysis should be instituted as soon as possible.

Oedema. One of the outstanding clinical symptoms of the nephrotic phase of renal deficiency in the patient described earlier, was the profound oedema. The distribution of nephrotic oedema in paraplegics and tetraplegics is similar to that found in non-paraplegic patients including the face (especially following recumbency during sleep), the legs, ascites, marked swelling of scrotum and penis and, in the terminal stage, pleural and pericardial effusion.

The underlying causes of oedema in renal deficiency are disturbances of local and renal mechanisms regulating the salt and water metabolism. The drain upon plasma albumin is demonstrated in these patients by the heavy albuminuria, resulting in alterations in the hydrostatic and colloid osmotic pressure, resulting in increased transudation of fluid from the intravascular into the interstitional space. Moreover, changes in the intrarenal autoregulatory mechanisms (de Wardener & Miles, 1952; Kintner & Pappenheimer, 1956; Seller, 1965), involved in the maintenance of glomerular and tubular function and renal blood flow, play an essential part in the disturbance of salt and water metabolism. A great deal of research on the micro-environments of the nephron has been undertaken in recent years with special reference to the functional role which the juxta-glomerular apparatus, with its various cell components and its afferent and efferent arterial and venous blood supply, plays in connection with the renin–angiotensin–aldosterone system in maintaining a glomerular–tubular balance (Hartroft et al., 1959; Hartroft, 1966; Tobian, 1966; Bull et al., 1966; Kirkendahl & Fitz, 1967; and others). However, there is still much to be learned in this very complex problem, and no definite conclusions can be reached at present regarding the intricate function of the hormonal system in relationship to glomerular–tubular balance.

Treatment

The treatment of oedema in the nephrotic phase of renal deficiency has, of course, to be considered in relation to all the other symptoms of renal deficiency. The improvement of anemia and albuminuria by full blood transfusions, special dietetic measures with reduced salt intake in cases of sodium retention, and the combating of infection will always take priority. In the case of extensive degrees of oedema with hydrothorax and ascites, the removal of fluid by mechanical means, such as trocar and Southey tube, may be followed by rapid improvement. Ascites is removed in semi-reclined position of the patient to facilitate the flow of the fluid. In order to prevent fainting resulting from the reduction of intra-abdominal pressure, a broad binder should be placed around the upper abdomen before the tapping, which should be tightened as the fluid escapes.

Diuretic drugs should be given with great caution and mercurial preparations are, of course, contraindicated in view of the damaged renal tissues. Peritoneal dialysis in combination with the conservative therapeutic measures has proved successful, as shown in the case described earlier.

HYPERTENSION ASSOCIATED WITH PYELONEPHRITIS AND AMYLOIDOSIS

This problem has been discussed in non-paraplegic subjects since the time of Richard Bright. Despite the fundamental experimental work of Goldblatt and his co-workers (1934), who demonstrated the importance of renal ischaemia in the pathogenesis of hypertension by constricting the renal artery in the dog, the problem of renal hypertension is still unsolved. Pickering (1955), in discussing the controversial literature on the relationship of pyelonephritis to hypertension, came to the following conclusion: 'The part played by chronic pyelonephritis in hypertension is most confusing and most challenging.' Clinical experiences on unilateral renal disease associated with hypertension and its disappearance or improvement following nephrectomy of the diseased kidney and, moreover, the histological findings of renal vascular stenosis in the removed kidney have been significant contributions for a better understanding of the pathogenesis of renal hypertension (Butler, 1937; Barker & Walters, 1940; Pickering & Heptinstall, 1953; Holley et al., 1964; Heptinstall, 1966). In recent years, experimental and clinical studies were concerned with the effects of changes in the renal artery blood flow due to renal artery stenosis on the renin–angiotensin–aldosterone system which, according to Brest et al. (1965), is, at least in part, operative in the mechanism of renal arterial hypertension. This view is in accordance with Genest's (1961) and Peart's (1965) work, who established that angiotensin II, the most important aldosterone-stimulating hormone, is a potent pressor substance which can significantly raise the arterial blood pressure.

This problem has recently been the subject of a Symposium on Hypertension held in Montreal by 84 research workers (Ed. Genest and Koiw, 1972) which dealt with the new advances made in the control of renin secretion and release, angiotensin I converting enzyme activity and immuno-assay methods for the measurement of angiotensin I and II. In addition, the disturbance of aldosterone regulation in early, uncomplicated benign essential hypertension and the 18-hydroxy-corticosterone secretion rate in early hypertension was also discussed. While these papers on experimental research will be undoubtedly of great interest to research workers on prevention and treatment of hypertension and chronic pyelonephritis in paraplegia, this highly complex problem is still far from solution. Irvine H. Page in his chapter 'The Remarkable Story of Hypertension' summed up his views on recent research as follows: 'Error is inevitable if you are creative and to err is human; to really foul things up requires a computer'.

Brest et al. (1965) also consider it likely that retention of sodium in the arterial muscle walls may intensify the vasopressor effect of the circulating angiotensin in the blood. On the other hand, Brest et al. consider the mechanism responsible for renal parenchymal hypertension to be much less well defined than that of renal arterial hypertension. Amongst the factors which are responsible for this discrepancy, they consider to be failure of kidneys to inactivate a pressure substance, deficient renal secretion of vasodepressor material and sodium retention. Their own studies indicate that excess of sodium rather than fluid plays the most important part in raising blood pressure, and salt restriction by diet or salt withdrawal by dialysis will improve renal parenchymal hypertension.

The greatly increased life-span of spinal paraplegics and tetraplegics after the Second World War naturally makes renal deficiency an increasingly important problem, whether this is caused by pyelonephritis with or without amyloidosis and/or hypertension. In a series of paraplegic patients, groups can be distinguished showing amyloidosis due to chronic sepsis, as a result of pressure sores and osteomyelitis, with relatively unimportant upper urinary tract infection; other patients will show renal impairment due to chronic pyelonephritis but no evidence of amyloidosis; yet another group will show the two conditions co-existing. Future studies should aim to define the relationships between renal amyloidosis, chronic pyelonephritis and hypertension in these various groups of patients. Regular blood pressure readings from the early stages in patients with pressure sores and in those with ascending urinary infection and throughout the later stages of these complications are essential. Diastolic pressure of 90–95 mmHg in young adults should be considered in accordance with Fishberg (1954) as abnormally high and should be the indication for detailed clinical and biochemical investigations, including blood urea, serum creatine estimation, creatinine clearance, electrolytes, renogram and rectal biopsy. Ophthalmological examination may also be helpful in the diagnosis of hypertension by revealing early retinopathy (see case P.R. in Table 22).

Tetraplegics with complete lesions are known generally to have a low blood pressure in sitting position, the underlying cause of which has been discussed earlier in this book (see page 295). Although we found on occasions increase of the pressure readings in lying supine position, these observations do not allow definite conclusions, and systematic studies comparing blood pressure readings in sitting and lying position in tetraplegics suffering from chronic ascending infection of the urinary tract, may be helpful in ascertaining persistent blood pressure changes due to renal pathology and/or amyloidosis in these high cord lesions.

Drug therapy

The early diagnosis of renal hypertension resulting from ascending infection of the upper urinary tract by various methods necessitating active and specialized management is now possible, and various therapeutic measures have been discussed. I have always been opposed to sedatives such as phenobarbitone, in particular for long-term therapy, because of their undesirable side-effects, especially fatigue and mental depression as they adversely affect the paraplegic's active life. There are now more potent anti-hypertensive drugs available which can be used advantageously, such as Rauwiloid (Cooper & Cranston, 1957), Inversine—mecamylamine hydrochloride—a ganglion blocking agent given in combination with Saluric, furthermore Esbatal-Bethanidine Sulphate, an adrenergic neurone blocking agent (Johnston, Prichard & Rosenheim, 1962; Boura & Green, 1963) and Aldomet, methyldopa (Cannon & Laragh, 1963; Hamilton & Kopelman, 1963 Johnson et al., 1966). Side-effects of these drugs can be minimized or altogether avoided by careful, individual selection of the cases suffering according to the degree of their renal hypertension. Aldomet is contra-indicated in cases with oedema.

CAUSES OF DEATH IN THE ACUTE AND CHRONIC STAGES

RENAL PATHOLOGY

In discussing the pathology of *postmortem* findings in 26 out of 458 traumatic lesions— 388 soldiers and 70 civilians (Guttmann, 1953), it was found that in 20 patients of our series, whose deaths were related to spinal cord injuries during the Second World War and the following years until 1950, the only or main cause was ascending urinary infection resulting in pyelonephritis and renal deficiency. Nineteen out of the 26 patients had suprapubic drainage at the time of death which was instituted elsewhere on the day or within the first few days following injury. In 5 cases the suprapubic drainage had been closed at varying periods before death, while only 2 cases never had suprapubic drainage.

The necropsy findings in all the 19 cases were uniform. The bladder, showing all signs of chronic infection, was contracted and adherent to the pelvis, being surrounded by a thick wall of fibrous tissue. The ureters were dilated, tortuous and adherent to the surrounding tissues and also embedded in dense fibrous tissue. The kidneys showed various degrees of hydro- and pyonephrosis and were also found to be embedded in a mass of fibrous tissue. Sometimes one of the kidneys was found to be in an extreme degree of atrophy and very small. These findings were associated in the majority of cases with amyloidosis of the kidneys and various other organs, but were only occasionally associated with hepatomegaly.

Tribe (1963) published the results of a more detailed analysis of 150 necropsies of paraplegics of our Spinal Centre, who died between 1945 and 1962. Twenty-eight patients died within 2 months after injury; of these, in 16, death was related to their paraplegia or tetraplegia. Respiratory failure in cervical lesions and pulmonary embolism in thoracic lesions (T5–T11) were the most important causes of death. The site of the venous thrombosis were the leg veins, in one case the pelvic veins. One of the cases died from paralytic ileus and another from pulmonary oedema due to overtransfusion.

One hundred and twenty-two patients died in later stages following injury, and in 71 death was related to paraplegia. Renal failure was the cause of 27 hypertension and all but 3 had pyelonephritis. Of 5 fatal cases of cerebral haemorrhage, 4 had hypertension associated with chronic pyelonephritis. In 11 of 13 chronic non-traumatic paraplegics renal failure due to chronic pyelonephritis was also the primary cause of death. Therefore, of a total of 84 cases where deaths were related to paraplegia 64 (76 per cent) died in renal failure, the underlying cause being chronic pyelonephritis.

This study was amplified by additional 70 cases, making a total of 220 necropsies, published by Tribe & Silver in 1969 in a monograph, which was concerned mainly with renal failure in chronic paraplegia. Of 174 traumatic and non-traumatic chronic cases related to paraplegia, 117 (97 traumatic and 20 non-traumatic) died from renal failure due to chronic pyelonephritis, the majority of them associated with amyloidosis.

Sixty of the 174 patients had hypertension (34·8 per cent), the diastolic pressure varying from 90 to more than 130 mmHg (the latter found in 25 cases). Of the 117 cases who died from renal failure due to pyelonephritis, 46 (38·5 per cent) had hypertension.

Paroxysmal hypertensive attacks due to autonomic hyperreflexia in lesions above T5 as a result of abnormal action of bladder or other internal organs, are not included in this series, as there is no proof that these attacks bear any relation to the development of persistent hypertension.

The age of the majority of hypertensive patients varied between 30 and 40 years. Cerebro-vascular incidents occurred in 7 cases. Hypertrophy of the heart (heart weight varying between 420 and 560 g) was found in 27 cases in this series, while in 19 cases the heart weight varied between 330 and 390 g. Forty-four varying degrees of left ventricular hypertrophy.

Numerous authors have given reports on the high incidence of renal mortality in paraplegics and tetraplegics. However, studies on the incidence of hypertension in chronic pyelonephritis following spinal injuries are still scanty and controversial. Following Reingold's paper (1960) on the pathology of selected cases of spinal cord injuries at the 9th Spinal Cord Injury Conference in V.A. Hospital, Long Beach, U.S.A., a discussion arose on the incidence of hypertension in renal disease, associated with pyelonephrosis. With one exception (Comarr) all other speakers felt that renal hypertension is a rare exception in these patients. Bors & Comarr (1970) found an incidence of 8·2 per cent of renal death with hypertension in their own cases. A more detailed analysis on hypertension in relationship to pyelonephritis and amyloidosis was given by Talbot (1965). Out of 43 paraplegics and tetraplegics upon whom autopsies were done, 35 had renal disease: 19 pyelonephritis, 3 amyloidosis only, 13 both. Of the 19 pyelonephritis cases 9, of the 3 amyloidosis only one, and of the 13 combined pyelonephritis and amyloidosis cases 6 had hypertension. Talbot's definition of hyerptension was systolic blood pressure of 150 mmHg and/or 100 mmHg diastolic blood pressure.

In our paper on comparative studies on endogenous creatinine and urea clearances in paraplegics and tetraplegics (Doggart, Guttmann & Silver, 1966) 18 out of 28 patients were suffering from chronic pyelonephritis. Table 22 gives the details of the clinical findings, from which it would appear that in 11 cases out of the 18 the pyelonephritis was associated with amyloidosis, and these patients had pressure sores, some associated with osteomyelitis. In the 11 cases amyloidosis was discovered by rectal biopsy, of these in one as early as 19 months after injury, in two patients it was found at *post-mortem*. Death occurred after 1–3 years in 4 cases after the diagnosis of amyloidosis had been made.

Hypertension was found in 8 of the 18 patients (44·4 per cent). in 5 of them diastolic pressure varied between 100 and 150 mmHg. Although, in the 3 additional patients who were of young age, the diastolic pressure was only 90 mmHg, this is considered as pathological in accordance with Fishberg's views (1954). One of these 3 (aged 32) had a systolic pressure of 150 mmHg, the second (aged 31) had a hypertensive retinopathy and the third (aged 27) with a blood pressure of 130/90 was oedematous with a proteinuria

TABLE 22

Patient	Age	Lesion	Time after injury	Relevant history	Creatinine		Urea	
					Serum (mg/100 ml)	Clearance (ml/min)	Blood (mg/100 ml)	Clearance (% average normal)
H.M.	48	C6 compl.	13 yr	Injured at 35. Severe pressure sores with osteomyelitis. Automatic micturition for next 12 years with normal I.V.P. but persistent infection. Epileptic fits at 47. Admitted at 48 with blood urea of 54 mg/100 ml, rising to 175 mg/100 ml. Amyloidosis diagnosed by rectal biopsy. Normo-tensive. Died at home.	3·6 2·9	6 7	144 103	8 12
G.W.	59	T2 compl.	6 yr	Injured at 53. Persistent urinary infection but normal I.V.P. Pressure sores with osteomyelitis. Oedematous; serum albumin 1·9 g/100 ml; serum globulin 3·65 g/100 ml. Proteinuria 4·9 g/24 hr. Amyloidosis (rectal biopsy). Normotensive. Maximum urine concentration 552 m.osmole/kg.	0·8 0·7	69 79	31 —	44 — ±
K.W.	32	T6 compl.	12 yr	Injured at 20. Immediate suprapubic cystotomy. Vesical stones. Pressure sores with osteomyelitis. Serum albumin 3·2 g/100 ml; serum globulin 4·1 g/100 ml. Proteinuria 7·5 g/24 hr. Amyloidosis (rectal biopsy). Maximum urine concentration 459 m.osmole/kg.	0·8 0·7	34 65	30 29	33 26

TABLE 22 (*continued*)

Patient	Age	Lesion	Time after injury	Relevant history	Creatinine Serum (mg/100 ml)	Creatinine Clearance (ml/min)	Urea Blood (mg/100 ml)	Urea Clearance (% average normal)
M.F.	32	T7 compl.	6 yr	Injured at 26. Pressure sores with osteomyelitis. Automatic micturition. At 31, oedematous; serum albumin 0·9 g/100 ml; serum globulin 200 g/100 ml. Proteinuria 12·8 g/24 hr. Positive Congo Red test; positive rectal biopsy. Died after subarachnoid haemorrhage. Amyloidosis confirmed.	3·8	19	99	—
P.R.	31	T7 compl.	10 yr	Injured at 21. Automatic micturition. At 26, hydronephrosis left, no secretion on right; bilateral reflux; diverticula of bladder. At 31, hypertensive retinopathy. Post-mortem diagnosis of renal amyloidosis.	5·2 4·9 9·3 10·1	10 8 2 2	67 70 109 156	11 12 8 4
G.M.	27	T10 compl.	8½ yr	Injured at 19. Pressure sores with osteomyelitis and a periurethral abscess. Suprapubic cystostomy performed. Hydronephrosis, hydro-ureter and diverticula. Oedematous; serum albumin 0·4 g/100 ml; serum globulin 2·4 g/100 ml. Proteinuria, 13·6 g/24 hr. Amyloidosis (rectal biopsy). Maximum urine concentration 528 m.osmole/kg.	0·7 0·8 0·7	86 65 73	30 29 38	— — 34
P.O'D.	48	T11 compl.	6 yr	Haemangioma of cord at 42. Pressure sores with osteomyelitis. Discharged at 45 with automatic bladder, sterile urine and bilateral hydronephrosis. At 48, B.P. 150/100. Proteinuria 2 g/24 hr. Amyloidosis (rectal biopsy)	2·8 2·9	15 23	99 66	11 20

W.C.	56	T12 compl.	19 yr	Injured at 37. Immediate suprapubic cystotomy. Infected urine. At 46, B.P. 175/110. At 52, nephrectomy for renal calculus; at 53, pressure sores; serum albumin 3·6 g/100 ml; serum globulin 3·7 g/100 ml. At 54, proteinuria 2·8 g/24 hr. Admitted terminally, confused and obliguric. Post-mortem amyloidosis.	6·8	3	100	—
G.A.	55	L3 incomp.	15 yr	Injured at 40. Pressure sores. Dribbling incontinence of urine. At 43, hydronephrosis. B.P. 220/150; at 45 indwelling catheter. Amyloidosis (rectal biopsy). Died at 55, chronic pyelonephritis and renal amyloidosis.	5·1	11	90	10
W.B.	43	Multiple sclerosis.	20 yr	Diagnosed as multiple sclerosis at 23. Unable to walk by 38. At 39, sores causing osteomyelitis. I.V.P. showed vesical calculus; serum albumin 2·1 g/100 ml; serum globulin 3·35 g/100 ml. Amyloidosis (rectal biopsy). Maximum urine concentration 577 m.osmole/kg.	0·5 0·4	81 72	24 18	77 —
T.H.	41	T12 compl.	19 mth	Admitted within 10 days of injury, urine rendered sterile; discharged with blood urea 41 mg/100 ml 252 days after injury. Readmitted 150 days later with residual of 20 oz, little secretion on I.V.P., infected urine, proteinuria; treated by tidal drainage. Amyloidosis (rectal biopsy).	1·7 1·3 2·0 1·7	44 67 50 56	81 36 46 62	24 44 — 29

of 13·6 g/24 hr and a serum albumin of 0·4/100 ml. These high incidences of hypertension in pyelonephritis and pyelonephritis associated with amyloidosis are in accordance with the results found by Tribe and Silver in their larger series.

In discussing the underlying histopathology of renal hypertension in pyelonephritis and amyloidosis, it would appear from all histological data available so far, that no clear relationship exists between the disturbances of the glomerulo-tubular system. There is general agreement amongst pathologists about the outstanding histopathological findings in chronic pyelonephritis and amyloidosis, associated with hypertension, such as endarteritis fibrosa with or without reduplication of the internal elastic laminae in arteries, proliferative glomerulitis, glomerular sclerosis, glomerular tuft necrosis and amyloid replacement of surviving glomerular tufts, etc. However, the same alterations of the renal tissues have also been found in chronic pyelonephritis and/or amyloidosis without hypertension. It remains, therefore, to be seen whether the solution of this problem will be found in refinement of histopathological techniques or by further elaboration of biochemical, perhaps immunobiological research.

(8) Cancer of the urinary tract

In the past this complication following spinal cord injuries was practically unknown because of the short duration of life of these patients. However, it has become a reality in recent years owing to the greatly increased life-span of paraplegics and tetraplegics after the Second World War. Therefore, this potential complication demands, in future, increasing attention by everyone concerned with the long-term management of these patients with regard to early diagnosis and early treatment. This applies, in particular, apart from paraplegics and tetraplegics with long-standing indwelling urethral or suprapubic catheters, to those who were subjected to cutaneous vesicostomy. Laskowski & Brantley-Scott (1965), who performed this operation on 45 patients, as introduced by Lapides (1960), found squamous metaplasia present histologically in 13 patients selected at random and cystitis glandularis in 2 of these cases. These changes are due to chronic irritation and environmental exposure resulting in metaplasia of the bladder epithelium to a mucus secreting glandular type of cystitis, which may cause development of malignancy of adenocarcinoma type. McIntosh & Worley (1955) reported 2 cases of adenocarcinoma amongst 25 cases of extrophy of the bladder.

Kawaichi (1960) reported 4 cases of bladder cancer amongst 1,600 paraplegic patients, 3 of transitional and one of squamous cell cancer. The ages of the patients varied from 36 to 49 years and the level of the spinal lesion ranged from T4 to L3. The diagnosis of cancer was made 18, 24 and 25 years after injury. Melzak (1966) reported 12 cancer cases (10 men, and two women) amongst 3,800 patients of our material, 11 of them involving the bladder and one the ureter. The average age of these patients was 51 years; the youngest 37, the oldest 68 years old. The level of the spinal lesions varied from C7 to S2. There was one cervical, 6 thoracic (T1–T12) and 5 lumbar-sacral lesions, 9 were complete, 3 incomplete. All patients had long-standing permanent bladder drainage by suprapubic (the majority) or urethral indwelling catheters. The cancer was diagnosed during life 13 to 42 years after injury, with the exception of one which was discovered *post-mortem.* The histological examination of our cancer cases revealed the following cell types: 4 transitional, 4 squamous, 3 mixed transitional and squamous and one papillary. The time of survival after diagnosis and treatment (cystectomy and cutaneous ureterostomy followed by deep X-ray treatment) varied between 7 days to $5\frac{1}{2}$ years.

Since 1965 regular cytological investigations have been carried out in paraplegics and tetraplegics, and Melzak reported in his paper of 374 urines examined, only one case proved positive and in 7 cases atypical smears were found.

Bors & Comarr (1971) found 15 cases of malignancy amongst 2,322 patients. The sites of the neoplasia in these cases were as follows: one urethra, eleven bladder, four kidney, one kidney and bladder. The average age of these patients was the fifth decade. The cancer was diagnosed 10 to 22 years after injury. No details of the histology are given.

The incidence of malignant tumours of the bladder and other sections of the urinary tract, published so far, is still too small to allow comparative statistics with those occurring within the non-paraplegic population in this country, and it remains to be seen whether or not the incidence is greater amongst spinal cord sufferers. It also remains to be seen what role chronic infection and long-standing use of indwelling catheters, especially those of rubber material, play in the aetiology of malignancy developing in the bladder in comparison to catheter-free paraplegics and tetraplegics.

CHAPTER 28.

DISTURBANCES OF INTESTINAL FUNCTION

Physiology and Pathophysiology

The complicated pattern of normal intestinal activity depends on pendular, circular and segmental movements of the various sections of the intestinal tract to establish mixing of the food with the gastric and intestinal secretion and to accomplish its digestion and absorption. There is a wide range in the speed of intestinal activity, which is highest in duodenum and jejunum, gradually slowing down towards the ileum, which is stimulated reflexly (gastro-ileal reflex of Hurst) to move its semi-fluid contents into the caecum, gradually filling the ascending and transverse colon. There, the absorption of salts and water takes place by the slow function of the haustra, until at certain long intervals, by a powerful mass movement of the transverse colon, the contents are transferred into the descending and pelvic colon. While all these processes take place without conscious awareness, the act of defaecation is initiated by conscious appreciation of an urge to defaecate ('the call to stool'), which is caused by afferent impulses to the sacral spinal centre and cerebral stations as a result of the filling and distension of sigmoid colon and upper rectum. Efferent impulses emanating from the sacral centre set up an opening mechanism, by evoking contractions of sigmoid and rectum and in turn relaxation of the rectal sphincters to allow the passage of faeces, which is assisted by straining—i.e. raising the abdominal pressure. Following emptying of the anal canal, a closing mechanism comes into action by contracting the levator ani to restore the everted mucosa, while contraction of the anal sphincter and relaxation of the tone of the colon takes place.

There are considerable variations of bowel habit amongst able-bodied individuals. Connell *et al.* (1963) found, in a statistic study on an industrial community, only 1 per cent of the population with bowel habits outside the range of three bowel actions per week, to three per day, while in 88·5 per cent the frequency ranged from 5 to 14 bowel actions per week. It is, therefore, essential for those concerned with the management of the spinal paralysed to consider the pre-paraplegic habit of these patients when analysing the intestinal abnormalities, especially in the stage of reconditioning.

Intestinal activity depends on a co-ordinated action of the various stations of the nervous system. The influence of the cerebral mechanisms on gastrointestinal activity is well known. Visual and olfactory impulses at the sight, smell or thought of food stimulate active flow of gastric juice and accelerate the digestive process, while disagreeable emotional states, such as fear, anger, worry, may result in complete depression of gastrointestinal activity. The act of defaecation also depends on cerebral influences, which, according to circumstances, may promote or inhibit the activity of the sacral spinal centre. In inconvenient circumstances, the inhibitory influence of the cortex will cause antiperistaltic action by increasing the tone of the anal sphincter, relaxing the colon. The contents move back into the colon and the desire to defaecate will disappear.

Hypothalamic influence on intestinal peristalsis and secretion has been reported by Beattie (1932), Beattie & Sheehan (1934) and others. Haemorrhages and ulceration of the gastrointestinal tract may occur as a result of acute lesions in the course of descending autonomic tracts from the level of the anterior hypothalamus to the level of the cervical cord.

The dominant nervous control of the gastrointestinal tract is divided into three systems: (a) Sympathetic ganglia and chain, which receive their impulses from the spinal segments Th5 to L2/3 via anterior roots. The thoracic and lumbar splanchnic nerves connect with the coeliac, superior and inferior mesenteric plexuses and, arising from the ganglia of these plexuses, postganglionic fibres travel with the blood vessels to the various parts of the gastrointestinal tract. (b) The parasympathetic control which is provided by the vagus for the stomach, the small intestines and the major part of the large intestines, while the sacral parasympathetic innervation, which originates in the sacral segments S2–4, innervates through the pelvic nerves the rectum and sigmoid colon. Parasympathetic fibres, especially from the vagi, also join the plexuses mentioned above and pass through them and end around ganglion cells in the mesenteric and submucosal plexuses of the intestinal wall (Fulton, 1945). The usual antagonistic action between sympathetic and parasympathetic innervation—the former reducing peristalsis and digestion, the latter increasing peristalsis and stimulating the production of digestive juices—may change into synergistic action in the control of gastrointestinal function, especially in conducting afferent impulses to the spinal cord. (c) Intramural autonomous innervation of the intestinal wall by the Meissner's and Anerbach's plexuses.

Changes in the peristaltic passage of food from the upper to the lower intestinal tract, its storage and solidification in the descending colon and sigmoid and finally intermittent defaecation from the sigmoid colon through rectum and anal canal are the inevitable results of complete as well as incomplete lesions of the spinal cord or conus–cauda equina. Since Lister (1858) demonstrated the inhibitory action of the sympathetic system on peristalsis in the rabbit, the physiology and pathophysiology of the various components of the intestinal tract have been the subject of intensive research (Masius, 1868; Gowers, 1877; Bayliss & Starling, 1900; Head & Riddoch, 1917; Hurst, 1921; Learmouth & Rankin, 1930; Denny-Brown & Robertson, 1935; Heslop, 1938; Sheehan, 1940; Munro, 1953; Floyd & Walls, 1953; Dagradi, 1953; Guttmann, 1959; Connell, 1962; Connell, Frankel & Guttmann, 1963; Melzak & Porter, 1964; Paeslack, 1965, 1967; Frankel, 1967; and others).

Studies in man have been concerned mainly with the rectal and colonic response to distension, since Masius (1968) and Gowers (1877) recorded reflex activity of the sphincter ani in response to rectal distension (Nathan & Smith, 1953).

My colleagues Melzak & Porter (1964) in their electromyographic studies on the external anal sphincter in 42 paraplegics and tetraplegics of Stoke Mandeville, found that with each increase of intrarectal volume the external sphincter at first responds by contracting. The rectal wall relaxes to accommodate the increased volume, but as soon as the rectal wall contracts the external anal sphincter relaxes until defaecation is complete.

Their findings, that the external anal sphincter shows continuous electrical activity and tonic contraction at rest, following transection of the cord above the level of the third lumbar segment, confirmed Floyd & Walls' (1953) electromyographic results, which showed conclusively that the human external sphincter ani is always in a state of tonic contraction during waking and sleeping hours. Bors & Blinn (1958), using needle electrodes inserted into the external anal sphincter and pubo-rectalis, also found constant muscle contraction at rest. These findings are not in accordance with Denny-Brown & Robertson's conclusions that 'the external sphincter ani is not tonic although it contracts reflexly and synergistically'. Melzak and Porter found the electrical activity and anal tonic contraction absent during the state of spinal shock and abolished following intrathecal alcohol block. The recovery of reflex activity of the external rectal sphincter from spinal shock is shown in Fig. 183 of one of their electromyographic findings.

Studies on the motility of the pelvic colon were undertaken by me in co-operation with Connell & Frankel (1963) on 26 patients with complete lesions of the spinal cord. The objects of these studies were (a) to determine differences in the resting motility of the colon resulting from injuries of the cord at different levels, and (b) to examine the effects of various stimuli as well as the effect of the intrathecal alcohol block. Table 23 gives the essential clinical data of the patients. All studies were made with the patient's relaxing on a bed in a quiet room, and the subjects were encouraged to read light literature. No food was allowed for 2 hr before the beginning of the study.

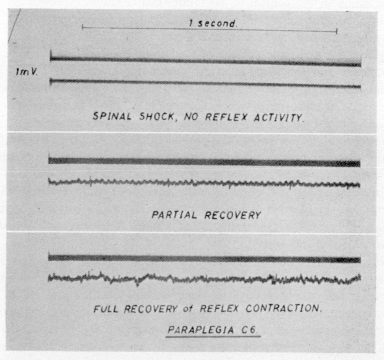

FIG. 183. Recovery of reflex activity of the external rectal sphincter from spinal shock. From Melzak and Porter (1964) *Paraplegia*, **3**, 282.

TABLE 23

Case no.	Age	Segmental level of cord lesion	Time since onset	Flaccid or spastic	Bowel function	Bladder function
1. J.H.	22	Complete C5 due to fracture dislocation C4/C5 vertebrae	10 months	Spastic	Spontaneous after suppositories	Co-ordinated automatic
2. A.B.	22	Complete C6 due to fracture dislocation C5/C6 vertebrae	3 years	Spastic	Digital evacuation	Disco-ordinated automatic
3. I.B.	21	Complete C6 due to fracture dislocation C5/C6 vertebrae	1 year	Spastic	Spontaneous after suppositories	Co-ordinated automatic
4. D.G.	26	Complete C7 due to fracture dislocation C5/C6 vertebrae. Active duodenal ulcer	6 years	Spastic	Digital evacuation	Disco-ordinated automatic
5. M.J.	22	Complete C7 due to fracture dislocation C6/C7 vertebrae	1 year	Spastic	Spontaneous after suppositories	Co-ordinated automatic
6. R.B.	24	Incomplete C6, complete T1 due to fracture C6 vertebra	1 year	Spastic	Spontaneous after suppositories	Co-ordinated automatic
7. T.M.	17	Incomplete C6, complete T2 due to fracture dislocation C5/C6 vertebrae	9 months	Spastic	Spontaneous after suppositories	Co-ordinated automatic
8. J.H.	22	Incomplete C7, complete T2 due to fracture dislocation C6/C7 vertebrae	5 months	Spastic	Spontaneous after suppositories	Co-ordinated automatic
9. L.H.	37	Incomplete C7, complete T3 due to fracture dislocation C7/T1 vertebrae	6 years	Spastic	Digital evacuation	Disco-ordinated automatic
10. D.B.	29	Complete T5 due to fracture dislocation T3/T4 vertebrae	5 months	Spastic	Spontaneous after suppositories	Co-ordinated automatic
11. H.S.	37	Complete T7 due to fracture dislocation T6/T7 vertebrae	5 months	Spastic	Spontaneous after suppositories	Co-ordinated automatic
12. F.C.	29	Complete C5 due to fracture dislocation C4/C5 vertebrae. Low intrathecal alcohol block five years before investigation	7 years	Flaccid	Digital evacuation	Atonic
13. L.S.	21	Complete C6 due to fracture C5 vertebra. Low intrathecal alcohol block two months before investigation	1 year	Flaccid	Digital evacuation	Atonic

TABLE 23 (continued)

Case no.	Age	Segmental level of cord lesion	Time since onset	Flaccid or spastic	Bowel function	Bladder function
14. J.B.	51	Complete T6 due to fracture T8 vertebra. Low intrathecal alcohol block eight years before investigation	10 years	Flaccid	Enema or digital evacuation	Atonic
15. D.S.	27	Complete T9 due to fracture T8 vertebra	6 months	Spastic	Spontaneous after suppositories	Co-ordinated automatic
16. T.D.	27	Complete T10 due to fracture T9 vertebra	9 months	Spastic	Spontaneous after suppositories	Co-ordinated automatic
17. T.C.	18	Complete T10 due to fracture dislocation T10/T11 vertebrae	9 months	Spastic	Spontaneous after suppositories	Co-ordinated automatic
18. H.T.	49	Complete T11 due to gunshot wound	15 years	Spastic	Spontaneous after suppositories	Weak disco-ordinated automatic
19. J.H.	50	Complete T11 due to haemangioma of spinal cord	1 year	Spastic	Spontaneous after suppositories	Co-ordinated automatic
20. H.H.	38	Complete T12 due to fracture dislocation T11/T12 vertebrae	9 months	Spastic	Spontaneous after suppositories	Co-ordinated automatic
21. R.A.	37	Complete T9 due to cordectomy performed for removal of astrocytoma	5 months	Flaccid	Digital evacuation	Autonomous
22. O.T.	58	Complete below T9 due to haemangioma. Bilateral cordotomy. Rhizotomy. Alcohol Block	7 years	Flaccid	Digital evacuation occasional enema	Atonic
23. J.P.	24	Complete T11 due to transverse myelitis	1 year	Flaccid	Digital evacuation	Atonic
24. K.P.	21	Complete T12 due to fracture dislocation T12/L1 vertebrae	5 months	Flaccid	Digital evacuation	Atonic
25. E.M.	46	Complete T12 due to fracture dislocation T12/L1 vertebrae	2 years	Flaccid	Digital evacuation	Atonic
26. J.E.	24	Complete L1 due to fracture L1 vertebra	10 months	Flaccid	Digital evacuation	Atonic

The technique adopted of recording intraluminal and colonic activity pressure was that of Rowlands *et al.* (1953) and Atkinson *et al.* (1957), using miniature balloons connected by fine polyethylene tubing to a metal capsule optic manometer of high sensitivity. Only in one patient (case 22) was a wireless telemetering capsule (Connell & Rowlands, 1960) used. The tubes and recording balloons, still attached to the manometer, were passed into the colon through the sigmoidoscope, which was then withdrawn. The recording tips were placed routinely at 15, 20 and 25 cm from the anus—i.e. they lay in the rectum and in the sigmoid at the recto-sigmoid angle respectively (Fig. 184). Respiratory and body movement were recorded by a stethograph around the upper abdomen and

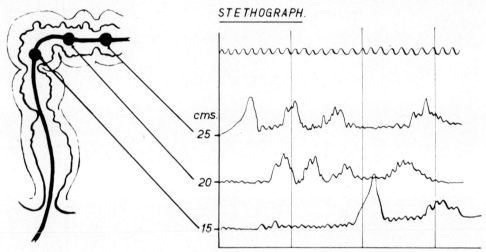

FIG. 184. Diagram illustrating method of recording. From Connell, Frankel and Guttmann (1963) *Paraplegia,* **1,** 102.

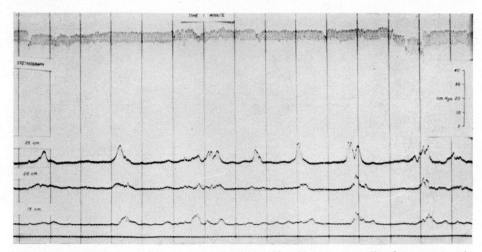

FIG. 185. Motility record from a normal subject. Simultaneous recording from 25, 20 and 15 cm from the anus. In this and other figures top trace is a stethograph calibration in 10 cm water divisions and verticals are 1 min intervals. From Connell, Frankel and Guttmann (1963) *Paraplegia,* **1,** 103.

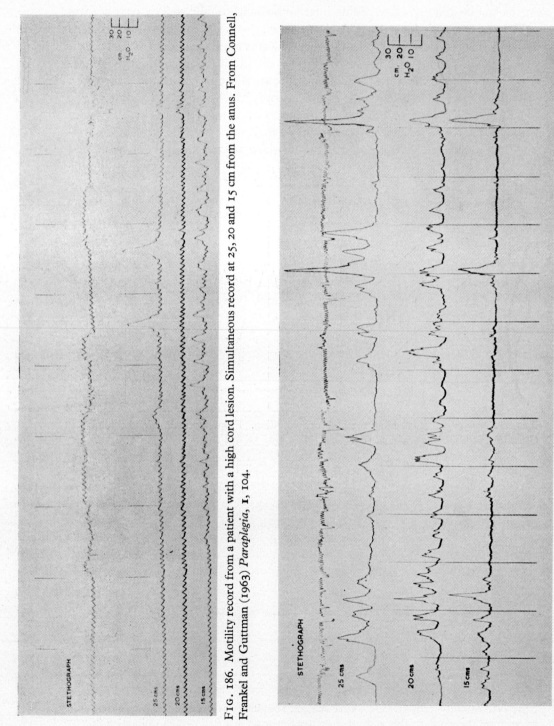

FIG. 186. Motility record from a patient with a high cord lesion. Simultaneous record at 25, 20 and 15 cm from the anus. From Connell, Frankel and Guttman (1963) *Paraplegia*, **I**, 104.

FIG. 187. Motility record from a patient with a complete lesion of the low thoracic cord with spastic paraplegia. Simultaneous

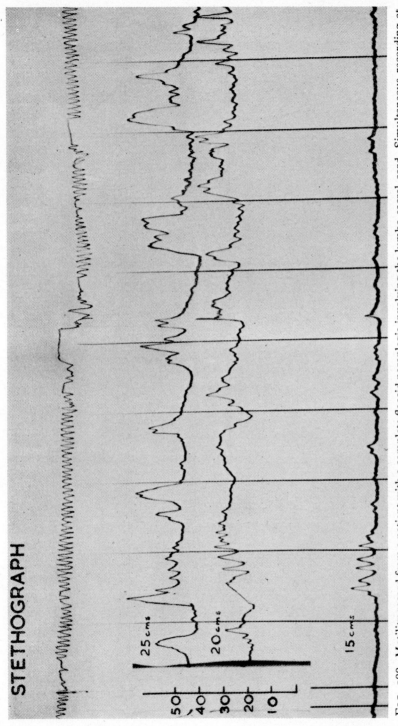

FIG. 188. Motility record from a patient with a complete flaccid paraplegia involving the lumbo-sacral cord. Simultaneous recording at 25, 20 and 15 cm from the anus. From Connell, Frankel and Guttmann (1963) *Paraplegia*, **1**, 106.

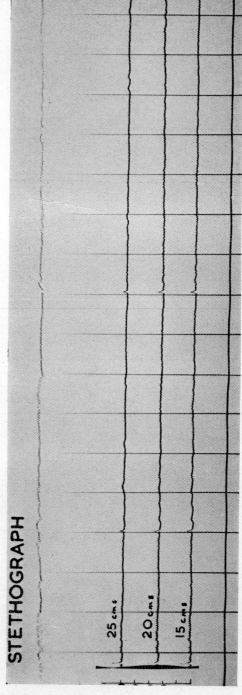

FIG. 189. Motility record from a patient with a cervical cord lesion with flaccid paralysis of the lumbo-sacral segments resulting from an alcohol block.

attached to a capsule manometer. Fig. 185 demonstrates motility record from a normal subject.

Sigmoidoscopy itself showed certain effects in nearly all cases. In the cervicals, when the sigmoidoscope reached 13 to 18 cm, there was reflex relaxation of the anus accompanied by certain remote autonomic reflex responses such as tingling in the face and throbbing headaches—symptoms which develop in these high lesions when their bowels are acting. Actually many of the cervicals defaecated during sigmoidoscopy. These effects did not occur in cervical patients who had had intrathecal alcohol block to abolish intractable spasticity. In flaccid lesions, there was no change in the atonic anus during sigmoidoscopy but the tone of the upper rectum and sigmoid colon was greater than in a normal subject at level of 15 to 20 cm and the patients as well as the normal control complained of periumbilical discomfort.

Fig. 186 illustrates motility records of patients with high cord lesion, low spastic lesion and flaccid lesion of the lumbo-sacral cord, in comparison with the motility record from a normal subject. High lesions showed, with one exception, concerning a patient with a complete C7 lesion who at the time of the study had an active duodenal ulcer, less colonic activity than the normal control and low cord lesions, and the amplitude of the waves was diminished (Fig. 187). In contrast, the records from patients with distal cord lesions showed increased colonic activity. There was difference in the percentage duration of activity between distal spastic and flaccid lesions, although the latter showed more irregular records (Fig. 188). Following intrathecal alcohol block resulting in destruction of the sacral centre and its parasympathetic innervation, sigmoid motility was minimal in every respect (Fig. 189). It would appear that, if the lesion affects mainly the lumbar segments, the sacral centre shows hyperactivity resulting in increased colonic activity. This indicates an inhibitory influence which the lumbar outflow exerts on colonic activity. Actually, an inhibitory centre in the lumbo-sacral region of the cord was postulated by Garry (1933) as a result of experiments in cats.

The effect of food was an increase in both percentage duration of colonic activity and in the amplitude of waves in 5 patients examined who had complete lesions of the cervical, upper and distal thoracic and lumbar cord. The increase in activity varied considerably from starting immediately or after latent periods up to 15 minutes (Table 24). The visual effect of food was studied in two patients, who were shown the meal but were not allowed to eat it for a few minutes. In one patient with a lesion below L1, there was an immediate and distinct increase in activity on seeing the meal, which was reinforced

TABLE 24. The effect of a meal on the duration of activity
in patients with spinal paraplegia

Subject	Level of lesion	Before meal (%)	After meal (%)
4	C7 (D.U.)	85	97
5	C7	33	55
7	T2	44	80
20	T12	87	95
26	L1	70	100

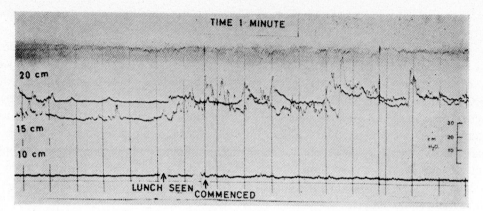

FIG. 190. The effect of a meal on the motility of the sigmoid colon in a spinal paraplegic (L1). (Patient No. 26). At first arrow patient was shown his meal. At the point indicated by the second arrow he began to eat. From Connell, Frankel and Guttmann (1963) *Paraplegia*, **1**, 110.

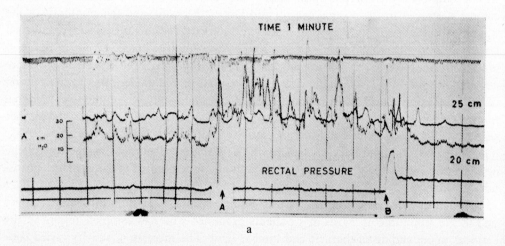

a

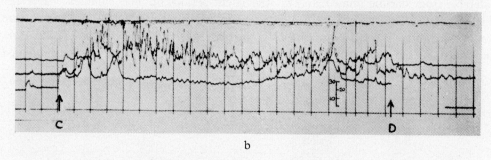

b

FIG. 191. Effect of moderate rectal distension on the motility of the pelvic colon. At the arrow A a soft rubber catheter tied to a latex balloon is passed into the rectum. At the arrow B, 100 ml of water are passed into the balloon resulting in immediate inhibition of the sigmoid activity. From Connell, Frankel and Guttmann (1963) *Paraplegia*, **1**, 111.

by the subsequent consumption of the meal (Fig. 190). In another patient with a Th11 lesion there was no effect on visual impulses, but the patient did not find the food appetizing. However, there was a definite response to eating.

Of special interest was the effect of distending the rectum on sigmoid motility, as found in 12 patients with complete lesion and levels ranging from C6 to L1. All 7 patients with spastic cord lesions (C6 to T12) showed a definite response which consisted in 6 cases of initial inhibition of sigmoid motility followed by a subsequent stimulation. The response was most marked nearest to the point of stimulation. Figs. 191a, b illustrate the responses to moderate and powerful rectal distension in a case of incomplete spastic lesions below C6 but complete below T2, with co-ordinated automatic bladder and bowel functions. In patients with cervical lesions, rectal distension elicited marked responses of other autonomic mechanisms, in particular cardio-vascular response, as described previously (Guttmann & Whitteridge, 1947), and in two cervical patients the study had to be terminated because of rise in blood pressure to high levels. The flaccid low thoracic and lumbar lesions and those cervical and mid-thoracic lesions who, following intrathecal alcohol block, became flaccid, did not show responses to rectal distension, and on filling the rectal balloon with larger amounts of water (200 ml) the balloon was extruded passively.

These studies demonstrate the important function of the lower sigmoid colon for the initiation of the defaecation reflex. It could be shown that stimulation of the bowel with sigmoidoscope resulted in relaxation of the anal sphincters and passage of stool. On the other hand, the usual response of the sigmoid to filling with a moderate amount of fluid (100 ml) was an initial inhibition of activity. Only when the rectal pressure greatly increased, following gross distension of the rectum due to a large amount of fluid (300 ml), did an increased sigmoid activity follow. This could be explained as the result of an intestino-intestinal reflex to prevent the forwards movement of more faeces into an already distended rectum (Connell, 1962). In this connection, it may be remembered that, in the small intestines of the cat, distension of one segment results in inhibition of neighbouring segments.

Clinical manifestations and treatment of intestinal dysfunction

Three main stages of intestinal dysfunction can be distinguished following complete or severe incomplete lesions of the spinal cord and conus–cauda equina:
1   absence or depression of gastrointestinal function in the stage of spinal shock,
2   the stage of automatic reflex activity or autonomous function of the intestines,
3   the stage of intestinal reconditioning.

The initial stage

The immediate effect of spinal cord transection on intestinal function in upper thoracic and cervical lesions is paralysis of the peristalsis, accompanied by faecal retention resulting from the atonic state of the whole intestinal tract, which represents the cardinal symptom in lesions of any level.

In patients with paralysed peristalsis, the bowel sounds are either absent or scanty on auscultation. Meteorism may develop fairly rapidly, but its degree varies, being usually absent altogether in lesions below T10. However, when present in upper thoracic and, in particular, cervical lesions, it always represents a serious complication, as it interferes with the function of the diaphragm and thus greatly increases the respiratory distress of the tetraplegic, which develops as a result of the paralysis of the intercostal muscles.

Such a patient needs constant supervision by both medical and nursing staff, and the early intramuscular injection of 0·3–0·5 mg of prostigmine at regular intervals (3 to 5 hr), combined with the introduction of a rectal tube, has proved a beneficial and even life saving measure.

In cervical and upper thoracic lesions, the paralysis of peristalsis may also involve the stomach, resulting in acute dilatation, which in turn increases the respiratory distress considerably. Gastric suction should be introduced as soon as this complication arises.

A further complication of the gastric involvement are mucosal haemorrhages and the development of acute gastric or duodenal ulcers called 'stress ulcers'. These stress ulcers have been observed in acute lesions anywhere in the course of the descending autonomic fibres, from the level of the anterior hypothalamus to the level of the cervical cord. The interruption of the vasoconstrictors in the spinal cord results in paralytic vasodilatation, leading to mucosal haemorrhage forming necrotic areas, eventually causing ulceration. How far stimulation of the vagus also plays a part in the development of stress ulcers is still a matter of conjecture, and it is possible that both mechanisms, paralysis of the vasoconstrictors on the one hand and hyperactivity of the vagus on the other, are responsible. If vomiting of the gastric juice or suction of the dilated stomach reveals more or less digested blood, blood transfusions may become an urgent indication. Patients who had previously gastric or duodenal ulcers may be particularly endangered.

The paralytic vasodilatation as a result of the paralysis of the vasoconstrictors also leads to the formation of oedema in all tissues, in particular the lungs. Therefore, intravenous transfusions of saline or glucose have to be restricted to prevent increase of the oedema, which could result in drowning the patient by excess fluid in the lungs.

The depression of the gastrointestinal function in the stage of spinal shock is, like the depression of the reflex function of skeletal muscles, the result of the sudden withdrawal of the central control. Consequently, the reflexes controlling defaecation are abolished and, as pointed out, there is complete faecal retention. Evacuation of the bowels in this stage should be achieved only by careful digital evacuation or by enema. However, the latter is not indicated in the first 2–3 days after an acute transverse lesion, as the intake of solid and even semi-solid food, as a rule, is greatly reduced, especially in high thoracic and cervical lesions. An enema of saline or soap solution in the acute stage is only indicated if digital examination reveals heavy accumulation of bowel content in the rectum, and it should be given carefully by an experienced nurse. Such an enema will at least remove the contents of a full rectum, and may also serve as stimulation to the sigmoid colon.

Sedatives and analgesics should, if possible, be avoided in the initial stage, as these drugs delay the development of the automatic function of the intestinal tract.

The second stage (automatic or autonomous function)

The return of peristalsis and bowel sounds varies from case to case but, as a rule, the first sounds appear within 2 or 3 days of cord transection at higher level, commensurate with proper management. The anal and bulbo-cavernosus reflexes, which at first are absent, will return early in cord lesions above the thoraco-lumbar junction, provided, no longitudinal damage affecting the spinal centre of defaecation has occurred. Once peristalsis has returned and the reflex activity of the isolated cord has started, intermittent automatic reflex defaecation occurs in cord lesions above the thoraco-lumbar junction. It is then the time to start planned defaecation.

Various factors may influence the establishment and efficiency of rectal reflex stimulation in the spinal man:

1 Positioning of the patient. Prolonged recumbency has certainly an adverse effect on the establishment of early and efficient reflex defaecation. During the Second World War, when the comprehensive management of spinal paraplegics and tetraplegics was not fully understood, this was conspicuous in paraplegics treated with prolonged recumbency in plaster casts. Some of these patients were admitted to Stoke Mandeville not only with over-loaded rectum but also with extreme faecal retention in all other compartments of the large bowels which had become hardened. These patients were often suffering from intermittent diarrhoea as a result of contractions of the overdistended colon and rectum (diarrhoea ex constipatione, diarrhoea paradoxa, overflow diarrhoea), and some of these patients were suffering from the effect of colonic distension on other autonomic mechanisms, as have been described as a result of bladder distension. However, this autonomic hyperreflexia as the result of colonic distension was found, as a rule, less pronounced as compared with the effects of bladder distension, owing to the greater elasticity of colon and rectum. Throbbing headaches may sometimes represent the leading symptom of intestinal distension. Regular turning day and night from the supine to the lateral positions facilitates bowel movement, whilst the patient is confined to bed. Exercises with chest expanders and gentle massage of the abdomen have also proved helpful in this respect.

2 The chemical and physical qualities of food certainly affect the rate of passage through the intestinal tract. Food of low residue, such as meat, rice, white bread, etc., progress more slowly than those with high residue, such as cabbage, bananas, animal and mineral fats; moreover, fruit juice, yoghourt and lactose act as mild laxatives.

3 The reflex activity of the isolated cord, both hypo- and hyperreflexia, may influence reflex defaecation. In lesions above T6, in which the abdominal muscles are involved in the spastic contractions of the muscles below the level of the lesion, these contractions may interfere with the propulsive activity of the various compartments of the intestinal tract, and may lead to increased activity of certain segments only. This in turn may lead to inadequate bulk being propelled to the distal colon. Moreover, it must be remembered that, in the stage of hyperreflexia, the tonicity of the external anal sphincter is greatly increased and, therefore, its resistance to the expulsive function of sigmoid and rectum is magnified.

Constipation in lesions resulting in destruction of the lumbo-sacral cord or of its spinal roots is of a different nature. In this event, the neural connections between the spinal centre and sigmoid colon and rectum are cut off, and these parts of the intestinal tract become autonomous. The paralysis is of lower motor neuron type, and the normal response of sigmoid and rectum to distension and the tonicity of the external sphincter is lost, the latter becoming patulous. The function of the levator ani is also impaired. There will be progressive accumulation of faeces which become hardened resulting in impaction. Moreover, owing to the complete loss of sensibility in the sacral area rectal incontinence is not uncommon. Defaecation in this type of paralysis depends on the volitional increase of intra-abdominal pressure and digital evacuation. During the second stage, as long as the patient is confined to bed, this will have to be executed by the nursing staff with the aid of suppositories and enemas. We have preferred to give the enema in a lateral position. It is recommended that the rectal evacuation, whether with or without enema, should be done preferably in the morning, either before or after breakfast, to initiate the regular habit of defaecation in the patient.

The third stage (reconditioning of intestinal function)

In this phase of readjustment, the full co-operation of the patient in the planned defaecation is of greatest importance to make the paraplegic socially acceptable, and the sooner his upright position and standing is established the better the result. It is important at this stage to carry out a thorough X-ray investigation of the gastrointestinal tract with the aid of contrast means. This will give information about any congenital or acquired abnormalities, such as enteroptosis, diverticulosis, megacolon, chronic gastric or duodenal ulcer, etc., which may have adverse effects on the reconditioning of the intestinal tract and need appropriate treatment. Unlike the bladder, the readjustment of the patient to his intestinal dysfunction can be accomplished in the great majority of cases, provided the patient's early instruction about his type of intestinal dysfunction and his systematic training to adjust himself to his intestinal disturbance is instituted. The aim is to establish a habit of regular and complete evacuation of the bowel once a day or every second day at a specific time. It has become a custom for these patients to evacuate the bowels every second day, but the patient and his attendant at home should really be advised to have his bowels open every day. Naturally, his pre-paraplegic habit of emptying the bowels will have to be taken into account. As a rule, the most suitable time for this procedure is the period after a meal in the morning, when the gastro-colic reflex acts as an excitatory stimulus to the peristalsis. In order to achieve a regular habit, enemas should be discontinued as soon as possible, and automatic reflex evacuation in cord lesions, if necessary with the help of mild laxatives and glycerine or bisacodyl (Dulcolax) suppositories, encouraged. Early return of the patient's upright position, as already stressed, is of great assistance. Moreover, in this stage of reconditioning, the patient must learn to utilize certain afferent stimuli, such as gentle massage of the abdomen, bending forwards to increase the intra-abdominal pressure or digital stimulation of the anal area. Stagnation of the contents of the lower intestinal tract, which not infrequently develops in later stages of cord lesions and may lead to constipation in these distal compartments, can be counteracted by stool softeners, such as mineral or vegetable oil or Dioctyl forte (sodium sulfosuccinate). The latter has proved particularly useful. The laxatives used at Stoke Mandeville are Sennacot tablets or granules, Cascara Elix, Syrup of Figs or Dubhalac liqu. (Lactulose), and their dosage as well as type has to be varied on occasions to achieve an optimal effect. Drastic laxatives should be avoided as far as possible, and liquid paraffin should be used only temporarily, because of its preventative action of carotene and fat absorption. In cervical lesions of higher level, evacuation of the bowels will have to be carried out by an attendant, preferably with the patient lying in lateral position, while tetraplegics below C7 and especially C8 have learned to open their bowels on the toilet.

In conus–cauda equina lesions, evacuation of the bowels depends on the severity of the lesion. In those cases where the parasympathetic connections to sigmoid and rectum are not completely interrupted, the peristaltic function of these intestinal compartments is still active, and the external rectal sphincter maintains its reflex function, although the external anal sphincter may be flaccid. Therefore, conditioned reflex function of these patients, as described above, is still possible. In more severe or complete conus–cauda equina lesions, where all connections between sacral cord and sigmoid and rectum are severed, rectal evacuation depends on the compensatory function of the intramural, autonomous innervation and the expulsive force of intermittent efficient intra-abdominal pressure by the action of diaphragm and abdominal muscles. The ability of the sigmoid to act as a reservoir is still present, and the efficient expulsive forces of abdominal pressure will evacuate the bolus into the rectum. However, digital evacuation by gloved finger will be necessary to avoid both constipation and incontinence. Colostomy, as recommended previously (Munro, 1952) to prevent rectal incontinence in these patients has not been found necessary in any of our conus–cauda equina lesions.

The development of haemorrhoids and anal fissures is a complication in later stages, in particular of conus–cauda equina lesions. While the latter is certainly the result of mucosal damage by careless and faulty digital evacuation, the former is the result of chronic constipation and prolonged strong abdominal pressure during faecal evacuation. However, this complication can, as a rule, be controlled by phenol injections, and only very seldom are more extensive operative procedures necessary. The same applies to the mucosal prolapse of the rectum as a result of intensive abdominal pressure and weakness of the levator ani.

Before the paraplegic or tetraplegic is discharged from hospital treatment, his attendants at home should receive information and guidance by the medical officer and nurse in charge of the case about the patient's intestinal dysfunction, to ensure his proper management after discharge.

CHAPTER 29

THE SEXUAL PROBLEM

Sexual disturbances, which inevitably follow a severe injury of the spinal cord, regardless of whether the lesion is complete or incomplete, constitute a complex problem in the rehabilitation of paraplegics and even more in tetraplegics. It must be remembered that, whatever the level and however severe the spinal cord injury may be, the urge to sexual relationship, the libido, continues commensurate with the patient's age and his or her pre-paraplegic sexual tendencies and activities. No mastery over physical disability can completely dispel that yearning for affection which is just as common in most severely disabled people as it is in the able-bodied. Therefore, the readjustment of the paraplegic to his sexual dysfunction and the adequate supplementation of his sexual drive is essential for his successful domestic and social resettlement. In this repect it is an important duty of the Medical Officer to give guidance to his male as well as female patients by discussing freely their sexual problems including advising in techniques of intercourse.

A. IN THE MALE

We have to consider here, in particular, the problems of potency and fertility. Both married and unmarried patients in the majority are naturally interested in their chances of reproductive activity. This information was found to be sometimes particularly important to patients of the Catholic faith or those who were engaged to Catholic girls. For, if their parents and, indeed, sometimes priests still adhered to the view, generally held for a long time, that paraplegics and tetraplegics were impotent and infertile, the people concerned met great opposition to marriage. Experience during the last 25 years has shown that such generalized prejudice is no longer acceptable.

The pathophysiology of sexual function

Normal sexual function depends on a co-ordinated activity of cerebral, spinal and peripheral components of the nervous system as well as on the condition of the anatomical structures of the reproductive organs themselves. Following spinal cord transection, one has, as with bladder and bowels, to distinguish three phases in the pathophysiology of the sexual organs: spinal shock, reflex return and re-adjustment.

Stage of spinal shock

In the stage of spinal shock, voluntary control is eliminated, as descending messages from the brain are blocked at the point of transection, as also are afferent impulses to the brain from the reproductive organs via the spinal cord at the point of transection. The erectional and ejaculatory functions are abolished. It is true that, in complete lesions, the penis becomes enlarged and more or less semi-erected, which is often misinterpreted as priapism, while actually this is a result of a passive engorgement of the corpora cavernosa due to the paralytic vasodilatation following the interruptions of the vasoconstrictor fibres in the antero-lateral tracts of the spinal cord. Priapism—i.e. complete and permanent erection—may occur in incomplete lesions in the acute stage if reflex function is present.

Stage of reflex automatism

Once the stage of spinal shock has subsided, the erection reflex becomes one of the components of the automatic functions of the isolated cord, taking part in the 'mass response' (Riddoch, 1917). In fact, it may appear, independent of cerebral participation, before the reflex responses of the skeletal muscles are fully developed. Tactile stimuli of varying type and intensity of the glans and around the penis, extending perineally or to either side of the medial surface of the thigh, or even stroking of the sole of the feet set up afferent impulses along the pudendal nerves to the 2nd–4th sacral segment, resulting in efferent responses, which run along the parasympathetic pathways causing increased blood supply and distension of the corpora cavernosa and corpus spongiosum. This will be associated with a reflex contraction of the bulbocavernosus, ischiocavernosus and the transverse perineal muscles, which are involved in the ejaculation reflex. Once the summation of afferent impulses during the process of erection is strong enough to elicit contraction of the seminal vesicles, stimulation of the prostate gland and the ejaculatory duct, resulting in ejaculation of the seminal fluid through the urethra is possible only by an associated reflex contraction of the internal sphincter complex of the bladder, which closes the bladder exit. Otherwise, as occurs following prostatectomy, the seminal fluid is ejected into the bladder. From all this, it is obvious how much seminal ejaculation in both complete and incomplete transections above the thoraco-lumbar junction depends on the integrity of a co-ordinated reflex activity of the various stations of the copulatory organs and how important it is to avoid their early local damage due to infection of the bladder.

Complete lesions

Reflex erection leading to seminal ejaculation in complete transverse lesions above the thoraco-lumbar junction, is rare; moreover, it also depends on the willingness and ability of the female partner to adjust herself to the paraplegic's position. If ejaculation in complete lesions occurs, this is without orgastic sensation, but in lesions above T5—in particular, cervical lesions—ejaculation is accompanied by stress phenomena of certain autonomic mechanisms (autonomic hyperreflexia), such as rise of blood pressure, bradycardia, sweating in face and headache. The paraplegic's gratification following ejaculation is certainly his pride in being able to satisfy the female partner. Moreover, successful ejaculation is followed by relaxation of the spasticity of the skeletal muscles. But there is no awareness of any somesthetic sensation of orgasm, especially in high lesions of the spinal cord.

Incomplete lesions

In incomplete cord lesions, various types of sexual dysfunction may occur depending on the severity of lesion. There may be dissociations between strength and duration of erection and power of ejaculation. Moreover, the associated closing reflex of the internal sphincter complex of the bladder may be impaired, resulting in ejaculation of seminal fluid into the bladder, or seminal urethral ejaculation is associated with discharge of urine.

Orgastic sensations may or may not occur in incomplete lesions, depending on whether or not there has been bilateral damage of the spino-thalamic tracts. In unilateral damage of the spino-thalamic tract, orgastic sensation is, as a rule, present although more or less diminished.

Excessive flexor—and especially adductor spasms—may be a great obstacle to penile penetration, even in incomplete lesions with good erection and ejaculation. Resection of the obturator nerve has proved, in our experience, to be most successful in removing this obstacle and ensuring satisfactory intercourse.

Cauda equina lesion. In cauda equina lesions, erection at will and reflexly is abolished only if the sacral centre between S2–S5 is destroyed, but seminal discharge may occur without erection if the lumbar component of the centre has escaped damage. However, some patients with incomplete or dissociated lesions of the cauda equina are able to get good erections at will, but either have at first no orgastic sensations or, in fact, experience discomfort and pain during ejaculation and are easily put off making further attempts. However, by further trial, the pain usually disappears and is replaced first by a sensation of warmth and later by some pleasurable sensation.

Sexual desire—dreams

There is a difference between the age groups as far as sexual desire is concerned. As one would expect, sexual desire is certainly more pronounced in the younger age groups, regardless of whether or not the individuals had been married or had had an active sexual life before their paraplegia or tetraplegia. In the writer's experience no great differences between males and females were observed in this respect, although in the manifestation of her sexual desire the female will be more passive than the male. This is evidenced by the greater interest of male paraplegics in sexual material, such as literature, pictures and photographs. It is not uncommon to find photographs or calendars of nude girls in various positions hanging on the wall of rooms occupied by male paraplegics living in hostels and other institutions. In this respect, there is really no difference between the paralysed and the able-bodied male.

An interesting point is the question of dreams, both day and night dreams, in paraplegics and tetraplegics. From personal interviews of both males and females it would appear that erotic dreams occur, especially in those who had sexual experiences before their spinal injury. In all the dreams reported, the individuals saw themselves as not paralysed. However, more experience on this subject is necessary to come to definite conclusions.

Sexual re-adjustment

The sexual re-adjustment of the paralysed is conditioned to a great deal by their desire, experience and sexual habits in their pre-paraplegic life, whether this applies to love play or actual methods of intercourse. It will also greatly depend on the co-operation and helpfulness of the partner. Individuals, who had been indifferent to sexual activity before their paraplegia, will hardly change. On the other hand, young married couples in particular, will be very eager to adjust themselves in one way or another to the new situation. Data published of the percentage of paraplegics and tetraplegics capable of intercourse vary (Bors, 1963; Jackson, 1972). Jackson recently found in 20 male paraplegic and tetraplegic athletes 85 per cent who had erections and 90 per cent who were able to carry out intercourse but only 35 per cent who had ejaculations and orgasm. However, these statistics do not classify these cases into complete and incomplete lesions.

It is much easier for a female paraplegic to satisfy her husband than for a male to prevent frustration of his spouse, if he gets only short-lasting strong erections or semi-erections or no erections at all. In those with short-lasting erection or semi-erection, attempts could be made to maintain the erection by a constricting device such as application of a rubber ring at the base of the penis, as recommended by Reuben (quoted by Jackson). However, many couples have found alternative methods of sexual intercourse by manual or oral stimulation and even by artificial penile appliances of plastic material.

It is obvious that in the sexual re-adjustment of spinal paraplegics and tetraplegics medical guidance must play a very important role. Once shyness and embarrassment on the part of the patient as well as of the medical attendant is overcome, the patient and his or her spouse will be only too pleased and grateful to discuss freely their sexual problems. The medical attendant can be of tremendous help, especially in young couples who had had no sexual experience before their paraplegia. The medical advice should include the most suitable time for and the positioning during intercourse, which may vary from case to case. Another important aspect in connection with intercourse is the function of the bladder in the individual case to avoid urination during intercourse. All this shows how important the proper assessment of potency and fertility is in these patients, which will be discussed in the following chapter.

The assessment of potency and fertility

Investigators have employed various procedures to assess potency and fertility in paraplegics and tetraplegics, which can be divided into two main groups:

(1) Questionnaire and personal interview technique

The investigators have, of course, to rely entirely on the statements of the individual by these techniques. Results obtained with these methods were reported by Bors in 1948 on 157 and in 1963 on 529 patients, Talbot in 1949 on 208 and in 1955 on 408 patients, Zeitlin *et al.* in 1957 on 100 and Tsuji *et al.* in 1961 on 655 patients. The latter authors stressed the difference between results obtained with the questionnaire technique and those during personal interview, by finding a higher percentage of erections and ejaculations recorded by the personal interview technique. However, there is general agreement amongst all these authors that the percentage of erections varying between 52–94 per cent were infinitely higher than that of the ejaculations 3–19·7 per cent. Intercourse capability varied between 23–33 per cent, orgasm 6–14 per cent, and reproductive results were the lowest (up to 5 per cent). Bors (1963) stated that while erection is more frequent with high lesions ejaculation occurs more often in those with low lesions. This is not, as will be shown later, in accordance with our experience.

(2) Direct examination of the ejaculate obtained

(a) *By prostatic massage.* This technique was used by Horne, Paul & Munro (1948). These authors found that the amount of ejaculate by prostatic massage could be increased with prior electric rectal stimulation—a method which was previously employed by Dexter, Lerner & Kaplan (1940) and by Joel (1941). However, Bors and co-workers were not impressed by the results obtained with this method in their own cases, which was in accordance with Kuhn's findings (1950).

Frankel *et al.* (1974) reported the effects of rectal intermittent electrical stimulation with up to 20 volts on blood pressure, plasma catecholamines and prostaglandins in a tetraplegic below C7/8. Electrical stimulation invariably resulted in autonomic hyper-reflexia including increase of plasma noradrenaline and large elevation of prostaglandin E.

(b) *By testicular biopsy.* Bors and co-workers studied biopsy specimens from testes in 34 patients with spinal cord injuries. They found that in all but 3 cases the biopsy revealed tubular atrophy while there was no disturbance of Leydig cells. Furthermore, with 2 exceptions, they found a correlation between testicular biopsy findings and the level of the spinal cord lesion. Lesions at or below T11 showed a lesser degree of testicular abnormality. The authors also correlated the biopsy findings with the result of sweat tests, using the Quinizarin method (Guttmann, 1937–47), and thus were able to study the relationship between testicular function and other components of the autonomic system. With 4 exceptions, a close relationship was found between testicular biopsy findings and the result of the sweat test. Lesser testicular changes were associated with normal sweating, while major testicular abnormalities were associated with impaired sweating. However, the 4 exceptions showed that there may be dissociation between these two components of the autonomic system. The disadvantage of testicular biopsy is that, for obvious reasons, it cannot be considered as a routine method in these patients and, moreover, it cannot give any indication of the function of the genital organs as a whole, nor does it give any indication of volume, sperm concentration, sperm motility and percentage of normal and abnormal forms.

(c) *By the intrathecal prostigmin assessment test.* My own studies on fertility in paraplegics and tetraplegics started in 1946, when I discovered an amazingly and selectively stimu-lating effect of prostigmine on the function of the reproductive organs following intra-thecal injection. It was previously known from the studies of Kremer & Wright on cerebral hemiplegia patients (1941) that intrathecal injection of prostigmine has a depressant effect on the skeletal muscles leading to hypo- or areflexia, unlike its stimulating effect on these muscles following intramuscular injection—hence generally employed in the treatment of myasthenia gravis. I, therefore, used intrathecal injection of prostigmine at the height of its depressant effect to determine the degree of flexion contracture developed as a result of intractable spasticity. In the course of this study, I found that a dosage of 0·25–0·3 mg was sufficient to elicit erections and ejaculations in traumatic paraplegics and tetraplegics, who hitherto were thought to be completely impotent and infertile. This test has been employed systematically ever since to assess the potentialities of erections and fertility in the spinal man, and the results on 34 and 90 patients respectively have been previously published (Guttmann, 1953, 1960). Recently, results on 134 patients at levels ranging from C5 to S4 were published, in whom over 180 tests were carried out (Guttmann & Walsh, 1970). One hundred and two patients had complete and 32 incomplete lesions. One hundred and four showed spasticity of various degrees and 30 were flaccid. The average age of the patient was about 28, the youngest being 18, the oldest 47. All patients were in satisfactory general condition at the time of the test and free from infected sores, but the great majority had some infection of the urinary tract.

Indications

The initial test was carried out to determine spermatic abnormalities, as it is well known that reduction of sperm concentration and reduced motility play an important role in male infertility. Both married and unmarried paraplegics in the great majority are naturally greatly interested in their chances of reproductive activity. Repeated tests were carried out:
1   to check the motility and concentration of sperms and their cytology,
2   to repeat the test with a higher dosage, when the first test revealed a negative result. In a few of the patients, the dosage had to be increased to 0·5, 0·7 and even 1 mg.
3   to check motility concentration and differential cytology following hormone treatment,
4   for the purpose of artificial insemination.

Methods and dosage

Because of certain undesirable side effects, especially vomiting, the patient has to refrain from solid food for some hours before the test and for 3 hours before injection the patient should not take anything by mouth. Before the test, a full neurological examination of the lower limbs is carried out and full assessment of reflexes and muscle tone has to be made. This is of special importance in more distal cord lesions, as there are often mixed forms of spasticity and hypo- or areflexia in certain parts of the lower limbs. This is particularly apparent in transverse lesions below T10/11, where the injury may also affect the conus and epiconus, or in higher transverse lesions which are combined with longitudinal damage.

Procedure. The patient is prepared in the usual way for a lumbar puncture and the test is carried out in a separate room. The drug used was neostigmin methyl sulphate

(Prostigmin—Roche), made up in 1 cm³ ampules each containing 0·5 mg, and a clearly marked 2 cm³ syringe is essential for the accurate amount of prostigmin injected.

After lumbar puncture (carried out in lateral position), the Queckenstedt test is carried out to ascertain the presence or absence of a subarachnoid block, as this has some bearing on the dosage. If there is no or only a partial block, 0·3 mg prostigmin is injected after first withdrawing 1–2 cm³ C.S.F. into the syringe to mix with the prostigmin. In high thoracic and cervical injuries, it is safer to start with 0·25 mg because of the rise in blood pressure in these high lesions during ejaculations, as a result of powerful contractions of the seminal vesicles and other ejaculatory organs, which may set up the same autonomic hyperreflexia as described previously by the forceful contraction of bladder and other internal organs (Guttmann & Whitteridge, 1947; Guttmann, 1954, 1969). If there was a complete block 0·3 to 0·5 mg was injected. In some cases where the initial test was negative and especially if the neurological examination indicated little or no effect on muscle tone and reflexes, the test was repeated, using larger doses of prostigmin provided there had been no untoward side effects during the original injection. Up to 1·5 mg prostigmine has been given in one exceptional case. After the injection, the needle is withdrawn, a dressing applied and the patient turned on his back with a pillow under his head. A suitable glass container with a screw cap is given to the patient with instructions to observe any erections and obtain any semen ejaculated. The examination of reflexes and muscle tone in the lower limbs is carried out repeatedly after the injection and recorded every ½–1 hour as this gives a good indication of the effect of prostigmin in each individual case. In distal lesions with areflexia, this information is, of course, not obtainable. It is important to measure pulse and blood pressure regularly during the test, especially in high thoracic and cervical lesions because of the possibility of exaggerated autonomic hyperreflexia due to seminal contraction during ejaculation. Moreover, in high thoracic and in particular cervical lesions a cystometrogram some time prior to the prostigmine test may give a clue about the threshold of irritability of the autonomic system.

The depressant effect on reflex function of the skeletal muscles (Table 25) started as a rule between 15 and 20 minutes after intrathecal injection, but there was usually a considerable delay—1 to 3 hours—before the onset of erections and ejaculations, which usually occurred at the height of the reflex depression. Once an erection had started, it continued in most cases for a considerable time, either intermittently or continuously, and sometimes it persisted for hours even after emissions occurred. In 2 low thoracic lesions (T10 and T12), with flaccid paralysis of the legs and one conus lesion, ejaculations occurred without erections.

The number of ejaculations varied considerably from patient to patient and also in different tests in the same patient. Only the minority of patients produced a single emission and as many as 7 or more were observed in some patients within a period of 2 hours. Table 26 shows number and percentage of positive ejaculations results in our 134 patients, divided into spastic and flaccid complete and incomplete lesions, and as can be seen in Table 27 the majority of negative results occurred both in spastic and flaccid lesions at levels between T10 and L4.

The volume of ejaculated seminal fluid varied considerably from patient to patient

TABLE 25. Effect of intrathecal prostigmin on reflex function

Case	Lesion	Reflex function before injection						Reflex function at time of ejaculation or at height of effect on motor function					
		K.J. R.	K.J. L.	A.J. R.	A.J. L.	P.R. R.	P.R. L.	K.J. R.	K.J. L.	A.J. R.	A.J. L.	P.R. R.	P.R. L.
1	C7 Complete	−	±	++	++	→	→	−	−	−	+	←	→
2	T5 Complete	+++	+++	+++	+++	←	←	−	−	?	±	↻	↻
3	T6 Complete	+++	+++	+++	±	→	→	−	−	(+)	(+)	→	↻
4	T6/7 Complete	+++	+++	+++	+++	←	←	−	−	−	((+))	↻	↻
5	T6/7 Complete	+++	+++	+++	+++	←	←	−	−	((+))	((+))	↻	↻
6	T7 Complete	+++	+++	+++	+++	←	←	−	−	−	−	↻	↻
7	T7 Complete	+++	+++	±	++	←	←	(+)	+	−	−	−	−
8	T7 Complete	+++	+++	−	−	−	−	(+)	+++	−	−	−	−
9	T9 Complete	+++	+++	+++	+++	←	←	(+)	(+)	(+)	(+)	→	→
10	T10 Incomplete	+++	+++	+++	+++	←	←	+	−	+	+	↻	↻
11	T10 Complete	+++	−	+++	+++	→	→	+	−	+	(+)	←	−
12	T10 Complete	+++	+++	+++	+++	←	←	−	−	−	−	−	−
13	T11/12 Complete	−	−	+++	+	(↻)	←	+	−	(+)	−	((↻))	−
14	L1/L2 Complete	+	+	−	−	−	−	−	−	−	−	−	−
15	L1/L3 Complete	−	−	+++	++	←	←	−	−	−	−	−	−
16	L2 Complete (Spastic)	++	+	+++	+++	←	←	−	−	−	−	−	−
17	L5 Complete	+	−	−	−	−	←	−	−	−	−	−	−
18	S1 Incomplete	−	−	−	−	−	−	−	−	−	−	−	−
19	S2 Incomplete	+	+	+	−	→	→	−	−	−	−	−	−

From Guttman and Walsh (1971), *Paraplegia*, **9**, 39.

TABLE 26. Prostigmin test

				Positive	Negative
Spastic 104 (77·6%)	Complete	75	(72·1%)	44 (59·7%)	31 (40·3%)
	Incomplete	29	(27·9%)	23 (79·3%)	6 (20·7%)
Flaccid 30 (22·4%)	Complete	27	(90%)	9 (33·3%)	18 (66·7%)
	Incomplete	3	(10%)	2 (66·7%)	1 (33·3%)
Total 134		134		78 (58·2%)	56 (41·9%)

TABLE 27. Prostigmin test

					Positive	Negative
Cervical (7·46%)	10	Complete	Spastic	3	1	2
			Flaccid	1	—	1*
		Incomplete	Spastic	6	6	—
			Flaccid	—	—	—
T1–T6 (22·38%)	30	Complete	Spastic	25	20	5
			Flaccid	2	1	1
		Incomplete	Spastic	3	3	—
			Flaccid	—	—	—
T7–T9 (22·38%)	30	Complete	Spastic	19	14	5
			Flaccid	1	—	1
		Incomplete	Spastic	9	5	4
			Flaccid (Polio)	1	1	—
T10–T12 (31·34%)	42	Complete	Spastic	19	7	12
			Flaccid	12	3	9
		Incomplete	Spastic	10	8	2
			Flaccid	1	1	—
L1–L4 (11·97%)	16	Complete	Spastic	8	2	6
			Flaccid	8	3	5
		Incomplete	Spastic	—	—	—
			Flaccid	—	—	—
L5–S4 (4·47%)	6	Complete	Spastic	1	—	1
			Flaccid	3	2	1
		Incomplete	Spastic	1	1	—
			Flaccid	1	—	1
Total	134			134	78	56

* Alcohol block.

TABLE 28

Name	Age	Date of test	Comp.	Incomp.	Spastic	Flaccid	Dose prostig- mine mg	Result emission	Volume cc	Count mill.	Motility per cent	Differential count
Sturg.	32	9.11.48	–	T12	+	–	0·4	1 – (Urine)	–	–	–	
								2 – (Urine)	–	–	–	
								3 – (Urine)	–	–	–	
								4 +	1·0	87	44	73% abnormal
								5 +	1·1	51	42	
								6 +	1·2	58	37	14% immature
								7 +	0·7	41	33	
Fro.	29	10.9.48	S1	–	–	+	0·5	1 +	1·0	4·5	23	Squamous cells + Testicular cells +
								2 +	1·1	3·1	20	Testicular cells +
								3 +	0·9	2	17	Testicular cells +
								4 +	0·5	2·3	18	Testicular cells +
								5 +	0·5	0·95	11	Debris
								6 +	0·3	0·6	9	Debris
								7 +	0·3	0·56	5	Debris
Harv.	27	2.2.48	C7/T1	–	+	–	0·3	1 +	1	73	2	Pus cells
								2/3 +	2	57	4	Pus cells and R.B.C.
								4/5 +	0·5	23	20	Pus cells and R.B.C.
								6 +	0·5	15	20	Pus cells and R.B.C.
Morg.	37	8.1.48	–	C6	+	–	0·3	1 +	1·5	45	60	–
								2 +	7·7	46	50	–
Craw.	23	12.10.56	T7	–	+	–	0·4	1 +	5·0	100	10%	
								2 +	2·5	100	(5%)	
								3 +	1·5	50		
								4 +	5	25	weak	
								5 +	<1	nil		–

and also in different tests on the same patient. In those cases who had several ejaculations, the volume of each emission became progressively less. However, sometimes the second or third emission was found to be larger than the first. This may be accounted for by the fact that in these cases there had been no ejaculation for very long periods before the tests, and it would appear that, in some of them, accumulated stimuli were necessary to set the whole mechanism of ejaculation into action.

In a number of cases, pH estimation of the seminal fluid was made which varied between 7–7·5. In one case a pH of 8 was found. In future, this test should be carried out systematically.

No relationship was found between volume and sperm concentration in the various subjects or in repeated tests on the same subject. Considerable variations were found, and the ejaculate may be just prostatic fluid with complete aspermia. Conversely, a small volume of seminal fluid may contain a much higher sperm concentration than a large volume.

The percentage of viable motile sperms was, as a rule, well below normal, especially in complete lesions, but in a small number of patients there were 50 per cent and more of viable sperms. Table 27 demonstrates examples of results obtained in 5 patients complete and incomplete, of various level, who during the test had more than one emission. It is known from fertility tests in normal subjects that, although a high motility of sperms is an

TABLE 29. Comparative microscopic results of seminal fluid in two prostigmine tests
cauda equina lesion (incomplete) below L5

Specimen	Volume		Count (millions, 1 cm^3)		Motility	
	13.2.48 cm^3	5.10.48 cm^3	13.2.48	5.10.48	13.2.48 per cent	5.10.48 per cent
1	0·5	1·0	11	50	5	70
2	0·5	1·0	12	49	10	70
3	0·5	5·0	111	116	40	50
4	4·5	1·0	90	57	40	50
5	1·0	1·0	122	47	30	40
6	0·5	2·0	142	3·6	30	20

Differential count: 13 February 1948
Specimen 1: 50 per cent abnormal forms (some tailless, some with two heads)
Specimen 6: 40 per cent abnormal forms (some tailless, some with two heads)
Differential count: 5 October 1948
Specimen 3: Head abnormalities = 49 per cent
Middlepiece and Tail abnormalities = 26 per cent
Total abnormalities = 55 per cent
Specimen 4: Head abnormalities
Specimen 4: Head abnormalities = 36 per cent
Middlepiece and Tail abnormalities = 29 per cent
Total abnormalities = 65 per cent

essential property of fertile spermatozoa, the ratio of motility provides only a rough index to the viability of the sperm population and its suitability for fertilizing the ovum (Harvey & Jackson, 1945).

Considerable variations were also found on detailed cytological examination in the percentage of normal and abnormal forms of sperms and other cells. The following case (case 17, Table 24) may serve as an example of detailed cytological examination, the more so as a comparison is possible between two tests carried out in this patient.

This patient was wounded in June 1944 and sustained an incomplete cauda equina lesion below L5. He had a cordotomy in October 1944, because of pain in right leg. Recurrence of pain recurred after 3 weeks although less severe. He had erections and nocturnal emissions 3 months after injury but lost emissions after cordotomy, however, he still had spontaneous erections. He was able to walk.

First intrathecal prostigmine test 17 February 1948, 0·3 mg. Second test 5 November 1948, 0·3 mg. He had 6 emissions on each occasion.

Table 29 shows the comparative microscopic results of seminal fluid in the two tests. Table 30 shows 6 patients with negative results in repeated tests in spite of increased dosage. It may be noted, however, that one single negative result does not necessarily signify permanent infertility, as improvement of reproductive function is possible. Actually, the prostigmine test may act as an induced stimulus on the function of the reproductive organs. Three of our patients with negative results became fathers later— one, an incomplete lesion below T7, even of twins. Although, for obvious reasons, some scepticism regarding paternity in these patients may be justified, the possibility of such achievement cannot be ruled out.

It has already been mentioned, that one of the reasons for the prostigmin test is to use the seminal fluid obtained for artificial insemination at the request of patients failing to get ejaculations during intercourse. The first 4 cases have been reported previously (Guttmann, 1960). They were all unsuccessful. However, the cause may not necessarily be with the paraplegic male. In one of the cases, the examination of the wife revealed an uterus bicornis and in another the wife was suffering from inflammation of the cervix. In 10 more cases, artificial insemination has since been carried out by Dr Walsh. In two cases, the wives conceived, but in one abortion took place after 3 months and in the other after 5 months. No information is available about the gynaecological conditions of these wives. Table 31 gives information about the number of artificial inseminations carried out in 5 cases and the findings of the seminal fluid in these cases. However, that this method can be used successfully has been shown by Dr R.Spira (1956), one of my former co-workers, whose paraplegic patient—a complete 7th thoracic lesion—fathered a child after three unsuccessful attempts by assisted insemination with the help of the intrathecal prostigmin test. This case also shows that improvement of fertility is possible in the paraplegic. Spira's patient was treated with Testosterone, 24 mg daily for 14 days and Gonadotrophin 1,000 units daily for 4 weeks. We, also, have given hormonal treatment combined with vitamin E 20 mg three times daily and in addition, in certain cases with weak erections with Potensan (Medo) 2–3 pellets 2–3 times daily. Although we have seen definite improvement of fertility, our results do not allow definite conclusions.

Recently Andres (1972) confirmed the effectiveness of the prostigmine test.

TABLE 30

Name	Age	Date of test	Level of lesion		Spastic	Flaccid	Dose prostigmine (mg)	Result
			Comp.	Incomp.				
Vid.	21	22.5.63 13.6.63	T6	−	−	+	0·4 0·5	−
Att.	43	3.10.66 31.10.66 29.11.66	T10	−	+	−	0·25 0·37 0·75	− −
Crock.	22	27.7.64 21.9.64	−	T10	+	−	0·3 0·5	− −
All.	30	5.4.62 2.5.62 20.11.62	−	T11	±	−	0·3 0·5 0·75	− − −
Win.	25	8.9.60 6.10.60 2.11.60	T12	−	+	−	0·3 0·5 0·75	− − −
Holl.	30	29.7.63 24.1.64	L1/3	−	±	−	0·3 0·6	− −

Name	Age	Date of prostigmine	Level Comp.	Incomp.	Spastic	Flaccid	Dose	Result No. of emissions	Total sperm	Motility per cent	Pus cells	Insemination	Result insem.
Den.	28	10.4.69		C6	Yes		0·25	+3	100 m.	< 5	RBC	+	–
									60 m.	16	+++		
		30.6.69		C6	Yes		0·25	+3	25 m.	20	no significant growth		
Cor.	30	12.4.65	T5		Yes		0·3	+2	45 m.	6		+	–
		11.6.65	T5		Yes		0·3	+2	50 m.	5		+	–
		12.10.65	T5		Yes		0·4	+2	not reported sl. active	< 5	+++	+	?3/12 abortion correspondence
		11.7.66	T5		Yes		0·45	+2	100 m.	10		+	–
		18.10.66	T5		Yes		0·4	+2	70 m.	7		+	–
		24.2.67	T5		Yes		0·4	+1	?	?		+	–
		19.6.67	T5		Yes		0·4	+2	?	?		+ with Dutch cap	–
Sym.	28	18.11.66		T6	Yes		0·25	+3	50 m.	10	+++	+	–
		11.2.67		T6	Yes		0·25	+5	45 m.	40	+++	+	–
		19.9.67		T6	Yes		0·25	+4/5	40 m.	20	+	+	–
Elm.	36	19.5.66	T7		Yes		0·3	–	some motile	(10) sl.	–	+	–
		7.11.67	T7		Yes		0·4	+1					
		24.10.68	T7		Yes		0·4	+3	65 m.	1	sterile	+	–
Reev.	29	3.3.56	T7		Yes		0·5	+4	330 m.	75 abnormal + 9 active			
	38	9.8.65	T7		Yes		0·45	+2	200 m.	20 fully			
		10.1.66	T7		Yes		0·45	+3	50 m.	10 slightly		+	–
		2.5.66	T7		Yes		0·25	+3	½ m.	5 slightly 10		+	–

Side effects on autonomic mechanisms

This chapter would not be complete without mentioning some undesirable side effects of prostigmin on the cardio-vascular system and other components of autonomic mechanisms. Headaches, sweating and vomiting may occur, regardless of the level of the lesion, and if vomiting becomes more marked, it may counteract the prostigmin's stimulating effect on the reproductive organs. It can be controlled by 1/100 Atropine. Only in 3 cases, was it thought wise to give an intravenous drip of saline to prevent dehydration. It has already been mentioned that, in cord lesions above T5 and in particular cervical lesions, violent contractions of the ejaculatory organs can set up that stress response of autonomic mechanisms described as a result of bladder distension (Guttmann & Whitteridge, 1947), resulting in exaggerated autonomic hyperreflexia with considerable rise of systolic and diastolic blood pressure. In one case, with complete tetraplegia below C7, the initial blood pressure of 90/70 rose during the ejaculatory stage of the test to 230/150. Immediate application of Pentolonium (Ansolysen) intravenously immediately reduced the paroxysmal hypertension. It may be noted that in this case a previous cystometrogram revealed a very irritable disco-ordinated automatic bladder, and an infusion of only 50 cm³ of fluid into the bladder elicited repeated and most powerful detrusor contractions. Therefore, it is advisable to carry out a cystometrogram prior to the prostigmine test in high cord lesions to ascertain the threshold and degree of irritability of autonomic mechanisms. Cerebral haemorrhages due to exaggerated autonomic hyperreflexia resulting in hypertensive episodes have been recorded following bladder distension and during the last stages of labour in high lesions (Thompson & Witham, 1948; Jung & Schmidt, 1962). We lost one tetraplegic with a complete C6/7 lesion. He had his first prostigmin test on 2 February 1948, when following injections of 0·3 mg the initial blood pressure rose from 120/85 to 150/90. Apart from vomiting, which was controlled by 1/100 Atropine, there were no undesirable side effects during 3 ejaculations. He got married, and in 1961 he asked for a prostigmin test for the purpose of artificial insemination. This was carried out on 15 September 1961. One and a half hours following injection of the same doses as previously (0·3 mg), he developed an epileptic fit and died later, as a result of a cerebral ventricular haemorrhage. At *post-mortem* an undiagnosed abscess behind the pancreas was also found. Recently, Rossier *et al.* (1971) studied in detail for the first time the cardio-vascular changes during ejaculations following prostigmin test, in a traumatic tetraplegic, by intra-arterial monitoring with simultaneous electro-cardiography and catecholamine estimation in blood and urine. Hypertension during ejaculation was accompanied by cardiac arhythmia, and a close relationship was found between the stress response of the cardio-vascular mechanisms and a rise in catecholamine levels. From all these and other author's observations the following conclusions can be made:

1   The widespread belief that patients with severe injuries of the spinal cord are completely and permanently impotent and infertile is no longer valid.
2   The distinct stimulating effect of intrathecal prostigmine on the sexual organs has opened new possibilities for clinical, physiological and biochemical research in a field

where imaginative speculation and deduction on scanty grounds rather than on well-founded evidence have prevailed.

3   A variety of types and degrees of reproductive deficiency can be distinguished through the intrathecal prostigmin test.

4   Future research on the chemistry of the seminal fluid may give clues as to the cause or causes of abnormalities of the morphology and function of spermatozoa. In this respect, the deleterious effect of bladder infection on the various stations of the reproductive system needs particular consideration.

5   The intrathecal prostigmin test can be utilized for artificial insemination. It is, however, essential that the female partner undergo a thorough gynaecological examination, including assessment of pH estimation of vaginal and cervix secretion and determination of the most suitable time for assisted insemination.

6   Blood pressure and pulse should be examined at regular intervals during the prostigmine test from the start, especially in cervical lesions, to counteract excessive autonomic hyperreflexia by appropriate measures (Ansolysen, etc.).

7   Patients, especially those with high cord lesions should be warned about undesirable effects of prostigmin.

B. IN THE FEMALE

The main aspects to be considered are the effects of cord or cauda equina on menstruation, pregnancy and labour. Studies on these problems have been published by Gertsmann (1926), Bors et al. (1950, 1960, 1963), Cooper & Hoen (1952), Talbot (1955), Guttmann (1956, 1963, 1964), Jung & Schmidt (1962), Robertson (1963), Comarr (1966), Göller & Paeslack (1970).

In this connection it is worth while remembering that van Wagenen (1933) found, following transection of the cord in the female primate, normal menstrual period present 5 to 6 days after the transection and thereafter normal periods at the usual intervals. Moreover, Goltz & Ewald (1896) succeeded in inpregnating spinal bitches which delivered normal litters of puppies.

Menstruation

In the great majority of our patients with complete or incomplete lesions at any level, there was either no or only temporary cessation of menstruation, the return of periods occurring from one to three months after injury. Only occasionally will the return of periods be delayed longer. Menstrual irregularities have been reported after spinal cord lesions, but the contrary may also occur—namely those patients with irregular periods before the lesion may become regular afterwards (Comarr, 1966).

Orgasm

Orgasm during intercourse following penetration of the penis is absent in complete cord lesions and those incomplete ones with bilateral section of the spino-thalamic tracts, but orgastic sensations may be aroused in complete lesions below T5/6 by tactile stimuli, especially in the erogenic zone of the breast, with erection of the nipples.

Pregnancy and labour

With the increasing number of marriages of paraplegic women in recent years, the problem of motherhood has become more acute. In the past, reports on pregnancy and labour in paraplegic women were very scanty (Gerstmann, 1926; Ware, 1934) but have increased in recent years (Jung & Schmidt, 1962; Hutchinson & Vasicka, 1962; Guttmann, 1963; Robertson, 1963; Jackson, 1964; Guttmann et al., 1965; Hardy & Warrell, 1965; Comarr, 1966; Rossier et al., 1969; Göller & Paeslack, 1970). Experience has shown that women with complete transverse lesions, even including tetraplegics, can become pregnant and deliver normal babies vaginally, and Caesarean section is indicated very rarely. The following case is an example: a woman of 21, while in the Army, sustained a fracture-dislocation resulting in a complete paraplegia below the 5th dorsal segment. Her bladder was treated by immediate suprapubic cystostomy. At a military hospital, she was found to be pregnant. Paraplegia as such was at that time considered to be an indication for terminating pregnancy, and this was carried out in her case at 16 weeks by abdominal hysterotomy. She was admitted to Stoke Mandeville in 1945, where she made an excellent rehabilitation and became one of the best sportswomen. After the war, she married a man with a traumatic cauda equina lesion. Twelve years after the injury, at the age of 33, she became pregnant and had 3 blood transfusions during that time because of anaemia with fainting attacks. Having regard to the permanent suprapubic drainage, which could not be discontinued because of her highly contracted bladder and chronic urinary infection, a classical Caesarean section was performed (Mr Struan Robertson) and a healthy boy was delivered, who is now 18 years old. One could hardly find happier and more grateful parents, and one could perhaps forgive them for imposing upon the poor boy the Christian names of the two medical attendants—Ludwig and Struan! The mother has continued her sportive activities in archery and took part in both national and international Stoke Mandeville Games including those in Rome and Tokyo.

In 1963, I reported on 27 babies—17 boys and 10 girls—born to 19 women with spinal cord lesions, three of them polios and 16 transverse lesions of the cord, amongst the latter 9 complete lesions at levels ranging from C7 to L1 following fracture-dislocations of the spine. Five of the paraplegics, amongst them 4 traumatic, had two children each after becoming paraplegics. No disturbances of the lactation, i.e. (a) the synthesis of milk secretion, (b) milk ejection, were recorded, but this problem needs further and more detailed studies in complete lesions below and above Th5, in particular in tetraplegic women. Three also had children before their paraplegia.

Two of the 27 babies were stillborn. One died in utero in a patient with a traumatic paraplegia below T5. This woman became pregnant again two years later and had a spontaneous premature delivery of a healthy girl. This courageous mother tragically died 1½ years later of an inoperable cancer of the bladder. The other stillborn baby was a breech birth at home to a woman of 20 with a complete transverse lesion below T12, who did not realize that she was in labour and did not send for the nurse until the baby was born. In fact, the husband discovered this after his return from work.

This case raises the question of the effects of pregnancy and labour on the sensory system. In 1926, Gerstmann reported a case of traumatic cauda equina lesion with motor paralysis below L1 and complete sensory loss below S2 in a woman who, two years after injury, was delivered of a child with normal labour pain. Foerster (1936) reported a completely painless delivery in a case of spinal cord transection at the level of T10 and came to the conclusion, in confirmation of Henry Head's views (1898) on the segmental innervation of the uterus, that afferent fibres from the uterus do not enter the cord above the 10th dorsal segment (Foerster, 1936). Our observations in complete lesions are in accordance with these views, and, indeed, the absence of nociceptive responses to uterine contractions made the diagnosis of the onset of labour difficult in these patients. Even in complete lesions at lower thoracic level, labour pain may be so diminished that the patient is unaware of labour, especially during sleep, even in the second stage, as shown in the case described above. Therefore, it is advisable to keep the pregnant paraplegic woman under careful observation at the expected date of delivery. About certain sensory responses during the final stage of labour in high lesions, see later.

Sometimes the bowel function may be upset and disorganized in paraplegics during pregnancy, and uterine contractions during labour may manifest themselves by bowel movement sensation. One of my former patients—an incomplete traumatic paraplegia below T6 whose first child was delivered by Caesarean section—became pregnant again 4 years later. The following is an excerpt from her vivid description of her pregnancy and labour.

'From the fourth month of pregnancy, the baby was leaning on my bowel, and as the months progressed I had less and less control on my bowel movements. On the night that the baby arrived, I woke up about midnight with the usual feeling that I wanted to have a bowel movement, except that after each peristaltic wave I came out in gooseflesh all over. After half an hour, I decided I would get up and give myself an enema but only got to the bathroom when I noticed a "show". At that moment the pain got very much worse, and I realized that these were labour pains and my husband rang for an ambulance. Three-quarters of an hour after arrival at the hospital, a boy of 7 lb 4 oz was born spontaneously.'

General care during pregnancy

General hygiene during all stages of pregnancy is even more essential in paraplegics than in non-paraplegics.

Anaemia during pregnancy has to be considered more seriously in paraplegics than in the able-bodied pregnant woman, as this complication results in lowering of tissue resistance to pressure and thus facilitates the development of pressure sores. The more 'pressure conscious' the paraplegic and her family have become during her clinical treatment by systematic education, the less is the danger, even in the presence of some anaemia, of developing pressure sores during pregnancy. This complication needs immediate adequate treatment. (For details see Chapter Pressure Sores.) It may be noted that in none of the patients described above did sores develop during pregnancy.

Blood tests should be carried out in pregnant paraplegic women at regular intervals. The conventional treatment with oral iron has its disadvantage in promoting constipation and thus increasing the intestinal dysfunction already resulting from the spinal cord lesions. The haemoglobin must not be allowed to drop below 80 per cent and the red cells below 4 millions and, as proved in some of our patients, blood transfusions are the quickest and safest method of restoring normal blood counts.

Care of the paralysed bladder during pregnancy is, of course, of paramount importance, in particular the avoidance of large amounts of residual urine. It was found in the cases described above that, during pregnancy, all trained patients, except the one who had a permanent suprapubic cystostomy, were able to continue their voiding mechanism, and only in the latest stages of pregnancy did difficulty develop and catheterization became necessary. There was no exacerbation of infection of the urinary tract, with one exception (the case of the woman with a complete lesion below T5 described who had a still-born child in the 32nd week and who had attacks of pyelitis during her pregnancy). This is the more remarkable as most patients, with the exception of the polio cases, had an infected urine at the time of pregnancy. Moreover, no renal or bladder calculosis or recurrence of calculosis developed in these women, including one case with a complete lesion below T5 and amputation of the right leg, who, as a result of treatment with an indwelling catheter for 4 months elsewhere, developed a severe bladder infection resulting in formation of two huge bladder stones, one lying on top of the other like millstones (see Fig. 192) and which were removed suprapubically (Dr Walsh) 3 years before pregnancy. There were no complications during pregnancy and on 17 March 1963 she gave birth to a healthy girl.

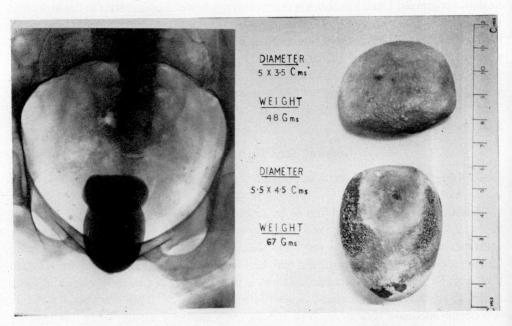

FIG. 192. From Guttmann (1963) *Proc. Royal Soc. Med.*, **56**, 383.

Reflex effects of uterine contractions on other autonomic mechanisms (the autonomic stress syndrome)

As one would expect, strong contractions of the uterus during labour, like other excessive visceral activity, elicit profound reflex responses in the cardio-vascular system and other autonomic mechanisms in cord lesions above T5/6. We first observed this in 1963 in a tetraplegic woman below C6 following fracture-dislocation of C4/5. During labour, when the head of the baby was deep in the pelvis, the first sign of autonomic hyperreflexia was an outburst of sweating on the left side of the face, associated with dilatation of the left pupil. Blood pressure rose steadily from 90/55 and the pulse fell, and about 10 min before delivery the BP reading was 180/100. Both pupils were dilated and there were outbursts of sweating on both sides of face and neck. The patient complained of frontal and occipital headaches of throbbing type, which coincided with each uterine contraction. Forceps were applied and during delivery the blood pressure rose to 190/100 and the pulse rate fell to 48/50. No irregularities of the heart rate were discovered by auscultation. After delivery of the baby and placenta, the exaggerated autonomic reflex responses ceased.

Since that publication (Guttmann, 1963), several more paraplegic women with complete and incomplete cord lesions were studied in detail during labour, amongst them two with complete lesions below T5 and T6. They confirmed the previous findings, that uterine contractions in advanced labour set up profound reflex responses in autonomic mechanisms, the most important being intermittent hypertension combined with bradycardia coinciding with the uterine contractions. One young woman with a complete lesion below the 5th dorsal segment, following fracture-dislocation of the spine, developed, in addition to the usual changes of the vascular system described above, profound cardiac irregularities at the end of labour. These were studied in detail electro-cardiographically and published elsewhere (Guttmann, Frankel & Paeslack, 1965).

Case report. Miss J.W. then aged 18, who had previously enjoyed good health, was a pillion passenger on a motor-cycle involved in a road accident on 11 May 1958. She suffered from:

1   Fractured skull, remained unconscious for 6 weeks.
2   Fracture-dislocation T3/4 (two weeks after injury had a laminectomy and spinal fusion) leaving a transverse spinal cord syndrome complete below T5.
3   Fracture of shaft right femur.

On 8 August 1958 admitted to National Spinal Injuries Centre, Stoke Mandeville Hospital, when her mental condition was good, she, however, remained rather talkative and excitable. She had a right abducens paresis which recovered and complete anosmia which had persisted. She had a complete spastic paraplegia below T5 segment.

She was treated and rehabilitated and was discharged home on 13 December 1958. Although the paraplegia remained complete below T5, she was independent, able to dress herself and get into and out of her wheelchair. Her urine was sterile and an intravenous pyelogram was normal. She had about 1 minutes warning of automatic bladder emptying; this warning consisted of tingling and sweating on her forehead; bowel action produced similar sensations.

She lived with her parents and took up full-time secretarial work until her marriage in 1962. She attended Stoke Mandeville for check-ups in 1960, 1961 and 1962, and on each occasion her neurological lesion was unchanged. Her urine was sterile and intravenous pyelograms normal. Her menstrual periods restarted 2 months after the accident and remained regular 5/28. (During intercourse she had no sensation in the lower part of body.)

Pregnancy

Last menstrual period 27 November 1962.

Expected date of delivery 4 September 1963.

The pregnancy was uneventful. The BP remained at 120/80 or less, and there was a trace of albumin on 23 July 1963; a sub-clinical urinary infection was treated with Furadantin.

As premature labour is anticipated in paraplegics, she was admitted to Stoke Mandeville Hospital on 8 July 1963. A vaginal examination on 15 July 1963 showed the cervix to be effaced, a further vaginal examination on 25 July 1963 showed no change. A further examination on 1 August 1963 showed the cervix to be 2 fingers dilated.

Labour

At 8 p.m. on 3 August 1963, regular uterine contractions every 5 to 7 min started. There were no abdominal sensations, but with each contraction the patient noticed tingling and flushing of the face. During contractions the BP rose from 120/75 to 130/80 and pulse rate dropped from 64 to 56. The cervix was still 2 fingers dilated. As it seemed that the patient was in early labour, she was transferred to Royal Bucks Hospital. During the next 7 days, irregular, mild contractions continued but there was no further dilatation of the cervix.

On 11 August 1963 at 8 p.m. uterine contractions became stronger and regular 1 : 8. With each contraction the BP rose to 150/100, the pulse dropped to 60, and at the end of each contraction the patient felt tingling, sweating, flushing of face and a burning feeling in the feet. Her cervix was 3 fingers dilated. Contractions continued through the night and by 11 a.m. on 12 August 1963 were regular and strong 1 : 3 with similar subjective sensations. A vaginal examination was performed and the membranes ruptured, the cervix was nearly fully dilated, there being only a 0·5 cm rim all round. During this vaginal examination, patient developed a frontal headache which persisted and became more severe until the baby was delivered. From this time on there were regular strong contractions 1 : 3. With each contraction the headache became more severe, there was sweating and flushing of the face and neck and she vomited several times. During the last half-hour of labour, each uterine contraction was accompanied by strong, rapid clonic spasms in the legs.

During the rest of labour, there was a progressive rise in BP and fall in pulse rate.

At 1.47 p.m., the BP had risen to 210/105 and the headache was severe. As the cervix was fully dilated the patient was catheterized (6 oz), an episiotomy was performed, forceps were applied (Dr A. Moolgaoker), and a healthy premature male infant weighing 5 lb 8 oz was delivered at 1.56 p.m. The placenta was delivered at 2 p.m. and the episiotomy was repaired. The headache was most intense during delivery, then disappeared, returned during delivery of the placenta, disappeared again and was replaced by a moderate pain in the back of the neck with slight stiffness which lasted 20 min.

No drugs were given, apart from an i.m. injection of 1 ml of syntometrine given with delivery of the anterior shoulder. No local anaesthetic was given for repair of the episiotomy; the insertion of each suture produced a strong contraction of the anal sphincter but there were no subjective sensations and no rise in BP.

Fig. 193 demonstrates the changes in blood pressure and pulse rate before, during and after delivery.

The cardiac irregularities developing during the various stages of labour could be recorded electrographically and were of special interest in this case. They were as follows:

At 1 p.m., during a uterine contraction, an irregularity of the pulse was first noted; clinically, this seemed to be due to extra-systoles. E.C.G. recordings started at 1.25 p.m. During the rest of the labour, a number of arhythmias were recorded, which are demonstrated in detail in Figs. 193a–g. Various arhythmias were demonstrated, starting with prolongation of the P-R interval with regular ventricular extra-systoles (Figs. 193a, b, c) followed by 2nd degree A-V block with A-V escape beats (Fig. 193e). On occasions, when there was only a moderate rise of blood pressure, a bradycardia with normal sinus rhythm was found (Fig. 193d). As the hypertension increased (1.52 p.m., Fig. 193f), 2nd degree A-V block returned and there were ventricular extra-systoles differing in shape and direction from those previously seen (Fig. 193c). During the actual delivery, the P waves disappeared and regular ventricular extra-systoles occurred firstly at every third beat (Fig. 193g) and later at every alternate beat (Fig. 193h).

As soon as the baby had been delivered, the electrocardiogram became normal, except that during the delivery of the placenta there were two more ventricular extra-systoles (Fig. 193i). The three standard leads after delivery are shown in Fig. 193g.

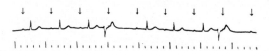

FIG. 193a. 1.28 p.m. Towards end of 1st stage of labour. One and a half hours after rupture of membranes. Lead I. P-R interval 0·28 seconds. Every third conducted beat is followed by a ventricular extra-systole which is followed by a compensatory pause. The arrows marking the P-waves show the fourth and eighth P-waves distorting the S-T segments of the extra-systoles.

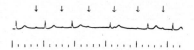

FIG. 193b. 1.30 p.m. Lead I. P-R-interval 0·32 seconds. P-waves marked by arrows. The third P-wave is not followed by a ventricular complex and the ensuing interval is terminated by an A-V escape beat, the S-T segment of which is deformed by the next P-wave.

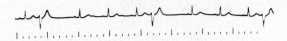

FIG. 193c. 1.31 p.m. Lead I. Every third conducted beat is followed by a ventricular extra-systole. In contrast with Fig. 2 the P-R interval is normal.

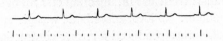

FIG. 193d. 1.38 p.m. Lead I. Bradycardia, rate 54 per minute with normal sinus rhythm during uterine contractions with moderate rise of blood pressure.

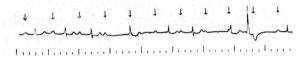

FIG. 193e. 1.52 p.m. Height of hypertension. Lead I. P-waves marked by arrows. The first P-R interval is 0·34 seconds, the next two are 0·4 seconds, the fourth P-wave is not conducted and the ensuing interval is terminated by an A-V escape beat, the fifth P-wave is hidden in the ventricular complex, thus the first part of the tracing shows 2nd degree A-V block 4 : 3. The sixth and seventh P-waves are conducted (P-R interval 0·4 seconds), but the eighth is not; the interval is again terminated by an A-V escape beat, the R-wave of which is deformed by the next P-wave (2nd degree A-V block 3 : 2). Following this, there is a ventricular extra-systole the S-T segment of which is deformed by the next P-wave. This extra-systole differs in shape and direction from those seen in Figs. 193a and 193c. From Frankel, Guttmann and Paeslack (1965) *Paraplegia*, **3**, 147.

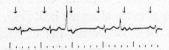

FIG. 193f. 1.52 p.m. Height of hypertension. Lead I. Two ventricular extra-systoles of different shape and size; the third and fifth arrows show P-waves distorting the S-T segment of the extra-systoles.

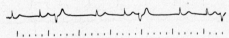

FIG. 193g. 1.55 p.m. During delivery. Lead I. No P-waves seen. Every 2nd supra-ventricular beat is followed by a ventricular extra-systole. The extra-systoles are again similar to those seen in Figs. 193a and 193c.

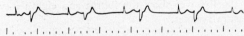

FIG. 193h. 1.55 p.m. During delivery. Lead I. No P-waves seen. Each supra-ventricular beat is followed by a ventricular extra-systole ('coupling' or 'bigeminus').

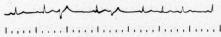

FIG. 193i. 1.59 p.m. During delivery of placenta. Lead I. Sinus rhythm, two ventricular extra-systoles.

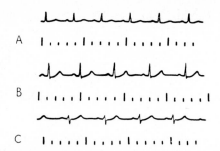

FIG. 193j. 2.32 p.m. 35 minutes after delivery of placenta. Leads I, II, III. Return to normal.

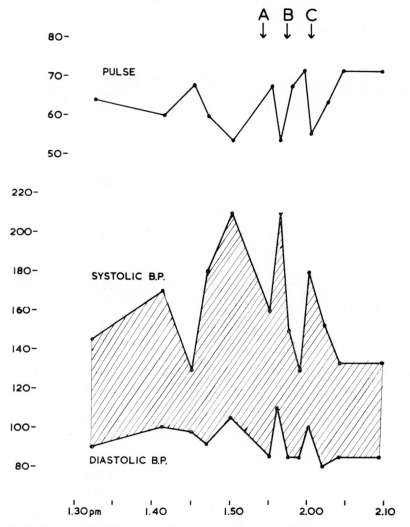

FIG. 193k. Demonstrates the rise of blood pressure and bradycardia coinciding with powerful uterine contractions. At A the forceps was applied, at B delivery was completed, at C the placenta was delivered.

Fig. 193k demonstrates pulse and blood pressure changes during the delivery of the baby and placenta.

MECHANISM OF CARDIAC IRREGULARITIES

In analysing the mechanism of the irregularities of cardiac rhythm observed in this case, it must first be pointed out that they are neither peculiar to pregnancy and labour in women nor to ejaculations in men with high spinal cord lesions, but are just another manifestation of exaggerated viscero-spinal reflex responses as an expression of the autonomic stress syndrome as described following distension of the bladder (Guttmann & Whitteridge, 1947; Guttmann, 1954). The difference in intensity and extent of the cardiac irregularities is explained by the difference in duration, frequency and intensity of the visceral stimulation. The increase in blood pressure as a result of the vasoconstriction, which in lesions above T5/6 involves the greater part of the vascular bed of the body, is most likely to be responsible for the observed bradycardia as part of a depressor reflex response aroused by the intact aortic and carotic sinus nerves on the one hand and the prevalence of vagal stimulation on the other. However, it seems likely that the stimulation of the autonomic innervation of the heart itself is the decisive factor of the irregularities of the heart rhythm. Whether and to what extent an increase of the level of catecholamines, locally and/or circulating, may contribute to the development and intensity of the cardiac arhythmias or may be even responsible as their initiator needs further studies.

In discussing this humoral factor, it must be remembered that irregularities of cardiac rhythm may occur during and immediately after the acute hypertensive paroxysms due to phaeochromocytoma. These arhythmias include extra-systoles and auricular fibrillations (Heglin Rand & Holzmann, 1937; Espersen & Jorgensen, 1947), atrio-ventricular block, dissociation with interference, and wandering pacemaker (Burges et al., 1936; Mortell & Whittle, 1945; Espersen & Jorgensen, 1947). Some of these arhythmias were interpreted by Raab (1953) as continued primary sympathetic and simultaneous secondary vagal stimulation.

It is also of interest to compare our findings on cardiovascular changes described during labour in women with cord lesions above T5/6 with those occurring in non-paralysed women during labour. Adams & Alexander (1958) found that, during uterine contractions, cardiac output increased by 19·7 per cent (dye dilution technique), and there was a rise in mean blood pressure from 94 to 120 mm. The electro-cardiogram during labour, unless non-paraplegic women are suffering from heart disease, shows no abnormalities, apart from extra-systoles in sympatheticotonic individuals.

In conclusion, the observations made on pregnancy and labour in women with severe lesions of the spinal cord are of great interest not only from a neuro-physiological point of view but, even more, from a practical gynaecological standpoint. In particular, the profound cardio-vascular reactions during the end of the first and second stages of labour resulting in hypertension, bradycardia, headaches and cardiac arhythmias, sweating and oculo-pupillary changes, etc., in women with cord lesions above T5/6 must be most carefully observed by both the medical and nursing attendants as they provide an important index of the progress of labour and the need for operative assistance. A rise of blood pressure above 180–190 systolic and 115 diastolic during the first or second stages of labour would appear to be an indication for expediting delivery by episiotomy, forceps or even Caesarean section, in order to avoid the danger of cerebral haemorrhages. In this respect, a case of complete cord lesion below T5 described by Jung & Schmidt (1962) is very significant. This woman developed intermittent hypertension with blood pressure rising to 230/110 mmHg with every uterine contraction. These hypertensive attacks were associated with 'dramatic convulsions and profound headaches'. Very soon, the intermittent rises of blood pressure were replaced by a slow, continuing rise to 230/145mm associated with vomiting. Although immediate Caesarean section was performed and a healthy boy was delivered, the mother developed a cerebral haemorrhage, which left her with a paralysis of the left arm, paralysis of ocular movements and a left facial paralysis. The authors explained the intermittent hypertensive attacks, which started following rupture of the membranes, when the child's head was just above the ischial spines, as a viscerospinal reflex response, in confirmation of Guttmann and Whitteridge's investigations on the effect of bladder distension on autonomic mechanisms, while the sustained rise of blood pressure was thought to be due to an acute rise in intra-cranial pressure due to hypertensive haemorrhage from a post-traumatic aneurysm. However, it may be stressed that cerebral haemorrhages as a result of intermittent hypertensive attacks in those high lesions due to excessive visceral activity may occur without the presence of cerebral aneurysms or other vascular abnormalities.

Recently, Göller & Paeslack (1970) reporting on cases of traumatic paraplegic women, who were pregnant at the time of injury and later gave birth to abnormal children, raised the question of whether or not the percentage of abnormal children born to traumatic paraplegic women was higher than that found in women who sustained other types of injuries during pregnancy. Only comparative statistics on a large scale would clarify this problem.

The married life of paraplegics and tetraplegics

One would expect that a disablement of a magnitude such as paraplegia or tetraplegia would set up in its wake difficult problems in the domestic resettlement of these severely disabled people, particularly in their marital adjustment. This is doubtless true to some extent. Nevertheless, it is an undeniable fact, that many subjects who were already married at the time of their spinal cord injury or disease, have continued their married life successfully for many years, and others have started their married life after having become paraplegics or tetraplegics.

Major statistical surveys on the marital lives of a particular number of paraplegics and tetraplegics are scanty. In 1962, Comarr of the Spinal Unit at Long Beach Veterans' Hospital, U.S.A., published a survey on 859 paraplegic and tetraplegic veterans of the U.S. Army and more recently Deyoe (1972) published a survey on 219 veterans of the U.S. Army.

In 1964 a statistical survey on the marital status of 1,505 living traumatic paraplegics and tetraplegics of marriageable age, treated at Stoke Mandeville was published

(Guttmann, 1964), 527 of whom were ex-service pensioners. There were 1,316 men and 189 women.

The marital status of these people before admission is given in Table 32, showing 674 (44·8 per cent), of whom 69 were women, married and living with their partners. This figure includes marriages both before and after injury, the great majority being after injury. A total of 777 (51·8 per cent), amongst them 99 women, were single, and

TABLE 32. Marital status of 1,505 paraplegics and tetraplegics before admission

	Paraplegics	Tetraplegics	Total
Men			
Married	467	138	605
Unmarried living with partner	8	3	11
Divorced or separated	7	4	11
Widowed	5	6	11
Single	528	150	678
Totals	1,015	301	1,316
Women			
Married	50	19	69
Unmarried living with partner	4	—	4
Divorced or separated	4	2	6
Widowed	3	8	11
Single	70	29	99
Totals	131	58	189

TABLE 33. Marriages after admission

Men Paraplegic men to:	Normal Women	Paraplegic Women	Total
Complete	141	9	150
Incomplete	85	2	87
Tetraplegic men to:			
Complete	13	—	13
Incomplete	20	—	20
	259	11	270
Women Paraplegic women to:	Normal Men	Paraplegic or Polio Men	Total
Complete	10	9	19
Incomplete	10	1	11
Tetraplegic women to:			
Complete	—	1	1
Incomplete	1	—	1
Totals	21	11	32

15 not included in the figure of 777 were known to be cohabiting. Before admission, 17 were divorced or separated and 22 were widowed.

Out of the 777 single patients in Table 31, 302 married after admission, the majority (267) being paraplegics. Table 33 shows the division of complete and incomplete lesions amongst the married paraplegics and tetraplegics in this group. The majority of para-plegic men who married normal women were complete lesions (141 out of 226), while the majority of tetraplegic men who married normal women were incomplete lesions (20 out of 33). No difference in number was found between complete and incomplete lesions in paraplegic women, who married normal men. Of our male patients, 11 married eight of our female paraplegics, while three more of our traumatic females married paralysed men not treated at Stoke Mandeville. If one adds the 302 of this group to the 674 who were living with their married partners at the time of their admission to Stoke Mande-ville, this brings the total of married paralysed out of the 1,505 under discussion to 976 (64·9 per cent). Amongst them were 192 tetraplegics.

Divorce

Table 34 gives data of divorce in these two groups after admission. The total of divorces of the two groups is 57 out of 976. If one adds the 17 already divorced before admission this brings the number of divorces out of a total of 1,015 marriages to 74 or 7·3 per cent.

TABLE 34

Married at time of admission to Stoke Mandeville Hospital		Divorced or separated after admission			
		Paraplegic	Tetraplegic	Total	%
Men	605	25	5	30	4·9
Women	69	5	–	5	7·3
	674	30	5	35	5·2

Married after admission to Stoke Mandeville Hospital		Married and divorced after admission			
		Paraplegic	Tetraplegic	Total	%
Men	270	16	4	20	7·4
Women	29	1	1	2	7·0
	299	17	5	22	7·36

Table 35 shows a statistic of children fathered by paraplegics and tetraplegics and those born to paraplegic and tetraplegic women and the number of adopted children. A total of 205 children were fathered by 108 paraplegic and tetraplegic men; 16 paralysed women, amongst them a woman with a tetraplegia below C6, bore 22 children. Fifty-nine paralysed men, amongst them four tetraplegics, adopted 79 children. It may be noted here, that in this figure 13 step-children of 11 paraplegics who married widows with children are also included. Of these 11 marriages, eight took place after admission to Stoke Mandeville.

TABLE 35. Children

Paraplegic	Fathers	96	Own Children	188
Paraplegic	Mothers	15	Own Children	21 (1 illegit.)
Tetraplegic	Fathers	12	Own Children	17
Tetraplegic	Mothers	1	Own Children	1
Totals		124		227
Paraplegic	Fathers	55	Adopted Children	73
Tetraplegic	Fathers	4	Adopted Children	6
Totals		59		79

In analysing the data given, it can be first stated that paraplegia as well as tetraplegia as such is not a hindrance to a happy married life. This applies to those who were already married at the time of injury as well as to those who married after their spinal cord lesions. Furthermore, it does not make any difference whether normal women married paraplegic or tetraplegic men (and this is no doubt the majority), whether normal men married paraplegic women or whether paraplegics married amongst themselves. Many stories of great devotion in this respect could be told. The fact that divorces in the group of those already married before their paraplegia are less frequent than in the group who married after tends to show that in the former group there has already been a basis of normal married life and companionship and, therefore, the loyalty of the normal partner is greater. In this connection. ten men and four women may be mentioned who, on admission, were known to have been cohabiting. Only two of these partnerships have broken up since; two paralysed men married their partners and the others are in *status quo*.

Motivation of marriage. The motivation which initiates normal people to marry spinal paraplegics appears to be in the majority of cases love and affection, but in some cases it has been loyalty to the man or girl to whom they were already engaged before the paraplegia or tetraplegia. Furthermore, with some women it has been a highly developed mothering instinct and in others no doubt financial security. The latter applies in particular to widows with young children but also to women who know that the prospective husband's pension or other income will provide a life of security. An extraordinary case is a married woman who became a bigamist by 'marrying' a tetraplegic service pensioner. She was not prosecuted for committing bigamy but was charged with stealing his money. The tetraplegic in question, far from being discouraged by this disappointment, has since married another woman and is living happily with her.

Divorce. This brings me to the interesting problem of divorce. At the time of the statistic, 22 paraplegics and tetraplegics of the 74 mentioned above had since remarried, thus bringing the total number remaining divorced to 52 or 5·1 per cent of the total number married. This, I feel, is infinitely smaller than one would expect in people with such a profound disablement. In fact, it is only slightly higher than the percentage of divorces among the general population in Great Britain, which according to the last census in 1961 was about 1 per cent. It is interesting to compare these figures with that of 412 out of 858 married paraplegics and tetraplegics given by Comarr in his statistics of 1962. The divorce rate after injury was 27–39 per cent. Although this figure is higher than that of the general population of the U.S.A. (26 per cent), it is below that of the population in Los Angeles, County of California (45–49 per cent), the highest in the U.S.A. However, the divorce rate of patients who were married for the first time after injury varied between 10 per cent for the non-military service-connected patients and 24 per cent for the military service-connected ones.

What are the motives for divorce? It can first be stated that revulsion to the paraplegia, as such was, as a rule, not found to be a significant reason for divorce, whatever the level and completeness of the lesion. Actually, one woman married to a man with a low cauda equina lesion who regained his walking abilities ran away with a man with a complete paraplegia below T11. In some cases, especially those where marriage took place in haste or when the normal partner was perhaps motivated by reasons other than love and affection—such as pity, financial reasons, etc.—when faced with realities the marriage broke up. Incompatibility was also a reason, especially in young and immature people who married hastily or in psychopathic individuals. For instance, one young woman who was already divorced from an actor before her paraplegia married a writer, but the marriage broke up after she became a paraplegic, when she fell in love with a R.A.F. officer with a very incomplete cauda equina lesion. She married the officer from whom, however, she became separated when her mental condition deteriorated. However, she has been married again for a number of years now. Another example is that of a Yugoslav paraplegic, who came to Stoke Mandeville and who, on return to his own country, left his normal wife to marry a British paraplegic girl, whom he met at Stoke Mandeville. They married and lived in Yugoslavia, but the paraplegic wife left him because she said he became intolerable. She returned to England, obtained a divorce and is now married to an able-bodied man. A further instance of incompatibility is that of a woman with a partial paraplegia who had a 17 year old daughter from her first marriage. She married a man 20 years younger than herself. Naturally, the marriage did not last.

Sexual frustration of the wife, regardless of whether it concerns a woman who had children by her husband before his paraplegia or after marrying a paraplegic, certainly accounts for divorce in some cases, especially if the normal woman becomes involved with another man and becomes pregnant. Sexual desire outside marriage has accounted for several of the divorces. One extreme case in this respect is that of a woman who, after having had no less than 11 children, left her paraplegic husband to live with another man. This may also apply to paraplegic women, although more rarely. One paraplegic woman left her husband to live with another man, by whom she had an illegitimate child. The most tragic case in this group is the case of a young tetraplegic woman with a lesion below C6—a former beauty queen—who was engaged at the time of her car accident. Her fiancé married her after her discharge from hospital and she had a child by him, but already at that time he had formed an association with another girl, who had also become pregnant by him. He left his tetraplegic wife shortly afterwards and married the other girl.

It has been our experience that paralysed women as well as paralysed men, whose partners have left them for one reason or another, have usually taken the situation well and, as already mentioned, quite a number have married again. There was only one exception—a psychopathic non-traumatic paraplegic who, although not included in these statistics, may be mentioned here. He had married a girl in haste and had become increasingly depressed by the unfaithfulness of his wife, and when she eventually left him, refusing to return, he committed suicide.

Children. Finally, a few words on the problem of children of paraplegics and tetraplegics. Our statistics on traumatic paraplegics clearly show that the generalized pessimism of many members of the medical profession regarding potency and sterility in paraplegic men and motherhood in paraplegic women is unfounded. In a previous paper (1963) —'The paraplegic patient in pregnancy and labour'—I have already discussed the question of motherhood of paraplegic women and have given evidence that, in spite of their severe disablement, they can bear normal children and look after them. Moreover, I have pointed out that confinement by Caesarean section should be limited to extremely rare cases.

With regard to potency and sterility, I refer to the previous chapter. As shown by the present statistics, it is obvious that men with complete and, in particular, incomplete lesions can sire their own children. Already in 1944, when the question of marriage of paraplegic soldiers arose, I could not accept the general attitude that paraplegics should be dissuaded from marrying, and the following case was a great encouragement in this respect. A young soldier with a cauda equina lesion below L5 was admitted with a suprapubic cystostomy from the battlefront. He had just been married before being called up to the Army, and after he received his severe injury he wanted to give his young wife a divorce, because he thought it would be unfair to her to remain tied to him. I persuaded him to wait until the suprapubic cystostomy was closed, which we succeeded in doing, and he made a good re-education of his bladder as well as an excellent adjustment to his remaining disability, being able to walk. He was sent home on leave, which he accepted with extreme reluctance, but after his return he was a dramatically changed man because he had realized that he could continue his marital activities. To conclude the story, he produced his first child within a year and on discharge home took up a job in a shoe-repairing department, having been a bricklayer before. One day I received a terse telegram, 'Twins, Sir—Bill'! Altogether, he had had four children.

As with some able-bodied married couples, it may take several years before pregnancy is achieved. In this respect, my first patient—a soldier with a cauda equina lesion below L2 on the right and L3 on the left, who was admitted on 3 February 1944—may be quoted. He, too, was admitted with a suprapubic cystostomy, which was successfully closed, and his urine became sterile. He was married just before the war, and his wife was very devoted to him. In 1954, he informed me very happily of the birth of a daughter. Unfortunately, the baby died a few months later of an intestinal obstruction.

Adoption of children. A very important achievement is that today, having regard to the great advances made in the rehabilitation of paraplegics and in restoring their working capabilities, adoption societies take a different and more co-operative view towards the adoption of children by paraplegics than they took previously. In this respect, it may be mentioned that we have patients in our material who were married before their paraplegia and had children. As the couples wanted more children and this could not be achieved in the normal way, they adopted children, and in all cases this has proved most successful. Even in these cases, the adoption societies have co-operated well.

In conclusion, if one accepts the three fundamentals for a happy marriage:

1 compatibility of personality and companionship
2 sexual satisfaction of the female partner
3 the production of children,

there is no doubt that the majority of paraplegics can fulfil the two first conditions. With regard to the third, the ability of paraplegic and even tetraplegic women to produce children is definitely greater than that of the paralysed man, although there is no doubt that a minority can sire their own children. How far this ability of the male partner can be improved by assisted insemination, with improved techniques of conservation of the paraplegic's own semen, remains to be seen by future biological research. Their marriages are, of course, subject to all the problems in marriages of the able-bodied; however, their divorce rate would not appear to be significantly higher.

In recent years, interest in the sexual problems and sexual rehabilitation of spinal paraplegics and tetraplegics has steadily increased and valuable studies on these subjects have been published (Jackson, 1972; Tarabulcy, 1972; Andres, 1972; Deyoe, 1972; Cole et al., 1973; Mooney et al., 1975).

CHAPTER 30

PSYCHOLOGICAL ASPECTS

A disaster in human life of such magnitude as a sudden transection or severe injury to the spinal cord, which throws the body completely out of gear, inevitably disrupts the psycho-physical entity of the organism resulting in pronounced effects on the paralysed patient's mind. This complex and challenging problem has been the subject of a number of studies, in particular during the last quarter of this century (Guttmann, 1945, 1953; Poer, 1946; Kennedy, 1946; Weiss & Bors, 1948; Negler, 1950; Michaelis, 1950; Wittkower *et al.*, 1954; Labhardt, 1962; Mueller, 1962; Bosches, 1963; Fordyce, 1964; Gunther, 1969).

I have made my studies on the mental behaviour of paraplegics and tetraplegics during and after the Second World War from individual interviews in my office, during routine activities in the ward, physiothrapy department, workshop and later in hostels and settlements, and last, but by no means least, on the sports field. Formal psychiatric interviews and specialized psychology tests were necessary only in very selected cases and specialist psychiatric treatment was very rarely indicated in this Centre. In my studies I found of invaluable help self-written reports by the patients about their reactions to the injury, including their reactions and attitude towards their family and other visitors. In this respect, a very significant remark about the frame of mind of people meeting paraplegics for the first time was the expression of one of our earliest patients—a priest wounded in 1943—who wrote: 'One of the most difficult tasks of a paraplegic is to cheer up his visitors.'

In the establishment of the psychological pattern in paraplegics and tetraplegics, the pre-traumatic personality, general mental ability, educational background, social standing, profession, age, as well as the severity and duration of the paralysis and the type and efficiency of the initial treatment following injury, were found to be essential factors. In this connection, the importance of the disastrous psychological effect of prolonged, enforced inactivity in hospital as well as later unsatisfactory housing conditions, sexual frustration, lack of suitable transport facilities and delayed employment cannot be emphasized too much.

The mental disorders observed can be divided into various groups, which, however, may pass indistinguishably into each other:

A. MENTAL DISORDERS RELATED TO THE SPINAL INJURY

(1) Disorders due to septic conditions

These are associated mainly with the infection of the urinary tract and pressure sores, and the most characteristic symptom is increased tiredness progressing to complete apathy, all too often misinterpreted as being 'unco-operative' or of 'bad type'. This was seen especially in traumatic paraplegics demoralized as a result of inadequate treatment and neglect, who were admitted with articular contractures, sores and urinary infection. They resented at first any active treatment and wanted to be left alone having resigned into their disability and with no will to live. Sometimes, sudden and unmotivated outbursts of irritability and rudeness may be the first sign of a pyrexial attack. Real toxic psychosis was found to be very rare. A man of 59 with a complete transverse lesion at T10 developed on three occasions, during acute deterioration of his sacral and trochanteric sores, a toxic psychosis of paranoid acoustic hallucinatory type, which promptly disappeared after excision of deep fascial sloughs with fat necrosis. The family history of this patient did not reveal any mental abnormalities. Most striking improvement of mental conditions, especially apathy, also followed blood transfusion in cases with anaemia due to toxic absorption.

(2) Reactive mental disorders

(a) *Stage of shock*

The sudden conversion of a vigorous person into a helpless wreck, naturally leads to severe psychological shock. The immediate effect is a state of daze in which clear thinking is retarded, if not completely abolished, and the flow of ideas is more or less slowed down. The traumatic paraplegic and even more the tetraplegic is, as a rule, incapable of realizing the whole extent of his disability. This stage may last for hours and days. Whether this can be explained by 'an unconscious protection against too massive or too rapid a perception of the traumatic and overwhelming reality' (Gunther, 1969) is a debatable point. Gunther attempts an interesting psychoanalytical theory of the mental alteration occurring during the acute trauma: 'During the stage of acute trauma, the patient withdraws all his emotional energy and interest from the outside world, thereby interrupting his relationship with it. This is probably an adaptation mechanism to maintain the integrity of the ego's original image of the body (and sense of self) in the face of an overwhelming disaster to the body and in the face of the loss of some of the normal sensory impact to the ego. This necessary protective adaptation of the ego at this stage is probably subject to little alteration by direct intervention from the medical personnel.' Our observations did not substantiate this theory that the interruption of the paraplegic's relationship with the outside world in the stage of shock following injury is due to his conscious or subconscious withdrawal of all his emotional energy and interest from the outside world to maintain the integrity of the ego's original image of the body. On the contrary, there are certain facts which do not seem to correspond with this psychoanalytical assumption. Patients may arrive at the Centre or hospital under the influence of drugs, such as morphia, which they have received during first aid and which add to their mental retardation caused by the traumatic shock. Moreover, the paralysed patient may be confused by the presence of phantom sensations, a not uncommon incidence, which he misinterprets as true feeling and active movements of the paralysed limbs. In tetraplegics, the mental retardation is intensified by oxygen deficiency as a result of the paralysis of the respiratory muscles resulting in profound lowering of the vital capacity of the lungs, and this mental retardation may deteriorate into confusion and unconsciousness, if the respiratory distress is not relieved quickly by appropriate measures. Paraplegics with associated injuries to the skull resulting in cerebral concussion may be unconscious for days and weeks, followed by a state of confusion.

(b) *Stage of realization*

The stage of psychological shock is followed by an early stage of shallow awareness of the disability and, in due course, by increasing realization of its extent. Some paraplegics exhibit anxieties already in this early stage of realization of their paraplegia, at first mainly concerned with the paralysis of their legs, and questions such as 'Will I walk again?' are by no means uncommon. Other patients avoid questions about the finality of their spinal cord lesion as if they are afraid to have full knowledge of the reality. In agreement with Nagler (1954) we found that they take refuge in an 'ostrich policy' as an escape reaction. They appear superficially reconciled and show co-operation with the medical, nursing and physiotherapy staff. In this frame of mind, the patient often reverts psychologically into childhood, by leaning on the doctor, nurse and physiotherapist as he did as a child on his mother, and he is quite content with the various passive measures of treatment. The full realization of his bodily plight begins really when more active co-operation is demanded of him and he becomes fully aware of his profound physical limitations and the implications for his future. It is mainly in this phase that a number of anxieties will become manifest, some of which are identical with those of other severely injured persons, such as fear of chronic crippledom, with all its restrictions in social activities and economic consequences, resulting in loss of earning capacity and thus becoming a burden to the family and everybody else. There are, however, in addition, anxieties of specific nature associated with paraplegia, in connection with the loss of control of bladder, bowel and sexual functions. To some patients, these are at first overwhelming barriers and may set up negativistic and provocative attitudes and breaches of discipline towards medical and nursing staff, while in others they may result in frustration, self-pity and self-centredness, associated with a sense of resentment against their fate and society. No doubt, most authors agree that the loss of control of sexual function constitutes a severe psychological shock in most paraplegics, regardless of whether married or single, the more so as the libido remains (see page 474). Although this stage of regression and denial can be overcome in the great majority of spinal paraplegics by empathy on the one hand and firm handling on the other on the part of the medical and paramedical staff, there are certain individuals who will develop more serious abnormal emotional reactions. It must be remembered, that one admits to a spinal unit individuals with a variety of constitutional psychological make-ups, including psychopathic individuals, who, as one would expect, may exhibit excessive emotional reactions. Trifling reasons such as having to wait their turn to be attended to for changing their urine bottles or being refused permission to get up may be exaggerated, leading to outbursts of excessive irritability and displays of temper, in which they may be quite capable of doing damage to others and themselves. In the writer's monograph of 1953, a psychopathic individual of paranoid-querulous type, with a traumatic paraplegia below T4 as a result of a motor-cycle accident, was mentioned who became quite negativistic in such a state of emotional dysbalance. He threatened to commit suicide by refusing to eat and drink, being well aware of the damaging effect of the restriction of fluid on his renal function, the more so as he had a congenital aplasia of one kidney and had to rely on the other already infected kidney. Any method of persuasion was of no avail, and only by firm handling and the introduction of fluid through a nasal tube as the last resort brought him eventually to his senses.

More serious are those patients who develop depression, resulting in all kinds of physical complaints including pain which may become an irrevocable fixation. In other cases of this type of regression suicidal tendencies may develop and actual suicidal attempts have been made. Fortunately, in our material the number of these patients is very small. This may be due to the fact that the patient's attention and concentration is directed immediately and constantly towards returning to a useful life by various activities at the Centre.

Another, though less common, reaction in the early stage of paraplegia is self-deception. A defiant attitude ('we can take it mentality') towards their paraplegia was found, particularly in young soldiers during and after the Second World War. Although this mental attitude towards the incapacitating effects of a paraplegia can be useful in obtaining enthusiastic co-operation in the early treatment, in later stages of rehabilitation it may lead to unrealistic and uncritical attitudes toward their physical limitations, naturally caused by the spinal cord lesion. They ignore instructions and advice from the medical or nursing staff, be these concerned with the prevention of pressure sores, with the speed of driving a motor vehicle or choosing a job or occupation for which they are unsuited, or falling head over heels in love and making unsuitable marriages, only to get divorced sooner or later.

Probably the most unfavourable mental reaction is indifference towards the severe disability resulting from the spinal cord lesion. These patients do not appear depressed or aggressive; they just do not care. Although such a patient will follow medical orders, he does so in a passive way without any initiative or sense of motivation. In agreement with other authors, we found this pattern of mental behaviour more frequently in patients with lower grade intelligence, but also in those who went through a long period of enforced inactivity either in hospital or institution. Such patients do not worry unduly about their disability but, although they do not show any direct aggression, they resent interference with the protection given to them in hospitals or institutions. If left to themselves without expert guidance they will easily deteriorate into 'professional' pensioners or charity cases.

B. MENTAL DISORDERS UNRELATED TO THE SPINAL INJURY

In a small number of our material, the spinal injury was self-inflicted. One soldier—a psychopathic individual—shot himself in the back to get out of the Army and sustained a complete paraplegia below T10/11. He was difficult to manage but eventually made a satisfactory rehabilitation so that he was given the opportunity to be admitted as a resident to the Duchess of Gloucester House to take up employment in light industry. He was full time employed, earned good money but was caught with others pilfering from his firm and was dismissed. He was given another chance and was re-employed by a firm producing lighters, but a few months later he was dismissed because of stealing some lighters. He left the Duchess of Gloucester House spontaneously, as otherwise he would have been dismissed as unsuitable for residency at this hostel, and returned to his family.

Only two patients (both with incomplete lesions and able to walk) had to undergo specialized treatment for chronic alcoholism. Recently one former patient who was full-time employed for many years died from acute alcohol poisoning.

Several psychotic individuals such as schizophrenics and others suffering from depression had tried to commit suicide by throwing themselves out of a window and sustained spinal fractures with spinal cord injuries. Sometimes, the traumatic shock may effect a remission of the mental illness. However, psychotic paraplegics need careful supervision by the nursing staff, as they may try to make another attempt and may become a danger to themselves and other patients. One case of schizophrenia who sustained a paraplegia tried to cut his throat with a knife he demanded from another patient. Fortunately, this was discovered immediately, and the self-inflicted wound which did not affect the large vessels of the neck was immediately sutured. Such psychotic patients should be transferred to a psychiatric department at a very early stage to receive specialized treatment.

Psychological treatment

When the paraplegic begins to realize the extent of his disability, it is the immediate task of both medical and paramedical staff to awake in the patient also the realization that he has still great forces of readjustment left in his organism which can be utilized and mobilized to overcome his disability, provided these forces of adaptation and repair are not counteracted by drugs, such as barbiturates, which interfere with clear thinking. The patient must be indoctrinated with the idea that spinal paraplegia is not the end but the beginning of a new scheme of life, which starts once he has come to terms with his physical defect. In our experience, this is greatly facilitated if the extent of the patient's definite physical defect and, at the same time, his possibilities of returning to his family and community as a useful and respected member is explained as soon as possible to both the patient and his relatives.

As pointed out above, it lies in the nature of such an overwhelming physical defect, as produced by a spinal cord transection, that the patient is inclined to be passive towards any treatment. Therefore, the sooner he is directed toward intensive and purposeful activity the easier his psychological readjustment and social re-integration will be achieved. In this respect, three measures have proved invaluable towards accomplishing this goal: active physical exercise, sport and work therapy. They have proved ideal methods to counteract abnormal reactions resulting in frustration, defeatism, resentment and isolationism and have been most invaluable in restoring the will to live with himself and with others and in developing his self-confidence, self-dignity and, most important of all, to make him aware of his responsibility towards his family and the community. Details of physiotherapy and work therapy are discussed in the respective chapters.

The creation of a cheerful atmosphere and good morale in the ward cannot be stressed too much. The whole unit must be deliberately impregnated with enthusiasm, for this inspires the patient to co-operate to the full and will help to re-organize his disrupted personality and thus restore the psycho-physical entity of the organism.

The psychological guidance of the paraplegic patient is, of course, primarily the responsibility of the medical officer in charge of the case. He has to create a close doctor–patient relationship, which will win the patient's confidence and make it easier for him to disclose his anxieties. On the other hand, he has to co-ordinate the work of his team of workers—nurse, physiotherapist, work therapist and welfare officer—concerned with the patient's management. Every member of the team must be familiar with the patient's personality and emotional reactions and conflicts. This will help to wean him from his initial passive attitude into an active role, in which he will learn to consider himself as the most important member of the rehabilitation team. Group exercises and team sport have proved invaluable in developing competitive spirit and comradeship and preventing a 'spoiled child mentality' (see Chapter on Sport).

A very important point in the psychological guidance is not only to make the patient aware of his capabilities by utilizing his existing and developing dormant talents, but also of his limitations caused by his physical defect. Only then will the paraplegic regain a psycho-physical harmony enabling him to cope with the demands of daily life, once he has left the protective life of the hospital.

Drug addiction and alcoholism, although in our material rare, can be most adverse to the patient's rehabilitation, and it demands great patience and firmness on the part of the patient's attendants to get him over these hurdles.

Equally as important as the psychological management of the paraplegic and tetraplegic is the psychological readjustment of the patient's relatives to the whole problem. They have to be instructed in detail by the staff, during their visits to the hospital, on how to deal with the patient sensibly and properly once he has returned home. They must not be overprotective but must learn when to assist and when to resist unreasonable demands. In particular and above all, everything should be done to help in the social re-integration of the paraplegic, by encouraging him to take up regular work and employment.

CHAPTER 31

CARE OF THE SKIN

The vital importance of maintaining a good hygienic condition of the skin and its organs from the very beginning of paraplegia and tetraplegia is now generally well recognized, though not always practised by both the patient and his or her attendants.

Cleanliness of the skin promotes better blood circulation by preventing clogging of the pores, thus facilitating the function of the cutaneous glands, which take part in the elimination of metabolic waste products of the body. In fact, it was found in this centre that, in cases with acute renal deficiency—for instance, after nephrostomy or during acute pyelitic attacks—the increased activity of the sweat glands represents an important auxiliary mechanism for the elimination of waste products. Scrupulous cleanliness is especially essential in those cutaneous areas which are easily saturated with urine and faecal matter, and the soles and heels should never be allowed to become scaly, but must be kept soft and clean, as this is an important measure for preventing ill-effects of pressure. Indeed, it is no exaggeration to say that the degree of cleanliness of the soles and heels is an excellent indicator of the efficiency of the medical and nursing staff concerned with the management of paraplegics. Fig. 194 demonstrates a paraplegic admitted to Stoke Mandeville with thick scaly skin on the soles of his feet demonstrating utter neglect.

The toe-nails also need careful attention and must be trimmed at regular intervals. Ingrowing toe-nails are not infrequent incidents in paraplegics and should be dealt with immediately. Not only are they a constant irritation to the peripheral nerve-endings

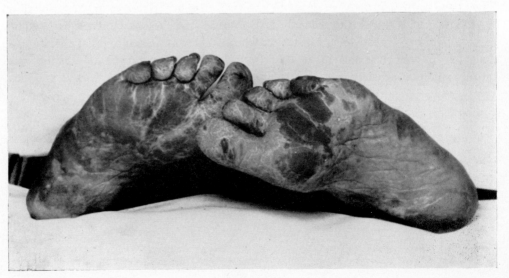

FIG. 194.

in the toes, thus increasing spasms of the paralysed legs, but by inevitably becoming infected they are a potential danger to the general condition of the patient.

ILL-EFFECTS OF HEAT AND COLD

The loss of sensibility in the paralysed part of the body includes the loss of appreciation of heat and cold. Objects, commonly used in daily life, may produce the most frightful burns in these cases. The hot-water bottle was found to be the main cause of burns in those paraplegics admitted with burns to this centre, and its use should never be allowed in these cases, even if protected by a cover. Instead, woollen bed-socks should be worn in bed in cold weather. The next on the list is the hot-water tap of the bath—especially in the case of ambulant patients. A paraplegic, before getting into the bath, should first make sure that the hot-water tap of the bath is completely turned off, and in bath-tubs for paraplegics it is preferable to have water taps situated in the middle of the bath instead of at the end. Wash-basins for paraplegics, which must be high enough to allow the wheelchair to be drawn up close to them, should have a bar on the floor to prevent the insensitive knees being burnt by the waste pipe when containing hot water. Spilling hot tea or coffee may result in scalding of the insensitive skin, and this is particular hazard for the female paraplegic when working with a kettle or saucepan from a wheelchair. This hazard can be best prevented or at least diminished by enlarging the space of the kitchen to facilitate better manoeuvring with the wheelchair and lowering the level of the electric or gas cooker as well as the sink to make work in the kitchen easier. One of our paraplegics developed severe burns of his feet in his car when the engine's heat made the metal under the front seat hot. Tetraplegics with sensory impairment in the fingers should always smoke with a holder to avoid burning. A further cause of burns in paraplegics is sitting too close to an open fireplace or electric fire, and when in such a position the limbs should always be protected. Precautions should also be taken in hot weather, when exposing the body to the direct sun in high thoracic and cervical lesions where the spinal heat-regulating mechanisms are impaired, as otherwise this may also have ill-effects.

Cold may also have ill-effects. Every paraplegic and tetraplegic with spasticity very soon becomes aware of the increase of flexor or extensor spasms when the paralysed part of the body is exposed to cold. Even more serious can be the effect of cold on the blood circulation in the distal parts of the lower limbs in certain cauda equina and conus lesions, which can result in permanent damage of the small vessels of the toes and feet as shown by their pinkish-blue colour and development of frost-bite. A useful precautionary measure is to prevent the legs being kept continuously in one position. Long woollen pants, woollen socks and warm, loose fitting shoes or fur-lined boots have proved beneficial, especially for those paraplegics engaged in factory work.

PRESSURE SORES

Definition and terminology

This condition is liable to develop in persons suffering from prolonged debilitating illnesses such as cachexia due to malnutrition, general shock following injury or burns, atherosclerotic vascular changes in old age, and lesions of the nervous system such as syringomyelia, multiple sclerosis and leprosy. In traumatic transverse lesions of the spinal cord, this has been considered throughout thousands of years as one of the inevitable complications, causing sepsis and early death. Although during the last quarter of this century this concept was proved as false, it still occurs in spite of all the advances made in this subject of medicine, not merely in the developing countries of Asia and Africa but, alas, in the so-called highly developed countries.

Various names have been used to describe this condition, such as trophic ulcers, decubitus, bed sores and pressure sores. In particular, the names bedsore and decubitus are misleading, as this condition may not only occur in bedridden patients but in any later stage of spinal cord lesions when the patient is wheelchair bound or able to walk. The correct name is undoubtedly pressure sore, for, from the results of all research, the statement can be made: *Where there is no pressure there is no sore.*

Mechanism

The mechanism underlying the causation of pressure sores in spinal cord sufferers has been a subject of many discussions in the old and modern literature (Brown-Sequard, 1853; Charcot, 1881; Riddoch, 1917; Trumble, 1930; Munro, 1940; Nissen, 1941; Guttmann, 1945, 1946, 1949, 1953, 1967; Dick, 1949; Exton-Smith & Sherwin, 1961; Kermani *et al.*, 1970; and others). The factors determining the formation of pressure sores can be classified as intrinsic and extrinsic.

A. INTRINSIC FACTORS

The most important intrinsic factor is the lowering of tissue resistance to pressure, which is most pronounced during the stage of spinal shock and flaccid paraplegia caused by the interruption of the spinal vasomotor pathways resulting in loss of the vasomotor control not only of the skeletal muscles, as is generally recognized, but also of the skin and mucosa. The loss of vasomotor control leads to a lowering of the tone in the vascular bed of the paralysed part of the body, especially the lower limbs. Therefore, a pressure which under normal conditions will not produce blockage of the blood supply resulting in ischaemia, will do so under these circumstances.

The second important intrinsic factor is the loss of sensation in the paralysed parts. Normally, afferent impulses arising from an area exposed to pressure, causing blockage of the blood circulation, elicit discomfort appreciated as numbness, pins and needles sensation and pain. These sensations, which are the earliest signs of impending ischaemia, normally readily initiate change of posture. Exton-Smith & Sherwin (1961) found the incidence of pressure sore in a group of 50 elderly patients to be directly related to the number of spontaneous movements they made during sleep. However, in transverse cord lesions, these sensations are abolished, and, if the patient's attendant ignores this most important fact and does not take appropriate measures to change the patient's position, ischaemia with all its deleterious consequences on the tissues inevitably occurs.

The third intrinsic factor is the anatomical arrangement of certain parts of the body

—i.e. the distance of bony weight-bearing prominences from the skin and the thickness of padding tissues such as fat and muscles between bone and skin.

The fourth intrinsic factor is the spasticity of the paralysed lower limbs, especially adductor spasms, which is responsible for the development of sores on the inner surface of knees and inner ankles as a result of producing shearing stress to the covering skin by continuous rubbing.

B. EXTRINSIC FACTORS

There are three extrinsic factors: pressure, maceration from exposing the skin to moisture (urine) and cold. Of these, pressure is of decisive importance, because causing blockage of the vascular supply represents the immediate cause in the development of sores. The degree and extent of the harmful effect of local pressure in paraplegia causing ischaemia of skin and deeper tissues are determined by its intensity, duration and direction. As to the direction, one must distinguish between purely vertical pressure and shear-stress, of which the effect of shear-stress is much more disastrous for its cuts of larger areas from their vascular supply. There can be little doubt that the forces resulting from shear-stress, acting parallel to the surface of skin and sliding the upper layers relative to the lower, play an essential role in determining the shape and size of a sore. In this connection, the disastrous effect of plaster casts and, in particular, plaster beds has already been mentioned.

With regard to the duration of pressure in producing death of tissues, Trumble (1930) found that a pressure of more than $1\frac{1}{2}$ lb per in^2 (about 80 mmHg) over a long period is likely to cause death of tissues.

Maceration of the skin by allowing the incontinent patient to lie in a wet bed may play an additional part in early decomposition and gangrene of the tissues once ischaemia due to pressure has developed.

Cold in later stages of paraplegia may facilitate the development of a sore due to vasoconstriction in the paralysed limbs.

Classification and localization

While pressure sores can develop in any part of the body which is exposed long enough to local pressure, in paraplegics one can distinguish between predilection places of sore development in the early stages and those in the late stages of paraplegia. The areas involved, as a rule, in the immediate and early stages are the sacrum (Fig. 195), trochanterics, ischium (Fig. 196), knees (Fig. 197), head of fibula (Fig. 135), heels and toes (Fig. 198) and, in patients lying on plaster beds or casts, also the spinous processes, ribs, and anterior and posterior superior iliac crests. Moreover, in patients placed in plaster, sores may develop at the edge of the plaster, even in the sensitive area, which of course are painful.

In later stages of spinal paraplegia, one has to distinguish between two groups of patients: (1) those who remain bedridden, for one reason or another, and (2) mobile paraplegics either in wheelchairs or walking with crutches and calipers. In the first group,

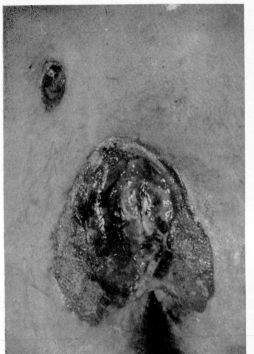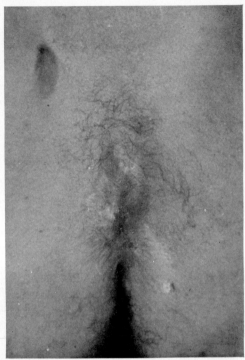

FIG. 195.

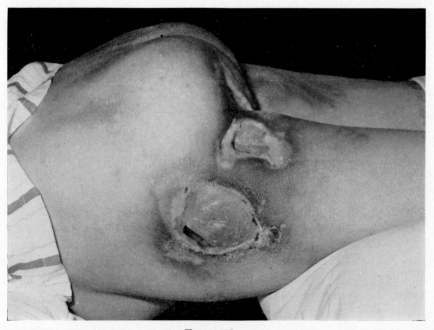

FIG. 196.

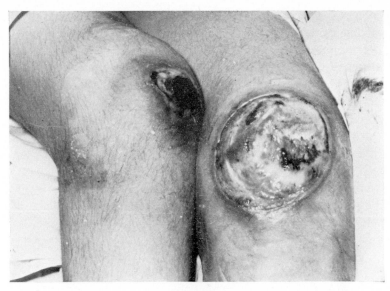

FIG. 197.

predilection places of sores, in addition to those already mentioned occurring in the early stages, are the patellae, inner surfaces of the knees, and inner ankles. Sores develop in these areas, particularly in cases with increased spasticity in which adductor and flexor spasms are predominant, and they are particularly dangerous because they easily penetrate into the knee and ankle joints. Special mention must be made of pressure in the trachea produced by tracheostomy tubes (see Chapter on Tracheostomy). Furthermore, a sore may develop at the inside of the nostril as a result of pressure from a nasal tube fixed by adhesive material against the innerside of the nose.

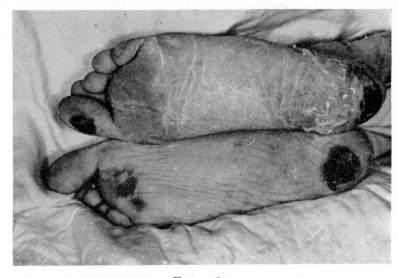

FIG. 198.

Predilection places of sores in ambulatory patients are the ischial tuberosities produced, in walking cases, mainly by weight-bearing calipers, but more frequently through
negligence on the part of the medical and nursing attendants by not instructing the
paralysed to relieve pressure by lifting himself at regular intervals or by the patient's
own negligence. Other predilection places in ambulant patients are the perineal area and
posterior surface of the penis (produced by urinals), the shins, outer ankles and fifth
metatarsal (produced by pressure against the wheelchair, motor-chair or car), and both
the dorsal and plantar surfaces of the toes, especially in cases of cauda equina lesion or
cord lesion where contractures of the toes occurred in the initial stages by faulty positioning.

From the mechanism and classification of bed sores given here, it will be apparent
that the old distinction between bed sores and pressure sores is a fallacy, as both result
from the same source—namely, pressure.

PATHOLOGY

The pathological changes in the cutaneous and subcutaneous tissues are determined
by the degree of ischaemia and the virulence and direction of spread of the inevitable
infection along the fascial plane or into the bone. Accordingly, it is possible to distinguish
the following stages in the development of sores.

1. **Stage of transient circulatory disturbance.** Pressure has been sufficient merely to
cause erythema of the skin, with some oedema, but without destruction of the tissues.
This pathological condition is reversible and promptly disappears if the pressure is
relieved and gentle massage applied.

2. **Stage of permanent damage to cutaneous tissues.** Various types of sores result
from this damage. One is characterized by erythema and congestion of the skin, which do
not disappear after relieving pressure but lead to induration and discoloration of the skin.
In another type, the superficial layers of the skin have been killed and may be excoriated,
exposing the exudating cutis vera. This type resembles an ordinary abrasion. In those
cases in which the dead epithelium remains intact, it is raised by exudation from the
cells of the cutis underneath, and a blister develops, which may be dark in colour if
haemorrhage has occurred (black blister). In a further type, deeper layers of the skin
may be involved, and this results in necrosis and formation of an ulcer after the slough
had been removed. The border of such an ulcer may become pigmented (Fig. 199).

3. **Stage of deep penetrating necrosis.** In this stage, the destruction also involves subcutaneous tissues, affecting fascia, muscle and bone. The necrotic and highly infected area
is usually surrounded by an inflammatory zone which will only disappear once the slough
is excised and the deep ulcer of the underlying fascia and muscle is exposed, as shown in
Fig. 200. This type of sore usually develops over sacrum and trochanters, and it may
assume enormous dimensions and grotesque shape. There are several varieties of shape:

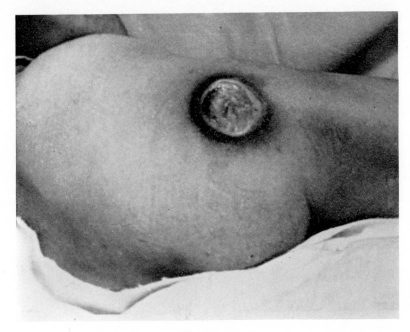

FIG. 199.

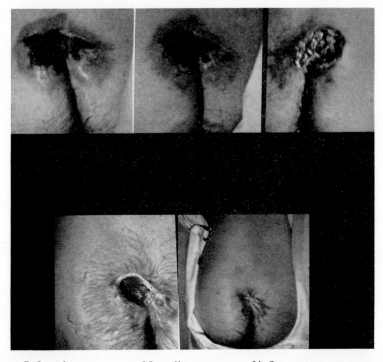

FIG. 200. Infected pressure sore. Note disappearance of inflammatory zone around sore after removal of slough.

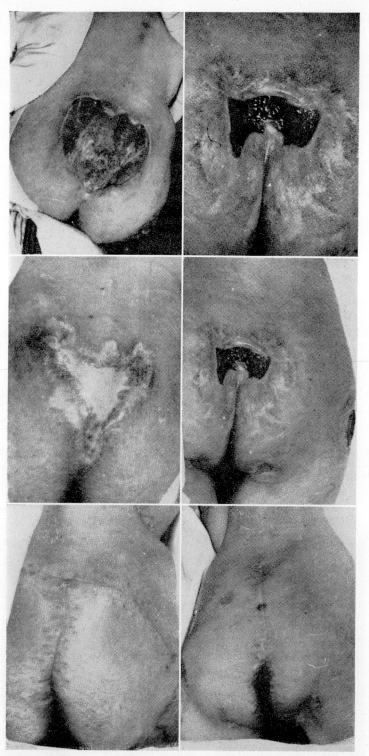

FIG. 201. Various shapes in sacral sores. (a) Triangular. (b) Trapezoid. From Guttmann (1955) *Brit. J. Plastic Surg.*, 7, 202.

triangular, quadrangular, trapezoid, and irregular (Fig. 201). Sometimes a large sacral sore may connect with sores over the ischial tuberosity, which may have developed simultaneously or at a later date (confluent sore) (Fig. 202). Often, the necrosis of the deeper tissues is more extensive than that of the skin, which accounts for the undermining nature of the sore.

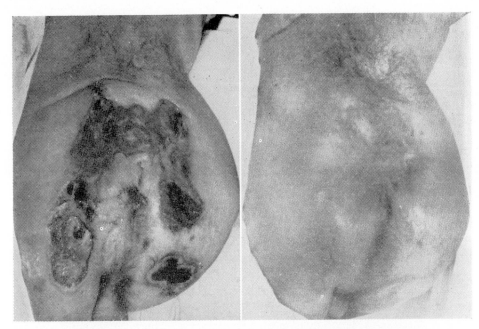

FIG. 202. From Guttmann (1955) *Brit. J. Plastic Surg.*, **7**, 200.

4. Sinus sore communicating with bursae. Trochanteric and, in particular, ischial sores also have the tendency to form deep sinuses, communicating with unilocular or multilocular bursae. The appearance of ischial sinus sores on the surface of the skin does not, as a rule, reveal the real size and extent of the connecting bursa or the resulting destruction of the underlying deeper tissues. Therefore, X-ray examination of the bony parts represents a most important routine examination in these cases, and moreover, contrast filling of the sinus (sinogram) has proved invaluable for the accurate diagnosis of the extent and direction of ischial sores (Fig. 203).

5. The closed ischial bursa. This represents a special variety of the ill-effects of pressure, found almost invariably in later stages of paraplegia, in ambulatory patients. As a rule, it develops as a swelling following acute trauma to the ischial region, such as bumping the buttocks or trochanters when the patient proceeds from his bed to his wheelchair or from his chair to a car, etc., but it may also develop without obvious acute trauma, due to continuous pressure. Aspiration of this swelling reveals bloodstained or just serous fluid, which usually recurs. X-ray following contrast filling will reveal a cavity of more or less elliptical shape (Fig. 204). If adequate treatment by rest in bed is not applied immediately and the patient is allowed to get up, the circulation of the skin covering the bursa will invariably suffer, resulting in ischaemia, necrosis, and formation of a sinus sore.

6. Cancerous degeneration of sores or scars. Gillis & Lee (1951) have drawn attention to the cancerous degeneration of long-standing sores and sinuses, and in their paper

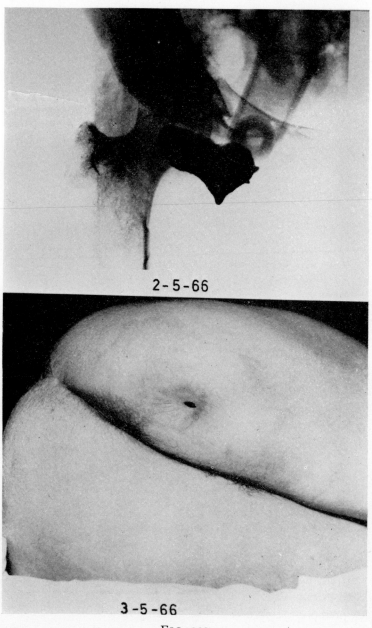

Fig. 203.

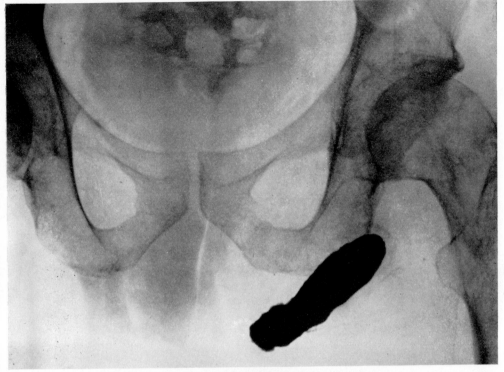

FIG. 204.

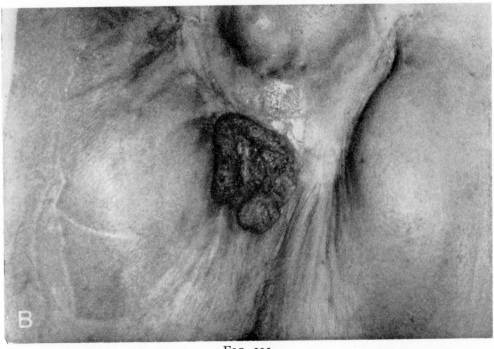

FIG. 205.

they mention two cases of cauda equina lesion from the First World War. Although this complication is a rare one in chronic sores, we have, amongst our material of several thousands of sores, one single incident of an epithelioma developing in the scar of a healed sacral sore (Fig. 205) which was excised by Dr Walsh and did not recur.

Complications following pressure sores

A. Infection: osteomyelitis, septicaemia

Sores always become infected, and, as already mentioned, in paraplegics they are, like the urinary infection, the commonest cause of sepsis and death. The infection is as a rule a mixed one of *Staph. aureus, B. strep. haemolyticus, Proteus, B. coli,* and *Ps. pyocyanea,* and will, if not counteracted from the very beginning, involve the deeper tissues and extend to the bone, causing periosteitis, osteitis, and osteomyelitis, with necrosis on the one hand and heterotopic bone formation on the other. Fig. 206 demonstrates two ischial

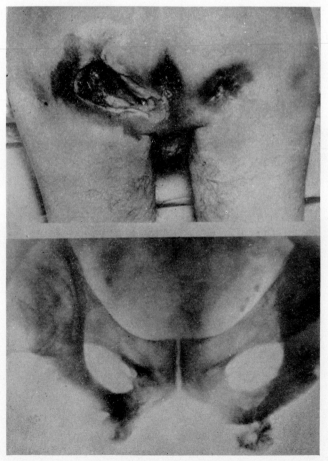

FIG. 206. Ischial sores with underlying osteomyelitis and ectopic calcification.

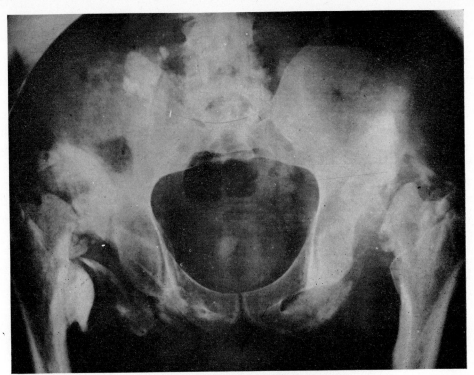

FIG. 207. Bilateral destruction of hip joints due to ischial sores.

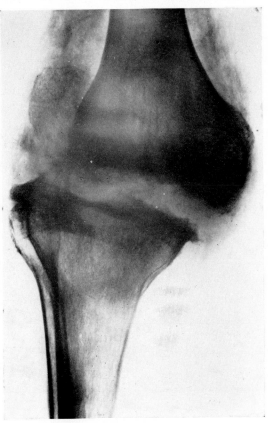

FIG. 208.

sores with underlying osteomyelitis. On the left side the ischial ramus is greatly destroyed and has a moth-eaten appearance, the right ramus is in an early stage of osteomyelitis, but both rami show ectopic bone formation as a result of the infection.

The great danger of developing osteomyelitis, following pressure sores of the trochanteric and, in particular, the ischial regions, cannot be stressed too much, having regard to the neighbourhood of the hip joints. In fact, in several patients admitted to the Centre, septic arthritis of the hip joints, with profound destruction of the acetabulum and head of the femur, was found (Fig. 207). In other cases, the septic arthritis involved the knee joints (Fig. 208). In cases with large sacral sores, the coccyx and part of the sacrum were found to be completely disintegrated and the ischio-iliac joint obliterated. Sores over the toes may also destroy joints (Fig. 209).

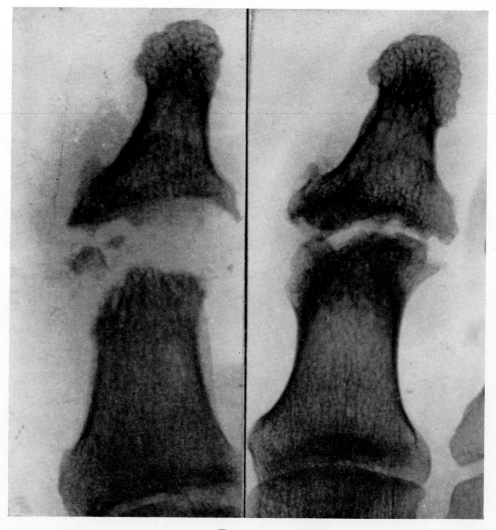

FIG. 209.

Of particular interest is the spread of infection in the sinus sores over the ischial tuberosity, and we can distinguish the extension of the infection in three directions:

a   Along the ischial ramus, the infection spreading, as a rule, in a lateral direction towards the hip joint, Fig. 207, although it may, very rarely, also spread medially towards the symphysis pubis.

b   Down along the posterior fascial compartments of the thigh, sometimes as far as the knee, in walking cases (Fig. 210).

c   Forwards into the region of the groin. This direction of spread is associated with prolonged and continuous nursing in prone position. The patient will develop a swelling in the groin, which will either perforate spontaneously or reveal pus on aspiration. The

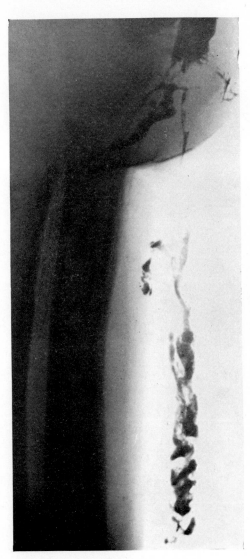

FIG. 210.

type of spread of infection is particularly dangerous as it is most obstinate to therapeutic measures.

d   A sinus developing from a trochanteric sore may spread into the anterior surface of the thigh, as shown by the sinogram in Fig. 211.

B. Nutritional effects

As one would expect, septic involvement of the bone naturally has its repercussions on the haemopoietic mechanisms, resulting in more or less severe anaemia. The tragedy in these cases is that, as a rule, the septic complications following pressure sores progress silently—a lingering or creeping type of sepsis without rise of temperature—and, moreover, if occasional flare-ups of temperature occur, these are often misinterpreted as due to ascending urinary infection. There is hardly any need to mention what disastrous effect

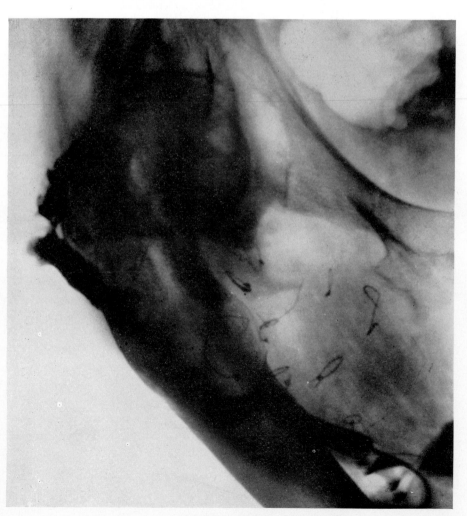

FIG. 211.

this septic condition has on the nitrogen balance of the patient. The drainage from sores results in continuous loss of protein. Poer (1946) found a daily loss of as much as 50 g of body protein as a result of drainage from sores. In fact, we have admitted paraplegics with pressure sores in such an extreme state of malnutrition that it could be compared only with that of inmates of Belsen Camp (Belsen type of paraplegic) (Figs. 6 and 7).

Treatment

General. In analysing the problem of treatment of pressure sores in paraplegics, it must at once be emphasized that local treatment of sores, whatever the method, will be of little or no avail unless it is correlated from the outset and throughout all stages of treatment, with the achievement of the best possible general condition. The importance of combating nutritional deficiency, the maintenance of nitrogen balance, and the treatment of anaemia, as some of the most important factors determining the rate of healing, cannot be stressed too much. In most of these cases with sores, repeated blood transfusions have to be given, and these, apart from high protein diets and vitamins, have proved to be the most efficacious way of dealing with anaemia and nutritional deficiency in these cases. It is necessary, in certain cases, to give at least one pint of full blood or, if undesirable reactions occur, packed red cells in saline at least once a week. There was one patient who came in with 17 sores who had as many as 81 blood transfusions during one year. All sores were healed and the patient discharged to his home. Cooper *et al.* (1950, 1951) claimed that testosterone improves the nitrogen balance because of its anabolic properties, and that this results in gaining weight and decreases the incidence of pressure sores in paraplegics. This has not been confirmed by other workers. Menion & Sheba (1961), using norethandrolone (Nilevar) in a double-blind trial on 395 geriatric patients, found no value in this drug for the prevention of pressure sores.

Local

(a) Prophylaxis. In discussing some of the main aspects of treatment mention must be made first of prophylactic measures. If the slogan 'Prevention is better than cure' has ever had any meaning, then it is in connection with pressure sores in paraplegics. Preventive measures should start immediately a paraplegia has occurred following injury, by removing hard objects from the patient's pockets, furthermore by padding bony prominences, counteracting traumatic shock, and, most important of all, by immediate transportation of the patient preferably to a spinal unit or hospital which can deal with spinal injuries. The immediate or very early admission of spinal cord injuries to a spinal unit has the great advantage that the whole set-up of such a unit, with its specialized medical and nursing staff, provides the best guarantee for the prevention of sores which, once developed, greatly delay the paraplegic's discharge from hospital and his rehabilitation to a useful life.

The cardinal prophylaxis is frequent change of posture, at least every 2 hours day and night, to relieve and redistribute pressure. The bony prominences over sacrum and trochanterics can best be safeguarded by placing the patient on pillow packs or, even better, on sorbo rubber packs (Figs. 73 and 74). Pressure to the heels can easily be prevented by placing pillows underneath the calves (Fig. 73b) avoiding those popular rings placed around the heels, whether made of cotton-wool, rubber, or other material. These were found to produce pressure sores, especially over the Achilles tendon, by shearing stress, rather than to prevent them. This is understandable if one remembers the course taken by the vascular supply to the heels, which can easily be interfered with by a constricting ring around the heels. It is unfortunate that, in the training courses of nurses, these 'halos' around the heels are still taught as the method of choice in preventing sores over the heels while their potential dangers are not considered.

As mentioned previously, in recent years the introduction of the Stoke Mandeville–Egerton electrically controlled turning bed has greatly facilitated the regular turning to prevent pressure sores and relieve pressure from established sores and thus promote healing. It may be stated that this is more difficult if not impossible to achieve with the Stryker frame, as the turning is only possible from the supine to prone position, in particular if a patient with a broken spine has sustained associated injuries such as fracture of ribs, haemothorax, etc., and has to lie in supine position for longer periods. The same can be said of the sheep-skin or the so-called ripple mattress (Gardner, 1948), where the pressure of the sets of compartments can be alternately inflated and deflated by a pump. Prevention or healing of a pressure sore will be best accomplished if the patient's position is changed from the supine into lateral position. To let the patient lie continuously or for periods longer than 2 hours in recumbent or lateral position will neither prevent nor heal sores penetrating into deeper tissues. Moreover, as already pointed out, the recumbent position is contrary to the principles of preventing stagnation and ascending infection of the urinary tract. Air and water mattresses have been abandoned, as they have not proved successful in preventing pressure on the bony parts.

As soon as possible, the paraplegic patient should be fully instructed in details about the dangers of pressure; indeed he should be indoctrinated with the idea that, as soon as he is transferred from a bedridden patient to the use of a wheelchair, prevention of sores or the break-down of a healed sore depends largely on his own alertness and watchfulness in frequently lifting himself, or, in the case of a tetraplegic, in shifting his position in the wheelchair from one side to the other.

Paraplegics with marked adductor spasticity should have a soft pad between the knees, the width of which must be adjusted to the degree of spasticity to prevent shear-stress between the knees.

Every evening before going to bed, paraplegics and tetraplegics should examine their buttocks for pressure damage with the aid of a hand mirror, or they should be examined by their attendants. To promote good circulation, gentle massage to the sacrum, buttocks and trochanter should be given. If the skin is harsh and dry it is well to use a mixture of olive oil and 50–60 per cent alcohol.

(b) Treatment of established sores. Once sores have developed, the principle of preventing pressure has to be enforced, and this represents the cardinal local treatment of sores. Furthermore, having regard to the fact that sores are always infected, early excision of sloughs, once they have developed and are demarcated, is necessary. If after removal of the cutaneous necrosis the underlying fascia is also found to be necrotic and appears to be infected, it should be incised and sufficiently excised to allow free drainage of the infected material. In many cases, underneath such a necrotic fascia, pockets of necrotic fat or abscesses will be found which have to be emptied. The immediate improvement of the patient's general condition, following such surgical transformation of a closed septic wound—a sore covered with slough is a classical example of a closed septic wound—into an open wound is always very striking. The old method, still advocated today, of leaving the slough untouched until it falls off by itself (Munro, 1952) or becomes liquified by various conservative procedures, is not only time consuming but most hazardous. It must be remembered that, in penetrating sores, the deeper tissues underneath the cutaneous slough are also necrotic and always infected. But, even if the deeper necrosis were to remain uninfected, the absorption of the dead tissues into the blood stream would in itself have toxic effects, manifested by listlessness of the patient, loss of appetite, bad taste in the mouth, and higher degrees of toxaemia may even lead to toxic psychosis. In one of my patients during the war, admitted with huge sloughy sores, the rapid disappearance of the psychotic symptoms following excision of the sloughs was most striking.

Following the excision of necrotic tissues and cleaning the surrounding skin, daily dressings are applied to the sores, using antibiotics in saline solution, varying in type and strength according to the type and severity of the infection. In our experience, dressings of streptomycin–saline ($\frac{1}{4}$–$\frac{1}{2}$ per cent) alternating with penicillin–saline have proved very effective to combat the local infection of the sore. Before the dressing is applied, the sore must be thoroughly cleansed with peroxide and saline.

Heavy chemicals are avoided in the local treatment, because they at least inhibit the growth of granulations and delay filling in of the defect resulting from the excision of the slough and may even cause direct damage to the tissues. Flavazole, 1 : 2,000, or, in very special cases of heavy proteus infection, 1 per cent in carbowax, is used for a few days. Once the infection of the sore has been checked by antibiotics or flavazole, wet dressings with sterile saline, weak boric solution (3 per cent), or Dakin's solution are substituted. In this early stage of healing—i.e. filling in the defect by granulations—dressings with greasy ointments of any kind, including paraffin, are strictly avoided.

Special attention has to be paid to the type of dressing used. The mere covering of the sore, especially sacral sores, with a thin layer of gauze which is fixed at the outer edges by thin strips of elastoplast is contraindicated for two reasons: first, such a dressing will never prevent reinfection of the wound by faecal matter and, secondly, it will crumple up and act as pressure to the granulating area and will thus not only delay the rate of healing but will, in fact, produce patches of necrosis in a healing sore manifested by patches of deep red or bluish discoloration. Therefore, after the wet dressing is applied, several layers of dry gauze is placed on top and the whole dressing is completely sealed off by porous elastoplast. Once the granulations have reached the level of the skin and epithelialization has started, this can be accelerated by pellidol ointment or, if the area is large, by seed grafts. With these procedures, sores of gigantic dimensions can be healed completely in a relatively short time (Fig. 212a).

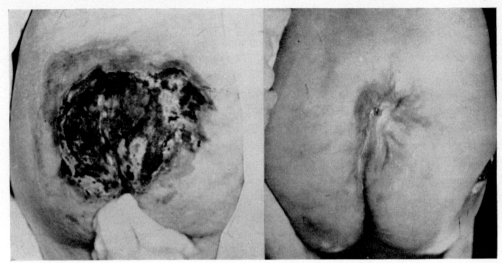

FIG. 212a. Large sacral sore healed by conservative treatment. Note relatively small healed scar.

HORIZONTAL DIMENSION = 18 cms. (7·1 ins)

VERTICAL DIMENSION = 15·8 cms (6·2 ins)

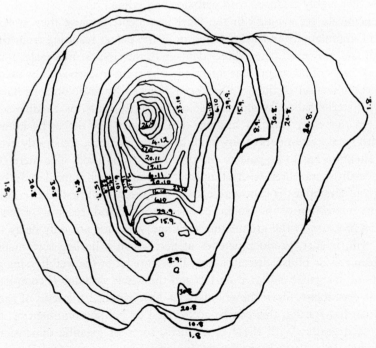

FIG. 212b.

EVALUATION OF TREATMENTS

The progress of healing can be assessed by photographs and by regular tracing of the sore with the two-film method (Guttmann, 1945). This is done by means of a sterile, decoated X-ray film or other transparent plastic sheath, which is placed over the sore and a second film which serves as a permanent record is placed on top. The outline of the sore is then traced on the top film with the date of the tracing. Tracings on the same film are repeated at regular intervals, every 4 or 6 days, and thus the speed and mode of healing can be determined by the change of size and shape of the sore. After complete healing the traced areas according to the dates are measured by means of a planimeter, a technique recommended by Carrel *et al.* (1918) for assessing the rate of healing of war wounds. Fig. 212b demonstrates the tracing and chart of the rate of healing of the gigantic sacral sore shown in Fig. 212c of a traumatic paraplegic. Such research would be

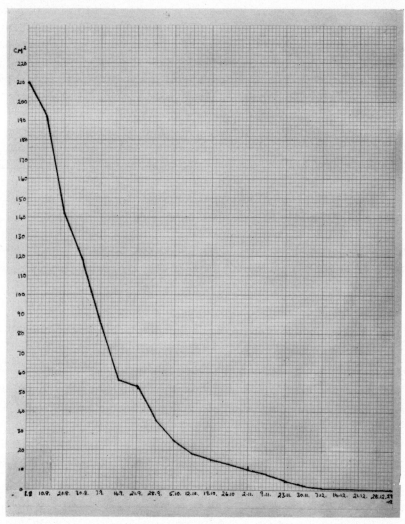

FIG. 212c.

most helpful in assessing the value of any local treatment recommended in the literature, such as poultices of carrots and turnips, linseed oil, bread (Paget, 1873), scarlet red, zinc oxide, tulle gras, or tincture of benzoine (Munro, 1940), fomentations (Riddoch, 1917), tannic acid (Latimer, 1934), aluminium, gold leaf (Gallagher & Geschichter, 1964; Oden, 1967), hyaluranidase (Davenport, 1962), animal collagen (Wanke & Grözinger, 1965; Stoop, 1970), negative air-ions (Ursu, 1970) and others. Unfortunately, most of these local procedures advocated do not give exact data and, therefore, comparative assessment of their value is impossible.

Amongst the various local treatments advocated, the ultra-violet treatment needs special mention, as it is still widely used by physiotherapists in the treatment of sores. From my own observations on pressure sores in paraplegics, I came to the conclusion that it has no advantage over any other local treatment unless at the same time the principle of avoiding pressure and the application of proper dressings, as outlined above, are strictly observed (Guttmann, 1970). It must be remembered that in pressure sores one deals with devitalized tissue. Therefore, a proper dosage of local applications of ultra-violet to the devitalized tissues is difficult and often impossible but there is no doubt that stronger doses have resulted in burns (personal observation).

The uncertainty of the value of so many local treatments has recently been aptly summed up by Dr Dollfus by quoting Dr Vilan of Paris, 'You can put anything you like on a pressure sore, except the patient'.

It has already been mentioned that one obstacle in the healing of pressure sores is intractable spasticity, particularly in complete transverse lesions of the spinal cord, which not only delays the rate of healing but makes later plastic repair of the sore difficult if not impossible. Major operations to deal with this complication, such as laminectomy with posterior or anterior rhizotomy to transform the spastic lesion into a lower motor neurone (i.e. flaccid) one, is, in these septic cases, most hazardous, as the profound surgical shock following such a major operation naturally increases the immediate danger to life of these often seriously ill patients. However, today such operations can be avoided altogether, as they can easily be substituted by intrathecal alcohol injections (Guttmann, 1953).

SURGICAL REPAIR

Epithelialization by pinch graft or 'postage stamp' grafts

The combination of surgical excision of sloughs and conservative management afterwards, as outlined above, has proved highly successful in our cases throughout the years. Sores of gigantic size and great depth could be healed and the resulting scar was, as a rule, a third of the original size of the sore (Fig. 112). As mentioned above, epithelialization of large sores over the sacrum can be accelerated surgically by skin grafts once the granulations have reached the level of the surrounding skin. We prefer pinch grafts to 'postage stamp' grafts as they take more readily. Pinch grafts are obtained by inserting the point of a wide-bore surgical needle into the skin of the donor area and removing a cone of the skin. Fig. 213 demonstrates the way of epithelialization following pinch grafts. The epithelium spreads irregularly from the centre of the pinch graft and confluent with the

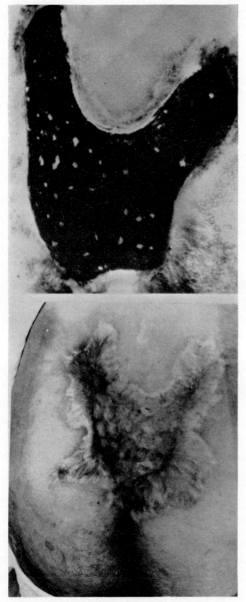

FIG. 213.

epithelium of its neighbours. The resulting final scar shows a cobblestone-like surface, unlike the smooth uniform scar of a sore which has grown more concentrically from the edges of the surrounding skin towards the centre of the sore (Figs. 201 and 202).

Treatment of skin surrounding large scars

Once a sore has been healed, it is important to adjust the surrounding skin and subcutaneous tissues to the remaining scar by proper massage to diminish tension which may lead to breakdown, especially in the centre of the scar where the blood circulation is particularly delicate and can easily be damaged by pressure or shear stress. This is also a very important pre-operative measure if plastic repair is contemplated, as the more pliable the surrounding skin has become the easier will be the approximation of the skin flaps following excision of the scar. We have always preferred to wait with closing skin defects with flaps until the sore is healed or at least in the last stage of epithelialization, because the size of the defect is greatly diminished by cicatrization.

Rotation and transposition flaps

A great variety of rotation and transposition flaps containing whole thickness of the skin and varying amount of subcutaneous tissue with or without addition of split skin grafts have been advocated for the surgical repair of large scars or sores, especially over the sacrum and trochanters (Barker, 1945, 1946; Conray et al., 1947; Osborne, 1955; Conray & Griffith, 1956; Blocksam, Kostrubala & Greeley, 1947; Bors & Comarr, 1948; Comarr, 1964; Bailey, 1967; Griffith, 1969). At the Stoke Mandeville Spinal Centre, the technique of glutaeal rotation flaps, as practised by Kilner and his school, has been adopted and carried out for many years successfully by my colleague J.J.Walsh (Fig. 201). This technique allows good approximation of the rotation flaps with the least amount of tension, and thus the whole scar is completely covered without forming a new open area which has to be covered with sliding grafts, as is often necessary following transposition flaps such as large thoraco-abdominal tubed pedicles as described by Conray & Griffith (1956), Bailey (1967) and others.

Trochanteric scars and ischial sores of smaller size are excised including removal of the osteomyelitic bone and closure by primary sutures can be accomplished in the majority of cases. The same applies to small sores over the buttocks.

Special mention may be made of two methods which I introduced some years ago for the surgical repair of special types of sores in the ischial area:

(1) 'Pseudo-tumour' technique for the removal of sinus sores

As already mentioned, the visible skin lesion in this type of sore is, as a rule, small and innocent in appearance, but it leads into a greater or lesser cavity adherent to the bone, and unless the wall of the cavity is excised in toto with the infected bone, such a sore will not heal. In order to facilitate the tedious dissection of such a flaccid bursa, the wall of which is often difficult to define, thus necessitating continuous working in a highly contaminated area, the cavity is first packed as tightly as possible with narrow ribbon gauze soaked in a brightly coloured antiseptic, usually flavine or flavazole, whereby the cavity is distended as much as possible and has the appearance of a tumour. The narrow opening in the skin is then closed with one or two sutures, and, through an elliptical incision, the whole mass of pseudo-tumour is dissected out of the surrounding tissues (Fig. 214). Contamination of the operation field is thus avoided. The pseudo-tumour adherent to the bone is then removed with the infected part of the bone (Guttmann, 1953). Only in selected cases has it been necessary to perform a complete ischiectomy—

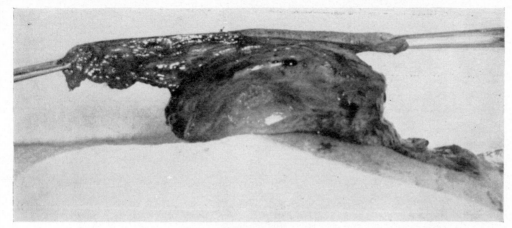

FIG. 214.

a procedure recommended by Bors & Comarr (1948). After removal of the distended bursa, the resulting cavity is closed by primary suture in several layers. With regard to suture material, catgut has proved unsuitable as it gives rise to abscess formation, but since it was substituted by steel wire or nylon our results in primary suture have greatly improved. The value of this method has been confirmed by other workers in this field (Bailey, 1967).

(2) Rotation-flap to diminish sensory loss in cauda equina lesions

In cauda equina lesions with saddle anaesthesia, ischial sores can be successfully treated by rotation flaps from the lateral, sensitive part of the buttocks. Such a procedure will diminish the anaesthetic area and to a certain degree restore sensation to pressure on the buttocks, thus making the patient aware of pressure. This has been achieved in the following case: in a patient with a cauda equina lesion below L4, who was admitted with profound distortion of the pelvis caused by lying for several months in a plaster bed where he developed two deep ischial sores, we succeeded in healing these sores completely by conservative means in two months. However, both sores recurred as soon as the patient was sat up, and indolent undermined ulcers resulted (Fig. 215a). At my suggestion, rotation flaps were performed by Mr Elliott Blake, one of Professor Kilner's colleagues, with the idea to diminish the area of sensory loss, in order to restore the feeling of pressure as much as possible and thus induce the patient to change his position. Fig. 215b shows the result several months later, clearly demonstrating that the aim of reducing the size of the insensitive area was achieved. There has been no recurrence whatsoever since the operation, which was carried out on 22 November 1944, and this patient has been employed full-time in a factory during the last 25 years.

Excision of ischium, trochanterics, head of femur and hip joint

These major operations may become necessary in certain cases of neglected trochanteric and ischial sores resulting in osteomyelitis. As already mentioned the infected bone has

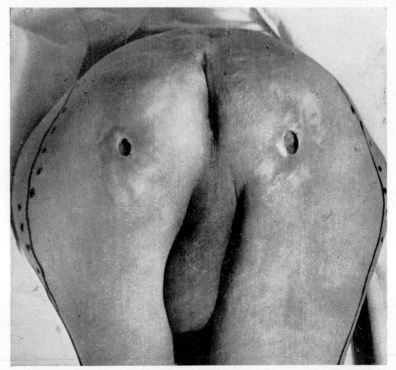

FIG. 215a. ———— line of anaesthesia, ... line of analgesia.

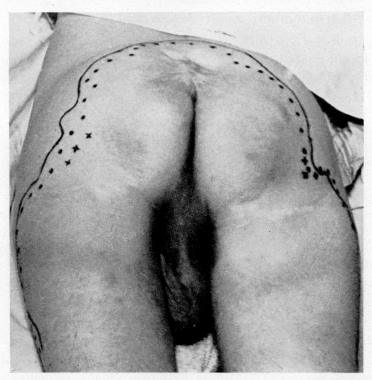

FIG. 215b.

to be removed, as otherwise the infection will spread further. Following removal of the infected trochanter there is, of course, the danger of a fracture of the femur underneath the trochanter later, especially under weight-bearing. More destructive is the operation if the infection, spreading from ischial or trochanteric sores, has affected the head of the femur involving the hip joint. Under these circumstances, the head of the femur has to be excised and the infected parts of acetebulum removed. Needless to say, systemic courses of antibiotics and blood transfusions before and after such operation are indispensable. Once the infection has subsided, it is sometimes amazing to what degree a new, though only incomplete, hip joint may develop. The regenerative forces of restoring a joint following healing of osteomyelitis as a result of pressure sores has been mentioned previously (Guttmann, 1953) and Fig. 209 show the restitution of a completely disinte-grated terminal joint of a big toe following healing of a pressure sore (in this case by conservative treatment).

Ectopic bone formation in soft tissues following ischial sores affecting the ischial ramus (Fig. 206) represents a relatively frequent complication, and, unless this is excised together with the infected ramus, the sore will not heal or will recur. However, total ischiectomy should be reserved for very selected cases, the more so as, following this operation there is a shifting of weight bearing to the other side, and there were a few cases where an ischial sore developed later on that side. However, this can be avoided, as Walsh found, by cutting a hole in the sorbo rubber cushion on the non-operated side which considerably relieves pressure when the patient sits in his wheelchair. Bilateral radical ischiectomy (Comarr, 1951) may have serious effects on the perineal urethra, and Comarr & Bors (1958) found perineal urethral diverticula in 58 per cent of cases following bilateral ischectomies. In contrast Arregui et al. (1965) do not mention this complication in their review on 94 patients, in whom 43 unilateral and 51 bilateral ischiec-tomies were carried out. Urethral damage following bilateral ischiectomy can be avoided if the ischiectomy is performed less radically—i.e. if the excision of the medial part of the ischial ramus is not extended too close to the symphysis.

Sores over the coccygeal area often tend to recur, and if the bone is infected a coccy-gectomy followed by primary suture will be necessary.

Sores over the knee may be very dangerous, once they have affected the knee joint (Fig. 208), and in this particular case because of causing septicaemia an amputation above the knee became imperative.

Sores over the shin usually heal conservatively by preventing any pressure on the sore or they can be treated by pinch grafts.

Chronic malleolus sore will only heal following resection of the infected bone.

Sores over the heels, which frequently occur due to inadequate care, will, as a rule, heal easily without surgery, apart from the removal of slough, as even the slightest pressure can be avoided in that area by the placing of two or three pillows underneath the calf. The heel and Achilles tendon will then be absolutely free from pressure whatever the patient's position may be.

Sores over the spine are now very rare since plaster casts and plaster beds were aban-doned, and I have not seen any for many years. During the war, they were sometimes found to be present over several vertebrae, and resection of spinous processes was necessary.

In tetraplegics below C5, occasionally a sore may develop over the elbow. Partial resection of the infected olecranon process and its bursa may be necessary.

PRE-OPERATIVE MANAGEMENT

There was a time when plastic surgeons were keen to perform rotation or transposition flaps in sores with active infection and were quite satisfied if the flap was taken by 50, 60 or 80 per cent. We always considered this as a 100 per cent failure as by such results an open septic wound was transformed into an undermined one. However, it is now generally agreed that surgical repair of sores in paraplegic patients should not be undertaken unless the active infection, in particular, of staphylococci and haemolytic streptococci, is controlled, the sore is healing and the general condition of the patient is perfect. Haemoglobin should be 85–90 per cent, red cells well over 4 millions. As the patient, following surgical repair of sacral and ischial sores, has to lie partly or entirely in abdominal position (Fig. 216) for several weeks he should get well accustomed to this position on sorbo-rubber packs before the operation. Of great importance is a thorough clearing out of the bowels on several subsequent days before the operation. The patient should be kept under antibiotic treatment one or two days before operation and this should be continued after the operation. If an extensive rotation flap is contemplated and heavy bleeding is expected, it is wise to start the operation with a slow blood transfusion to avoid surgical shock.

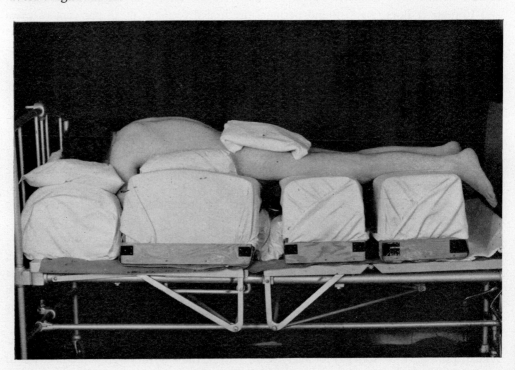

FIG. 216.

POSTOPERATIVE CARE

A plastic operation, as any other major surgical procedure, may easily have an adverse effect on the unstable vasomotor control of these patients, and pulse and blood-pressure need careful attention in the first few days after operation. Blood transfusions are often necessary to counteract prolonged surgical shock in these patients. Haematomas have to be removed immediately and can be voided by suction through a fine multiperforated polyethylene tube following operation. Flexion of the hips is not allowed for three weeks after complete healing of the ischial and trochanteric sores, after which time passive flexion is started and gradually increased to a right angle, until flexion produces no tension of the skin whatsoever. The patient is usually not allowed out of bed until 4–5 weeks after operation.

Pressure consciousness

Finally, no healing of a sore, whether by conservative or surgical procedures, will be successful if the patient has not been instructed about the dangers of pressure and how to avoid it. In other words, the patient has to be made absolutely 'pressure or sore conscious', and this is the most important pre-condition in the prevention or recurrences of sores and thus in the successful rehabilitation and industrial resettlement of paraplegics. The paraplegic who is employed, must never forget to lift himself at regular intervals even when sitting on a 4-in sorbo-rubber cushion, which should never be covered with stiff rexine. Clothing and footwear has to be chosen carefully to avoid rubbing or pressure to the tissues, especially to malleoli and toes. The urinal has to be in a proper position to avoid pressure or friction in particular to the penis. As paraplegics with complete lesions are insensitive in their paralysed limbs, they must take care not to knock their legs against hard objects when transferring themselves from the wheelchair to the car and vice versa. 'Look before you leap' means to a paraplegic more than a proverb, especially for those with healed sores. Tetraplegics should avoid prolonged pressure on the elbows when resting their forearms too long on the arm rest of the wheelchair or on a mattress—when lying prone in bed. Tetraplegics below C6 who can propel themselves in their wheelchairs should have a soft leather pad over the palm of the hand to prevent pressure to the insensitive ulnar area of the hands.

Amputations

Not very long ago surgeons (Lindenberg, 1953; Street, 1958; Chase & White, 1959; Felix, 1959) performed amputations on patients with transverse lesions of the spinal cord as a preventive measure to the development of pressure sores, or these operations were carried out indiscriminately in paraplegics suffering from sores in the paralysed limbs which could have been healed by adequate conservative or surgical treatment or even on the grounds, that without their 'useless' legs, they will be more mobile. During the Second World War the writer saw such mutilated victims, amongst them a tetraplegic, who had a bilateral amputation above the knees performed some time after his injury. The tragedy in this case was that he made a considerable recovery from his cord lesion, but as a result of the amputation he was unable to sit. In two other patients with transverse lesions even high amputations with exarticulation of the hip joint were performed because of penetrating pressure sores. In a case with marked spasticity of the legs the right leg was amputated above the knee because of a sore penetrating into the knee joint. As a result the patient developed such a profound flexion contracture of the hip that the stump became firmly fixed to the abdomen, indeed a shocking sight. The writer has always been strongly opposed to these mutilating procedures, carried out indiscriminately (Guttmann, 1961).

Amputations of limbs in transverse lesions of the cord should have the same strict indications as accepted in non-paralysed patients:

1   Vascular obstruction of a large artery resulting in stoppage of blood flow and gangrene of the limb below the obstruction due to any acute or chronic vascular afflictions such as thrombangiitis obliterans.

2   Severe congenital or acquired deformity of one or both legs combined with contractures. In 1959 a report was given about a 17 year old girl with spina bifida with profound deformity of both feet who, in spite of full function of the quadriceps on both sides, since early youth was chair-bound. Following bilateral amputation below the knees and fitting with appropriate prostheses she was able to stand and walk for the first time in her life. The same result was achieved in another case of spina bifida—a man aged 40 in whom, because of profound deformity of the right foot, an amputation below the knee was performed (Guttmann, 1959).

3   Certain compound fractures of long bones involving disruption or other severe damage of large vessels.

4   Severe osteomyelitis of the ankle joint, which cannot be healed by conservative treatment, to restore walking capability in conus–cauda equina lesions.

CHAPTER 32

CLINICAL MANAGEMENT OF SPASTICITY

The heightened reflex activity of the isolated cord, following transection or severe lesions in continuity resulting in violent flexor or extensor spasms and rigidity of the muscular system below the level of the lesion, represents one of the most incapacitating of complications and is a formidable obstacle to the rehabilitation of paraplegics and tetraplegics. However, with the advances made in a better understanding of the factors promoting and, in particular, preventing excessive spasticity, and consequently the introduction of selective modern techniques of treatment, this complication has lost much of its dread.

The management of spasticity consists of a combination of conservative and surgical procedures according to type, severity and extent of the heightened reflex activity. Nurses and physiotherapists have to play a most essential part in dealing with this problem.

A. CONSERVATIVE TREATMENT

1. Elimination of factors lowering the threshold of spinal reflex activity

A number of intrinsic and extrinsic factors may act as nociceptive stimuli to the unrestrained activity of the isolated cord. Distension of any internal organ in the paralysed area, particularly the bladder, is one of the most important violent initiators of reflex spasms. It is obvious that the smaller the capacity of the bladder (as found in contracted bladders following suprapubic cystostomy and prolonged indwelling catheter drainage) the smaller the amount of urine necessary to elicit the reflex response of the skeletal muscles and the more frequent the spasms. Of equal importance is distension of the rectum and colon through stagnation of faeces. Indeed, the beneficial effect of the evacuation of an overloaded rectum on the intensity of reflex spasms is often remarkable as also is the prevention of stagnation of the faeces in the higher parts of the colon by the administration of adequate laxatives. Furthermore, intervening infection—in particular urinary flare-up or toxaemia from pressure sores and, last but by no means least, anaemia—also lowers the threshold of reflex activity of the damaged spinal cord. Frequently, the increased spasticity of the paralysed limbs was found to be the first sign of active urinary infection, long before the temperature rose and other symptoms appeared. Moreover, the successful treatment of these infectious conditions has often resulted in a decrease in the intensity of flexor spasms.

Another factor conducive to reflex spasms is the irritation of sensory organs in contracted tendons and joints. In non-paralysed persons, the irritation of these sensory organs is appreciated as pain. In complete and also severe incomplete transverse lesion of the spinal cord, sensation is lost in the paralysed area, but nevertheless the afferent impulses arising from the contracted joints or tendons remain just the same and act as strong afferent stimulus to the isolated cord, thus increasing its unrestrained activity.

Passive movements from the start are essential measures and are most effective in the prevention and treatment of excessive spasticity. The effect of passive movements on the relaxation of spastic muscles is increased by placing the patient in a continuous bath of a constant warm temperature while these movements are carried out under water.

It was found that alternating passive movements of paralysed spastic legs, produced by cycling action in a pedal exerciser worked with the arms, has a remarkably relaxing effect on spasticity. The writer's design of such an exerciser for paraplegic patients (Guttmann, 1949) is described in detail in the chapter on physiotherapy. The relaxing effect of this pedal exerciser, which represents mainly a fatigue effect, lasts several hours and in some cases even throughout the day, and this naturally gives great relief to the spastic paraplegic patient. Thus, in accordance with Riddoch's observations (1917) that fatigue has a depressant effect on spasticity, we utilized the fatigue effect on the spastic patient to facilitate his activities in the wheelchair or walking in parallel bars or on crutches. Another method to relieve spasticity is that of continuous tetanizing of muscle groups by low voltage currents (Lee *et al.*, 1950; Vogel *et al.*, 1955). However, this method did not become popular.

2 Utilization of postural reflexes

The effect of posture on the flexor and extensor reflex response has already been mentioned. While, in the supine position, the flexor reflex response of hips and knees is predominant, in the prone and upright position it is the extensor reflex synergy. Following my physiological studies in the spinal man, I have systematically used the earliest possible standing position of paraplegics in parallel bars as a means of overcoming the exaggerated action of the flexors of hips and knees. It was found that, with training, the change from the flexor to the extensor synergy could be greatly accelerated, sometimes even to such an extent that standing and walking in parallel bars without the aid of any artificial support to the legs was possible. In high thoracic and especially cervical lesions, the extensor synergy of the trunk and lower limbs could be greatly enhanced by placing the patient for several hours into prone position.

3. Effect of drugs on spasticity

For many years, there has been a constant search for a drug which would have a long lasting, relaxing peripheral effect on spasticity without having undesirable side effects on the whole organism. From all personal observations and publications of many authors, it can be concluded that so far such a drug does not exist. This applies to Curare (Tubo-curarine), Myanesin (Tolserol, Mephenesin), Chlormezzanine (Trancopal), Equanil (Metrobamate), Flexine (Zoxazolamine) and Prostigmin, the latter by mouth or intramuscular injections (Schlessinger, 1946; Elkins & Wegner, 1946; Guttmann, 1946; Weiss *et al.*, 1956; Carter, 1959; Ganz, 1959). Myanesin first described by Berger & Bradley (1946) as a muscle relaxant in animals has been widely applied in past years in the treatment of rigidity and spasticity, but toxic reactions such as haemoglobinuria and thrombophlebitis at the site of the injection were observed (Pugh & Enderly, 1947). We have used most of these drugs on our own patients but found that, while these drugs may have a depressant effect on the spastic muscles, they also affect the muscles of the normal part of the body as well as producing undesirable psychological effects. Amongst the drugs examined, Tigloidine, a tiglic acid ester of the atropine series, advocated by O'Rourke et al. (1960) in spastic paraplegics has proved quite useless in our own patients. In recent years, Valium (Diazapem), an analogue of Librium (Chlordiazepoxide), has been widely used in this and other countries (Dejak & Lowry, 1965; Neill, 1965; Wilson & McKecknie, 1966; Kerr, 1966; Nathan, 1970; and others). In a discussion held at the annual meeting of the International Medical Society of Paraplegia in 1966, there was general agreement that Valium has definitely a relaxant effect on spasticity in small doses without affecting too much the patient's general condition. However, it may lead to drug addiction like Librium if used in prolonged medication and higher doses (Jousse, Frankel, Guttmann & Walsh, 1966). Maglio (1966), who treated paraplegics, tetraplegics and haemiplegics with Valium in doses of 40 to 50 mg, found that alcohol is an absolute contraindication when Valium is used, and Kerr (1966) found, in doses of 16 to 24 mg daily, drowsiness and a feeling of slackness of the limbs in incomplete lesions as the main side effects. Corbett et al. (1972) carried out at Stoke Mandeville a double blind cross-over trial of Valium against Amytal and Placebo on 22 spastic paraplegics. Observations were made by 6 independent observers. It was found that Valium was significantly more effective than Amytal and Placebo and there was a low incidence of side-effects.

With regard to the effect of Prostigmin, there is no doubt that intrathecal injections of Prostigmine 0·3 mg has a profound but only temporary relaxant effect on the skeletal muscles (Kremer, 1941; Guttmann, 1953), and I have used this first in cases with intractable spasticity combined with profound contractures of hip and knee joints to determine the degree of contractures whilst the depressant action of this drug on the skeletal muscles was at its height. With regard to its action on the reproductive organs, see chapter on sexual function.

B. SURGICAL PROCEDURES

(1) On the spinal cord or spinal roots

(a) Laminectomy and myelolysis—cordectomy

In the past, laminectomy and myelolysis has been performed by many neuro-surgeons to relieve spasticity. However, there is no doubt that this procedure cannot be the answer, having regard to the many factors involved in the pathophysiology of the isolated cord, and, in fact, most surgeons with experience would now agree that this operation can only achieve temporary, if any, relief.

Cordectomy (MacCarthy, 1954) represents a very destructive operation and would be justified only in certain intramedullary tumours but not in traumatic lesions of the spinal cord.

(b) Posterior rhizotomy

Foerster, in 1911, reported on the beneficial effect of posterior root sections in 81 cases of spastic paralysis of various aetiologies—among them four cases of traumatic paraplegia, but in only two of which proved this operation to be effective. Freeman & Heimburger (1948) tried this method in two cases without success, which is in accordance with the experience of previous authors (Kreuz, 1932; Lehmann, 1936; Tarlov, 1966). My personal experience of posterior rhizotomy, gained at Foerster's clinic and later in my own department at the Jewish Hospital, Breslau, is in accordance with these authors. In spite of excellent initial success in spastic cases, recurrence of spasticity occurred, despite extensive posterior rhizotomy from L1–S3 (Guttmann, 1931). This is understandable, if one remembers that in selective posterior rhizotomy the input from the remaining posterior roots will sooner or later compensate the lost afferent impulses of the divided roots.

(c) Anterior rhizotomy

Munro advocated anterior rhizotomy for relieving intractable spasticity (1945, 1948). He suggested division of the anterior roots from T12 to S2 and reported satisfactory results in numerous cases in transforming the spastic lesion into a flaccid lower motor lesion. He recommended electrical stimulation of the sacral roots prior to their resection while cystomy was carried out in order to preserve satisfactory bladder function. Martin & Davis (1948) resected as high as T10 and they and Elkins & Wegner (1946), Maltby (1945), Freeman & Heimburger (1947) and others confirmed Munro's views. Dick (1949) mentions seven cases of the Spinal Unit, Winnick, where anterior rhizotomy was performed by Sutcliffe Kerr from T10 to S1 with the result that spasticity was abolished in several cases and the bladder capacity increased. However, in 5 of the 7 cases, the sexual erection reflex was abolished. Mayfield (1945) and Kennedy (1946) stressed the point that anterior rhizotomy is indicated in selected cases only—a view with which I agreed (Guttmann, 1946, 1953). Recently, Sutcliffe Kerr (1966) reviewed 30 cases (23 males, 7 females) in which he performed this operation, 19 of them being traumatic cord lesions above T10. In all cases, the spasticity was more or less relieved in the legs. Sutcliffe Kerr does not claim that this procedure is necessarily superior to other methods of prevention and treatment of spasticity but points out that it can be a useful procedure in certain circumstances. The operation may be indicated in a patient who is desperately ill from extensive pressure sores or urinary infection or is suffering intolerably from frequent spasms and yet may be in good general condition. Other authors mentioned certain disadvantages with this procedure which deserves serious consideration:

1 Identification of the spinal roots is not always a simple matter, as pointed out by Botterell, Macdonald & Mackenzie (1946). The difficulty of root identification is obviously increased in more distal cord lesions, when injury to the spine has more or less resulted in spinal deformities and alterations in the topographical relations.

2 If not only the leg muscles but also the abdominal muscles, such as in mid and upper thoracic as well as cervical lesions, are involved in violent spasms, a very extensive

laminectomy or two laminectomies are necessary in order to divide all the anterior roots necessary to denervate these muscles.

3 It must be pointed out that, in chronic traumatic paraplegics, laminectomy represents a destructive operation which weakens further the stability of the spine and the back muscles so vital for the restoration of the paraplegic's upright position and independence. Moreover, postoperative shock, which inevitably follows laminectomy as in any other major operation carried out under general anaesthesia, has always to be taken into consideration. However, there is no doubt that in those years, anterior root section was a breakthrough in the radical elimination of intractable spasticity.

(2) Surgical procedures on peripheral structures

Tenotomies, myotomies, muscle transplantations, partial or complete resections of peripheral nerves, and osteotomies have been practised in the treatment of spasticity, mainly by orthopaedic surgeons, for many years. They have proved most effective in many instances provided proper selection of the individual procedures was made and the operation followed up by purposeful conservative treatment. From all personal experience, the writer has no doubt that procedures on peripheral structures should be given preference to destructive operations on the spinal cord or intrathecal injections of alcohol or phenol, especially in incomplete lesions with satisfactory bladder and sexual function. The choice of the procedure depends on the degree and type of spasticity and the ascertaining and evaluating of those individual muscles or muscle groups which are predominant in the heightened reflex activity. In certain protracted cases, a combination of two or more procedures may be necessary to achieve the desired results. In the following only the common operations are mentioned.

(a) *Elongation of the Achilles tendon—Tenotomy of toe flexors and/or tibialis posterior*

These operations are indicated if the plantar flexors of the feet and toes are predominant in the increased reflex activity and, in particular, if contractures have developed due to faulty positioning of feet and toes during the stage of spinal shock and violent flexor contractions have developed later. It is important to combine the elongation of the Achilles tendon with subcutaneous tenotomy of the flexors of the toes if these muscles are contracted. In some cases, plantar flexion synergy is associated with marked inversion of the foot; therefore, the elongation of the Achilles tendon should be combined with tenotomy of the tibialis posterior which is a strong supinator of the foot. The relaxant effect of the elongation of the Achilles tendon on the whole flexion reflex activity is sometimes very striking.

As to technique, the patient is placed in prone position in such a way that the feet and ankles hang freely over the lower end of the table. This allows assessment of the proper angle of 85° of the feet's position following elongation of the Achilles tendon and prevents over-correction in dorsiflexion. Once the tendon is exposed, all layers of the tendon sheath have to be thoroughly dissected and retracted, but the elongated tendon must afterwards be covered completely by the sheath with fine silk sutures.

Of the three incisions used of the tendon—frontal (vertical), oblique and Z-form—I previously carried out the vertical technique but the Z-form has become the most popular. For the suture of the edges of the divided tendon, either finest silk or stainless steel sutures are used. Great care must be taken when applying the dressing and well padded splint that the position of the feet at 85–90° angle is maintained and pressure to heels must be strictly avoided during the following weeks. Standing and walking should, normally, not commence before three weeks after operation. It is then the task of the physiotherapist and the patient to ensure full weight-bearing on the whole plantar surface of the feet.

Tendon transplantations for the correction of severe spastic pes equino-varus, by transferring part or the whole of the tibialis anterior tendon on to the extensor digitorum or, in cases of severe spastic equino-valgus, transferring the peroneal tendons on to the extensor digitorum, have rarely been necessary.

In the past resection of two-thirds of the branches of the gastrocnemius muscle, the dorsal branch of the soleus and the innervation of the toeflexors (Stoffel's operation) has been used for elimination of the increased plantar flexion reflex activity and contractures. However, this operation has had only temporary effects, and the end results have been as disappointing as the selective resection of the spinal roots.

(b) *Resection and/or elongation of knee-flexors*

Prolonged approximation of the knee-flexors during the stage of spinal shock by keeping the legs in semi-flexion often leads to tendinous contractures and in increased flexor spasms once reflex automatism has developed. Unless the contractures can be overcome by conservative means (see chapter on Physiotherapy), resection of inner hamstring tendons with or without elongation of the biceps femoris has to be performed to restore standing and walking.

(c) *Resection of the obturator nerve and myotomy of the ilio-psoas*

The most incapacitating part of the reflex flexion synergy are violent hip flexor and adductor spasms, often resulting in contractures if not counteracted from the beginning. These complications not only make standing and walking impossible but greatly interfere with the sexual activity of paraplegics and tetraplegics, especially those with incomplete lesions where potency and fertility is preserved. If adductor spasms are predominant, the intrapelvic, extraperitoneal resection of the obturator nerve, as introduced by Selig (1914), is the method of choice, and in our material has proved the most effective treatment of this complication. Fig. 217 shows the effect of this operation in a severe though incomplete transverse lesion below T5 with profound adductor spasms which not only made walking most difficult but also greatly interfered with sexual intercourse. Following bilateral intrapelvic obturator resection walking capability greatly improved, and the patient was able to carry out his marital activities with full satisfaction to his wife and himself. This method is infinitely preferable to the subinguinal, extrapelvic resection, as the obturator nerve has already branched off into its peripheral ramifications, nor has myotomy of the adductors proved a suitable method in these cases. Crushing or only partial resection of the obturator, which is still recommended (Griffith, 1969), has generally proved unsatisfactory and of only temporary value in these patients, as there is recurrence of violent adductor spasms as soon as the nerve has regenerated. Michaelis

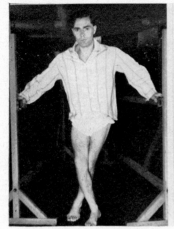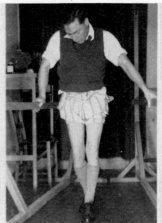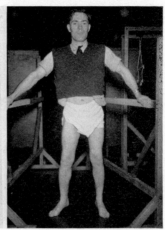

FIG. 217.

(1965) reported on 78 paralysed patients of our Centre, in whom he had carried out 102 obturator resections with excellent results and no failure. In addition to abolishing the adductor spasms and contractures, this operation had a considerable relaxant effect on the whole spasticity of both lower limbs. In young adults without adductor contractures, unilateral obturator resection may be quite sufficient to remedy excessive adductor spasms. For, bilateral resection in these cases may result in marked over-correction, and later in abduction contractures.

In severely spastic patients, the prevalent adductor spasms and contractures are greatly aggravated by profound flexor spasms and contractures of the hips. Tenotomy of the iliopsoas below or above the obturator membrane and with or without detachment of the minor trochanter has not proved satisfactory in our cases. The method of choice to correct flexion contractures of the hips has been proximal tenotomy of iliopsoas, which can be combined with obturator nerve resection at the same operation. Michaelis (1965) reported permanent, complete correction of the contractures in 11 out of 14 patients with profound spasticity and extreme flexor contractures of the hips. In one case, a myotomy of the oblique externus abdominis had to be added to the iliopsoas myotomy on the right side, because sudden spasms of this muscle tended to throw the patient off balance when standing or walking.

C. RELIEF OF SPASTICITY BY CHEMICAL BLOCKING

(1) Phenol or alcohol blocks of peripheral nerves and motor points

In recent years, reports have been published on relief of spasticity and contractures by blocking peripheral nerves and motor points with chemical agents, such as phenol and alcohol (Lacombe *et al.*, 1966; Weiss *et al.*, 1966; Cain *et al.*, 1966; Apolinario, 1966: Khalili & Betts, 1967). This method to eliminate the predominant spastic muscles is used mainly in incomplete lesions with good voluntary or reflex bladder and sexual function.

The technique is simple. The peripheral nerve or motor point is first located externally, using a surface monopolar electrode. A needle electrode coated with teflon, except for its tip, is then inserted and an electric stimulator is used to identify the respective nerve fibres or motor point. The needle is in the desired position when the least intensity of the electric current elicits the maximum contraction of the muscle to be blocked. Some authors inject first a test solution of 1–2 ml of 0·5 to 1 per cent procaine or xylocaine before injecting 2 ml of 40 or 60 per cent alcohol (Lacombe *et al.*) or 0·3 to 0·5 ml of 2, 3 or 6 per cent aqueous phenol solution (Apolinario, Cain, Khalili). There is immediate relief of spasticity of the muscle innervated by the blocked nerve fibres. The duration of the beneficial effect varies, and repeated injections at varying intervals are often necessary to achieve longer lasting results. From all these observations, it can be concluded that these peripheral nerve and motor point blocks are of considerable value in reducing spasticity in selected cases, especially if surgical procedures for one reason or another are not contemplated.

(2) Intrathecal alcohol or phenol blocks

It is well known that chemical agents injected intrathecally for spinal anesthesia or for relief of pain due to malignant tumours may result in paraplegia.

In early 1946, I studied the effect of intrathecal injection of alcohol into the thoraco-lumbar junction of the cord for transforming the spastic paraplegia into a flaccid motor lesion in complete cord lesions with intractable spasticity and flexion contractures of the legs. Although, at first, only small doses (1 to 2 cm^3) of 80 per cent alcohol were used, the immediate effect in abolishing the most violent flexor spasms and giving relief to the patient was most striking, and the first results were reported at the Neurological Section of the Royal Society of Medicine (Guttmann, 1946). However, it was found that the effect was only temporary, and, in due course, larger doses (6–10 cm^3 at the maximum) were injected intrathecally to block the spinal roots of the cauda equina, as this procedure is technically simpler than the blind, intra-medullary injection. Canadian and American authors (Gingras, 1948; Sheldon & Bors, 1948) confirmed the striking effect of the alcohol block on intractable spasticity, using larger doses (10–15 cm^3), and, in due course, the intrathecal alcohol block has been widely used by other workers in this field. The idea of this procedure was to replace the surgical procedures on the spinal cord, previously mentioned, by the chemical relief of spasticity, in particular in those patients with intractable spasticity suffering from septic conditions due to pressure sores, where larger operations necessitating laminectomy and general anaesthesia would constitute too great a risk.

Technique. The patient is placed in lateral, tail-up position (40°) having regard to the lighter specific gravity of the alcohol, to avoid its running too far headwards. A lumbar puncture is performed, without anaesthetic, as a rule, between the first and second or second and third lumbar vertebrae, using a fine needle. Only in special cases, where excessive abdominal spasms are present in addition to the intractable spasticity of the lower limbs is the puncture performed between the 11th and 12th dorsal vertebrae. 2–3 cm^3 of cerebro-spinal fluid is withdrawn, followed by slow injection of absolute ethyl alcohol (1 cm³ per minute). The total amount of the injected alcohol depends on the time of the disappearance of reflexes—the first being the sole and ankle jerks—and the development of total flaccidity. This can be achieved in the majority of cases following injection of 6 cm³. It is essential that an assistant records, following testing, the details of transformation of the spastic lesion into a lower motor neuron lesion. Following injection, the patient is left for about 3 minutes in the same position and then, maintaining the tail-up position, is very slowly turned to the opposite side so that the alcohol can circulate and block the opposite spinal roots. After 5 minutes, the patient is turned slowly on to his back, where he remains for several hours. The tail-up position can be discontinued, as a rule, after 2–3 hours.

The absorption of ethyl alcohol from the subarachnoid space

Earlier work on the absorption of substances from the subarachnoid space in man was mainly concerned with the absorption of 2 ml of 10 per cent sodium iodide solution in the urine in cases of cerebral syphilis and schizophrenia (Guttmann, 1929). It was found that onset and duration of the excretion could be greatly delayed.

Katzenelbogen (1935) came to the conclusion from animal experiments that there are two pathways of absorption, one directly into the venous blood and the other indirectly into venous blood by the way of the lymphatics. Aird & Seifert (1952) assumed that the absorption of alcohol from the subarachnoid space takes place very rapidly, but these workers did not offer any experimental evidence to substantiate their assumption. Eggleton (1942) showed that ethyl alcohol administered orally is rapidly absorbed and can be found in the blood, cerebral spinal fluid and urine within a few minutes of its administration. It seemed, therefore, worth while to investigate this problem following intrathecal alcohol injection in complete lesions of the spinal cord, which the writer in co-operation with Robinson, the biochemist of Stoke Mandeville Centre, carried out (Guttmann & Robinson, 1956).

Method and procedure

The Cavett method was used to determine the absorption in blood and urine (Kent-Jones & Taylor, 1954). No fluid intake was allowed for 2 hours before and for at least 2 hours after the intrathecal injection. Urine specimens were collected by means of an indwelling catheter and blood specimens by finger prick. The urine specimens were tested by Rothera's method, and in all experiments blank determinations were carried out on blood and urine specimens collected immediately before the alcohol injection. It was usually found that there was blank value equivalent to about 10 mg of alcohol in urine and about half that value in blood.

Results (Fig. 218a, b, c)

In all cases, alcohol could be detected in the blood within 15 minutes and in urine within 40 minutes of injection. Sometimes, the alcohol found in the blood within 5 minutes and in the urine within 20 minutes. Alcohol was not found in the urine later than 5 hours after the injection. This is in interesting agreement with the results of Eggleton who, using very much larger oral doses of alcohol, found that excretion was complete in 5·5 hours.

The blood alcohol concentration rose and fell much more rapidly than urine concentration. In view of this very rapid rise and fall in the blood alcohol concentration, blood specimens were collected every 5 minutes for the first hour after injection in order to determine the time of the alcohol's first crossing the CSF/blood barrier. In 3 of 9 cases in whom blood alcohol determinations were done, a double peak was observed in the graphs of blood alcohol against time.

Eggleton showed that the increased diuresis following oral ingestion of alcohol showed marked variation in response in different subjects. This is also true to the response to intrathecal alcohol. Eggleton also showed that the diuresis was in proportion to the amount of alcohol injected. Since the amount of alcohol given to our patients intrathecally could not be varied over a wide range, no observations could be made in this respect. However, we found that in several of our cases the renal secretion was found to be suppressed during the first hour or two following the first intrathecal injection.

The outstanding result of this study is the rapid absorption of alcohol from the subarachnoid space into the blood stream and thence into the urine. The maximum values in the blood were already obtained within the first hour following injection and in one case even within the first 20 minutes. Another interesting point is the observation in several of our cases of a decrease in the rate of secretion of urine in the first hour or two after alcohol injection. It may be speculated that this depressant effect on the renal function may be the result of the acute transformation of the spastic lesion into a lower motor neuron lesion.

Clinical effects

The effect of the alcohol block is illustrated in Fig. 218d in a case of profound intractable spasticity in flexion and adduction. In this case it was extremely difficult to carry out an intermittent catheterization because of the very pronounced adductor contractures which had developed as a result of the adductor spasticity. Fig. 218e demonstrates the minimal abduction which could be attained in spite of great muscular effort on the part of the attendant. The complete relief of the intractable spasticity of the legs following alcohol block was very striking, as seen in Fig. 218f. In all cases, whether flexion or extension spasticity, the intrathecal alcohol block has proved very effective in making the life of these unfortunate sufferers more comfortable and worth while living, and in particular in tetraplegics, it immensely facilitated the nursing of the patients.

In thoracic and cervical lesions, the relief of spasticity in the trunk and abdominal muscles greatly helped to restore the upright position of the patient. In those cases in which the muscle spasms were associated with pain, the effect of the alcohol block was sometimes dramatic (see Chapter on Pain). Of special importance was the beneficial result in the treatment of the uninhibited hypertonic bladder (Fig. 219a), in particular the contracted bladder, which all too often was the main cause of widespread reflex responses of both the skeletal muscles and autonomic mechanisms (autonomic hyperreflexia). In fact, in cases where the cystogram showed a contracted and sometimes grossly deformed hypertonic bladder, this was the main indication for the alcohol block.

In these cases, the injection was performed between the 3rd and 4th lumbar vertebrae and immediately transformed the spastic automatic bladder into a hypotonic autonomous bladder with greatly increased capacity, as shown in Fig. 200b, which allows closure of suprapubic cystostomy or discontinuation of indwelling catheter drainage and proves essential in the treatment of urinary reflex incontinence (see Fig. 164). It is obvious that the intrathecal alcohol block in such cases, where the disco-ordinated and contracted spastic bladder and the intractable spasticity of the legs are transformed into a flaccid lower motor neurone lesion within a few minutes, is infinitely preferable to a laminectomy and radical anterior and posterior rhizotomy from T10 to S5, with all the paraphernalia of a major and long lasting operation, as advocated by Meirowsky, Scheibert & Hinchey (1950). Moreover, the establishment of a flaccid motor paralysis greatly helped in the healing of pressure sores and, in particular, facilitated plastic repair. Finally, in spastic cases developing pathological fractures of long bones, for instance of the femur, the alcohol block facilitated proper alignment by osteosynthesis. Another beneficial effect of the alcohol block was found in cases with spasticity of the legs associated with most troublesome outbursts of hyperhidrosis. Fig. 220a shows a patient with a complete traumatic transverse lesion below T12, who was suffering from spasms and almost constant profuse sweating over both lower limbs which made his life miserable. Following alcohol block sweating in the lower limbs was greatly diminished and practically abolished below the knee at the end of the sweat test, while the proximal parts of the body showed profuse sweating (Fig. 220b).

Undesirable side effects and contraindications. The most undesirable side effect is the loss of sexual reflex activity which may be permanent. Therefore, the intrathecal block is contraindicated in cases of incomplete lesions with severe spasticity, where the sexual function, in particular, erections are maintained. It is also contraindicated in lesions with satisfactory reflex or voluntary function of the bladder. In such cases, operations on peripheral nerves or muscles or peripheral nerve or motor point blocks with alcohol or phenol are the methods of choice. Another drawback to the intrathecal alcohol block is the flaccid paralysis of the rectum, and great care must be taken to avoid constipation by manual evacuation, combined, if necessary, with enemas and laxatives.

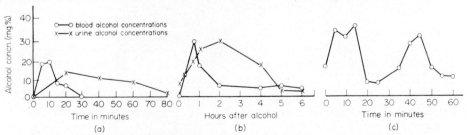

FIG. 218. ○——○ blood alcohol concentrations; ×——× urine alcohol concentrations. (a) Patient was a man aged 26, with a complete transverse spinal syndrome below T2. 8 ml of alcohol were injected between T12 and L1. (b) Patient was a woman aged 43, with a complete transverse spinal syndrome below T5. 6 ml of alcohol were injected. (c) Double peak in the concentration of alcohol in the blood. The patient was a man aged 29 years with a complete transverse spinal syndrome below T6. 8 ml of alcohol were injected between T12 and L1.

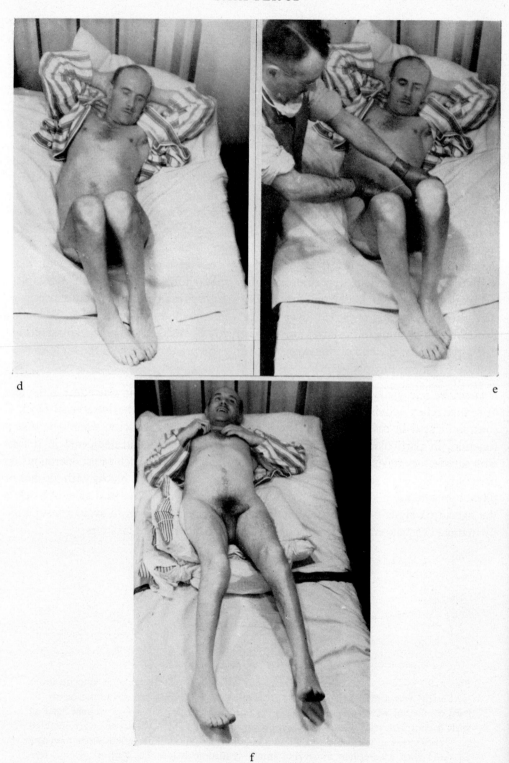

d   e

f

FIG. 218.

It was found, even following larger doses of intrathecal alcohol injection, that in some cases spasticity was not completely abolished or returned after certain periods. If the reflex activity is only mild or moderate this is by no means a disadvantage. A repetition of the alcohol block is indicated only if the spasticity again becomes uncomfortable to the patient, which, in the writer's experience, is rather uncommon.

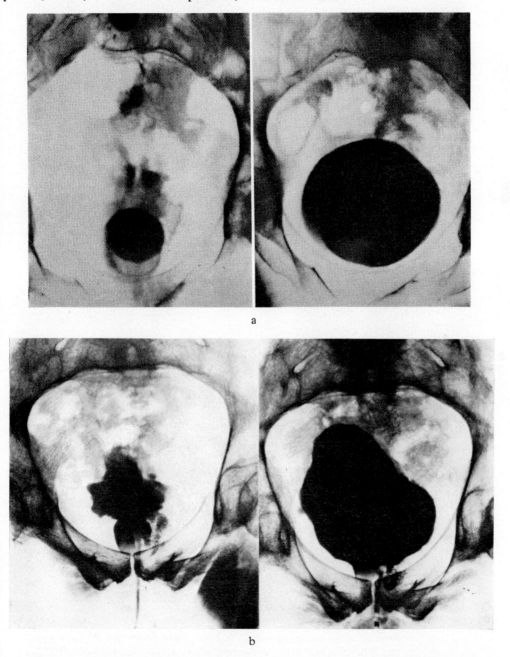

FIG. 219. Patient before and after alcohol block with grossly deformed contracted bladder. (Complete transverse lesion below T11/12.)

Intrathecal phenol block

Since Maher's publication (1955) on the beneficial effect of phenol injections to relieve pain in incurable cancer, intrathecal injections of this chemical have been used for relieving spasticity in paraplegia (Nathan, 1959; Kelly & Gautier-Smith, 1959; Liver-

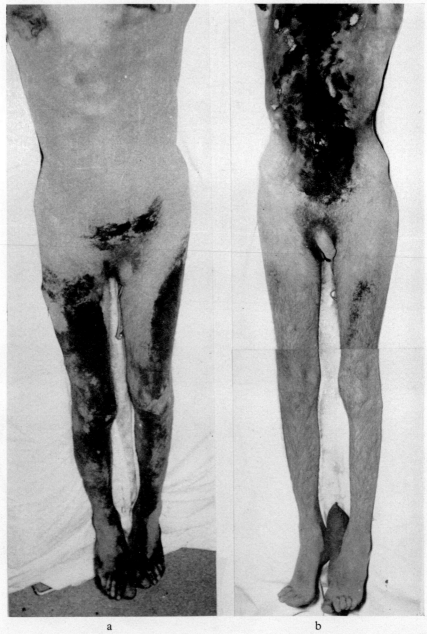

a   b

FIG. 220. (a) Profuse spontaneous sweating in both lower limbs before intrathecal alcohol block. (b) Thermo-regulatory sweat test after alochol block shows almost anhidrosis in lower limbs (Guinizarin Method).

sedge & Maher, 1960; O'Hare, 1962; Griffith, 1969; and others). It has been suggested that the phenol injection can be used unilaterally and far more selectively as a chemical rhizotomy in incomplete lesions than is possible with alcohol because of the hypobaric value of alcohol. This can be achieved if the patient, following injection, is left for some time and up to 2 hr lying on the side to be blocked. Animal experiments on the effect of phenol (Nathan & Sears, 1960) showed a differential blocking effect of 5 per cent phenol solution in myodil and 0·5 and 0·1 per cent aqueous solution on the various action potentials, by stimulating peripheral nerves and recording from anterior and posterior roots of the cat. These authors found that phenol blocks the various fibre groups of a nerve root in the same order as do standard local anaesthetics, in that 'C' Fibres are blocked first and the fastest conducting 'A' Fibres are blocked last. When phenol solution is placed in contact with a spinal root for a certain time, it may produce irreversible block of 'C' Fibres, while the block of Alpha Fibres is reversible. Weiss *et al.* (1966) suggested that phenol may be so selective, that only the Gamma Fibres are interrupted. However, these authors did not give any experimental proof of their statement. However, before contemplating phenol or alcohol injections for intractable pain it is worthwhile to try intrathecal injections of isotonic iced saline as suggested by Savitz and Malis (1973).

Technique. The patient is placed on the X-ray table lying on the side to be blocked and tilted forward about 20° with a pillow placed under the pelvis. An X-ray is taken across the table to ascertain how much tilt of the table is necessary to cover the desired area with the phenol solution. O'Hara followed Kelley's procedure to sterilize the phenol in glycerine, and 20 per cent concentration is selected to reach the anterior roots. The best results were achieved following intrathecal injection of 1·5–2 cm³ of this solution. Cain (1965) is using 7·5 to 10 per cent phenol in glycerine solution for the initial injection in patients with complete cord lesions. Comparison of therapeutic results obtained using equal concentrations of phenol in glycerine and phenol in pantopaque (R) or myodil revealed greater relief of spasticity and longer duration of effectiveness using glycerine. Liversedge & Maher (1960) attributed this difference of efficacy to a slower release of phenol from myodil and to the globular emulsive form of pantopaque compared with glycerine's direct contact with the spinal roots. However, Griffith (1969) preferred phenol mixed with 5 cm³ of pantopaque, as it allows the injection to be performed under fluoroscopic control. The spinal roots treated by this solution are from T10 caudally. If the patient is kept lying on his side for 6 hours the roots of the opposite side, as claimed by Griffith, are not affected and the chemical rhizotomy remains confined unilaterally only.

Fair, good and excellent results in abolishing spasticity of the lower limbs with intrathecal phenol injections have been reported by various authors. However, the writer does not agree with the sometimes too optimistic views expressed regarding sparing bladder and sexual function following 'selective' phenol injections, having regard to cases admitted later to Stoke Mandeville with definite and long lasting bladder paralysis. The writer agrees with Cain (1965) that very careful consideration must be given to patients with incomplete spinal cord lesions, who have appreciation of sensation or motor control in their lower limbs, and he recommends for these patients tenotomy, neurectomy or peripheral nerve injection, in accordance with the writer's indication of intrathecal alcohol blocks in incomplete lesions of the spinal cord.

CHAPTER 33

SURGICAL RECONSTRUCTION OF THE TETRAPLEGIC HAND

The greatly increased life span of traumatic tetraplegics has no doubt widened the scope of reconstructive surgery of the lower motor neuron paralysis of muscle groups of hands and fingers which, hitherto, was confined to victims of polio and peripheral nerve lesions, and several authors have described techniques of reconstructive surgical procedures in tetraplegics (Thompson, 1942; Napier, 1956; Wilson, 1956; Street, 1958; Riordan, 1959; Fowler, 1959; Nickel *et al.*, 1963; Lamb, 1963, 1972; Zancolli, 1965; Lipscomb *et al.*, 1965; Freehafer, 1967, 1969; Sarrafian, 1969; and others).

From all experience certain conclusions have been drawn:

There is no single solution to surgical reconstruction and each case should be considered individually.

The careful study of the patient's personality and the degree of readjustment to his muscular deficit by mobilization of natural forces of adjustment is as essential as the detailed analysis of the actual neurological defect. From my personal experience on a very large number of traumatic tetraplegics below C6/7 there is no doubt that these patients can readjust the function of their arms and hands with or without aids to a considerable degree, enabling them to carry out daily activities, such as self-dressing to some extent, combing the hair, cleaning the teeth, shaving with an electric shaver, feeding, typing, writing, using the telephone and taking part in certain sports, etc., provided the extensor carpi radialis longus and brevis and the brachioradialis are of good strength. Naturally, in these cases we have already in the early stages of their paralysis encouraged them: 'If you can't use one hand, use both hands' (Guttmann, 1969).

It must also be remembered that only a very small percentage of tetraplegics are suitable for reconstructive surgery to improve the muscular function of their hands and fingers for certain daily activities. According to McSweeney (1969) and Bedbrook (1969) in only 5 per cent of the clinical material is constructive surgery applicable. On the other hand, Lamb in a recent paper (1972) reported about 113 cases which he treated in a period between 1958–69 of whom 25 patients had reconstructive surgery (22·16 per cent).

Another important point to be considered before contemplating reconstructive surgery is the time, which has elapsed since the spinal cord injury. It is a well-known fact, that in incomplete cord lesions, muscle groups which initially show complete paralysis may recover to more or less considerable degrees; this applies, in particular, to brachioradialis, triceps, pronator teres, extensor carpi radialis longus and brevis and flexor carpi radialis. Opinion varies amongst authors regarding the time when tendon transfers are indicated. From my own personal observations no reconstructive surgery appears to be indicated before $1\frac{1}{2}$–2 years after cervical cord injury. This will give the tetraplegic patient enough time to assess his own capabilities in compensating his neurological deficit in hand and fingers, and at the same time will allow the medical attendant to assess properly the chances as well as the risks of tendon transfers.

There is general agreement that in all operative procedures the mobility of the wrist joints is of the greatest importance.

In analysing the various levels of complete spinal cord lesions the following have to be considered:

C5/6 lesions. At this level all muscles of the forearms and hands including brachioradialis and pronator teres are paralysed, or the brachioradialis is only very weak. The only muscles of good or moderate power are the deltoid and biceps. To restore extension of the wrist, which is so important for some daily activities in this type of tetraplegia, cock-up splints, as devised by Nickel and his co-workers, can be used beneficially. Alternatively, a fusion of the wrist joints in moderate extension can be contemplated, and in one of our cases has proved of benefit.

Lesions below C6. In these cases, the function of the brachioradialis and pronator teres is preserved to varying degrees, while the extensors of the wrist, in particular the extensor carpi radialis brevis, are either weak or paralysed. In such a case, the brachioradialis, if of strong power (at least 4), can be connected with the tendons of the extensor carpi radialis brevis and thus the radial deviation as a result of the over action of the extensor carpi radialis longus can be corrected, and full extension of the wrist restored. By full extension of the wrist, passive flexion of the fingers on the metacarpophalangeal and interphalangeal joints results, and this enables the patient by exercises to acquire some degree of grasping power.

Opposition of the thumb may be obtained by fixing the proximal end of the opponens to the distal part of the ulnar, thereby, the extension of the wrist will pull the thumb into some degree of opposition. However, a number of workers in this field prefer the permanent stabilization of the thumb in opposition through a metacarpal bone block between the first and second metacarpals. The first metacarpal is brought into abduction and flexion as well as medial rotation, and this position is fixed by the bone graft which is taken from the iliac crest.

Lesions at and below C7. In these cases the flexor carpi-radialis is active. Lamb (1972) potentiated the natural tenodesing effect of the long flexors, when the wrist is dorsiflexed by transferring the extensor carpi-radialis longus through a large window cut in the interosseus membrane above the pronator quadratus to the flexor digitorum profundus. The branchioradialis was transferred to the flexor pollicis longus. The extensor carpi-radialis brevis was left to dorsiflex the wrist. Lamb carried out this operation in 13 patients of whom 11 were improved. However, no details were given of the type of improvement in these cases, particularly C7 where the flexor carpi-radialis is working (Group 4 of Lipscomb). This muscle was used by Lamb as the motor for the abduction–opposition of the thumb muscle by using a free tendon graft from the palmaris muscle.

In lesions at C8, the interossei and lumbricales are still paralysed and so are the abductor pollicis brevis and opponens. Various surgical procedures of the intrinsic muscles of the fingers have been recommended (Fowler, 1959; Riordan, 1959; Zancolli, 1965). However, it is still very questionable whether these procedures have been really beneficial to improve the functions of these muscles in tetraplegics, and unless the patient needs these muscles for specific fine movements these surgical procedures in tetraplegics are really unnecessary.

CHAPTER 34

PRINCIPLES AND TECHNIQUES OF PHYSIOTHERAPY

The role of the medical and physiotherapy staff

One of the predominant activities of the specialist in charge of a spinal unit and his senior medical staff is the planning and personal supervision of the physical treatment of his patients. For, upon their knowledge of each case and their functional and psychological analysis of the patient's disability, depend indication, duration and modification of the various forms of physiotherapy. In every case, a constructive programme has to be devised, and never is the physiotherapy department called upon blindly for 'physiotherapy, massage or remedial exercises', just to make the patient feel 'that something is being done'. For each instance, the physiotherapist in charge of the case must receive detailed instruction about the patient's disability and the treatment to be applied, which must be carried out in concert with that of the other members of the team: the nursing staff, physical training instructor, occupational therapist, and vocational training instructor, for all these personnel also take part in the physical restoration and psychological readjustment of the paraplegic and tetraplegic. On the other hand, physiotherapists have to take part in certain procedures which are usually considered as the prerogative of the nursing staff, such as the proper positioning of the paralysed in the acute stages and, in particular, assisting in overcoming respiratory distress and lung complications of tetraplegics. With her specialized knowledge and experience, she can greatly assist the patient to accomplish his satisfactory return to the community. For, by her regular contact with the patient, she learns problems which may have not been revealed to other members of the team. Therefore, she can act as a vital link in the chain of communication and can pass on important information to the medical officer in charge of the case and to other members of his team, which is so helpful for a successful rehabilitation.

It has been our experience throughout these years, that the physiotherapists connected with the physical restoration of spinal cord sufferers have become deeply interested in and even fascinated by the daily problems of their cases. This has, no doubt, developed as a result of the establishment of a regular, weekly session, nick-named 'Circus', in the Physiotherapy Department, held regularly by the Director of the Centre and his whole medical staff. At these sessions, every patient is seen, and details of progress and treatment discussed with the physiotherapist in charge of the case. Throughout the years, societies of physiotherapists and remedial gymnasts, as well as the speciality of physical medicine as a whole, have benefited greatly from the new approach to the treatment and rehabilitation of traumatic spinal paraplegia. Their rather passive and palliative approach of the past towards these patients has been replaced by a programme of purposeful activity and dynamic rehabilitation. The fundamental change which has taken place in the attitude of the physiotherapist towards paraplegic patients is best evidenced by quoting from an article—'Looking Back'—written in 1949 by a former physiotherapist of this Centre for *The Cord*, **2**, 33–35, the journal of British paraplegics: 'Such small and disheartening knowledge as we had of the occasional paraplegic treated during our training in no way encouraged us to hope that we should come into further contact with them'. But, she concludes: 'From the days of dread of having to go and move some wretched immobile paraplegic's toes, hoping to avoid embarrassing questions, yet remain falsely optimistic, one can now with confidence sum up the probable picture and thoroughly enjoy the years spent in helping him to become an individual—independent, mobile and reasonably fit'. In recent years, it has become routine for many physiotherapy training schools to send their students to this Centre for lectures, and throughout the years numerous physiotherapists from many countries came to Stoke Mandeville to be trained in our methods. Moreover, post-graduate courses in physiotherapy in spinal paraplegia are held every year by the senior medical staff and physiotherapy staff, formerly under the leadership of Miss D.Bell and since her retirement, most efficiently under that of Miss I.Bromley, Superintendent Physiotherapist.

Techniques

Details of the principles and techniques of physiotherapy as introduced and developed in this Centre since 1944, have been published elsewhere (Guttmann, 1946, 1949, 1967; Hobson, 1956) and they are here summarized and supplemented. Moreover, Miss E.P.G.Hobson (1956), a former physiotherapist of this Centre, published a short monograph on 'Physiotherapy in Paraplegia'.

The two fundamentals in the physical treatment of paraplegics and tetraplegics are early start and continuity until the maximum of benefit is accomplished. The chief objects to be pursued are as follows:

1. Physiotherapy applied to the paralysed parts of the body

This comprises:

a   Prevention and treatment of contractures and atrophy (correct positioning, passive stretching, passive and auto-assisted movements).
b   Electrotherapy in lower motor neuron lesions.
c   Management of the respiratory disturbances in tetraplegia.
d   Treatment of spasticity (see special chapter on Spasticity).

(a) In the early stages, the physiotherapist has to assist the nursing staff in keeping the paralysed limbs in proper position, in order to prevent continuous adduction, flexion, internal rotation of the legs, drop foot, claw toes, and pressure to the neck of the fibula. In particular, the customary practice of placing a 'donkey' underneath the knees should be avoided, as it produces flexion of knees and hips which, if continued for long periods, inevitably leads to contractures of the flexor muscles of the knees and hips, which in turn encourage and increase flexor spasticity once the period of flaccidity in cord lesion has ceased.

Passive movements of all joints of the paralysed limbs should be carried out at least three times daily and, if possible, more often in the acute stage of paraplegia to promote better circulation in the paralysed limbs and prevent oedema and contractures. However, flexion and abduction movements should be carried out gently and with care. Maximal abduction and flexion of the hip over 90° should be avoided in the stage of flaccidity during the spinal shock period, as brisk and too extensive passive movements may lead to haemorrhages in the tissues around the hip joints which may facilitate the formation of para-articular ossification. Moreover, there is also the danger of producing fractures or dislocation of the femur in cases with lower motor neurone lesions resulting in atrophy and osteoporosis. In incomplete cord and cauda equina lesions, auto-assisted movements should be started within the first few days after injury, and the patient should be encouraged to improve the function of partly paralysed muscles himself as often as possible during the day, after having been instructed about the technique by the physiotherapist.

Contractures of paralysed muscles in lower motor neuron lesions

While, in general, care is taken to prevent drop foot and contractures of the Achilles tendons, in many cases of conus–cauda equina lesion the paralysed toes were found in profound flexion contracture (Fig. 221). It is obvious that such a complication greatly delays rehabilitation of paraplegics, as not only is it impossible to commence standing and walking exercises while the toes are in this condition, but there is an increased danger of pressure sores occurring, as soon as the patient is allowed to stand. Contractures of the knee joints in semi-flexion or extension may also develop in flaccid paraplegia, due to faulty positioning. In some patients admitted to this Centre with conus–cauda equina lesion or anterior horn lesions—for instance, following poliomyelitis—extension contractures

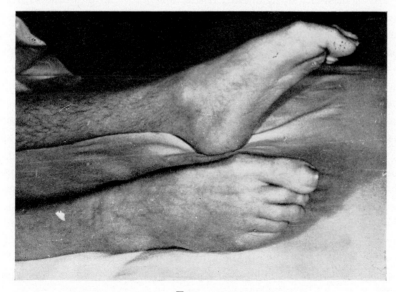

Fig. 221.

of the knee joints had been deliberately produced elsewhere, in order to 'facilitate standing and walking'. However, this method has proved to increase rather than diminish the paraplegic's disability, as it makes sitting in a wheelchair, motor tricycle or car most difficult or even impossible and may diminish the chances of re-employment. The most incapacitating contractures in lower cord lesions are flexion contractures of the hips, resulting in backwards distortion of the pelvis. These contractures develop if the patient is allowed to lie for too long in lateral position with flexed hips and knees. In anterior horn lesions, involving the trunk and shoulder muscles, faulty positioning of the patient is responsible for the development of scoliosis, even if the lesion is symmetrical. This applies in particular to children and adolescents. I have seen the most gruesome forms of scoliosis and flexion contractures of the lower limbs on polio victims during my visits to the African countries, and Professor Huckstep of Kampala, in particular, has drawn attention to this condition (1968).

Care and treatment of the paralysed hand and fingers in tetraplegics

This has been a neglected subject for many years, caused mainly by delayed admission of traumatic tetraplegics to Spinal Injuries Centres, but also by inadequate measures taken in the acute stages in Spinal Units, to prevent oedema and contractures of the metacarpophalangeal and interphalangeal joints. As a result of the interruption of the vaso-constrictors in these high lesions, the vaso-motor control is crippled and oedema develops below the level of the lesion, including hand and fingers. Collagen is deposited in the oedema fluid, and if the oedema is not overcome by frequent movements of the wrist, metacarpophalangeal and interphalangeal joints and fixing the arm and hand for some periods in vertical position to counteract oedema by physiotherapist as well as nurses and instructed visitors, the deposited collagen becomes transformed into fibrous tissue and loss of elasticity of ligaments, fasciae and joint capsules follows, resulting in contractures. This mechanism has been well described by Sharrard (1967). In this connection it may be mentioned that in elderly tetraplegics oedema followed by contractures of the metacarpophalangeal and interphalangeal joints sometimes develops in spite of regular and intensive physiotherapy by passive movements. The mechanism of this complication is still obscure but in some of these patients this can be prevented by bringing the arm into vertical position.

It is essential that before physiotherapy to the hand and fingers is commenced, a detailed assessment of all muscles of the upper extremity is carried out. This applies, in particular, to complete lesions of the cervical cord at C6 and below C6 and C7 where varieties in the muscular deficit occur due to the multi-segmental innervation of the forearm, hand and finger muscles. Attention has already been drawn to the prevention of flexion contractures of the forearm as the result of the paralysis of triceps, which can be absolutely avoided by proper positioning of the forearm in extension to counteract the overaction of the strongly acting biceps in these patients. In certain lesions at or below C6 the extensor carpi radialis longus may be active while the brevis is paralysed. Therefore, the hand will be pulled in extreme radial abduction, if faulty positioning of the hand is not prevented.

Furthermore, in this type of lesion pronation contracture of the forearm may develop, if the forearm is left lying continuously or for long periods in pronation.

In complete lesions below C6 the hand should not be left lying flat on the bed, as this invariably leads to extension contractures of the wrist and fingers. Palm rolls or palmar pads are usually employed to avoid contractures of the metacarpophalangeal joint, but these are only effective if they allow flexion of that joint well beyond 45°. Our Occupational Therapy Department has constructed a type of 'Boxing Glove' splint which has proved most effective in producing maximum flexion of the metacarpophalangeal and interphalangeal joints. This can be combined with a wrist 'cock-up' splint, as advocated by Cheshire & Rowe (1970). If contractures of these joints are prevented, the prehensive effects of the wrist extension by strong action of the extensor carpi radialis longus and brevis on the paralysed long finger flexors can be considerable in helping the tetraplegic to grasp objects with some power. If the wrist extensors are weak artificial splints as developed by Nickel and his colleagues (1963) and Freehafer (1969) have proved of value in specific cases.

Hand in hand with proper positioning and regular frequent passive movements of all joints, not just twice or three times a day as is usually done, but every half an hour by the patient himself, goes the education of the patient to utilize the remaining function of muscles and joints to mobilize and develop re-adaptive movement patterns (trick movements), which will enable him to become relatively independent in some of his daily activities. This re-education of the patient is, of course, intensified as soon as he is up in his wheelchair by the combined operation of the physiotherapist and occupational therapist. Reconstructive surgical procedures can be of value at a later date in selected cases to improve the function of hand and fingers (see Chapter on Surgical Reconstruction of the Tetraplegic Hand).

Contractures in upper motor neuron lesions

Permanent fixation of paralysed limbs in any position must also be avoided in transverse lesions of the cord above the thoraco-lumbar junction as they are serious complications to spasticity.

In spastic lesions involving the upper limbs, as a result of cervical injuries above C5, contractures usually develop in adduction of the arm and pronation of the forearm. These can be avoided by proper positioning of the arm in abduction and of the paralysed forearms in supination, in the initial stages. Once developed, they are difficult to overcome, but auto-assisted movements, using a simple device, have proved to be most helpful in hemiplegia or tetraplegia as a result of cerebral injury. This is demonstrated in a case of traumatic triplegia, following gunshot injury of the head, resulting in profound adduction and pronation contractures of the left arm (Fig. 222). A splint is fixed to the dorsal surface of the hand, fingers and forearm, by a bandage, thus keeping the hand and fingers in extension. Metal rings, which are soldered to the radial border of the splint, are connected to a rope passing over a pulley fixed over the patient's head. According to the position of the pulley, a pull on the free end of the rope by the patient with his normal arm, or by his attendant, will either abduct the paralysed arm or supinate

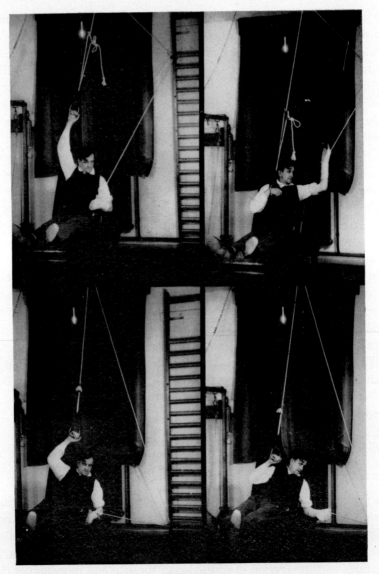

FIG. 222.

the forearm, or produce simultaneous movement of both. This simple device can also be used by bed patients.

Contractures of normal muscles

Contractures may also develop in normal muscle groups, due to their unrestrained action over their paralysed antagonists following lower motor neuron paralysis. This was found in cases of conus–cauda equina lesions—particularly those below L3, where contractures of the hips, with distortion of the pelvis, easily develop, due to the unrestrained action of the intact muscles—namely, quadratus lumborum, iliopsoas, quadriceps, adductors, and internal rotators—if the proper positioning of the patient has been neglected in the early stages, but also later on, if the patient has given up standing exercises and sits the whole day in his wheelchair. These contractures are often very painful on passive or active movement, and the disfigurement may be grotesque, as was seen in a young woman of 22 years, who contracted transverse myelitis and was admitted to Stoke Mandeville $7\frac{1}{2}$ months after onset of the illness. The neurological signs were those of an incomplete lesion below L3. However, these symptoms were overlaid by flexion contractures of the knees and most severe flexion contractures of the hips, resulting in subluxation of the right hip and extreme lordosis, with backwards distortion of the pelvis, as the result of prolonged, faulty positioning in bed (Fig. 223a and b). The reduction of such multiarticular contractures is difficult and demands great patience and endurance on the part of both the patient and the physiotherapist. Correct positioning and passive movements alone are generally ineffective in reducing long-standing and excessive contractures, and these procedures need to be supplemented by passive stretching for longer periods. This can be carried out as follows:

1 Flexion contractures of the hips and knees are best reduced by stretching while the patient is in supine position or by placing the patient into prone lying position, either in bed or on a plinth, with the aid of pillows, well-padded slings and straps.

2 Adduction contractures of the legs are best treated in lying or half-lying position for increasing periods on the plinth, with the legs maintained in abduction over each side of the plinth by weights attached to well-padded slings around the knees. When such patients sit in their wheelchairs, the knees should be kept well apart by placing firm pads of increasing size between the knees.

3 For the reduction of extension contractures of the knees, the sitting position over the end of the bed or plinth or in a wheelchair is preferable. Protective pillows are placed in front of and behind the legs, below the knees, and a strap is then placed around the legs and fixed to the legs of the plinth or bed or to the lower part of the wheelchair. The strap is gradually tightened, thus increasing the degree of knee flexion.

4 For the reduction of fixed lordosis, with flexion contractures of the hips resulting in backwards distortion of the pelvis, suspension of the patient in hanging position has proved most effective (Fig. 223c and d). The patient is suspended in the hanging apparatus by a corset fixed round his trunk. He may support himself in parallel bars, while being pulled into suspension. At first, some patients may have difficulty in tolerating the hanging position and have to be closely supervised. The period of suspension is commenced with 5 min and gradually increased to half an hour or longer. As a rule, the weight of the body is sufficient to stretch the contracted muscles of the spine and hips, but in certain cases, weights have to be fixed to the legs to increase the stretch.

The physiotherapist has to be warned to carry out all passive movements and stretching procedures with great gentleness and care, in order to avoid fractures, especially of the femur, as the development of osteoporosis has always to be borne in mind, in paraplegics.

Special attention is drawn to abduction contractures of the arms, due to over-action of the normal deltoid, and, in particular, to flexion contractures of the forearms, due to overaction of the biceps and brachioradialis muscles, occurring so often in cervical

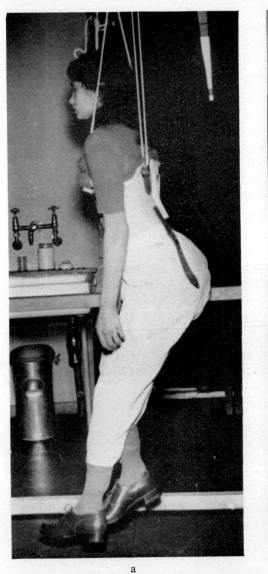
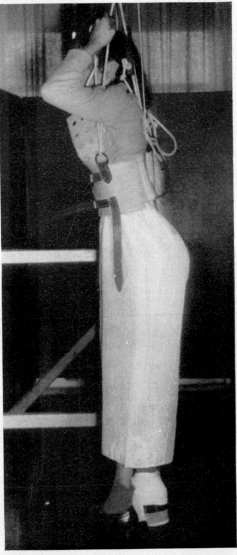

a   b

FIG. 223. (a) Patient at 16.2.1949. (b) Patient at 18.10.1951. (c) Patient at 16.2.1949.
(d) Patient at 18.10.1951.

injuries below C6. The unrestrained action of the biceps, as a result of the lower motor
neuron paralysis of its antagonists, the triceps, is particularly dangerous, as it leads to
most incapacitating contractures of the elbows and thus greatly increases the tetraplegic's
disability. This contracture, which is still accepted by some members of the medical
profession as an inevitable anomaly of the upper limbs in mid-cervical lesions, can easily
be avoided if, from the beginning, care is taken that the patient lies with his forearms
extended, and is not allowed to lie with the arms across his chest. See Fig. 6, also showing
the great improvement after intensive daily passive stretching and placing the forearm

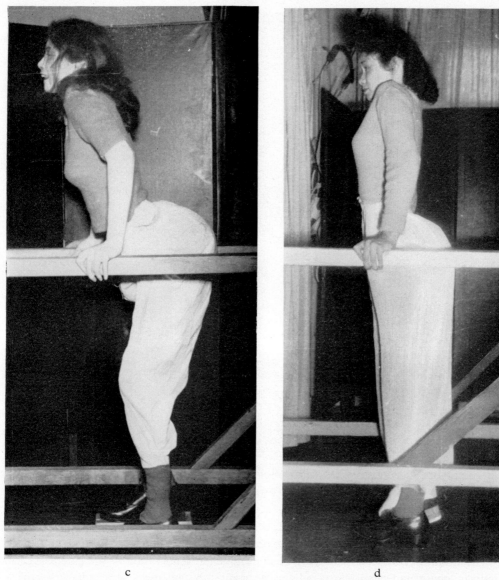

c   d

FIG. 223.

in extended position by well-padded straps and, later on, by a triceps brace, as seen in Fig. 6, on the left arm.

In view of the possibility of at least partial recovery of function of the triceps in these cases, owing to the individual variability of its multi-segmental innervation, the importance of preventing further damage due to over-stretching by the overaction of the biceps is emphasized. By systematic auto-assisted exercises, combined with daily electrical stimulation of the triceps, its function may recover to such a degree that extension of the forearm against gravity and resistance may become possible. This increases the tetra-plegic's independence immensely and enables him to lift himself, use his wheelchair,

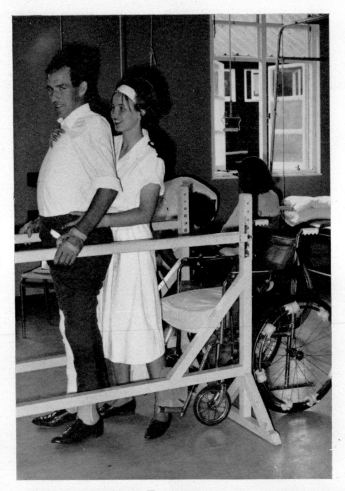

FIG. 224.

take up work and, as shown in Fig. 224, even stand and walk a short distance in parallel bars or on long crutches assisted by the physiotherapist.

Mention may also be made here of the segmental innervation of the extensor carpi radialis longus and flexor carpi radialis. As a rule, the extensor carpi radialis longus is found to be functioning in lesions below C6 and is particularly strong in lesions below C7, producing radial abduction of the hand. As the extensors and flexors of the fingers are paralysed in these lesions, the unrestrained action of the extensor carpi radialis longus may lead to extension and radial abduction contracture of the wrist, with consequent flexion contractures of the fingers.

The most deleterious type of contractures due to plaster beds, in which the patient had lain for months, has already been mentioned. Men, who had recovered from cord or cauda equina symptoms, were frustrated for many months or years, because of the super-imposed contractures of the joints and of the distorted pelvis, developed as the result of this enforced fixation. But, even such severe contractures can be overcome by well-planned, continuous physiotherapy, which consists of a combination of stretching, passive movements and suspension therapy with slings and pulleys.

(b) **Electrotherapy.** In certain groups of paraplegics with lower motor neuron lesions such as those of cervical roots, cauda equina or anterior horns, daily electrotherapy has been included in our programme from the start but entirely as a substitute for active exercise of the denervated muscle groups—i.e. the individual muscles or muscle groups are exercised by the electrical stimulation.

This problem has been the subject of controversy since John Reid, in 1841, described the beneficial effect of the galvanic current in denervated muscles. The therapeutic importance of electrotherapy was at first over-rated, and used indiscriminately for all sorts of afflictions, and this resulted later in scepticism, criticism and even complete repudiation of its value. At the time of the outbreak of the Second World War, many clinicians and experimental workers, both in Great Britain and abroad, condemned the use of electrotherapy in lower motor neuron lesions. This view was based on Langley & Kato's widely accepted but unproven theory (1915) that atrophy of denervated muscles was a fatigue phenomenon, caused by ceaseless fibrillations, and it was, therefore, assumed that further activity of denervated muscles by electrical stimulation would even be harmful (Tower, 1939). This theory was not confirmed by later workers in this field. Solandt & Magladery (1940) found no correlation in electromyographic studies between the degree of fibrillation and the rapidity of muscle atrophy.

In my own experiments, both in man and animals, in which no attempt was made to avoid fatiguing denervated muscles by electrical stimulation, neither was an increase in atrophy found nor was the beneficial effect of electrical exercise prevented. It would appear that the criterion chosen by investigators, whose results suggested that galvanism was ineffective (Langley & Kato, 1915; Molander et al., 1942; Doupe, Barnes & Kerr, 1943) or even harmful (Chor et al., 1939) was influenced by inadequate techniques such as application of weak current, ineffective dosage of stimulation (10 to 30 contractions only), in particular by insufficient frequency of treatment (three times a week), or fixation of the limbs in plaster casts, which by pressure merely added local damage to the denervated muscle fibres.

Experiments on rabbits, undertaken in the early stages of the Second World War by me, in co-operation with E. Guttmann, the relationship between onset, strength, duration and frequency of direct galvanic stimulation of denervated muscles after crushing as well as primary and secondary suture, following severance of the peroneal nerve, were studied. It was found that daily application of galvanic exercises of 20 to 30 minutes duration, with a current strength sufficient to elicit powerful contractions delayed and diminished atrophy in denervated and re-innervated muscles. The earlier the treatment was started, following denervation, the greater was the effect. After a maximal treatment of 1 hour daily, beginning the day after denervation, it was found that the muscles lost only 17 per cent in weight in 60 days, compared with a loss of 59 per cent of the untreated muscles. Most important of all, a good contractile power of the treated denervated muscles was preserved throughout the whole treatment, as compared with the untreated side. Clear differences were also revealed in the macroscopic appearance at biopsy as well as in the histological

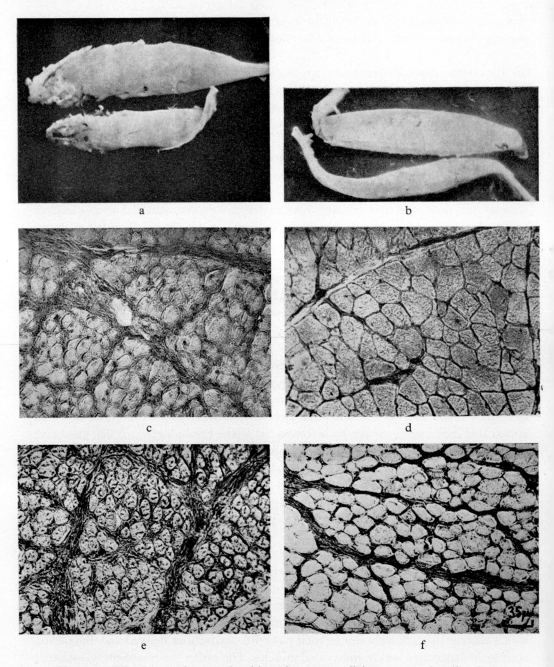

FIG. 225. Tibialis anterior muscles (*a*) and extensor digitorum muscles (*b*) of the treated and untreated legs of rabbit 957. Galvanic exercise of the left leg was begun 7 days after operation and was continued for 60 days. Cross sections of untreated (*c*) and treated (*d*) muscles of rabbit 957. Cross sections of untreated (*e*) and treated (*f*) muscles of rabbit 909. Treatment was begun 3 months after operation and was continued for 60 days. From Gutmann, E. and Guttmann, L. (1944) *J. Neurology, Neurosurgery and Psychiatry*, **7**, 7–17.

findings between treated and untreated muscles, as shown in Fig. 225. Larger muscle fibres and definitely lesser degree of fibrous tissue formation between the muscle fibres were found in the exercised muscles. Although the galvanic exercise did not affect the time of onset of recovery, following nerve suture, the strength and degree of motor recovery was higher in the treated muscles (Gutmann & Guttmann, 1942, 1944). These results, which are in accordance with those of Fisher (1939) and Hines *et al.* (1942, 1943), have been confirmed by Jackson (1945) in patients with ulnar nerve lesions and combined median and ulnar nerve lesions due to war injuries. Moreover, she also confirmed our findings, that daily electrical exercise of denervated muscles gave better results than if this treatment was given only three times a week. Of particular interest is Jackson's confirmation (1945), that immobilization of the affected limb appeared to increase the rate of wasting when galvanic exercise was not given.

Technique

Daily electrical exercise is started as early as possible, following lower motor neuron lesion in paraplegics and tetraplegics (about 5 days after injury), and is applied in gradually increasing number of contractions, starting with 50–100 per session of 15 minutes. In due course, as many as 600–800 and more contractions are applied to paralysed muscle groups during one session of about 30–45 minutes. This treatment is given at least once a day, if possible twice daily. Care is taken to elicit powerful muscle contractions, separated by rest periods of a few seconds. In the early stages of lower motor neurone lesions, the denervated muscles still react to direct faradic stimulation, and this type of current may be used; it has, however, to be substituted by galvanic or sinusoidal current in later stages, as soon as R.D. has developed. In root and anterior horn lesions, not associated with sensory disturbances, galvanism strong enough to elicit powerful contractions is painful and poorly tolerated, especially if only small sized electrodes are used. In such cases, sinusoidal and other forms of current should be used. Ionization effects which may be caused by unidirectional current by balanced-pulse galvanism, as recommended by Wickham (1948). The ionizing effect of a square-wave stimulus of relatively high amplitude is avoided by a following stimulus of opposite polarity with subliminal amplitude but of prolonged duration. The skin has to be thoroughly moistened with warm water. Since the skin resistance decreases during electrical exercise, the same vigorous contraction can be obtained by progressively weaker current strength. Hard water should be avoided as it may deposit insoluble calcium in the tissues underneath the cathode, and common salt may be mixed with the water. R.H.S.Holbourn and I suggested as an even better solution for preventing skin burns: 25 g of Na_2HPO_4 and 12 g of NH_2PO_4 in 1 litre of water being diluted with 5 to 10 times its volume before use.

The electrodes should not be restricted to one position but should be repeatedly altered, to avoid local damage by burning the underlying tissues; thus the current is directed to various parts of the muscle. As mentioned before, if depolarized impulses are used the danger of burning is greatly diminished. However, the danger of burning the skin can altogether be avoided, if the active electrode is moved and stroking stimulation along the whole length of the muscle is applied. This technique is particularly important

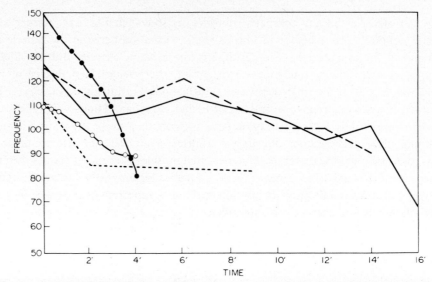

FIG. 226. Deltoid examined in free sideways extension of the arm. Action potential frequency in various normal subjects on fatigue resulting from identical working performance.

in the electrical exercise of denervated large muscles, such as triceps brachii or gastro-enemius. This stroking technique also guarantees the inclusion of all muscle fibres in the exercise. Some intelligent patients were taught to carry out the electrical stimulation of the muscles themselves, which saves the physiotherapist's time.

It may be emphasized that the totally or partially denervated muscle needs a similar individual training by electrical exercise as does the normal or recovering muscle by active exercise. In this connection, attention may be drawn to a previous study on chronaxy (Altenburger & Guttmann, 1928) on fatigue of normal muscles, such as deltoid and quadriceps, examined under identical conditions, which revealed a definite, individual variability in the reaction of these muscles to fatigue, as shown in Fig. 226. Yet, whatever the individual differences in muscle behaviour, from all my experience I have come to the conclusion that the fear of over-fatiguing denervated muscles by frequent electrical stimulation has been grossly exaggerated in the past and has led all too often to quite useless application of electrotherapy, such as 10 contractions only. Daily electrical exercise following nerve suture or lesions in continuity which may regenerate, should be continued until re-innervation and voluntary function of the muscles occur, so that active exercise by the patient himself becomes possible. This naturally varies according to the type and severity of the lower motor neuron lesion and, in particular, on the active co-operation of the patient once re-innervation of the muscles has occurred.

As an example of the value of systemic electrotherapy in a cervical root lesion, the following case may be quoted: A naval rating, aged 37, sustained a complete lesion of the left 5th cervical root, as a result of a fall from a bicycle, resulting in a degenerative paralysis of the deltoid muscle, with complete R.D., as a result of a fracture of the 6th cervical vertebra. In this case, daily electrical stimulation was started 8 days after injury, with gradually increasing number of contractions up to 800 per session of $\frac{1}{2}$ to $\frac{3}{4}$ hour. One hundred contractions were followed by a short period of rest. Nine months after injury, there was a first faint flicker of function in the posterior portion of the deltoid. The patient gradually improved, and 14 months after injury there was a weak faradic response in the anterior and middle portions of this muscle. One month later, he was able to abduct his left arm to 70°, with his forearm in flexed position. Seventeen months after injury, he could lift the whole extended arm above the horizontal and maintain it there for 1 or 2 seconds. He gradually improved, until he was finally able to lift the whole extended arm above the horizontal against resistance and keep it in this position for a very long time. The profound atrophy of the deltoid muscle gradually improved, but there remained a definite difference in its size as compared with the normal side. However, throughout the stage of denervation, the deltoid retained a good contractile power, in response to galvanic stimulation (Guttmann, 1949).

In conus–cauda equina lesions, electrotherapy is given in selected cases only and mainly to restore or improve the function of partially denervated muscles, in particular those which are important for standing and walking—i.e. quadriceps and glutaei. This is given, especially to the quadriceps in cauda equina lesions below L2–L4. It has been our experience with these injuries that if they are complete below L4, the paralysis of the extensors and plantar flexors of the feet and toes as a rule remains permanent, and it is, therefore, a waste of time to apply electrical stimulation to these muscles, as the paralysis of these muscles can easily be compensated by simple toe-raising springs. Only in partial root lesions of L4/L5 should electrotherapy be tried.

(c) **Management of respiratory disturbances in higher dorsal and cervical lesions.** The higher the cord lesion the greater the patient's dependence upon the action of the diaphragm and accessory muscles for his major respiratory function. This applies, in particular, to cervical lesions above C7. In order to increase the vital capacity of the lungs, the patient must be taught to exercise at short intervals the remaining respiratory muscles, especially sternomastoid and trapezius, to the fullest possible capacity, and maximal apical inspiration must always be encouraged, as well as diaphragmatic breathing. As has been mentioned before these patients are particularly endangered, if they develop congestion of the lungs. The physiotherapist's main role in these cases is basically the same as that for any other acute chest condition, in that she helps the patient to cough and expectorate mucus accumulated in the larynx, trachea and lungs. The importance of a close co-operation between nursing and physiotherapy staff in these acute cases cannot be over-emphasized, as each is dependent on the good will of the other. As the patient is turned by the nursing staff at regular intervals, the physiotherapist must know the time of these turns and must fit in her work accordingly—the more so as the respiratory treatment in these cases has to be carried out frequently.

Technique

It is better to treat such a patient for short periods but often, rather than give him two or three long sessions, which may be too tiring for the patient. It is necessary to elevate the foot end of the bed and tilt the patient's head down which greatly facilitates draining the chest more fully from the lower lobes. In this connection the Stoke Mandeville–Egerton turning and tilting bed greatly facilitates the work of the physiotherapist.

In order to improve the function of the diaphragm in cervical lesions, the physiotherapist must fix the diaphragm with her hands by applying pressure during expiration, in order to compensate for the loss of abdominal muscles which normally, by their resistance, facilitate the action of the diaphragm. As the physiotherapist places her hands over the lower lobe and on the lower chest wall, the patient takes a deep breath in, and, as he breathes out with forced expiration, the physiotherapist vibrates the chest wall, giving maximal pressure at the end of each expiration. After this has been repeated several times, the physiotherapist then tells the patient to breathe out as far as possible and then to cough, trying at the same time to expectorate the loose mucus from his chest. As he coughs, she slides her hands down from the lower rib cage, so that she can give pressure over the upper part of the abdomen, in order to replace the function of the paralysed abdominal muscles. It may be noted that, in transverse lesions of the cervical and upper thoracic cord, although the intercostal muscles are completely paralysed, their tone recovers to some extent, in later stages, and, once the spinal cord below the level of the lesion regains its automatic function, these muscles may become active by reflex action and participate in the act of respiration (see Chapter on Respiratory Complications).

In addition to the technique of facilitating expiration and preventing congestion of the lung, the physiotherapist's important task is to mobilize, exercise and overdevelop the auxiliary respiratory muscles, in particular sternomastoid, trapezius, levator scapulae, platysma and scaleni to improve the upward movement of the chest and thus increase the antero-posterior diameter of the chest. The patient has to be encouraged to carry out these exercises as often as possible during the day.

Glossopharyngeal breathing, also called 'frog' breathing or 'gulping' has been used as a substitute for breathing in high cervical lesions due to poliomyelitis, in which there is a paralysis or weakness not only of intercostals and diaphragm but also of the levator scapulae and trapezius (Pool & Weerden, 1973). It makes use of the function of the mouth and throat muscles to act as a pump, to force air into the lungs. A special technique of this type of breathing has been described by Clarence W.Dail (1951). However, this technique is now rarely used, as it is replaced in these high lesions by tracheostomy.

The physiotherapist has also important functions in the management of the tetraplegic after a tracheostomy has been performed and, like the nursing staff, must, therefore, be familiar with the technique of the respirator and the suction technique through the tracheostomy tube. The danger of vigorous and excessive suction causing adverse vagal and vasomotor reflexes resulting even in heart arrest has already been mentioned (see Chapter on Respiratory Complications).

Sudden respiratory and heart arrest may occur during the execution of passive movements of the paralysed legs or during the turning procedure of the patient, caused by an embolus. Therefore, the physiotherapist, like the nursing staff, must be familiar with the technique of artificial respiration, which she must commence without delay and continue until members of the nursing and medical staff arrive on the scene. It has been the vigilance and immediate action of some of our physiotherapists which saved the life of such patients.

(2) Adaptation therapy of normal parts of the body

General principles of compensatory training

These are carried out, from the early stages, in conjunction with passive movements, proper positioning, electrotherapy, etc., with a view to overdevelopment of those muscles, which are essential for a patient's upright position and readjustment of postural and vasomotor control of these cases.

Overdevelopment of arm, trunk and abdominal muscles

The most important muscles to be exercised in spinal cord lesions above T7 are the latissimus dorsi, trapezius, rhomboidei, teres major, serratus anterior, pectorals, and last but by no means least, the triceps—and, for distal cord lesions, also the abdominal and long back muscles. Compensatory training of these muscle groups is important for the following reasons:
a   the combined operation of these muscle groups will greatly improve the balance and mobility of the trunk;
b   the combined operation of these muscle groups will restore the paraplegic's capability to walk between parallel bars on crutches, by means of pelvic tilting or by promoting swinging movements of the trunk. The knees are fixed with light bivalved walking plasters and, later on, with calipers, keeping the feet at the correct angle by means of simple toe-raising springs; thus, the paralysed legs are used as stilts;
c   training of the abdominal muscles is also of great importance for the re-conditioning of the bladder and for the restoration of the sexual function of the paraplegic.

Techniques

The following are special methods which have been developed at Stoke Mandeville to achieve compensatory training effects:

Resistance and suspension exercises

Auto-assisted, resistance exercises of the upper limbs are introduced in the early stages, while the patient is still in bed, with the aid of simple springs unit (chest expanders) and ten pulls or more are made by the patient every half an hour to an hour. This immediately encourages the paraplegic to activity, and it is the co-operation of the nursing staff and physiotherapist to ensure that these chest-expander exercises are carried out regularly by the patient.

Later on, exercises in suspension and against resistance by means of pulleys and weights are added, as introduced and developed by Mrs Guthrie-Smith (1943). These have been an important contribution to physical readjustment in certain stages, and the Guthrie-Smith apparatus has proved invaluable for these exercises. Fig. 227 shows a patient with a complete lesion below T3, conveniently suspended in such a position as to allow movements unhampered by friction or weight of the paralysed body, doing

suspended exercises in such an apparatus. The arms are elevated and the hands are
holding on to the upright bars. In cervical lesions with paralysis of the flexors of the fingers
the hands may either be bandaged on to the bars, or the patient will hook his wrist or
elbow round the bars, giving himself a fixed point from which to work. Care must be
taken that the pelvic sling does not produce friction to the sacrum, especially in the
presence of scars from healed sores, and a pillow must be placed between the patient
and the sling. Patients wearing a rubber urinal must be suspended with legs lower than
the pelvis, in order to prevent back-flow of urine from the urinal into the trousers.
In patients with severe flexor spasms, the legs will have to be kept in extension by well-
padded splints. The patient first learns to swing his pelvis from side to side, by action
of the shoulder muscles and pectorals and, particularly, trapezius, latissimus dorsi and
triceps. The same effect can be achieved by suspension exercises, once the patient can
sit in a wheelchair. His arms are suspended in abduction by an elbow sling and overhead
rod, to which a spring is also attached, and he can exercise his shoulder muscles against
resistance. Furthermore, the power of the back and abdominal muscles can be increased
by suspension exercises in sitting position, on a plinth. In due course, the back muscles
and pectorals may reach a state of hypertrophy which is sometimes quite grotesque, as
seen in Figs. 228a and b in a case of complete transverse lesion below T6.

Fig. 229a shows the contracting latissimus dorsi in its whole length in a case of complete transection below T3. Note the hypertrophic latissimus dorsi bulging out below the
axillae in Fig. 229b.

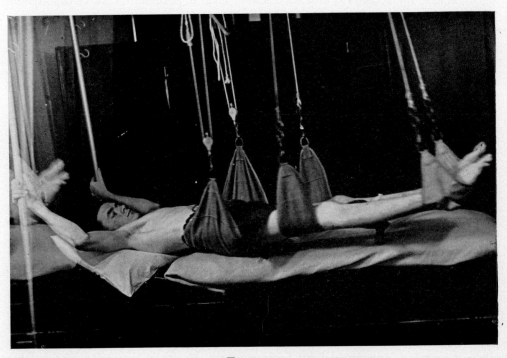

FIG. 227.

The Stoke Mandeville bed-cycle

As a result of observations, that alternating passive movements of the paralysed legs have a beneficial effect on spasticity by relaxation, the writer designed in 1946 a pedal-exerciser for promoting self-activated exercises by the paraplegic to relieve the work of the physiotherapist (Guttmann, 1949). This apparatus, which was later constructed and manufactured by Standard Sales Ltd, 113 Newington Causeway, London, S.E.1, was originally designed for patients still confined to bed but is now used in physiotherapy departments in various countries as an essential piece of equipment for patients needing

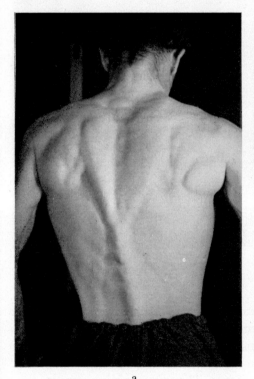 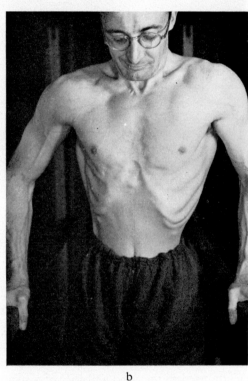

a   b

FIG. 228.

this type of physiotherapy. It is operated by the patient in lying position and has a wide application in the treatment of paralysed patients. Through the medium of interconnected hand- and leg-operated cranks, a variety of effects can be achieved with this bed-cycle. It improves the power of the arm and trunk muscles, it greatly improves the blood circulation in both the normal and paralysed parts of the body, it has proved invaluable in overcoming contractures, and lastly it has a beneficial effect on spasticity by causing fatigue in the spastic muscles. In patients with partial paralysis in arms and legs and dissociated forms of paralysis, the apparatus is beneficial in improving the strength of the weak muscles as well as recovering muscle groups.

The device consists, in principle, of two standard-type bicycle cranks suitably mounted

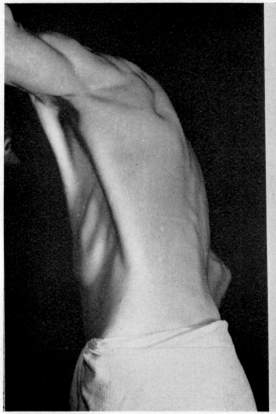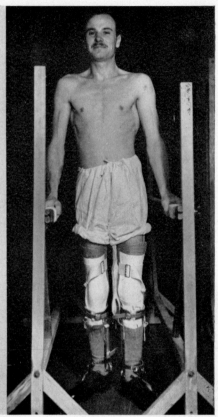

a   b

FIG. 229.

and connected by cycle chains through a standard three-speed gear, modified by the
addition of a second sprocket to take the second chain. The iron frame supporting this
bicycle device, is built in such a way as to give complete clearance for the knees when
the machine is in operation. The frame is held in clamps, mounted on supports which are
rigidly fixed to the head and foot of a standard bed. The frame is fitted with two hubs
which carry brakes and can apply a load to either the hands or feet, singly or combined,
as required. The load is adjustable by a screw and can give a load up to 12 lb. The pedals
of the driving cranks, used for the hands, have the webs removed, and a spindle form of
hand-grip is fitted instead. On the foot pedals, the webs have been retained and are used
for holding a metal boot to which the paralysed legs are strapped. The boot is made of
$\frac{1}{16}$ in. iron and the sole is bolted to the pedal and hinged at the heel to a curved gaiter,
which fits snugly around the calf of the leg; the whole is leather covered, and straps are
provided to secure the feet and legs. All parts which come in contact with the patient
are felt-padded. The foot and leg supports are adjustable, both as to the distance between
the feet and to support behind the calf—the latter to prevent adductor spasms. A speedo-
meter and mile counter are incorporated in a position, which can be seen by the patient,
to observe the duration and speed of the movements. The revolution counter is fixed on

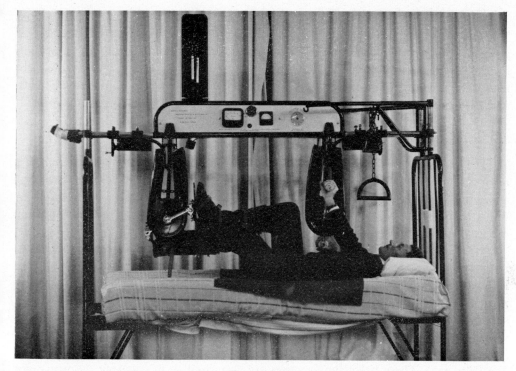

FIG. 230.

the foot pedal, and by calculation it has been found that 360 revolutions of the feet equal a mile along the road. Moreover, there is also a pre-selected clock device incorporated, which enables the physiotherapist in charge of the patient to select the duration of the exercise without being in attendance during the exercise.

While this apparatus has proved its value throughout the years for the physical restoration of paraplegics, certain adjustments were necessary to convert it into an Ergo-Dynamometer for our studies on the physical effects of graduated exercises on paraplegics. The necessary modifications have been carried out by my former Senior Research Assistant Dr N.C.Mehra in co-operation with Mr A.Dudley, an engineer. The original milometer has been converted to a tachometer, showing revolutions per minute and total number of revolutions in a given time. A dynamo, a milliampermeter and a voltmeter have been incorporated which constitute the dynamometer. The work output on the instrument at zero external load can be calculated in watts. Furthermore, a series of 7 different coloured lights have been introduced. The current is supplied by the dynamo, and the different coloured lights appear in succession at a definite number of revolutions per minute as the rate of revolutions varies. The patient is instructed to keep to a particular light in accordance to the desired rate of revolution. This enables him to keep an approximately uniform speed. Moreover, balances of different capacity can be substituted, giving friction loads up to 25 lb. They are mounted on adjusting screws which vary the friction load. The work output can now be calculated in foot-pounds per minute by a special formula. Fig. 230 shows the apparatus in action.

(3) **Restoration of posture and vasomotor control**

The loss of postural sensibility in complete transverse cord lesions above T10 represents a serious complication, for it makes it difficult and in higher lesions above T5, impossible for the paraplegic to maintain his equilibrium in sitting and standing position. It is the task of the physiotherapist to develop that new pattern of postural sensibility, which was discussed in the chapter on Postural Control. There are three stages in this treatment.

Technique

1   The first stage consists of exercises of the patient in a sitting position in front of a mirror, during which the arms are raised in various directions, whereby the paraplegic and tetraplegic learns to compensate for the loss of postural sensibility of the trunk by visual control. This visual-motor feed-back is a most essential factor in the production of a new pattern of postural control, to enable the paraplegic to develop his sitting balance. At first on raising one arm a swaying response follows immediately, but with continuous balancing exercises under visual guidance this swaying response diminishes, because he learns to shift the centre of gravity necessary for the maintenance of balance when he moves his arms, and thus learns to appreciate his position in space. Gradually, commensurate with the development of the new pattern of postural sensibility, he will be able to sit with his arms raised and eyes closed and keep his equilibrium (Fig. 231a and b). Already, at this stage, sport, especially archery, has proved an excellent remedial exercise (Fig. 232). These balancing exercises are also essential in restoring the vasomotor control in tetraplegics with the aid of an abdominal binder to prevent hypotension by too much accumulation of blood in the abdominal vascular bed.

2   The second stage in postural readjustment is learning to maintain balance by catching and throwing a ball or heavier object such as a sandbag. Group exercises have proved very valuable at this stage (Fig. 233). Sports such as table tennis, throwing the javelin or club and shot putting can be usefully employed.

3   The third and final stage in restoring balance consists of rapid alternations between free movements of the arms against resistance, as practised in punch-ball (Fig. 234) or fencing exercises in the wheelchair, whereby variations of movements and diversities of situations occur. In this stage, wheelchair basketball has proved invaluable, for the diversities of situations caused by the movement of the ball, on the one hand, and the movement of the opponent on the other, have proved of paramount importance for promoting the new pattern of postural control in the paralysed. Swimming has also been usefully employed for the restoration of postural control in both paraplegics and tetraplegics. The paralysed part of the body, especially in higher cord lesions, has the tendency to float in the water, due to its greater buoyancy (Fig. 236). Therefore, the paraplegic when using the breast stroke will at first experience difficulty in keeping head and shoulders above water and must develop a new postural control in the water. One of the most extreme examples of postural reconditioning through intensive training is one of the writer's former patients who, in the Second World War, lost his left arm in the upper third of the humerus and then developed after the war a complete paraplegia below T3 as a result of transverse myelitis. He was previously a keen swimmer and insisted on trying

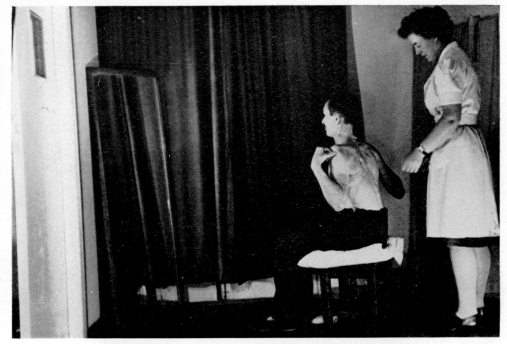

a

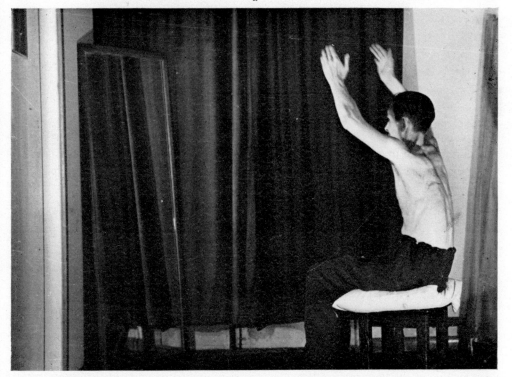

b

FIG. 231. Balancing excerises in front of a mirror.

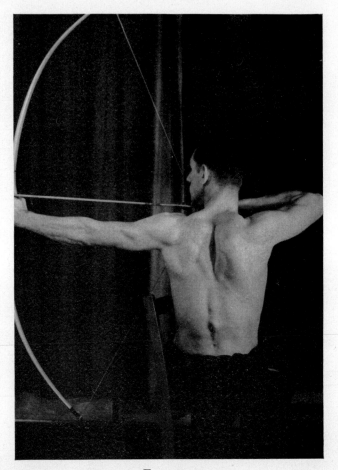

FIG. 232.

swimming again. He succeeded, using his right arm alone, with the result that he was able only to swim in a circle like a fish with one fin. In due course, he was provided with a frog-arm to the stump of his left arm, which enabled him, after training under supervision of his physiotherapist, to swim straight. At a later stage of training, his postural adjustment had improved to such an extent, that he was able to swim in an almost straight line using the stump of his left arm without the frog-arm.

The effect of fully restored posture and locomotion is well illustrated by a patient with a complete cord lesion below T9 (Fig. 235).

Hydrotherapy

The employment of water for the well-being of the individual in general and for hygienic and therapeutic purposes in particular is as old as man himself. The beneficial and recreational value of being immersed in the medium of water is already apparent in the lusty kicking of the baby, and is later demonstrated by young and old through manifold playful activities afforded by swimming pools and many other bathing facilities.

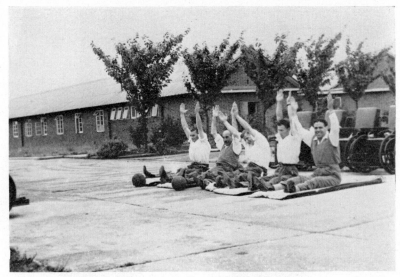

FIG. 233. Group Exercises.

In the rehabilitation of paraplegics and tetraplegics, water therapy and training for water sport play a very essential part, and a swimming pool of adequate size—preferably 25 m in length—should be one of the essential equipments of a spinal injuries centre. The former Ministry of Pensions took up the challenge and, in spite of severe economic stringencies in Great Britain as a result of the Second World War, provided the facilities

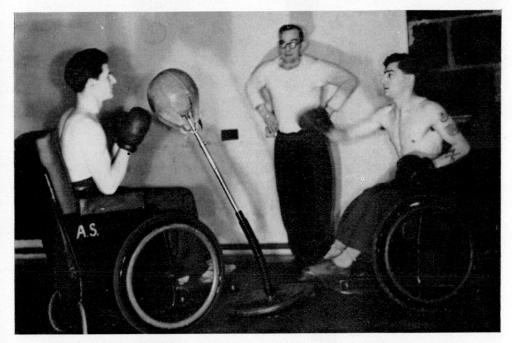

FIG. 234. Physiotherapy, punch ball exercises in the gym, paraplegic patients.

Start

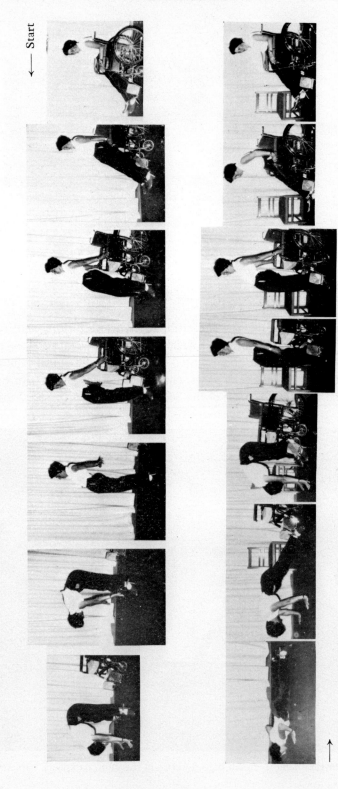

Fig. 235. Posture and locomotion demonstrated by a fully rehabilitated patient with a complete spinal cord lesion below T9.

of a 10 m swimming pool for the Stoke Mandeville Centre in 1952–53 (Figs. 239, 240). The pool has an electric hoist to which a stretcher can be attached to lower tetraplegics into the bay of the pool, where the physiotherapist, standing within the encroachment of the bay, in the form of a Hubbard tank, can give passive movements to spastic or contracted legs and arms. There is, in addition, another hoist to which patients can be transferred from the wheelchair and hoisted into the water. Paraplegics, more progressed in their rehabilitation, can hoist themselves from their chair into the water with the aid of handles attached to a chain. Moreover, the pool is also provided with steps and double rails for paraplegics, who are able to walk into the water. The temperature of the chlorinated water of the pool, which is circulating continuously, varies between 82–85°F, and regular bacteriological tests are made to ensure sterility of the water. This pool is still used every day with great satisfaction to all concerned, but, naturally, spinal centres set up in recent years in various parts of the world, have more or less modified this pool according to their purposes.

Emphasis is laid in paraplegics on active hydrotherapy to utilize and mobilize all that is left in the sensory-motor system. Therefore, passive procedures, such as the so-called under-water therapy by douches and other elaborate forms of jets, which is so popular in countries of the European continent, should not be used as hydrotherapy for the paralysed. Swimming represents one of the most natural forms of remedial exercise and has proved invaluable in restoring the paraplegic's co-ordination, strength, speed, endurance and self-confidence and also in counteracting spasticity. In the contest with himself to improve his performance, the paraplegic and tetraplegic learns to overcome fatigue— a predominant symptom in the early stage of rehabilitation. Moreover, swimming has

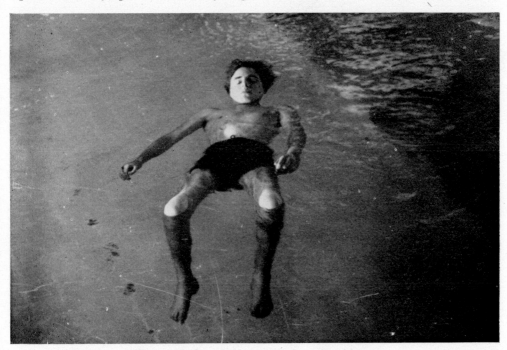

FIG. 236. Greater buoyancy of paralysed legs.

proved invaluable for the development of movement patterns, which promote a new
postural control in the water. As mentioned above, the paralysed part of the body has a
tendency to float in the water due to its greater buoyancy (Fig. 236). Therefore, the
paraplegic, when using the back-stroke and, in particular, the breast-stroke, has to use his
trunk and arm muscles to hyperextend his back in order to keep his head above water.
The time of adjustment to the water, naturally, varies according to the level of the lesion,
age and whether or not the individual was a skilled swimmer before his spinal cord injury.
Paraplegics, who were skilled swimmers before their spinal cord lesion, can adjust themselves to the water in a very short time—sometimes in a few minutes. Actually, one of my
former patients, who sustained a complete paraplegia below the waist as a result of a
fracture-dislocation of the spine through falling from a rock into the sea and hitting
another rock during the fall, instantaneously adjusted himself to his new condition, and
thus saved his life by swimming breast-stroke ashore using his arms only. Another
patient—an officer—who was thrown into the water when his ship was torpedoed during

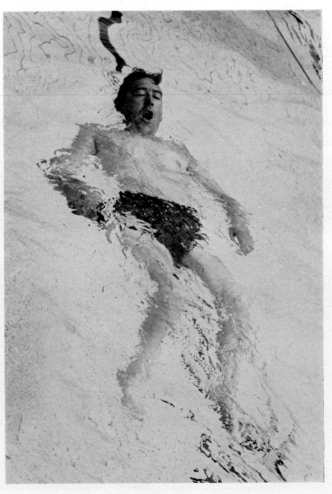

FIG. 237.

the Second World War, received his paraplegia while in the water through a shell. He immediately adjusted himself and using his arms saved his life by swimming ashore.

While the back-stroke is used in the initial training, as being the easiest stroke, paraplegics even with higher lesions, including distal cervical lesions, can also become skilled in breast-stroke and crawl. Fig. 237 demonstrates back-stroke in a tetraplegia below C6/7 (note the buoyancy of the paralysed legs) and Fig. 238b crawl executed by two paraplegics.

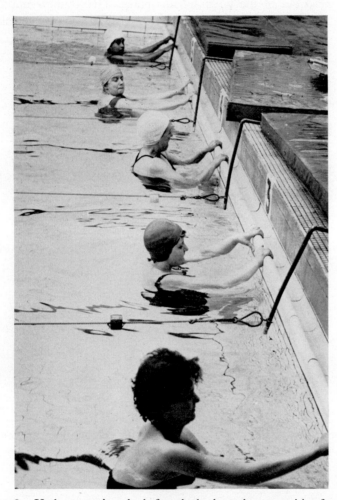

FIG. 238a. Under starter's order before the back-stroke competition for ladies.

Crawl presents a special problem in complete paraplegics. As the legs cannot be used to stabilize the body, the body will rotate with each stroke of the arm. In back crawl, this can be overcome to a certain extent by a sculling action with the arm which is in the water (Fig. 238). However, by achieving greater skill the sculling can be abandoned. The problem of rotation also exists for the front crawl. It is well known that able-bodied swimmers also rotate their bodies in the water but this is less pronounced because rotation of hips and pelvis can be prevented by the action movements of the legs. In paraplegics and tetraplegics the whole trunk and pelvis will rotate as the paralysed legs cannot counteract the rotation of the pelvis (Fig. 238). This is particularly conspicuous in tetraplegics due to the paralysis of most of the trunk muscles. Only in exceptional cases of tetraplegia at the level of the 7th or 8th cervical segment will the paralysed be able to use the crawl. Such tetraplegics are trained to swim two or three strokes face down in the water, then lengthen the stroke and at the same time hyperextend the back and bring the head out of the water for air intake. This training improves the vital capacity of the lungs and by the time they leave the Centre they may be able to swim one

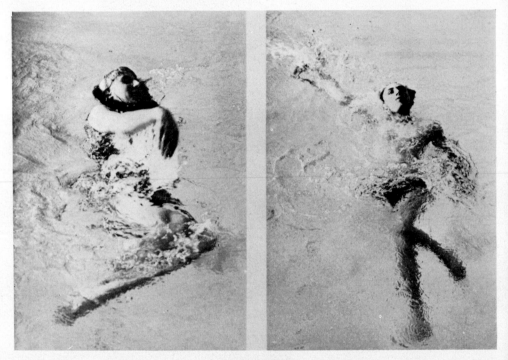

FIG. 238b. Crawl.

length of the 10 m pool face down. During swimming competitions the competitors start in the water holding on a starting rail, as shown in Fig. 238a. Fig. 239 shows a tetraplegic below C7 with paralysis of all finger muscles, who became very efficient in underwater swimming.

The problem of adjustment of the very young needs special mention. We have commenced training in swimming with children from the age of 3. Paralysed children on the whole greatly enjoy swimming lessons. Fig. 240, a boy of 3½ during his early training who, after 4 months, was able to take part in a competition of children. However, some paralysed children—like able-bodied of their age—show terror at first when lowered into the water and cling tightly around the neck of their physiotherapist. It needs great patience, firmness and perseverance on the part of the instructor to overcome this anxiety and at the same time to teach the paralysed child to swim.

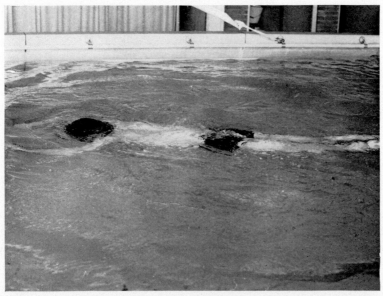

FIG. 239. Breast stroke by tetraplegic (C7), head under water, spine and body in one line after training.

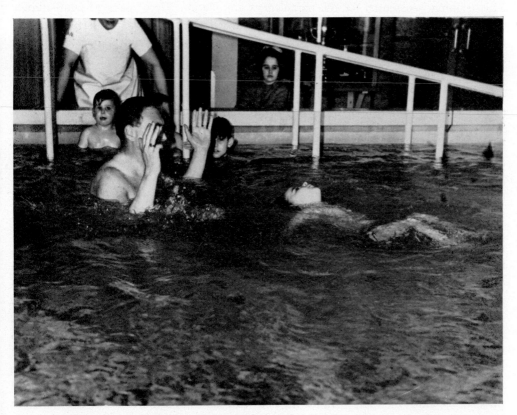

FIG. 240. Training in swimming of a paralysed child under the age of 5.

Exercises to restore independence

SELF-DRESSING

To prepare paraplegics for future independence, self-dressing exercises are included in our programme, as soon as they are able to raise themselves from the lying to the vertical position. They are taught and encouraged by both the physiotherapist and nursing staff to dress themselves in the minimum of time. This procedure includes hoisting themselves from their beds on to their wheelchairs, either with or without the aid of a chain handle fixed over the bed. In due course, paraplegics will develop their own most suitable individual technique, especially with regard to putting on their trousers, socks and shoes. It was found that a well-trained paraplegic, paralysed at or below T10, should be able to dress himself completely (without putting on his calipers) in about 5 minutes, higher lesions between 8 and 18 minutes. Timing of these patients during the dressing exercise by the physiotherapist or nurse is important for promoting punctuality in their routine daily activities in the ward and attendance at the physiotherapy department and workshop, and this is a useful preliminary for their employment later.

TRANSFER FROM BED TO WHEELCHAIR, FROM WHEELCHAIR TO CAR, ETC.

This training is essential for the paraplegic's ambulation. Here again, physiotherapist, occupational therapist and nursing staff have to share in the training and assist the patient until he becomes proficient in this, by no means easy performance. Knocking the hip against the armrest of the wheelchair, or the ankles or feet against the footrest of the wheelchair or the edge of the floor of the car must be avoided to prevent bruises and sores. Transfer from bed to wheelchair or wheelchair to the bath, toilet or car and vice versa should always be carried out without haste and under strict visual guidance. The phrase 'Look before you leap!' should become engrained in the paraplegic's brain, as this will be the best prevention of bruises, traumatic bursae and last but by no means least, fractures of the legs. A few of our paraplegics fractured legs, by sheer carelessness, when transferring themselves from the chair on to the toilet.

The technique of transferring from wheelchair on to the bed, toilet, bath or car and vice versa naturally varies according to the level of the lesion, age, individual aptitude and skill of the patient on the one hand, and type of bed, wheelchair, toilet, bath, motor tricycle or car on the other, and in due course, every paraplegic has to adopt by training, his own favourite routine. Some prefer, when transferring from bed on to the wheelchair, to have the chair parallel to the bed, while others have the chair standing at right angles to the bed. The easiest and safest procedure for beginners is, to have the chair fixed by its brakes alongside the bed. The patient, sitting as near to the edge of the bed as possible, should hold with one hand the handle of the movable bedpole and with the other support himself on the farside armest of the chair. He then lifts his body on to the seat of the chair and afterwards moves one paralysed leg after the other with his hands on to the footrest. At a later stage, the paraplegic may dispense with the handle of the bedpole altogether and push off the bed with his extended arms. The transfer from bed on to the wheelchair and vice versa is greatly facilitated, and knocking of the hip

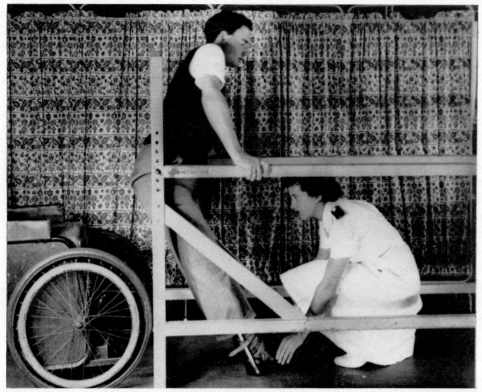

FIG. 241a. Prevention of slipping.

avoided, if wheelchairs with detachable armrests are used. This is particularly essential in assisting transfer of tetraplegics from wheelchair into a car. This can be facilitated by placing a short board between the chair and the seat of the car, on which the tetraplegic can slide into the car. Another point, which should be remembered when transferring from wheelchair to the toilet, car, etc., is to avoid bumping down on the toilet seat or car seat, because of the danger of causing bruising or a deep haematoma of the ischial region or scrotum. For tetraplegics with paralysis of all arm and hand muscles, hoists greatly facilitate the transfer of the patient from bed to the wheelchair or from wheelchair into the bath (Fig. 260).

Standing exercises

As soon as the power in trunk and arm muscles, as well as the patient's postural and vasomotor control in sitting position have sufficiently improved, as a preliminary to ambulation, the paraplegic has first to learn to get up from his wheelchair on to the parallel bars, keep his balance in standing position and get back slowly into his chair. These activities, which the able-bodied would perform subconsciously, are rather a strenuous undertaking for paraplegics—especially those with high lesions. Supervision and help from the attendant are needed until the patient is able to perform this activity unaided (Fig. 241a).

On getting up in the parallel bars, the patient has to lean forward and place his hands along the bars as far in front of his body as possible. Furthermore, he must place his feet on the ground, with legs kept in extension by calipers or walking plasters, at such an angle as to prevent them from slipping forwards during the act of pulling himself up on to his arms. In due course, paraplegics with strong arm muscles can acquire the technique of an athlete in getting on to the parallel bars—i.e. swinging their feet forward along the floor, pushing up quickly on to their arms and swinging their feet backwards.

Balance in standing position without corsets is at first maintained under visual guidance—i.e. by placing a mirror in front of the patient, so that he can correct his postural disturbance, until the new scheme of postural sensibility along the normal back muscles, mentioned previously, is sufficiently developed. Paraplegics with low and mid-thoracic lesions may eventually learn to keep their balance in standing position by supporting themselves with one arm only on the parallel bar and throwing and catching a ball or sandbag with the other hand. Balancing exercises in standing position are also helpful for improving the patient's confidence and skill when later he graduates to the use of crutches. When standing with crutches, he leans on one crutch and lifts the other forward, sideways and upward.

Paraplegics with complete lesions above T_5, where the splanchnic control is crippled and consequently the circulatory adaptation to sudden change of posture is inefficient, may complain about a feeling of giddiness and fainting, during their first standing exercises. Therefore, the paraplegic should be warned not to get up too quickly and, moreover, the period of standing in these cases should be increased only very gradually. In due course, the patient learns to overcome the circulatory disturbance by contracting his back muscles or by deep inspiration.

The great therapeutic value of daily standing and walking exercises, and the need for the paraplegic to continue these permanently at home, after leaving hospital, should always be stressed. In particular, their beneficial effect in the restoration and maintenance of a good blood circulation, in promoting a satisfactory renal and bladder function, in overcoming spasticity, and in preventing contractures of hip and knee joints and obesity should be fully explained to the patient and his attendants, the more so as some patients have the tendency to discontinue standing exercises at home.

Paraplegics with spastic lesions, who have developed a preponderance of extensor spasms, may be taught to use them advantageously for standing without the aid of appliances. In this connection, attention may also be drawn to the beneficial effect of weight-bearing on bone growth by standing exercises in paralysed children.

In the beginning of standing exercises, the physiotherapist's position in relation to that of the patient is important to control his dysbalance. She should stand behind the patient holding one hand over the iliac crest and her other round the chest wall (Fig. 224).

Sitting down from the standing position has also to be learned, under supervision. This should be done slowly, to prevent the legs from slipping forward, and at first the physiotherapist has to assist by holding the feet and pressing them to the floor (Fig. 241a). In particular, the patient must be taught to avoid sitting back into his chair with force, and knocking his ischium against the chair. In lesions above T6, a second physiotherapist or orderly may at first assist the sitting down procedure by standing at the patient's side holding one arm and hand round the front of the patient's waist and the other hand gripping the back of the patient's trouser waistband.

Preliminary exercises to walking

These consist in mobilizing the pelvis and are of particular importance for the four-point gait. The patient is taught to tilt the pelvis alternately right and left upwards, in lower lesions with both the abdominal and trunk muscles, in lesions above T6 mainly with latissimus dorsi and trapezius. The patient practises alternate right and left pelvic tilting, standing in parallel bars and keeping his body as upright as possible. These tilting exercises have proved most essential for increasing the strength and action of the abdominal and trunk muscles as well as triceps. While carrying out pelvic tilting, the patient is taught to swing the leg forwards and backwards and by standing parallel to one bar, to swing the legs sideways. Furthermore, he has to learn to place his feet accurately on the floor. This is particularly important in spastic lesions with preponderance of plantar flexor spasms or contractures, and to overcome these he has to stand with the full weight of the body on his heels.

Walking

In most paraplegics, even those with complete lesions of the upper thoracic and lower cervical cord, walking capabilities can be restored to variable degrees. Walking exercises are started in parallel bars, and the patient is taught to walk forwards, backwards and also has to learn turning in parallel bars, which in itself is an excellent balancing exercise, especially in transverse lesions above T10 (Fig. 241b). He then continues in a walking frame, before graduating to crutch walking. The writer's own design of a walking frame for paraplegics and tetraplegics is equipped with hand-brakes on either side, which increases safety and stability of the frame and gives the paraplegic greater confidence, particularly in the beginning of walking exercises outside the parallel bars. Moreover, it enables the paraplegic in the course of his training to walk not only in a forward direction but also, by putting on one brake only, to turn towards the side of that brake, which in itself helps to improve his postural control. Furthermore, the frame is equipped with a seat with wedge-shaped cushion for resting during the exercise (Fig. 242). In all these exercises, time and distance are gradually increased. Naturally, the walking capabilities of a paraplegic, especially those with higher lesions, will always remain limited, but, however small it may be, it greatly increases his range of activity and independence at home and place of employment.

Types of gait

Amongst the various types of walking, the following are taught as routine at Stoke Mandeville:

Four-point gait. The patient moves his left hand forwards, along the bar, then swings the right leg through by tilting the pelvis upwards. He now transfers the body-weight on to

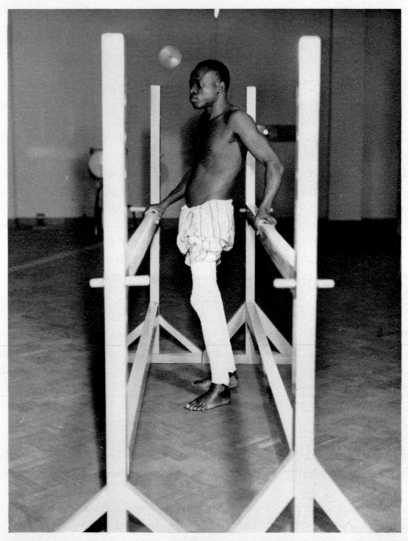

FIG. 241b. Turning in parallel bars.

the right leg, moves his right hand forward and swings his left leg through, by tilting the left side of the pelvis upwards. Attention has to be paid to placing the feet accurately on to the floor, so that the full weight of the body rests on the standing leg. Although locomotion is slow in this type of gait, it is by far the safest, when walking with the aid of arm or elbow crutches (Fig. 243).

Swing-to gait. This gait is preferable for patients with mid- or high-thoracic lesions and accelerates walking in lesions below T10. Their hands, placed on the parallel bars or grasping crutches, are moved forward simultaneously, and the body then lifted and pulled forwards a short distance. The feet and legs always remain behind the level of the

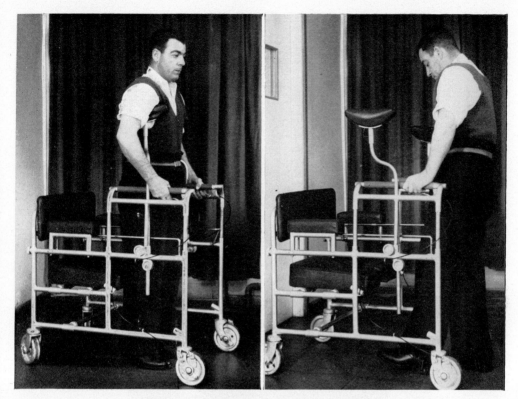

FIG. 242. Stoke Mandeville walking frame.

arms and crutches. This posture guarantees a firm triangular base and prevents over-balancing in forward direction.

Swing-through gait. This type is especially used in cord lesions at the level of T9 and below and represents the quickest form of locomotion. The arms and crutches are moved forward, and the body is then swung through in front of the arms and crutches, the hips and spine being held in hyperextension (Fig. 244). Then the arms and upper trunk are swung forward simultaneously, so that a firm triangular base is established, and then the legs and body are swung forward again. However, in higher lesions, especially those with spasticity of the abdominal muscles, the swing-through gait may entail the risk of throwing the patient off balance by sudden abdominal spasms resulting in a 'jack-knife' forwards movement.

Walking sideways, backwards and up and down stairs. Once the paraplegic has gained skill and confidence in forward walking on an even surface, he is taught to walk over small obstacles, such as sandbags or blocks, in order to be able to negotiate kerbs and, as a preliminary, to walking up steps and stairs. Furthermore, he has also to learn to walk sideways and backwards, as a preliminary to getting into and out of his wheelchair and negotiating corridors, toilet, etc., unaided.

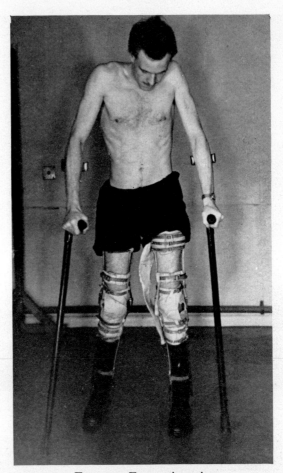

FIG. 243. Four-point gait.

Many houses and, in particular, public buildings, have steps at their entrances and—alas—it will still take many years to persuade authorities and architects to build or adjust houses and public buildings (see later) to enable disabled persons, especially the paralysed, to have easy access to them. Therefore, it is still essential to train paraplegics to negotiate steps and stairs. The technique to walk upstairs depends (a) on the type of stairs—i.e. whether they have one or two banisters or fixed handrails, (b) on the type and level of the lesion. Therefore, in every case the physiotherapist has to train the patient to develop and practise the technique of walking upstairs and downstairs most suited to his or her particular disability. Naturally, paraplegics with distal cord lesions and strong abdominal muscles will be able to walk upstairs by holding on to the handrail or banister with one hand and the other on his crutch, and then lift his feet up individually from step to step, or if this is too strenuous, lift the whole body. He will also have to find out, whether it is more convenient to walk upstairs forwards or in a backwards position. Paraplegics with weak or paralysed abdominal muscles will, of course, have greater difficulties. Some have learned to sit on the step with the back to the stairs and a cushion strapped to the seat and will then lift themselves on to the next step with their arms.

Abnormal gait patterns in spinal cord and cauda equina lesions

The spastic gait. The spastic gait is subject to considerable variation, according to the degree of pyramidal tract lesion, and in certain cases to the associated lower motor neuron involvement in both complete and incomplete transverse spinal syndromes. The main characteristic of the spastic gait is loss of the essential element in human locomotion, namely alternating stepping. Normally, while the standing leg supports the body, the other is flexed at hip and knee, raised from the ground, swung forward, and placed in a suitable position to receive and carry the weight of the body. In the severely spastic gait, the flexion phase is more or less abolished, and the legs are rigid in extension and adduc-

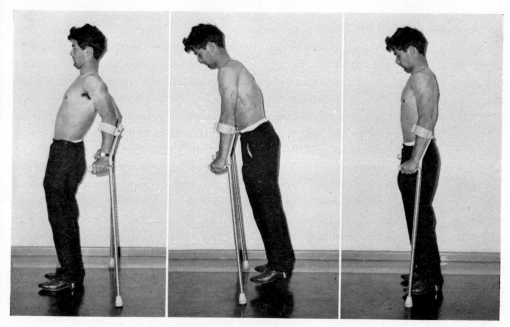

FIG. 244. Swing through gait. Complete paraplegia below T11.

tion. One leg is dragged after the other and each is brought forward with a movement of circumduction. During the phase of circumduction, the body is tilted forwards and sideways, in order to counterbalance the swinging leg. In hemisection of the spinal cord (Brown–Séquard syndrome), the difference in posture of the body during the walking movement of the normal and the spastic leg is particularly striking. In milder forms of spasticity in incomplete spinal cord lesions, hip and knee flexion are possible to varying degree.

The spastic foot during walking is inverted due to predominant action of the tibialis anterior and posterior, and its outer border shuffles along the ground. Conversely, under certain circumstances, the action of the peroneal muscles is preponderant due to weakness of the tibialis anterior as a result of a superimposed lower motor neuron lesion, and consequently the foot deviates into eversion. The result is flattening of the longitudinal arch and development of a flat foot with valgus deformity. If this deformity exists bilaterally, 'Charlie Chaplin' type of gait may develop. In cases where spasticity of the plantar flexors of foot and toes is predominant, the patient has difficulty in placing the foot firmly on the ground, and as a result of the overaction of the long flexors the toes drag along the ground. This is particularly apparent when the patient walks without shoes.

Analysis of the spastic paraplegic or paraparetic patient's total body movement by the medical attendant, in co-operation with the physiotherapist, will serve as a basis for the choice of the most suitable techniques to restore or improve the patient's walking capability. Other factors which have to be considered in the assessment of gait, especially in complete cord lesions, are for what purpose the gait is required and how far it is practical.

The training should be started in parallel bars in front of a mirror to establish a new pattern of gait under visual guidance, and walking on elbow crutches should not be started until the patient has overcome the hip extension, adduction and circumduction movement of the legs, as well as the forward and sideways tilting of the body. In extension and adduction spasticity, auto-assisted exercise on the Stoke Mandeville bed-bicycle often has a relaxing effect, as a preliminary, to the walking in parallel bars or on crutches in promoting flexion of hips and knees. Another useful method in this respect is walking exercise in a heated swimming pool, and relaxing of the extension-adduction spasticity can be achieved by preliminary passive movements of the legs given by the physiotherapist. Certain paraplegics with strong extensor spasms learn to turn them to good use by standing and walking on them without calipers in parallel bars and deliberately provoking contractions of the latissimus dorsi. When relaxation of the extensor group occurs and knee flexion is imminent, the patient braces himself, and by this manoeuvre the pull, which the latissimus dorsi exerts on the pelvis, serves as a strong afferent impulse to initiate the extensor response of gluteal muscles, hamstrings and quadriceps. Some paraplegics with complete mid-thoracic lesion were able to walk several lengths of the parallel bars without assistance, and thus regain relief and a sense of well-being from stretching their bodies and holding the upright position. Above all, the resulting relaxation of their spasticity may last for several hours (see also Chapter on Spasticity).

The ataxic gait. The term 'ataxic gait' presupposes that the patient is able to walk but that his gait is unsteady and he has difficulty in keeping the equilibrium of his trunk. The underlying cause of ataxia is either involvement of cerebellar pathway or damage to the posterior columns or posterior roots. In spinal cord lesions, we have to deal mainly with the latter cause. In incomplete lesions of the spinal cord, the damage of the neural elements may only involve the posterior column tracts or—more frequently—it is combined with the damage of the pyramidal tracts. In cauda equina lesions, the damage of the posterior roots may also be in the foreground of the clinical symptomatology. Unlike cerebellar ataxy, the ataxy based on the loss of posterior column sensibility increases when the patient walks in the dark or has to close his eyes (Romberg sign). Moreover, there is hypotonia of his muscles if there is no additional damage to the pyramidal tracts. The patient walks by widening his base, and the loss of postural sensibility in the muscles and joints of the hips, legs and feet interferes with his stepping movements, which become irregular, and the feet are not properly placed on the ground. His unsteadiness, due to loss of postural sensibility in the trunk, is particularly obvious in turning movements.

Physiotherapy of the ataxic gait is based on the pioneer work of Frenkel-Heyden (1900) on the compensatory training in tabes dorsalis, and spinal specialists as well as physiotherapists should be fully familiar with the details of his technique of compensating for the loss of postural sensibility under visual influence. Here again, as described in the foregoing section on the spastic gait, walking exercises in front of a mirror are indispensable. Patients with this type of incomplete spinal cord or cauda equina lesions will usually be able to walk on one, or in more severe cases, on two sticks. It may be noted that in combined pyramidal and posterior column lesions, as is the case in multiple sclerosis and combined degeneration of the cord in pernicious anaemia, the patient is much worse in the dark, as he has great difficulty in controlling his spastic legs and feet.

The swaying-shambling gait. This type of gait is the result of unilateral or bilateral paralysis of the gluteal muscles in cauda equina lesions or polio. The essential features of the abnormality of movement patterns in this condition differ, depending on whether the paralysis affects the gluteus maximus or medius.

The gluteus maximus gait. The characteristic feature is the backward thrust of the trunk, causing the line of gravity to fall behind the centre of the hip joints, and thus acting as an extension force to prevent jack-knifing of the hip joints. The gravity is balanced by the tension of the ilio-femoral ligament. The backward swaying gives the gait a clumsy appearance, and difficulties arise, especially on fast walking as the steps are shortened due to the backward swaying. The task of the physiotherapist is to train the patient to raise himself from hip-flexion to the upright position in parallel bars and later on sticks with the aid of trick movements. As long as biceps and quadriceps are strong, the paralysis of the gluteus maximus can be compensated. However, with additional weakness or paralysis of the quadriceps, walking without long calipers and short corsets stabilizing the hips is impossible. Furthermore, flexion contractures of the hips as a result of the gluteus maximus paralysis have to be counteracted by early hip extension exercises.

The gluteus medius gait. The characteristic feature is sideways swaying, producing a shambling type of gait. This muscle normally abducts the leg and fixes the pelvis by securing the rim of the pelvis against the trochanter. Moreover, this muscle also rotates the leg inwards. Therefore, unilateral paralysis of this muscle results in considerable deformity of hip and leg. The pelvis drops and the leg on the side of the paralysis assumes, during the swinging phase of gait, an adductory position, combined with outward rotation of the foot. The abnormal movement pattern during walking is an alternating shift of the body to the sound side during the swinging phase of the leg and to the affected side during the supporting phase of the involved limb. In bilateral paralysis of the gluteus medius, the waddling gait is greatly increased and resembles that of a congenital dislocation of the hip. The gluteus medius gait can be greatly improved by long

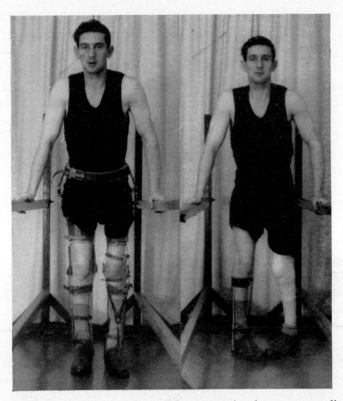

FIG. 245a. Paralysis of external rotators. After correction by proper appliance (left).
On admission (right).

calipers with pelvic band or short corset provided with hip joint hinges, which allow flexion
of the legs but prevent adduction and external rotation. In incomplete paralysis of the
gluteus medius, intensive exercises in slings and abduction exercises carried out in lateral
position combined with walking exercises in front of a mirror may improve the condition
greatly. Contractures of the adductor muscles must be avoided.

The gait in paralysis of the external rotators. In dissociated cauda equina lesions,
L4–S1, the paralysis may involve mainly the external rotators of the leg especially gemelli,
pyriformis, obturator externus and internus and quadratus femoris, and the resulting
deformity is internal rotation of the legs and feet, which is particularly cumbersome
in bilateral lesions as shown in Fig. 245a. Long calipers with hip joint hinges which allow
flexion of the hips and outward rotation but prevent internal rotation (Fig. 245b) will
remedy this abnormal gait.

The high-stepping gait in paralysis of the dorsi flexors of the feet. The inability
to dorsiflex the foot resulting in a paralytic drop foot, is a characteristic feature of cauda
equina lesions below L4/5. The patient compensates this inability by increased flexion
of the knees and hips, in order that the dropped feet clear the ground. The resulting

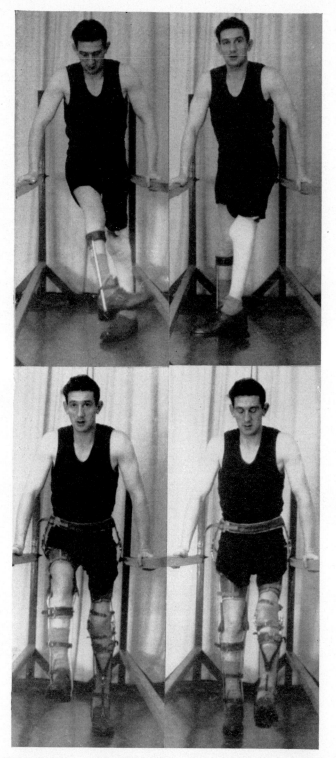

FIG. 245b. Walking before admission (top). Paralysis of external rotators in a case of conus-cauda lesion. Walking after correction with long calipers and pelvic band which prevent internal rotation.

abnormal movement pattern is a high-stepping gait. Neglect leads to flexion contractures of the feet and toes which may result in pressure sores, especially in the plantar surface of the big toe. Proper toe raising springs, or in certain cases Lambrinudi's arthrodesis, will counteract this complication and the high-stepping gait.

CHAPTER 35

WALKING APPLIANCES AND
MEANS OF TRANSPORT

TRAINING SPLINTS

These are indispensable for the vast majority of severe incomplete or complete spastic
lesions of the spinal cord. Before prescribing proper calipers, bivalved splints made from
plaster or Paris are used. These splints are made individually by our physiotherapists, and
care is taken to ensure that the edges of the anterior shell well overlap the posterior one
to prevent any friction of the soft tissues between the two shells. Five to six bandages
of plaster of Paris are sufficient for making the splint, which, of course, must be padded.
The splint, which reaches from mid-thigh to mid-calf is fastened by a crepe bandage.
The splint is also provided with a toe-raising spring to ensure dorsi-flexion of the foot.
These training splints have proved invaluable throughout the years, and certain patients
for whom, from one reason or another, calipers from steel or duraluminium were not
prescribed, took their splints home to continue their standing exercises in them (Fig. 241).

WALKING CALIPERS

Non-weight-bearing calipers only are used at Stoke Mandeville for distal and mid-
thoracic lesions. They are used for providing stability of the paralysed legs, but at the
same time they must be as light as possible, and the weight of each caliper for adults
must not be greater than 4 lb. The metal side bars are made from duralumin or specially
light steel. Duralumin is used mainly for young adults or children. The leather top and
calf cuffs are fastened by straps, which is time saving for putting on and taking off the
brace. The automatic self-locking knee joint is the Hoffmann type with supporting knee-
cap, and the strap catch enables the patient to unlock or lock the brace easily without
assistance. Only in very spastic cases with increased flexion spasticity is some assistance
necessary to lock the hinge. We prefer the ring lock knee hinge to the pawl lock knee
hinge, as the latter, when the hinge is unlocked, tends to damage the trousers. The metal
side bars fit into sockets in the heel of the shoes. A simple toe raising spring is attached
to a lug or D-ring on the shoe to avoid foot drop. Patients with inversion or eversion of the
foot need T-straps attached to their calipers (Fig. 246). When the tibialis anterior and
posterior muscles are paralysed and the foot, due to the action of the peroneal muscles,
turns into a valgus position, this may be prevented by means of an outside steel and inside
T-strap. In a case with paralysis of the peroneal muscles, the varus deformity of the foot
is corrected by an inside steel and an outside T-strap. An associated equinus deformity
may be controlled by an additional drop foot stop or a toe-raising spring (see above).

Whatever type of appliance has been prescribed, it is the duty of the spinal specialist
as well as the physiotherapist to ensure the proper fitting of the appliance as soon as it is

delivered by the maker. Particular care has to be taken to ensure that those areas of legs and hips such as trochanters, epicondyls and malleoli, are completely free of pressure from the caliper, and ill-fitting appliances should be returned immediately to the maker for re-adjustment.

Paraplegics walk with the aid of arm or elbow crutches. Therefore, shoulder and arm muscles must be strong enough to ensure this task. If the triceps muscles are weak, a posterior gutter splint must be attached to the crutches to stabilize the arms. Patients using elbow crutches or sticks may complain at first of paraesthesia, aching or cramp in the palm of the hand and, in particular, in the thenar muscles, as a result of pressure. Periods of rest should be included, and the patient should exercise his hands. Long arm crutches may produce too much pressure in the arm pits, resulting in irritation or pressure palsy of parts of the brachial plexus. As there are now various walking aids of tripod type available, the physiotherapist may choose one of them at one stage or another for restoring the walking capability of paraplegics. Fig. 246 demonstrates the type of leg brace which for many years has proved satisfactory for paraplegics.

In certain cases, it becomes necessary to attach the caliper to a pelvic band or short leather corset, and in these cases a hip joint hinge connects the caliper with the pelvic band or corset which allows flexion and some abduction of the leg. However, pelvic bands and short corsets are ordered only after careful consideration in selected cases with deformity of pelvis or spine. This is contrary to the practice of authors in U.S.A.,

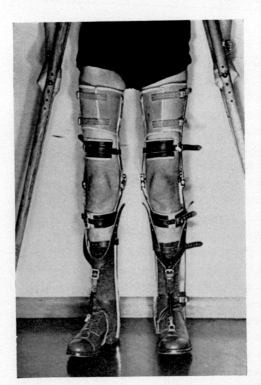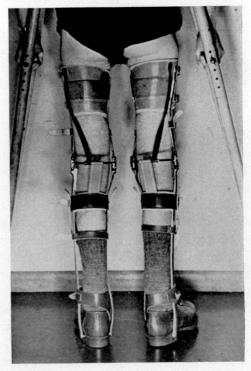

FIG. 246. Non-weight-bearing calipers.

who believe it is better to use too much bracing and then reduce the braces to the proper size. It is not my experience, that the addition of more extensive bracing has ever conveyed to the patient the feeling of failure nor is it much easier technically, as has been argued, to cut down braces to a lower level than to start with small braces and build up, if needed (Betts & Rosen, 1969).

In certain individuals with spastic incomplete lesions, the overaction of the quadriceps may produce hyperextension of the knee, resulting in genu recurvatum. To avoid this complication, the provision of a long caliper without locking knee joint hinge but with a pad behind the knee to stop hyperextension, has proved very beneficial.

MEANS OF TRANSPORT

WHEELCHAIRS

For the paraplegic's and tetraplegic's locomotion, a wheelchair is indispensable and represents the most essential equipment to promote their independence and social reintegration into the community. The time has passed when the paralysed with function of their upper limbs had to spend their lives in rigid and clumsy 'bathchairs' or even in wicker-bodied invalid carriages. Changing demands, commensurate with the advances made during the last quarter of this century in the rehabilitation of spinal cord sufferers, have resulted in developments in the design and construction of wheelchairs. Following a Symposium on Wheelchairs, organized by the Polio Research Fund and held under my chairmanship in November 1963 in London (published in 1964 in the *Journal of Paraplegia*, **2**, 20–70), in which medical experts, representatives of the Ministry of Health, engineers, manufacturers and wheelchair users took part, much information has been correlated in assessing design requirements, which has resulted in intensifying research on this subject in this country and abroad (Nichols *et al.*, 1966; Agate, 1967; Scott & Mason, 1966; Lewin & Brettgard, 1968). At that time, the National Health Service alone purchased, at an average annual rate of 13,000 wheelchairs, and, during 1962–63, 23,000 wheelchairs were issued, of which 16,000 were loaned to new patients of various disabilities. The total number of wheelchairs issued at that time was approximately 67,000 (Jolly, 1964). There is no doubt that these figures have increased ever since. Naturally, this large number of wheelchairs given free on permanent loan by the National Health Service to severely disabled persons of various disabilities, must have some bearing on cost. Therefore, the Ministry's endeavour is to evolve wheelchairs, which on the one hand will meet the needs of the majority of invalids and on the other lend themselves to bulk production methods, such as the model 8 series, described in its *Handbook of Wheelchairs* (Walker, 1964). In this connection, it is debatable whether model series 1, 3 and 9 described in the handbook are really necessary for bulk production, even if one considers disabilities such as cerebral palsy, arthritis, cerebo-vascular disease, multiple sclerosis, etc. However, as far as wheelchairs for spinal paraplegics and tetraplegics are concerned, the Ministry does not reject the prescription of the Everest and Jennings wheelchair as far as Stoke Mandeville Spinal Centre is concerned, although it is not included in the new handbook of the Ministry, if the consultant considers this as the most suitable general purpose wheelchair for his paralysed patients (Guttmann, 1964).

Wheelchairs for spinal cord sufferers can be divided into three main groups:

1 Rigid-framed wheelchair for indoor use only. These should be used for exceptional cases only.

2 Hand-propelled general purpose folding wheelchairs for use both indoors and outdoors, which are also suitable for transit.

3 Power-driven wheelchairs for tetraplegics with extensive paralysis of both upper limbs.

In the following, only groups 2 and 3 are discussed in some detail.

Hand-propelled general purpose folding transit chair

This type is used by a great majority of paraplegics but also by tetraplegics with lesions below the 6th cervical segment. It enables the paralysed to move independently about indoors and outdoors, including to and from his place of employment, studies, entertainment, sporting activities, etc., when travelling in his motorized conveyance. Therefore, such a chair must have certain qualities which are indispensable: stability, reliability, easy accessibility, light weight, easy manoeuvrability and good performance and, last but by no means least, good appearance. The latter point is very important from a psychological point of view, and it is significant that paraplegics (and other disabled persons) instinctively prefer a wheelchair which has the least appearance of an 'invalid' chair. In my view, no colour-painted wheelchair can compete in this respect with a chromium-plated one.

With regard to stability, it must be admitted that the lighter the wheelchair the greater the difficulty in securing stability. However, it has been proved that modern all-purpose folding wheelchairs of 36 lb weight can maintain adequate strength to ensure satisfactory stability. Moreover, a weight between 35 and 38 lb greatly helps the paraplegic to lift and stow the folded chair into his motorized tricycle or car unaided. The width of the folded chair should not be greater than $10-10\frac{1}{2}$ in. Easy manoeuvrability of the wheelchair is essential. Therefore the overall width for adult's wheelchairs should, as a rule, not be more than 25 in to allow free passage through doorways, the average width of which is 28 in, and along corridors. A wheelchair-narrower, to diminish the width of the chair by 3 in, should be one of the requirements of a general purpose chair, even at the cost of increasing the weight, to enable passage through narrow doorways in ships, bathroom, lift, etc. (Denley, 1964; Guttmann, 1964). Wheels, handrims and castors are also important factors for the paraplegic's and tetraplegic's mobility in his wheelchair. At Stoke Mandeville, we have for many years advocated 24 in for the large wheels at the back, as they ensure correct upright position and facilitate negotiation of kerbs and steps. For tetraplegics with paralysis of the fingers and who have to rely on the extensors of the wrist, large wheels at the back provide a better leverage for self-propelling with the extended wrist (Walsh, 1964).

The type of tyre on the wheels may vary in accordance with the condition of the floor. On concrete road and other hard surfaces, for instance basket ball pitches on sports grounds, narrow solid tyres are preferable, while pneumatic tyres are more suitable on soft ground or loose gravel. Non-porous inner tubes with efficient valves do not, as a rule, require inflating more than two or three times a year.

The Ministry has previously provided wooden handrims which, however, proved to be unsatisfactory because of easy splintering. They have been replaced by nylon-coated steel. Moreover, aluminium alloy or plastic material is also suitable and may diminish the weight. For tetraplegics with paralysis of the fingers, the adjustment of capstans facilitates self-propelling. These patients need protection of the palm of their hands by a soft leather appliance.

Castors should not be less than 7 in for the small front wheels and should run on well sealed ball bearings. Castors of smaller diameter, especially the 5 in castor, are less satisfactory, as they run into difficulties in negotiating carpets, loose rugs and other small obstacles such as kerbs. We have always preferred the 8 in spoked castor, as fitted to the Everest-Jennings and Vessa chairs, to the 7 in solid castor of the Ministry's chair, as the latter in spite of its smaller size is heavier than the former.

The footrest of an all-purpose folding chair must be divided and able to be folded upwards to facilitate getting into and out of the chair. Moreover, it should be adjustable for height to suit individuals of varying sizes. Another advantage is to be able to swing each section of the footrest outwards, which reduces the overall length of the footrest and facilitates easy operation. To prevent the feet from slipping off the footrest in patients with troublesome spasticity, special adjustments are necessary, consisting of a rim on the back where the heel of the shoe rests in combination with a strap across the foot.

The backrest for paraplegics with lumbar and thoracic lesions should not be higher than 20–22 in, but the chair should be constructed to take a clip-on extension to increase the height of the backrest which will give adequate support for patients with higher lesions. Only tetraplegics above C6/7 will need a higher backrest permanently, some of them even with head support. Moreover, semi-reclining and reclining fixtures may be necessary to be included in the construction of the chairs for these high lesions.

Armrests should be easily removable and well padded to ensure easy transfer to and from the wheelchair, thus avoiding injury to the insensitive hips and buttocks. Only certain types of distal spinal cord lesions without disturbance of sensibility, such as polios, do not need detachable armrests. Armrests in which the upper front angle is cut out, called 'desk' or 'domestic' armrests, to allow the chair to be brought up close to a desk or table, are in many cases preferable to the conventional straight armrests.

Wheelchairs for paraplegics and tetraplegics must be provided with a 4 in sorbo-rubber cushion, which is most essential for preventing pressure sores. In recent years, electrically controlled ripple cushions (Talley Surgical Instruments Ltd, London) have been advocated for preventing pressure sores in paraplegics. These are justified only in tetraplegics with paralysis of their triceps muscles, as all other spinal paralysed can and should lift themselves at regular intervals to relieve pressure from their buttocks, and counteract the development of contractures in hips and knees. The disadvantage of such an electrically controlled ripple cushion is the increase of weight of the chair through its battery.

Proper brakes are most essential components of hand-propelled wheelchairs. They can be fitted either independently on either side and operated by a separate handle, or one brake can be operated by a lever fitted on one side with cable operation to the opposite wheel, which ensures simultaneous action of both brakes. The latter arrangement is, of course, essential for people with paralysis of one upper limb, who operate their specially constructed wheelchairs with one arm propulsion. There is still room for improvement of design of wheelchair brakes.

From all my experience with various designs of wheelchairs during the last 30 years, I consider the Everest-Jennings model, manufactured in this country by Zimmer Orthopaedic Ltd, Bridgend, and the more recently developed Vessa folding chair (Queen Mary's Hospital, Roehampton, London), as the most suitable wheelchairs for paraplegics and tetraplegics at present on the market. Both chairs can be provided with extra attachments for special requirements. The Vessa general purpose chair has the advantage of being lighter than the Everest-Jennings general purpose chair and is also cheaper, but less durable than the Everest-Jennings chair. Recently, Zimmer Ltd have also produced lightweight wheelchairs (35–$39\frac{1}{2}$ lb).

The prescription of a wheelchair is the responsibility of a senior physician or surgeon in charge of a spinal unit. It is highly recommended that Spinal Injuries Centres be provided by the authorities concerned with sets of various designs of wheelchairs both for adults and children, as this greatly facilitates the prescription of an appropriate chair for the patient in accordance with his individual requirements. For special cases, especially those in full-time employment in factories, a second wheelchair may be prescribed which, as a rule, is granted by the authorities of the Health Service in this country. Physicians and surgeons concerned with the treatment of paraplegics and tetraplegics should realize that these patients need their chairs as early as possible during in-patient treatment, to become efficient in its use in the shortest possible time during their daily activities. Although there has been some improvement in the delivery of wheelchairs, there are still unnecessary delays which are caused

1   by late prescription by the medical officer in charge of the case

2   delay by the administrative office in forwarding the application form of the medical officer to the regional authorities of the Health Service

3   delay in the regional office of the Health Service in placing the order with the manufacturers

4   despatching the wheelchair from the factory.

When a new wheelchair is delivered, several trial runs should be carried out during the first few days to ascertain whether the chair is mechanically faultless. This applies as much to fitting of screws, ball-bearings and bolts as to the function of the brakes and the performance of the chair at speed. In particular, any deviation of the chair at speed from the straight direction on removing the hands from the wheels must be reported immediately to the makers. Serious damage to the chair must be reported to the Ministry's authorities, so that the paraplegic can be provided with another chair pending the return of his repaired wheelchair.

The Ministry of Health is responsible for all repairs and replacements due to fair wear and tear or due to circumstances beyond the user's control, but the user will be expected to meet the cost of any repairs or replacements caused by misuse or neglect.

The day-to-day maintenance of the wheelchair is the responsibility of the user, and it is in his own interest to keep the chair in good running order, regularly cleaned and well lubricated. This is so very important for maintaining the paraplegic's independence and working capability.

Special mention should be made of the wheelchair problem in the many economically restricted countries in the world. There are hundreds of thousands of spinal cord sufferers in Africa alone as a result of polio, tuberculosis, transverse myelitis and traumatic lesions following fractures of the spine, stab wounds and gunshot injuries, let alone victims of other disabling afflictions, who are in need of suitable wheelchairs. Yet, wheelchairs designed and manufactured in Europe and U.S.A. are unacceptable by the developing countries in Africa and Asia for two reasons: firstly, they are too expensive to be made available for a large number of paralysed and other severely disabled people; secondly, these chairs are, as a rule, unsuitable for use in the bush and on the rough conditions of the roads, especially during the rainy season; thirdly, local repair of the chair is at present practically non-existing. In recent years, attempts have been made to design and construct wheelchairs at low cost which can stand up to these tropical conditions. In this respect, R.Huckstep, former Professor of Orthopaedic Surgery at Kampala University in Uganda, has carried out pioneer work. He designed a wheelchair which can be manufactured locally by semi-skilled labour from easily available material and which is strong enough to stand up to rough ground, sand, dust and water. The cost of the chair (without sorbo-rubber cushion) is only £8 (1968), as compared with £30–£50 (1968) for modern wheelchairs manufactured in Europe and U.S.A.

Electrically propelled wheelchairs

In recent years, various types of electrically propelled indoor and outdoor wheelchairs have been designed for tetraplegics who, on account of their severe paralysis of both upper limbs, are unable to use hand-propelled wheelchairs and are dependent on the help of others to be moved about in their wheelchairs. For patients under the Health Service, these power-driven wheelchairs can be supplied free on loan on the recommendation of a hospital consultant. Most of the conventional indoor wheelchairs can be adapted to an electric wheelchair by the provision of a small electric motor and a joy stick acting as control. For instance, the Everest-Jennings Power Drive Wheelchair is supplied with two 6 V batteries and a special $7\frac{1}{2}$ A heavy-duty battery charger for fast overnight charging and for tetraplegics with complete or severe paralysis of deltoid, biceps and triceps but with some function of the fingers, with a control panel which gives finger-tip control over speed and direction. The chair turns in its own space, which is of great advantage in confined spaces. The disadvantage of the original power drive chair was, that the joy-stick was operating against four micro-switches and, therefore, one had only on/off control. Jerkiness occurred by speed acceleration, affecting the tetraplegic's arm causing oscillation. This was obviated by a special device, developed at my suggestion by Mr R.G. Maling in the former electro-medical research unit of the Stoke Mandeville Spinal Centre, which allows proportional control over speed and smooth performance (Guttmann & Maling, 1965). Fig. 247 demonstrates this device controlled by hand in a tetraplegic girl

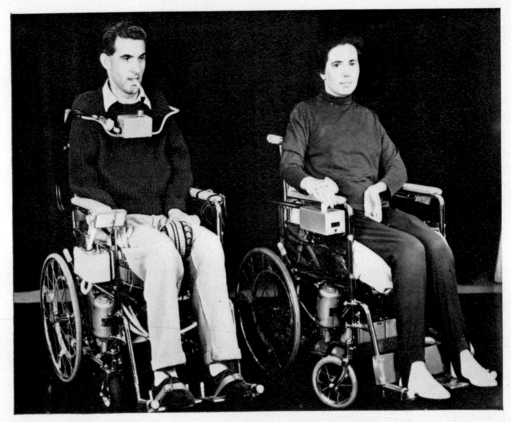

FIG. 247.

with a complete lesion below C5, while the other patient, a tetraplegic below C4 with paralysis of all muscles of both upper limbs, controls the device by breath. Recently, Mr A.Dudley, an engineer, working in co-operation with my successor Dr J.J.Walsh, has continued research on the Zimmer's Power Drive chair and the A.C. Cars Ltd 'Epic' chair, Mark 2 (Model 102). He designed an electric simulator consisting of a compact box with a multi-pin socket fitted at each end into which the operating control is plugged. The simulator contains its own power source in the form of a P.P.4 battery. Controls for arm, chin, head and breath are available according to the tetraplegic's individual handicap. Dudley's device has recently been accepted by the Ministry, as its price is low, for electrically powered wheelchairs issued by the National Health Service. However, it has not yet proportional speed control, but research to achieve this is in progress.

HAND AND POWER CONTROLLED TRICYCLES

Hand-propelled tricycles for severely disabled people have been in use for hundreds of years. As an example Fig. 248 demonstrates a tricycle for propulsion by hand-operated pedals which a German paralysed watch-maker from Nürnburg constructed himself in 1652, and Fig. 249 shows a tricycle with worm-drive control of Connt of Gruyere

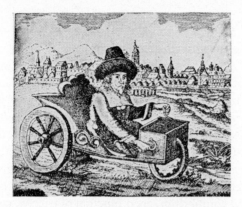

FIG. 248.

from Switzerland which was constructed for him in the middle of the eighteenth century. In due course, improved designs of these vehicles have been developed in various countries. In Great Britain, the Ministry issued some years ago two types of tricycles without weather protection, one controlled by lever propulsion for patients with full use of their arms (model 33 of the new handbook) and the other for propulsion by hand-operated pedals (models 29 and 30). These types of unprotected transport are today hardly used by paraplegics let alone tetraplegics—not even their motorized version.

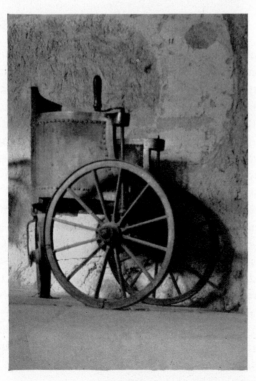

FIG. 249.

Weather-protected motor propelled tricycles

Commensurate with the steadily increasing numbers of employable paraplegics, the construction of all-weather protected motorized tricycles has become imperative. Actually, in the course of the last 20 years, considerable improvements have been made in the design of this means of transport, which is still widely issued for paralysed people under the National Health Service. The most modern power controlled tricycle issued for paraplegics under the N.H.S. are: Model 70 of the Ministry of Health's handbook, manufactured by Invacar Ltd, Thundersley, Essex, and A.C. Ltd, Thames Ditton. This waterproofed vehicle is automatic and provided with a wide sliding door on either side to allow easy access. It can be driven by paraplegics of any level but only by incomplete cervical lesions with good equilibrium, good function of triceps, wrist extensors and long flexors of the fingers. The disadvantage of this conveyance is the inability to carry passengers, and the paraplegic driver is deprived of companionship. Naturally, the paraplegic has to undergo tuition in the use of the motorized tricycle, which is provided at the expense of the N.H.S. by the British School of Motoring. At the end of the training course, the patient has to pass a driving test, as applies to car drivers, before being entitled to use the vehicle in traffic, and the regulations of the road apply to him just as much as to car drivers. The paraplegic must remember that a motorized three-wheeler is not a racing car, and he is strongly advised to remain always below the allowed maximum speed.

MOTOR CARS

This naturally represents the ideal form of transport for both paraplegics and tetraplegics. In Great Britain, Canada and U.S.A. hand-controlled motor cars were granted by the state already in the 'forties to paralysed and other severely disabled ex-service pensioners. Civilian paraplegics and tetraplegics were not entitled to a free issue of motor cars under the N.H.S. However, the most recent regulation of the Department of Health and Social Security in Great Britain makes a private car allowance also for paraplegic and tetraplegic civilians and other severely disabled persons. The annual allowance is £100 paid quarterly in advance. No additional allowance is made towards the purchase or modification of a car. The car must be registered and insured in the applicant's name and he must possess a full driving licence. Recipients are exempted from payment of vehicle excise duty. A hospital consultant's recommendation is necessary for the private car allowance as it is necessary for obtaining a powered three-wheeled vehicle. Cars are not supplied under the N.H.S. as a general rule, but may be supplied in place of a three-wheeler, amongst other disabled persons, to double amputees or defects of the locomotor system such as the spinal paralysed or persons whose walking ability is sufficiently restricted to bring them in the above categories, but are not employed, may be provided with a vehicle to enable them to carry out the duties of a household including shopping. Cars instead of powered three-wheelers can be supplied in the following circumstances:

1   jointly for two such persons who are relatives and who live in the same household, provided that one at least will be able to drive;

2   for a disabled parent, able to drive, who for a substantial part of the day is in sole
charge of his/her young child;
3   for a disabled person able to drive, who lives with a blind relative;
4   for an eligible disabled person suffering from severe haemophilia.

The cars supplied are taxed and insured by the Department and are replaced free of
charge when required unless the replacement is necessitated by the user's negligence.
The user is responsible for maintenance and repairs but an annual allowance is paid
towards this.

There are various types of conversion to hand-control, both mechanical and servo-
assisted. In Great Britain, Reselco-Invalid Carriages Ltd (London, W.6) have done
pioneer work in the development of hand-controls, and their design has been accepted by
the Ministry for cars which have adequately wide doors to allow easy access for the
paraplegic. The lay-out of the Reselco Conversion control is one of great simplicity.
The clutch and accelerator controls have the form of two 'L'-shaped levers, back to
back forming a 'T' fitted at about 3 in. below the rim of the steering wheel in the 'three
o'clock' position. The brake has the form of a push-on, spring-off lever at the driver's
left hand.

Getting into and out of the car may present problems to the paraplegic, and training
given in this respect by the physiotherapist should already start, whenever possible,
during the later stages of rehabilitation at the Spinal Centre. Some paraplegics prefer
to slide along a board from their wheelchair to the car seat. Although this has the disadvantage of being somewhat time consuming, it obviates the necessity for swinging the
whole body weight into the car. However, the majority of paraplegics learn to enter the
car by lifting themselves from their chair on to their car seat, using a handle fitted just
above and inside the driver's door. Tetraplegics above C8 need, as a rule, the help of at
least one strong attendant for their transfer from wheelchair to car. Not so long ago, it

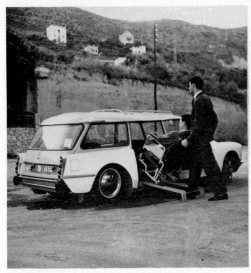
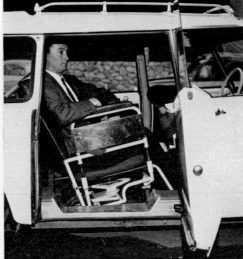

FIG. 250.

would have been inconceivable that a tetraplegic would be capable of driving a hand-controlled car. Today, thanks to advances made in the rehabilitation of these high lesions, tetraplegics, at least those of C8 and C7 level, have proved to be quite able to drive a hand-controlled car after having passed their driving test to the satisfaction of the examiner. This is one of the finest examples of how the human mind can overcome what seemed to be an unsurmountable physical handicap. For high tetraplegics who are not able to drive a car themselves and need an attendant, cars or vans are now available of the type shown in Fig. 250 which enable them to travel to their place of work or with their families. The tetraplegic (C5) illustrated in Fig. 250, not only returned to his business but became the founder of the first Spinal Injuries Centre in Spain (Barcelona).

PUBLIC TRANSPORT

There is still a great need for adjustment of public transport to the requirements of the paralysed. This applies, in particular, to the railways. Paraplegics still have the greatest difficulty in entering compartments and often find it easier to travel in the guard's van where they may have to travel together with a pig or other animals, indeed a very unsatisfactory and degrading situation. Therefore, some adjustments to the carriages is necessary for wheelchair users to facilitate their travel by train.

Travel for paraplegics and other wheelchair users by air has, generally speaking, been made easier in recent years. However, some airlines still have difficulties in accommodating these severely disabled people, and, in particular, there is not always a lifting device available at airports to facilitate the carrying of the paraplegic into their aeroplane seat.

The least adjusted public transport facilities are ships. Thousands of paraplegics today are respected citizens through their work and other social activities. They are taxpayers, as any able-bodied person. Yet they are still confronted with difficulties when contemplating making a cruise on one of the ocean-going liners as part of their recreation. It is really high time that modern shipping lines adjust their ships to the accommodation of wheelchair bound disabled persons.

CHAPTER 36

SPORT

In 1944, very soon after the inception of the Stoke Mandeville Centre, I introduced sporting activities as an essential part of the medical treatment. I felt that, in a country where sport in one way or another is part of the life of most people, it would be an omission not to include this important pastime and recreation in the rehabilitation of the spinal paralysed. The first report on the effect of sport on these patients was published a year later (Guttmann, 1945). It was proved that sporting activities were most essential in the physical readjustment of these patients and in preventing boredom of hospital life, and above all it paved the way to a fuller and more enjoyable life for these disabled people. From the physical point of view, sport proved of immense therapeutic value in restoring the disabled person's strength, co-ordination and endurance. Moreover, sport, being the most natural form of remedial exercise, was successfully used as a complement to the conventional methods of physiotherapy to restore activity of mind and self-confidence in the paralysed. The great advantage of sport over formal remedial exercise lies in its recreational value, which is a motivating force in the enjoyment of life. Recreation thus becomes an important factor in achieving the psychological equilibrium, so necessary to the severely disabled person in coming to terms with his physical defect. The final and probably the noblest aim of sport for the paralysed in a wheelchair is to help him regain contact with the world around him. By instilling self-discipline, competitive spirit, self-respect and comradeship, sport restores and develops mental attitudes, that are essential for any successful social re-integration. Actually, in certain games such as archery, bowling, snooker and table tennis, the paralysed and amputees are capable of competing with the able-bodies, and the same applies in swimming for amputees and the blind. There are many sports which can be adjusted to the paralysed; in fact, the first team game I introduced in 1944 was wheelchair polo, soon followed by the more suitable and exciting wheelchair basketball. In due course, other sports followed, such as archery, skittles, bowling, fencing (both foil and sabre), field events (javelin—distance and precision—shot put and club throwing), weight lifting from the supine position and wheelchair racing and slalom. Figs. 251–255 demonstrate some of the sports practised by paraplegics.

Archery is the ideal sport for strengthening the arm and trunk muscles and improving respiratory and cardiovascular functions. The pullweight of the bow varies between 36 and 42 lb for men and 25–38 lb for women, children, naturally, are using lighter pullweights. Today, wheelchair archers are competing in the F.I.T.A. Round, the internationally recognized longest distance in archery (90, 70 and 50 m, each shot with 36 arrows), and several paraplegics have won the F.I.T.A. Star (by scoring more than 1,000 points). Moreover, archery has great fascination, as the archer accomplishes everything by his own judgement and strength and nothing is mechanized for him.

A combination of darts and archery, called Dartchery, was introduced as a special wheelchair sport. While the pattern of the target is that of a dart board, the target is enlarged to a diameter of 2·6 ft in size to fit on an archery boss. The minimum shooting distance is 15 yards (Fig. 251).

Using a 4 channel electromyograph I studied with my colleague Dr Mehra, the alternating muscle groups mainly involved in archery and dartchery on 9 male paraplegic subjects with complete lesions at levels ranging from C6 to T12 (Guttmann & Mehra, 1972). Four actions were studied in the course of archery exercise:

1. First draw (I.D.): consisting of loading the arrow on to the bow and pulling the bow string 1 or 2 in to establish the right position for shooting.
2. Horizontal draw (FDH): The holding arm (in right handers the left) is raised to the horizontal and the bow string is pulled with the opposite right arm to full extension.
3. Vertical draw (FDV): The left arm holding the bow is raised over the horizontal and the bow string is drawn to full extension with the right arm.
4. Releasing the arrow.

The muscles examined electromyographically were: Trapezius (Trap.), Rhomboids (Rhom.), Latissimus dorsi (Lat. Dors.), Pectoralis major (Pect.), Serratus Anterior (Serr. Ant.), Biceps (Bic.), and Triceps (Tric.). Fig. 252a demonstrates the results obtained in a case of T12 lesion as compared with the result in a case of C7 lesion with acting triceps (Fig. 252b).

The lowest electrical discharge occurred during loading and first draw, while the maximal discharge was found during horizontal and in particular vertical draw. In all cervical and also high thoracic (T3) lesions trapezius and rhomboids showed particularly marked electrical activity indicating the importance of these muscle groups in bracing the shoulders in these high lesions. In contrast the electrical discharge in latissimus dorsi and serratus anterior was practically absent. That the biceps on the drawing right arm and the left triceps on holding the bow in extension show high electrical discharge is obvious. Of interest is that on sudden release of the arrow there was an immediate intensive electrical discharge.

The most dramatic results of training are seen in wheelchair basketball players. The degree of neuro-muscular co-ordination and endurance they can achieve is almost unbelievable. They have mastered the techniques of passing, catching, and intercepting the ball, while racing down the court; a crash into an opponent's chair is an automatic foul. It is no exaggeration to say that the paraplegic and his chair have become one, in the same way as have a first-class horseman and his mount. Fig. 253 shows a scene during a basketball match. Incidentally, this is a sport where the paralysed has an advantage over the able-bodied (as the writer and his medical and physiotherapy staff found out for themselves), as the able-bodied, due to his different pattern of co-ordination, has the tendency to move his legs while trying to catch the ball from his opponent, causing him to lose his balance and fall out of his wheelchair.

It may be noted that sporting activities have not been confined to the paraplegics but have been extended also to tetraplegics. There is no reason why a tetraplegic with a lesion below C6/7 with a good extensor carpi radialis and weak triceps but paralysis of

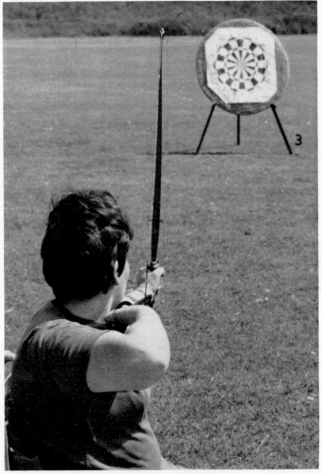

FIG. 251.

the fingers, cannot be trained in table tennis, with the paralysed fingers fixed by a bandage to the table tennis bat (Fig. 254). Such tetraplegics can also be trained in archery, the release of the arrow being performed by the extension of the wrist which releases a hook, fixed with the bandage on to the palmar surface of the right hand, while the paralysed fingers of the left hand are fixed to the bow by a bandage or leather appliance as demonstrated in Figs. 255a and b, and Fig. 256 shows our children's group during one of their training sessions. Their ability to swim has already been discussed in the chapter on Hydrotherapy.

It is beyond the scope of this short survey on sport for the paralysed to go into details of all the techniques and rules of the games. Rules for the individual sports have been worked out throughout the years and are compiled in a special book called 'Handbook of Rules of the Stoke Mandeville Games for the Paralysed' (Guttmann, 1959).

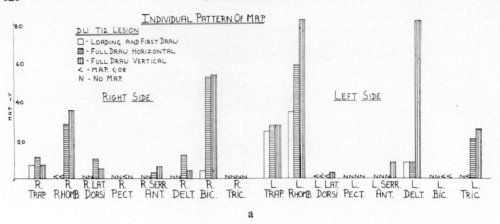

a

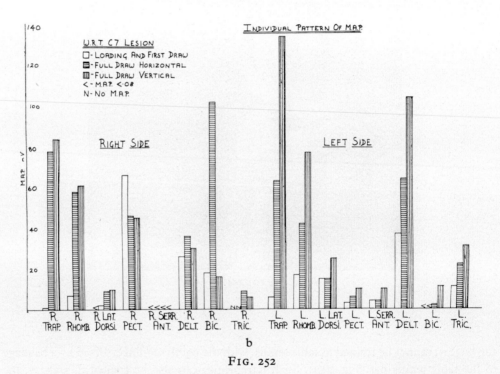

b

FIG. 252

THE STOKE MANDEVILLE GAMES FOR THE PARALYSED

With all the benefits that clinical sport conferred on male and female paraplegics and
tetraplegics of various ages, during their in-patient treatment at the Centre, it was only
logical that their sporting activities be expanded after discharge from hospital into a
national and possibly even an international sports organization. So, on 28 July 1948, the
first Stoke Mandeville Games for the Paralysed were founded. The number of competitors was small—only 16—and all were ex-servicemen and women, paralysed from war
wounds or fractures. This event coincided with the opening of the Olympic Games in
London, which gave me an idea which I voiced at the 1949 Stoke Mandeville Games. At

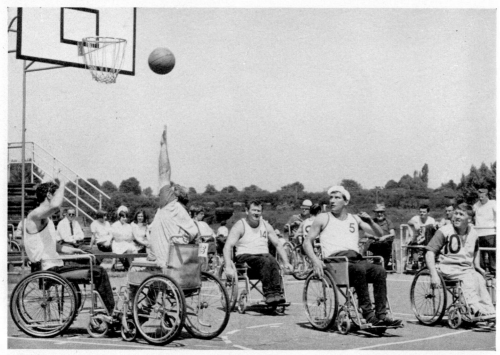

FIG. 253.

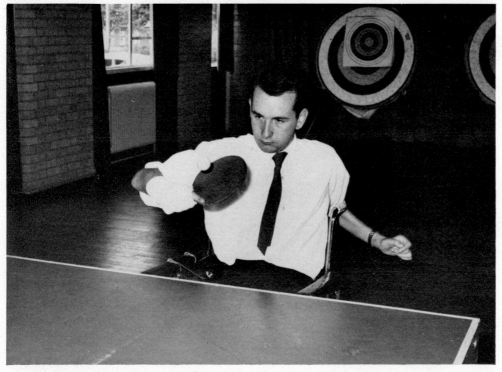

FIG. 254. Tetraplegic below C6 at table tennis.

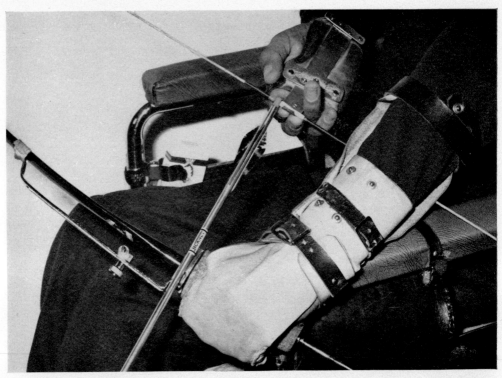

FIG. 255a.

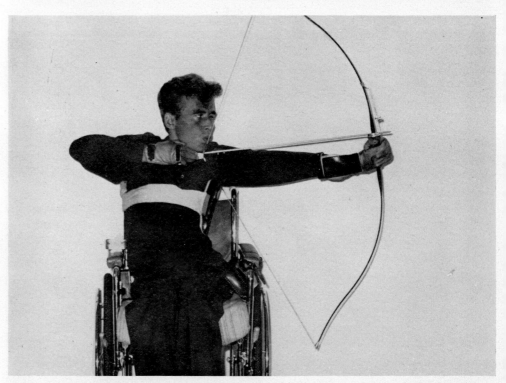

FIG. 255b. Archery appliances for tetraplegics. Note in Fig. 255a the hook fixed to the palm of the hand enables the tetraplegic to pull the bow with biceps and deltoid. The arrow is released from the hook by extension of the wrist.

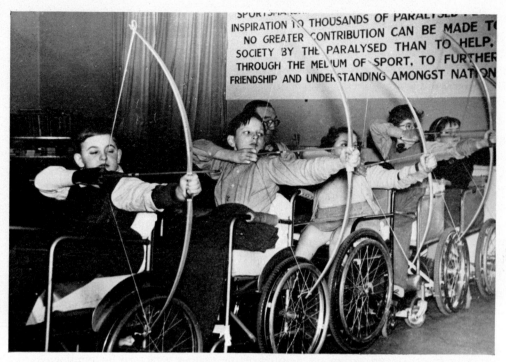

FIG. 256. Training of children in archery

the prize-giving ceremony, looking into the future, I expressed the hope, that the time might come when this unique sports movement would be not merely an annual national sports festival but would spread to other countries, becoming truly international and achieving the status of the paralysed person's equivalent of the Olympic Games (*The Cord*, 1949). Few of those present shared this conviction, yet only three years later a small team of paraplegic ex-service men from the Netherlands came to Stoke Mandeville; thus the year 1952 was the start of an ever-growing annual international sports festival for the spinal paralysed. Year by year, the number of sports events and the number of nations taking part have increased, and so has the standard of the competitions. In 1957, no fewer than 360 competitors came by air, land and sea to participate in the Stoke Mandeville Games. As an equivalent to the Olympic Committee, the International Stoke Mandeville Games Committee was formed as the governing body of these Games.

The International Stoke Mandeville Games take place every year in July, at the Stoke Mandeville Sportsground, and every fourth year, the Olympic year—if possible, in the country of the Olympic Games. It was 1960 that brought the real fulfilment of this dream. For the first time, these Games followed closely upon the Olympic Games in Rome, when 400 paralysed sportsmen and sportswomen and 300 escorts represented 21 countries. Competition was under Olympic rules and took place in one of the Olympic stadiums. This was a great success not only as far as the standard of the competitions and records were concerned but, of no less importance, in educating the public that sport is not the prerogative of the able-bodied, but that people with a disablement of such magnitude as spinal paraplegia can become true sportsmen and sportswomen in their own right. After the Games, the late Pope John XXIII addressed the 400 competitors and 300 escorts during a special audience, held in the Vatican City. His appraisal of the philosophy of the Stoke Mandeville Games, which the reader will find at the opening of this book, can hardly be better expressed. It may also be mentioned in this connection, that during the 1956 Olympic Games in Melbourne, the Fearnley Cup was awarded to the organization of the Stoke Mandeville Games by the Olympic Committee, an award given for outstanding achievement in the service of the Olympic ideals.

It was during the Winter Olympic Games in Innsbruck 1976 that the International Olympic Committee decided that 'the Olympic Movement will in future give its patronage to the Stoke Mandeville Paraplegic Games which is a fine and fitting gesture to many gallant people'. This is indeed a realization of a dream!

In 1964, the Games were held in the Olympic stadium at Tokyo, following immediately upon the Olympic Games, where 335 competitors representing 23 nations came together to compete in friendly rivalry. The Games were opened by the Crown Prince of Japan. The interest of the Japanese Government, the municipal authorities of the metropolis and the public as a whole was overwhelming. During the course of these Games, more than 100,000 spectators were counted, and members of the Imperial family and other leading personalities attended daily. These Tokyo Games had far-reaching social consequences. The Japanese Government, having recognized the accomplishment of paraplegics in sport, set up within six months of the Games a factory for employment of paraplegics and other severely disabled, which is run on purely business lines, something hitherto unknown in that country. At present, there are four such factories, called Japan Sun Industries under the directorship of Dr Nakamura, a former pupil of Stoke Mandeville.

The 1968 Games took place in Israel, as the Mexican authorities were not able to organize these Games in connection with the Olympic Games. Seven hundred and fifty competitors and over 300 escorts came to the Holy Land, representing 28 countries. It was significant for the spirit of the people of that country, being themselves engaged in a struggle for their own survival, that they opened their doors for this event in the field of sport and humanity, which involved the organizing Israeli Committee and the Government in great financial efforts. The opening ceremony took place in the sports stadium of the University in Jerusalem attended by 25,000 people. It was opened by the Deputy Prime Minister, Mr. Ygal Allon, as the Prime Minister was ill. In the evening, delegations of all nations taking part were received by the President of the State of Israel. One of the highlights of these Games was a pilgrimage of all competitors and escorts to Nazareth, where they were welcomed by the Arabic Mayor of Nazareth and the Jewish Mayor of Upper Nazareth, and where Archbishop Isidoros of the Greek Orthodox Church gave the blessing on behalf of all religious denominations—indeed a unique event of unity of mankind.

The XXI International Stoke Mandeville Games in the Olympic year of 1972 were held in Heidelberg, Germany, before the Olympic Games in Munich, and 1,000 paraplegics and 400 escorts represented 45 nations. The number of competitors could have been doubled had more accommodation been available. The City and University of

Heidelberg, the German and American Army Authorities and, in particular, the Industrial Rehabilitation Centre (Berufsförderungswerk), where all the participants were accommodated, really competed with each other to make this Olympiade of the Paralysed a resounding success. The Games were opened by the President of the German Federal Republic, and many other leading members of Government and Community visited the Games. The standard of performance was high, and many world records were broken. Above all, a true Olympic spirit prevailed throughout the Games, so very different from the unfortunate events, which were to assail during the Olympic Games in Munich later in the month of August 1972. These events were a tragic demonstration of how exaggerated nationalism, politics and commercialism can make a travesty of the Olympic ideals and jeopardize the whole future of that great sports movement of the Olympic Games. The 1976 Olympiad for the paralysed will take place in Toronto, Canada.

Who would have thought, 25 years ago, that these severely disabled could travel thousands of miles to hold sports festivals? Yet, today they do so, not only for their own enjoyment, but to the enthusiastic response of thousands of able-bodied spectators.

For a number of years following their inception, the paraplegic games were financed and fully supported by the Aylesbury Hospitals Management Committee, which also administers Stoke Mandeville Hospital. However, it was the Paraplegic Sports Endowment Fund, a voluntary organization, registered under the Charities Act and founded in 1954, which built several huts for the accommodation of the visiting teams and financed the sending of paraplegic British teams abroad. In recent years, the administration of the Games have become separated from the Hospital Authorities, and the British Paraplegic Sports Society has been entirely responsible for the administration, in particular, when the Ministry of Health, as the owner of the large sports grounds, agreed to lease this land to the Fund for a 'peppercorn' rent.

In 1968, the Fund agreed, at the writer's instigation, to build a large Sports Stadium for the Paralysed and Other Disabled on these sports grounds. For some years, it was my dream to build such a stadium for the following reasons: (1) Most of the existing sports stadiums in this and other countries are unsuitable for the access of severely disabled, especially those in wheelchairs, because of architectural barriers. (2) Moreover, if severely disabled are able to carry out their sport in these stadiums, they are usually allowed only on certain days and hours and are segregated from the other sports community, as there is still the deeply ingrained prejudice that sport of the disabled may be embarrassing to the able-bodied. (3) It became necessary to make our Games independent of the weather.

The Stoke Mandeville Sports Stadium (Fig. 257a), consisting of a huge sports hall (100–120 ft), with a gallery for spectators, several smaller rooms, one for 3 snooker tables, another for 6 table tennis tables, a conference room, an olympic swimming pool of 25 m, with 6 lanes, dressing rooms, widened toilets, lift, a dining hall for 250 wheelchair users, accommodation for 80 escorts and several rooms for administration, has been built within one year, and its cost defrayed mainly from voluntary contributions but also with grants from the Government, the Borough Council of Aylesbury and the County Council of Buckinghamshire. It was officially opened on 2 August 1969 by H.M. Queen Elizabeth II during the 1969 International Games (450 competitors from 29 countries) (Fig. 255) and has been in full use ever since. While the disabled (physically or mentally) have

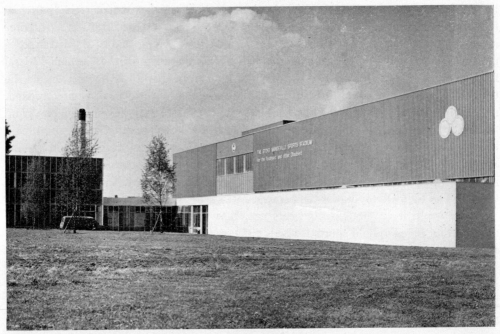

FIG. 257a.

always priority, this stadium has also opened its doors for sport to certain sections of the community, such as school children and sports clubs, to promote a better understanding between the able-bodied and disabled and help the latter in their social re-integration into the community. There is, of course, easy access for wheelchair users to enter the stadium and within the various rooms, and it is gratifying to note that the set-up of this stadium has been a guide to architects engaged in the building of other sports stadiums for the common use of able-bodied and disabled.

The success of the Stoke Mandeville Games has led to a steady increase in interest in sport amongst the paralysed, and as a result two offshoot sports events, on a small scale, have been established in recent years: the British Paraplegic Commonwealth Games, which were held first in 1962 in Perth, Western Australia, and later in Kingston, Jamaica (1966) and in Edinburgh, Scotland (1970); furthermore, the Pan-American Games, held first in 1966 in Winnipeg, Canada, 1968 in Buenos Aires, Argentine, and in 1970 in Kingston, Jamaica. However, the games of the paralysed have also been an incentive to sporting activities among other types of disabled. As a result, the British Sports Association for all Disabled (B.S.A.D.) was founded by the writer in 1960, and annual multi-disabled sports events are held at Stoke Mandeville Sportsground, where amputees, blind, cerebral palsy and spinal paralysed compete in certain games against each other and in others in their own sections. Throughout the year, the following annual sports events are held: in May an annual sports event for 5–16 year old multi-disabled juniors, in October for multi-disabled adults, in June the annual National Paraplegic Stoke Mandeville Games and at the end of July the International Paraplegic Stoke Mandeville Games.

In addition, organizations for the disabled, such as the British Limbless Ex-Service-men's Association, Polio-Fellowship and the British Spastic Society, have held their annual games at the Stoke Mandeville Stadium. Moreover, throughout the year, and particularly from February to October, training weekends on various sports are held by paraplegic sports clubs, and paraplegics take part during the week in table-tennis and indoor rink bowling league matches with the able-bodied. Twice a week, patients from the nearby mental hospital, at Stone, have swimming sessions and twice a week mentally retarded young adults from two residential schools also have swimming sessions. Once a week, patients from the National Spinal Injuries Centre, who are in the later stages of their in-patient treatment, come to the stadium with their physical instructor and physiotherapists, to receive training in various sports. Three times a week, an organized play group of physically handicapped and mentally retarded children under 5, with their mothers, have a morning session at the stadium. Last, but not least, every fortnight a group of elderly physically handicapped from Aylesbury also take part in games. This survey gives an idea of the sporting activities of the disabled at Stoke Mandeville Stadium, in concert with the able-bodied, which has fundamentally changed the whole concept of sport.

The B.S.A.D. has been recognized by the Government and the Sports Council as the governing body for all disabled in this country and receives financial support

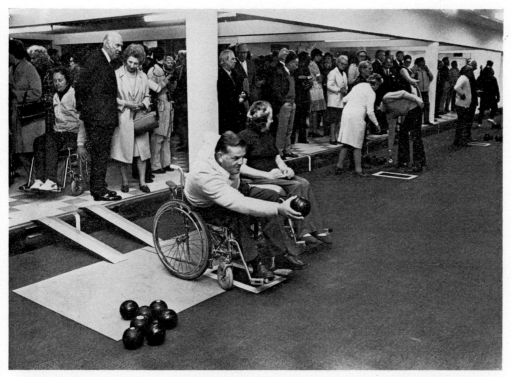

FIG. 257b. Opening of Lady Guttmann Indoors Bowls Centre, Stoke Mandeville Sports Stadium for the Paralysed and Other Disabled. See special ramp for players in wheelchairs.

from the Government as any other governing body of sports organizations for the able-bodied.

In 1974, the 6-rink Lady Guttmann Indoor Bowls Centre was added to our sports facilities for the disabled as well as for the able bodied, especially elderly people. This bowling green is in use daily and competitions are held between the able bodied, amputees, blind and paraplegics. The wheelchair bound disabled reaches the green by means of a small ramp, and a special mat is laid on the green to prevent damage by the wheelchairs. Paraplegics play with the able bodied as much on equal terms as they do in archery which, naturally, helps in their social re-integration with the community. Fig. 275b demonstrates bowling by a paraplegic at the opening ceremony of the Bowling Centre.

CHAPTER 37

RECREATIONAL ACTIVITIES AND
SCHOOL EDUCATION

Various recreational activities, to combat boredom in hospital, such as concerts, lectures, cinema shows and visits to exhibitions, were included in the programme of rehabilitation of these patients, who were also encouraged to take the initiative in organizing various recreational activities. A chess club was formed amongst the patients, and in 1944 a choir was started by the writer under the leadership of a voluntary conductor. At Christmas, the paraplegics were the carol singers of Stoke Mandeville Hospital, which was not only a great encouragement to other severely disabled people but gave themselves a feeling of contributing to the enjoyment of their fellow patients, which helped their own morale. In the summer of 1946, the 'Choir on Wheels' performed most successfully at a public concert in the hospital concert hall.

A few of our former patients have shown interest in the piano. As, however, they were

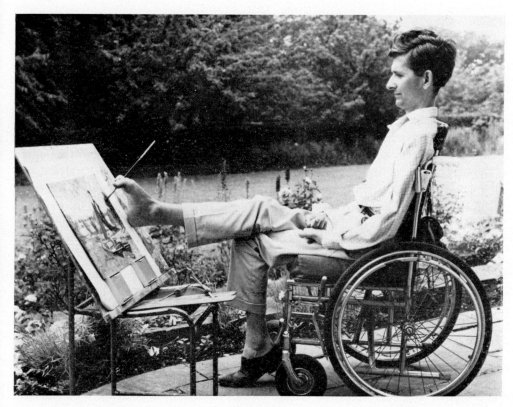

Fig. 258.

unable to use the pedals, one of the patients designed an ingenious device which enabled the paraplegic to operate the pedals with his elbow.

Also, at one stage, a dramatic society, formed among the patients, produced and acted a dramatic play, 'Libel', with great success. One of the main characters in this play was played by a tetraplegic with a complete transverse lesion below C6. The producer was a girl suffering from poliomyelitis with complete paralysis below the chest.

Art classes are still being held at Stoke Mandeville, which have proved invaluable to mobilize dormant talents in painting and other crafts. Any art medium promotes a great feeling of accomplishment, and amongst the various types of art, painting is very important as it provides also a good exercise for finger movements, wrist and arm. This is of particular importance for tetraplegics, who have either complete or partial paralysis of their fingers and learn trick movements to hold the brush in the hand. Some of those who have complete paralysis in the fingers have learned to paint with the brush held between the teeth (mouth painting). Certain cases of polio who are completely paralysed in the upper limbs have learned to paint with their toes (foot painting) as shown in Fig. 258. Painting is indeed a very rewarding occupation for high spinal cord lesions, as it increases the patient's awareness to his surrounding world and the beauty of nature. (See also Chapter of Industrial and Professional Resettlement.)

SCHOOL EDUCATION

Throughout the years, our paraplegic children were given regular school education by a teacher, appointed by the Ministry of Education (Fig. 259). Children have daily lessons in school and are, of course, divided into classes according to age. Education is already started with children below the official school age and has taken the form of playgroups.

In recent years, a play group movement has been started as a 'do it yourself' nursery school, were children with their mothers gain benefit. There is no doubt, that these playgroups are of benefit to cerebral palsy children and spinal paralysed children such as spina bifida, below school age, and mothers should be encouraged to enrol their children in these playgroups. At the Stoke Mandeville Sports Stadium for the Paralysed and other Disabled, such a playgroup has been set up, and sessions are held three times weekly. This project has proved most successful and of great benefit also to the mothers.

The writer has always been most anxious, that paraplegic children of school age should continue their education, wherever possible, in ordinary classes of ordinary schools, in order that they may integrate with able-bodied children and may have the same chance to attain the highest scholastic achievements. There is still great need to adjust ordinary schools to disabled children in wheelchairs, by arranging easy access, by having classrooms on the ground floor where they can receive their education together with able-bodied children or by having lifts built in multi-storey schools. Another very important point is to enlarge one or two toilets for the use of children in wheelchairs and also adjust the desk to the height of the wheelchair.

The same facilities should also be given in universities to students in wheelchairs. They should have easy access to lecture rooms, laboratories, libraries, etc., and also proper facilities for using toilets, if necessary by widening doorways and increasing

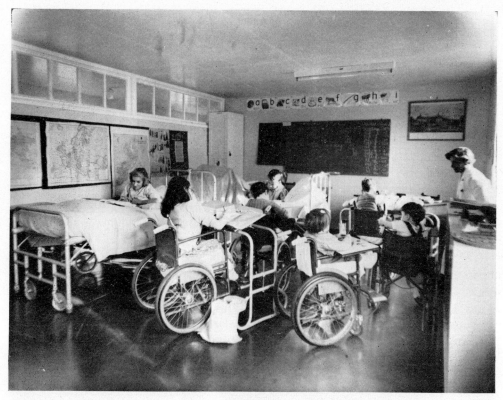

FIG. 259.

space within the toilet. In this respect, Professor Nugent of the Illinois University in the U.S.A. has been pioneering for many years with excellent results.

Spinal paraplegic children should not, as a general rule, be admitted to special schools for disabled to be mixed with cerebral palsy children with mental defects. There has been an increased understanding of this principle in recent years, but that was not always so, and to give an example the following case may be mentioned: a boy with a complete transverse lesion below T10 was placed, after discharge from the Spinal Centre, in a special school for disabled, where he was quite unhappy. He was a bright boy, and when the writer was approached by the boy's father steps were taken to place the boy in an ordinary school, where the headmaster was most co-operative. In due course, this boy gained a scholarship in mathematics to Reading University and from there he won a scholarship to Trinity College, Cambridge, where he passed his Ph.D. in mathematics with flying colours. He obtained an appointment as lecturer in mathematics at Nottingham University and became married, and from there he won a Fellowship to Princeton University in the U.S.A. At present, he is lecturer at San Francisco University. This boy, had he not been given the opportunity of a normal education might now have been perhaps a second class clerk in an office. There is still a good deal to be done by educating authorities to separate the purely physically handicapped child from the physically and mentally handicapped.

CHAPTER 38

OCCUPATIONAL THERAPY—REHABILITATION BY WORK

From the beginning, it was realized at Stoke Mandeville that a satisfactory rehabilitation of paraplegics—i.e. their restoration to useful and socially accepted citizens—could only be achieved, if their physical readjustment went hand in hand with their re-adaptation to work adjusted to their permanent disability. This principle was introduced from the start as part of the medical treatment and was, therefore, supervised by the Director in charge of the unit and his medical staff.

The work of the occupational therapist, like that of the physiotherapist, is of great importance in the physical and psychological readjustment of both paraplegics and tetra-plegics. Their work also consists to a great extent in exercises to strengthen the remaining muscle groups above the level of the lesion. This applies in particular to tetraplegics. These patients can be divided into three categories:

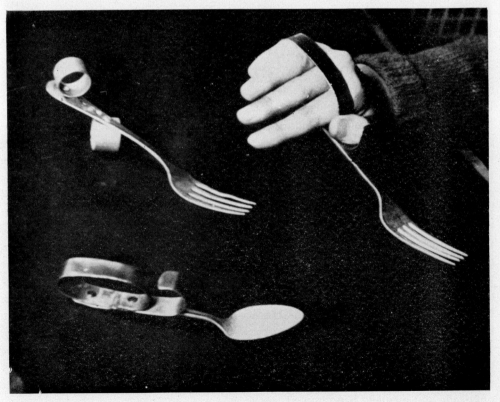

FIG. 260.

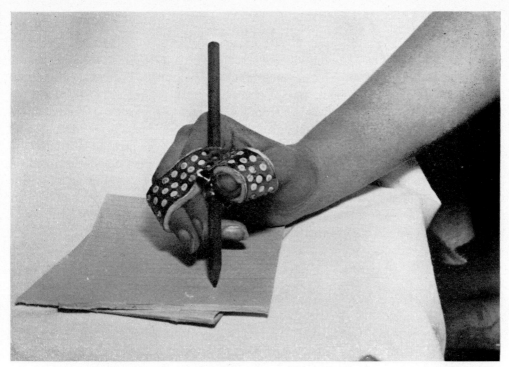

FIG. 261.

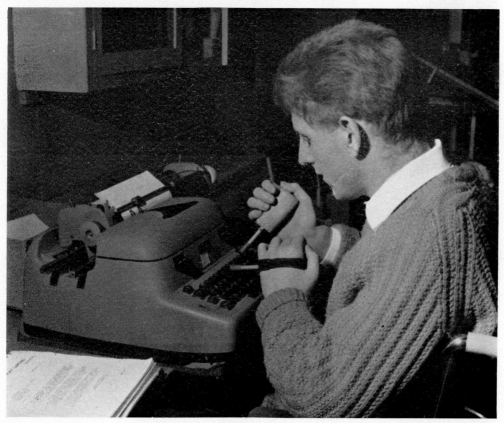

FIG. 262.

1   Those with wrist extensors for whom simple gadgets are required to enable them to turn pages, feed themselves, use a comb, toothbrush, help them to dress themselves, at least the upper part of the body, hold a pen and pencil, etc., and control an electric typewriter. These make their lives easier and more useful. Figs. 260 and 261 demonstrate some of the gadgets used by tetraplegics at the Occupational Therapy Department of the Centre which are simple and light. These gadgets, such as a plate buffer which clips on plate edge to give support when picking up food, a light plastic splint adapted for fitting with different implements for use with a toothbrush, or the same splint with a simple rubber ended stick for typing or page turning, make it possible even for complete lesions below C6 to carry out daily activities. Fig. 262 demonstrates a complete lesion below C6, using an electric typewriter with both hands.

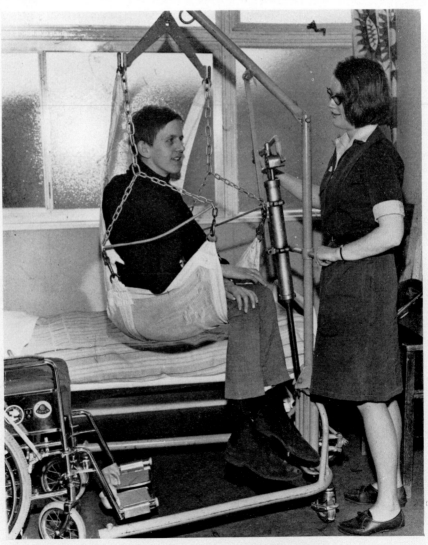

FIG. 263. Mobile hoist for tetraplegics at home.

2 Those tetraplegics without wrist extensors but with good functioning biceps and partial functioning triceps can use these appliances with the aid of a cock-up splint.

3 The very high tetraplegics without function of any muscles of the upper limbs can now use the POSSUM or another similar electronic apparatus as mentioned in the chapter on Historical Introduction. Moreover, tetraplegics, when at home, will need a mobile hoist (Fig. 263) which has proved of great help to their attendants to lift them from their beds into their wheelchairs and vice versa and also for the transfer of these patients to the bath and toilet.

The work of the occupational therapist should be in close co-operation with that of the physiotherapist as one profession complements the other.

Rehabilitation by work whereby emphasis has been laid on early vocational training can conveniently be classified in the following stages:

(1) Work therapy in the early stages

Naturally, in the early stage of treatment when the patient is still bedridden because of his fractured spine and his complications, work first starts in the form of simple handicrafts, as taught and supervised by the occupational therapist. Everybody concerned with occupational therapy for paraplegics must clearly understand that this is by no means occupation merely as a diversional measure. It is used immediately to restore the lost power of concentration and to revive initiative in order to shift the psychomotor capabilities of the paraplegic from the paralysed to the normal parts of the body. This type of work is invaluable in developing the mobility and dexterity of fingers and arms, upon which the future earning power of the paraplegic depends, therefore, this represents already the first step in the paraplegic's industrial rehabilitation. The objects to be pursued in this work are punctuality, skill and speed, and it is up to the occupational therapist to instil these principles into the patient. It should be noted that several patients who showed particular interest and ability in leatherwork, needlework or rug and toy making have actually continued this work later on and have started a business on their own at home. For others, the skill achieved in making leather handbags proved useful in their training later for shoe repair and woodwork.

In certain cases, specific pre-vocational training was introduced even in the early stages following injury, by correspondence courses in commercial art, accountancy, banking and law. In a previous publication (Guttmann, 1946) mention was made of the first man to pass his examination in law at the Centre, 10 months after his injury. He was a young officer who was admitted in June 1944 from the battle-front with a gunshot injury in the right lung, causing a large haemothorax, and through the spine resulting in a complete paraplegia below T11/12. He was encouraged to start his studies while laid up in bed. Fourteen months after injury, he entered Oxford University as an undergraduate, and at that time he was provided with a special grant from the Ministry of Pensions to employ an attendant to take him, sometimes on his back, to tutorials through the narrow stairways of the College. Four terms later, he was elected secretary of the Law Society at his College, and in the summer of 1947 he passed his final examination and 2 months later was employed in a legal department.

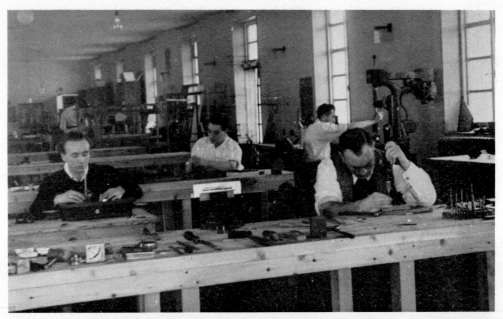

FIG. 264. Retraining, precision instrument class.

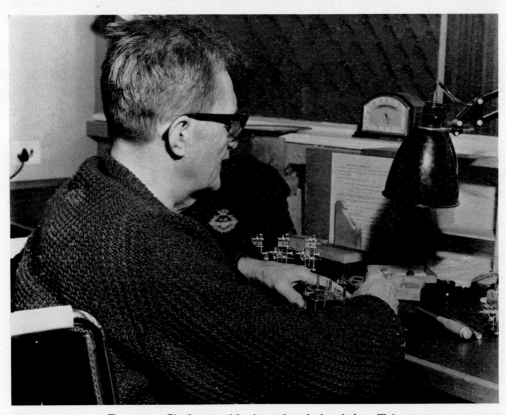

FIG. 295. Clock assembly (complete lesion below T4).

Work therapy in later stages

As soon as the paraplegic or tetraplegic is up in a wheelchair, he has to attend regularly either the occupational therapy department or workshops. The former Ministry of Pensions, who administered Stoke Mandeville Hospital until it was taken over in 1950 by the Health Service, agreed to put pre-vocational training in hospital, as part of the medical rehabilitation, on a wider basis by providing workshops for woodwork, cobbling, precision engineering with hand operated lathes (Fig. 264), clock assembly (Fig. 265),

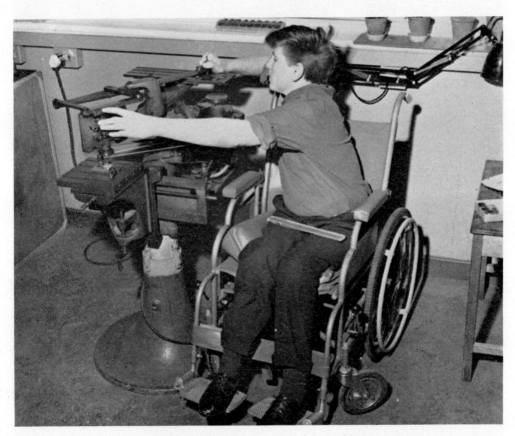

FIG. 266. Training on engraving machine.

engraving (Fig. 266), draughtsmanship and typing. Pre-vocational training in hospital has been particularly useful for tetraplegics with partial or complete paralysis of their finger muscles. Fig. 267 shows a tetraplegic below C6/7 using both hands to carry out woodwork with a handsaw and Fig. 268 shows a tetraplegic with complete paralysis of all fingers—the only wrist muscles working being the extensor carpi radialis longus and brevis—engaged in inlay work, producing beautiful wooden bowls. He attained such skill that after discharge from the Centre he took this work up as a home occupation earning good money. Fig. 266 shows a young boy of 16 being trained in the use of an engraving machine. In more recent years, training in computor and teleprinting was added to the variety of skills. The work is graded and correlated to the physical improvement of the patient and, of course, his intellectual ability and personality. The medical staff must take an interest in the progress of the patients, and regular reports given by the instructors are most helpful in assessing progress. As in the case of early work therapy, emphasis is laid on the patient's punctuality, dexterity and speed. Sometimes it has been necessary to switch patients from one occupation to another.

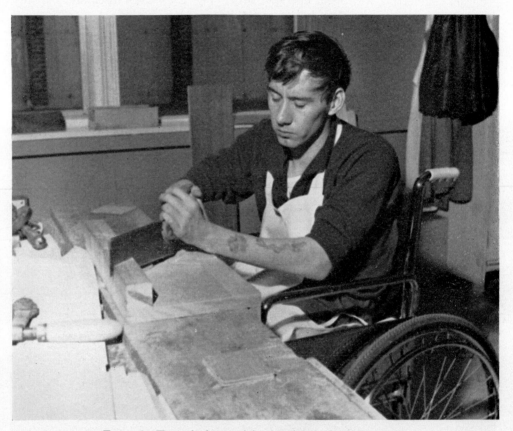

FIG. 267. Tetraplegic practicing handsaw using both hands.

For female paraplegics a kitchen equipped with furniture including a cooker, adjusted to the easy reach of a wheelchair user is part of our O.T. department to enable female paraplegics to adjust themselves to housework including cooking (Fig. 269).

Naturally, it was not to be expected that everyone would make full use of the various facilities offered. In numerous cases, especially those who had long spells of sepsis and those admitted in later stages from other units or hospitals, where they had been kept in prolonged enforced inactivity, it took some time to arouse the patient from his state of frustration, apathy and inertia to which he had resigned himself. Such patients needed continuous guidance and encouragement from the medical officer and nursing staff as well as the instructors to ensure steady progress. Moreover, other factors such as education, temperament and individual inclination towards work have to be taken into consideration. Obviously, a spinal cord injury does not necessarily transform a previously workshy individual into a first-rate conscientious worker. Furthermore, it does not necessarily follow that every paraplegic who has taken up pre-vocational training in a particular subject will carry on with the same occupation when he returns home or is transferred to a hostel or permanent settlement. Circumstances were sometimes found to be unfavourable for carrying on with the same occupation, for which the patient was trained at this Centre. However, from all experience gained in the many years, it can be concluded that early vocational training in hospital has proved invaluable in restoring

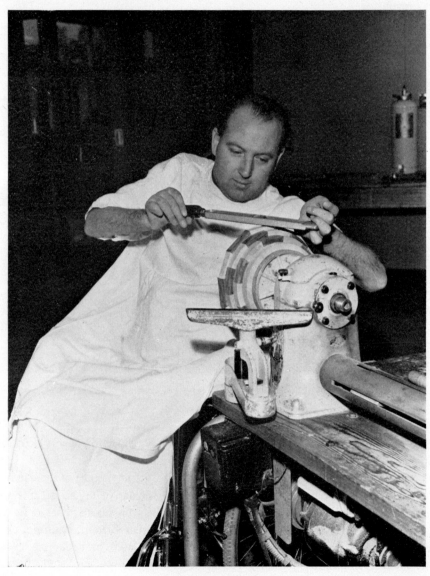

FIG. 268.

activity of mind and competitive spirit and is a most important step towards the social re-integration of paraplegics. Most of the patients have shown keen interest in pre-vocational training, and many made tremendous efforts either to adjust their former trades to their permanent disability or to take up training in a new occupation. It may be noted that, in some modern Spinal Injuries Centres, such as in the Ludwig Guttmann–Kurt Lindemann Haus at the Orthopaedic University Clinic, Heidelberg, and the Accident Hospital, Murnau, theoretical and practical facilities are introduced for full industrial training, culminating in nationally recognized examinations.

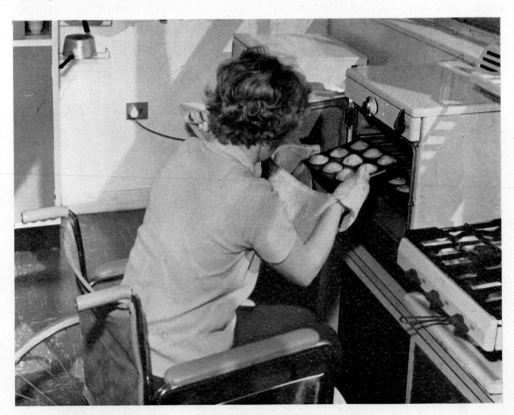

FIG. 269. Paraplegic housewife at work.

In some instances, the whole educational level of a patient has been raised by pre-vocational training. This we have seen in regular soldiers, bricklayers, coalminers, jockeys, etc. From the numerous examples the following case may be mentioned:

L.V. was admitted to Stoke Mandeville on 2 May 1951 at the age of 27. He had left school at the age of 10, following a riding accident. At the age of 11, he became a stable hand and an apprentice jockey, and at the age of 12 he won his first flat race. In due course, he became one of the outstanding jockeys in Great Britain, winning, amongst other races, the Scottish Grand National. Three months later, he broke his spine in a riding accident, resulting in a paraplegia below T5. When he was admitted to the Stoke Mandeville Centre $3\frac{1}{2}$ months after the injury, he was thoroughly demoralized, revolting against his fate and the world and at first refusing treatment, as he wanted to die. Gradually, he became interested in sport, and it was that which restored his will to live and his self-confidence. He became an outstanding archer by continuous concentration in this sport, and very soon he captained a team to compete in Berlin in an international contest for the disabled.

His professional ambition was then to become a secretary in a racing stable, but he had first to improve his very scanty education by correspondence courses in elementary arithmetic and reading. In addition, he received clerical training in the administrative office of the hospital, and from there he won his diploma as a clerk. A chartered accountant in Aylesbury accepted him on probation without salary. There, he became interested in accountancy, and in due course by hard work and concentration he passed his examinations as an accountant and was employed. His ambition grew commensurate with his experience, and in 1961 he set up his own practice in Aylesbury, with phenomenal success. With the increasing practice, he took a partner and employed in his staff two accountants, two assistant accountants, two typists, one computer operator and one articled junior accountant. His final ambition was to set up a training establishment for paraplegics in accountancy, but—alas—this life of tremendous accomplishment, from an almost illiterate jockey to a chartered accountant in spite of his high paraplegia, was cut short by a road accident in 1969, in which he was killed.

As early as 1944, an experiment was carried out in Aylesbury by arrangement with a local factory with the first six rehabilitated paraplegic soldiers, still inpatients at Stoke Mandeville, to find out whether paraplegics would be able to work side by side and in competition with able-bodied workers in a factory. They had to be at the factory by 9 o'clock in the morning, to work until 12.30, when they returned to the hospital for lunch, and to continue work from 2 to 6 p.m. Although this work was rather monotonous, it proved to our satisfaction that paraplegics could be successfully placed in factories side by side with able-bodied people. This experiment proved invaluable as an incentive to the Ministry of Labour and employers in changing their attitude regarding the employability of disabled people in wheelchairs. In due course, the Ministry of Labour set up Industrial Rehabilitation Centres in various parts of the country, where disabled people, including paraplegics, could receive further training and placement in industry. Such industrial rehabilitation centres have also been set up in other countries, the most well known being the Joseph Bulova School of Watchmaking in New York, under its Director Mr Ben Lipton, the Johannes Straubinger-Haus, in Wildbad, Germany, under its Director, W.Weiss, set up the Caritas Association, and the Berufs-förderungswork in Heidelberg under its Director, W.Boll, which was very instrumental for the success of the XXI International Stoke Mandeville Games in Heidelberg.

Domestic resettlement

(1) In the paraplegic's own home

The great majority of paraplegics and tetraplegics have returned to their own homes to live with their family within the greater community. Table 41 and 43 (page 661–3) gives details about the domestic resettlement of the writer's statistic of his first 3,000 patients.

This achievement, no doubt, represents the most satisfactory form of domestic re-settlement for paraplegics and should be aimed at as much as possible. Before their final discharge, most patients are sent home first on leave in order to give them as well as their relatives the opportunity to readjust themselves to the new scheme of living. At one stage in the development of this Centre in 1945, the British Legion placed an old rectory in Aylesbury at our disposal, which was converted into a 'home' in order to give married and unmarried paraplegics, whose homes were not suitable for their reception, the opportunity to spend several weeks with their families in an atmosphere similar to that in their own homes. During their stay at 'Walton House', the men remained under the medical supervision of the hospital, and wives and parents were instructed in the efficient handling of their paralysed husbands and children.

This temporary domestic resettlement was discontinued as soon as other voluntary organizations, the Government and, in particular, local authorities were in a position to readjust the patients' own homes to their wheelchair lives. The principal requirements for the adjustment of homes for paraplegics and tetraplegics can be summarized as follows:

Outside requirements. The entrance gateway and the concrete pathways should be level and wide enough to take a wheelchair easily. Steps should be eliminated and replaced by sloping paths.

A garage should be attached to the house, wide enough to admit a car and a wheel-chair, to enable the paraplegic to get into and out of the car. Today, this is a condition under which a paraplegic may receive a motorized conveyance under the regulations of the Health Service in Great Britain. It is highly recommended that the garage doors are opened electrically with the aid of an electronic 'eye'.

Doorways and hall. Entrance should be level, or a step leading to the entrance should be very low. Doorways and hallways need widening to allow easy access for a wheelchair. Locks placed high in the door may need lowering. Handrails may be necessary in a hall or passage to allow easy access and turning of a wheelchair into the living-room, kitchen, toilet and bathroom, the door-frames of which should also be widened. The bottoms of doors and wall corners should be protected with metal plates to avoid damage by the wheelchair. Sliding doors have proved invaluable. The height of windows, cooking stoves, sinks, cupboards, wash-basins, latches and electric light switches should be adjusted to the height of the wheelchair users.

Bathroom. The height of the W.C. and wash-basin should be level with the height of the wheelchair, and the W.C. be provided with handrails to facilitate transfer from the chair on to the W.C. Moreover, an overhead chain and grip may be necessary. The wash-basin must be high enough to enable the wheelchair to go underneath. However, the metal waste-pipe should be protected to prevent the insensitive knees and legs from being burned by running hot water.

One of the exercises to restore a patient's independence is transferring from wheel-chair to bath and vice versa, which is taught by physiotherapists in co-operation with occupational therapists. Usually, a paraplegic with mid or low thoracic lesion, sitting in his chair, can place his legs over the edge of the bath and lift himself into the bath by using a handle on a chain hanging over the bath. The process is reversed for getting out of the bath.

To facilitate the use of baths for paraplegics we have developed an apparatus originally presented by John Bell and Croyden which has proved to be useful.

This consists of a seat with back support, both covered with latex rubber, placed on cylindrically shaped bellows inflatable by water pressure through simply connecting the apparatus with a rubber or plastic hose to the bath tap and lifting a metal lever,

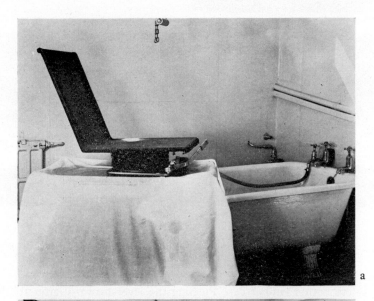

a

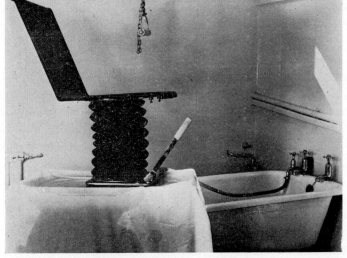

b

FIG. 270a, b. Bell and Croyden hoist.

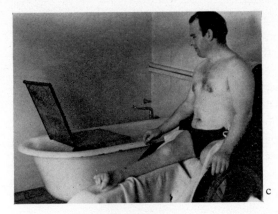

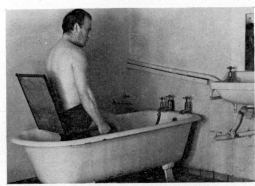

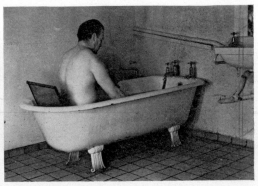

FIG. 270c, d & e. Bath hoist in action.

covered for safety with a rubber cap. Pushing the lever forward, after the bellows are full, and putting it into a slanting position makes the seat stable and at a level with the bath edge and wheelchair seat. Little strength will now suffice to move from the wheelchair seat on to the apparatus seat.

By pressing the lever down the seat will immerse gently into the water under the patient's weight. After completing the bath all that the patient has to do is to lift the lever and he will be raised again. A pressure of 15 lb per square inch, which is the normal mains pressure, is sufficient to raise a weight of 35 stones to the level of the top of the bath. Then the patient has to place his legs outside and lift himself into the wheelchair.

The whole apparatus is made from light alloys and materials able to resist corrosion.

Figs. 270a–e demonstrate the apparatus and its use.

Bedroom. Bedroom and bathroom should be preferably on the ground floor with easy access from one to the other. If this is not possible, a lift should be installed to enable the paralysed in his wheelchair to use the rooms of the first floor. Windows should be low enough to be operated from the wheelchair. The height of the bed should be level with the height of the wheelchair. The electrically controlled Stoke Mandeville turning bed may be installed for high thoracic and cervical lesions to facilitate turning during the night.

In recent years, housing authorities have become more aware of the fact, that the difficulties in adapting houses for wheelchair users could be obviated without affecting normal usage by different design of houses. Actually, many of the existing houses of paraplegics cannot be properly adapted and they and their families have to be rehoused. Local authorities have, therefore, built houses of bungalow type in increasing numbers for these severely disabled people. There is no doubt that the need for proper housing facilities for paraplegics and tetraplegics is an ever-increasing problem, having regard to the increasing number of medically rehabilitated spinal cord sufferers, ready for their social re-integration into society, in particular, employment, which is increasing from year to year.

Although the community responsibility in this respect has improved in recent years in this and other highly developed countries, there is still much to be desired. This applies especially to the adaptation of many public buildings such as railway stations, airports, schools, universities, museums, theatres, cinemas, sports stadiums, exhibition buildings, etc. Not only is access for wheelchair users to many of them difficult or impossible from an architectural point of view, but these barriers are increased by certain fire regulations. Only recently, one of the writer's former paraplegic patients, outstanding through her social and sportive activities, intended to visit with her husband a building exhibition, when they were confronted with a sign: 'Dogs, Prams and Wheelchair Users not allowed!' Another paraplegic—a former officer, wounded in the last war and now himself an architect—who recently wanted to visit a building exhibition, was also refused entry because of the existing rigid fire regulations which in their present rigid form are really intolerable. One can only hope that the passing of the Chronically Sick and Disabled Persons Act, 1970, will accelerate the breaking down of these architectural and social barriers. In this connection, a re-thinking about the existing rigid fire regulations and emergency exits in public building is overdue.

(2) In special temporary or permanent residential settlements

The existing facilities of residential settlements for paraplegics and tetraplegics in Great Britain has already been mentioned.

There are paraplegics and, in particular, tetraplegic civilians who for one reason or another are not able to return to their own homes or prefer to live in hostels or permanent residential settlements. As the number of tetraplegics is increasing year by year, the need for residential hostels is ever increasing in Great Britain and many other countries. Mention has already been made of the hostel for tetraplegics of 30 beds built at the writer's instigation as a pilot scheme in 1964 within the precincts of Stoke Mandeville, but this scheme has not yet been extended by the authorities concerned to other parts of the country. However, other countries have adopted this scheme, and from all those seen by the writer, those in Melbourne and, in particular, in Perth, Western Australia, are the finest examples. The hostel for tetraplegics in Perth is combined, like that at Stoke Mandeville, with sheltered employment facilities.

Industrial and professional resettlement

Even in the writer's first statistics of traumatic paraplegics of the Second World War, 139 out of 186 (74·7 per cent) discharged to their own homes were gainfully employed, the majority of them (68·4 per cent) in full time work (Guttmann, 1953). This satisfactory result was continued throughout the years, and Table 44 (page 664) shows the employment statistics of the writer's first 3,000 patients.

In evaluating the type of industrial and professional resettlement, several groups can be distinguished, some of which may be mentioned here:

(a) The first group consists of paralysed who, before their injury, had already been employed in skilled, semi-skilled or unskilled occupations and have succeeded in going back to their former trades in spite of their severe disability.

The very first patient of this Centre (H.C.) is an example of this group. He was wounded in 1943 and was admitted to the Centre on 3 February 1944 with a conus–cauda

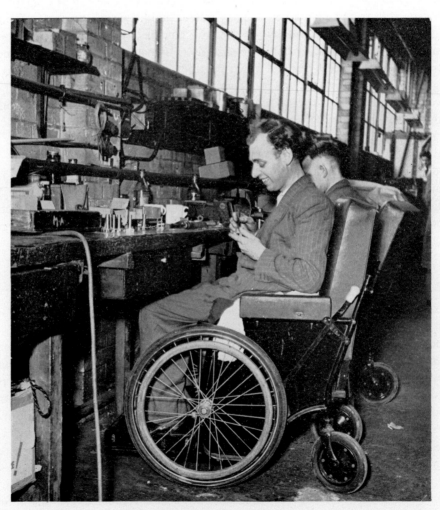

FIG. 271. Assembly work in factory.

equina lesion below L2/L3, with suprapubic drainage and a deep pressure sore over the left buttock. In due course, he developed in addition a para-vertebral abscess. Before joining the army he had been employed in a factory as a glove maker. As a preliminary to his industrial rehabilitation, he started needle and leather work while bedridden, and later he became a member of that working party mentioned earlier on which the first experiment in industrial employment was made. He was also trained at the Centre in cobbling. After discharge on 2 May 1946, he almost immediately returned to his former job, and the factory provided him with proper facilities to enable him to carry out his work from his wheelchair. He worked full time and his absence from work has been negligible. He changed his domicile and went to another part of the country but is still full time employed.

Other patients of this group, who were engaged in clerical work previous to their injuries, had, of course, little difficulty in carrying on with the same or similar work after their discharge from the Centre. Some of them have even succeeded in returning to their former jobs with higher qualifications, having worked for and passed examinations whilst in the Centre. Many paraplegics who, before their paraplegia, were engaged in semi or unskilled work in factories have found employment in industry in assembly work, light engineering, watch and clock repairing, etc., working side by side and in competition with their able-bodied co-workers. Fig. 271 shows two former patients engaged in light engineering in a factory in London.

As an example, a man with a complete paraplegia below T11, associated with amputation of the left leg following gunshot injury, may be quoted, who previous to his war injury was employed in a bank. He was advised to prepare, by means of a correspondence course, for a higher qualification and, in due course, successfully passed his examination. When his condition was satisfactory enough for him to be transferred to our convalescent home, Chaseley, Eastbourne, arrangements were made there for him to start part-time work as vocational training at a local branch of his bank. He now lives in a specially built bungalow in Amersham and drives several miles every day to his bank where he has been employed for 23 years.

Another outstanding example of this group is a surgeon from Budapest who was outstanding in pediatric surgery. He sustained a traumatic paraplegia below T11 in 1963, at the age of 56. Four months after injury, he was admitted to Stoke Mandeville in a pretty hopeless condition. However, he made an excellent readjustment to his complete paraplegia, including walking on elbow crutches. He was firmly encouraged to take up surgery again, and with great reluctance he agreed to try. Four months after his discharge from Stoke Mandeville, he sent us photographs of his first operation (megacolon), which he performed in standing position having designed a special support. Figs. 272a, b, c shows the various stages of being transferred to the theatre, scrubbing up, etc. He constructed a special frame with a support in front to prevent falling over and an orderly pushed him to the washroom and theatre, as shown in Fig. 272. In his letter he wrote 'I enclose photographs of my first operation after my paraplegia. This happened to be the day of my 57th birthday, a very happy occasion.' There are several doctors paralysed as a result of spinal cord injuries or disease, who are now directors of spinal units or general rehabilitation centres and doing outstanding and devoted work in this speciality.

Another example is a tetraplegic from Barcelona, Spain, who since his tetraplegia, has been outstanding in his social activities for the community (W.G.-G.). In spite of his profound disability (complete tetraplegia below C5), he returned to his previous leading position in the sherry business of his family. During his inpatient treatment at the Centre, he became interested in the designing of spinal units. After return home, he re-built a dilapidated hospital for venereal diseases, which was offered to him by the Spanish Government, and became the founder and chairman of the Board of Management of the first Spinal Injuries Centre in Spain, in his home city of Barcelona which increased within 5 years from 20 to 80 beds.

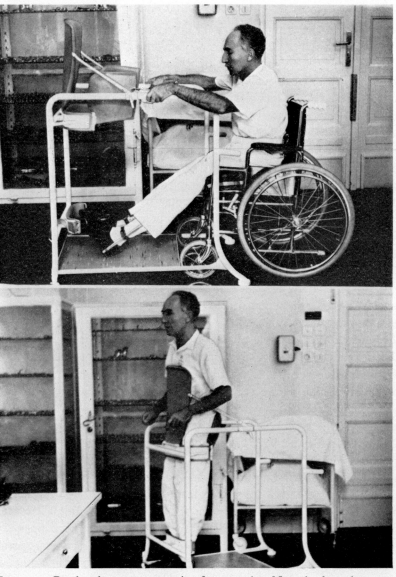

FIG. 272a. Paralysed surgeon preparing for operation. Note the frontal support to maintain balance.

(b) This is a group of paraplegics who, owing to their permanent disability, were not able to return to their former jobs but succeeded in getting different jobs in their former trades. As an example is a man who, previous to his injury, had worked in a chemist's shop and had sustained a complete paraplegia below T6. He became employed by one of the largest pharmaceutical firms in this country as a proof reader and making abstracts from various medical and pharmaceutical journals. In co-operation with his son, he set up a small factory for making optical lenses. He has been full-time employed since 1946.

Another example of this group is a priest with a complete paraplegia below T7 due to gunshot injury in the war. He overcame the critical condition in which he was admitted and became an excellent example to other paralysed in his ward. He took up his priesthood again after the war and is still continuing his ministry part-time, and in addition he is also employed in marking examination papers.

(c) This group consists of paraplegics and tetraplegics who were not able to return to their former occupation, such as regular soldiers, officers, bricklayers, coalminers, etc., and had to be trained to other jobs.

Mention has already been made of a former bricklayer who was trained at the Centre in cobbling and leatherwork and has been in charge of a section in a shoe-making factory for over 20 years.

A young naval lieutenant, with a complete transverse lesion below T12 took up a

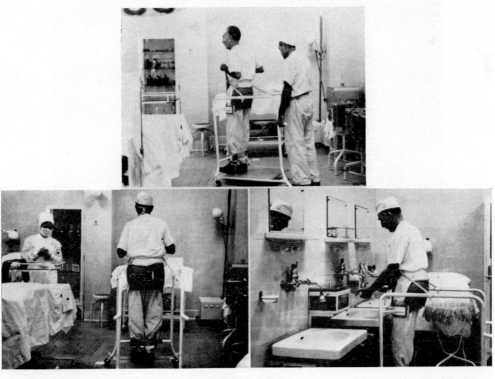

FIG. 272b.

correspondence course in agricultural science. He has been full-time employed for the last 24 years by the Bucks. Agriculture Executive Committee and is an established civil servant for many years (R.M.).

One of the most outstanding examples in this group is Major D.A. who, before the war, worked in his old-established family firm of theatrical costume makers which, however, did not excite him very much. In 1944, while serving in India, he developed severe polio which left him with a considerable residual paralysis of both legs. In spite

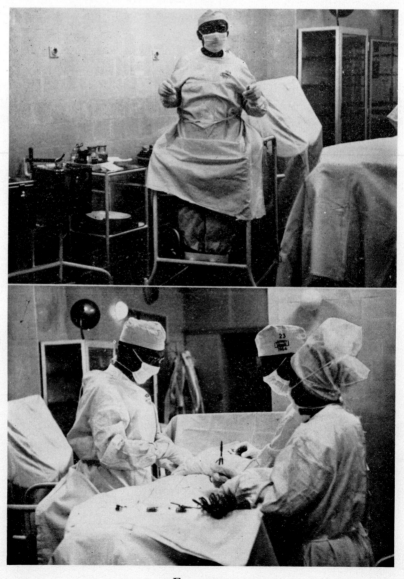

FIG. 272c.

of his disability, he was destined to become one of the outstanding and dynamic personalities in the British film industry. The incentive to become a film producer occurred in
the Spinal Centre, when he was watching an unpretentious film about 'A Day in the
Life of Mrs Roosevelt's Pet Dog'. Through his former occupation and, in addition,
encouragement from his father-in-law, he established contacts with the world of entertainment. In spite of his physical handicap, he worked with tremendous drive and energy
to win a place in the top class of producers, which he achieved through, amongst other
productions, the film 'Reach for the Sky', which tells the story of the famous R.A.F.
pilot in the Second World War, Group Captain Douglas Bader. In 1956, Major Angel
won the British Film Academy Award. As a side line to his busy life, he is engaged in
various charities, and for many years has been a very active member of the Board of
Management of the Paraplegic Sports Endowment Fund.

(d) This group consists of paraplegics who, at the time of their injuries, were either
totally untrained or whose training had been interrupted by the war.

As an example, a young man who, at the age of 22, sustained a transverse myelitis
in 1946 resulting in a severe although incomplete spastic paraplegia below the waist
while serving in a submarine in 1945. When admitted to the Spinal Centre in September
1947, he had pressure sores, severe urinary infection as a result of suprapubic cystotomy
and was quite demoralized due to enforced inactivity in the previous hospital. It was
gratifying to see how this young man, after his sores were healed and his urinary infection
controlled, changed from being one of those headaches to the medical and nursing staff
into a splendid, co-operative patient once he started training in our precision instrument
workshop. He was the first patient to take up draughtsmanship and soon satisfied his
supervisor so much that the Ministry of Works agreed to train him in their training
college at Worcester. He passed all his examinations with flying colours and has been
employed full-time as a draughtsman in one of the London offices of the Ministry of
Works, driving several miles in his own car from his home to his office, and is now a
senior draughtsman in charge of a department. There, he met another 'graduate' of Stoke
Mandeville, a girl who was admitted at the age of 21, 5 years after having sustained a
complete paraplegia below T11 at the age of 16. She, too, was trained in draughtsmanship
as a tracer, went through the same training college and was employed in the same
department in London as a tracer. She is one of the outstanding paraplegic sportswomen,
particularly in table tennis and bowling, and has taken part in all international contests
with great distinction. In recognition of her sporting achievements she received the
British Empire Medal some years ago. These two became married and John B. became
the Founder Chairman of the Stoke Mandeville Paraplegic Athletic Club.

We discovered artistic talents in several of our patients, who were encouraged to
develop these talents. In some cases, they received voluntary help and tuition during
in-patient treatment from professional artists. Some have taken up an arts profession after
leaving the Centre.

An example is Jim L., now aged 41, who, before he was called up to the Army, was
an apprentice in cabinet making. In 1953, he was wounded in the Korean War and
sustained a complete paraplegia below T3. He developed his dormant artistic talent in
painting and sculpturing and after leaving the Centre received training from a professional

sculptor. He is now a very successful painter and sculptor. He dedicated a very good sculpture of a paralysed shot putter to the Stoke Mandeville Sports Stadium for the Paralysed and Other Disabled (Fig. 273). He summarized his own views of his achievement very aptly: 'I reckon it took the combined forces of the adversity of paraplegia, the "university of Stoke Mandeville" and a generous dose of traditional Scottish stubborn pigheadedness to develop my latent talent'. In addition to his artistic occupation he is the editor of the magazine of the Scottish Paraplegic Association. Fig. 274 shows him at work.

Another example in this respect is C.R., an officer who, in 1944, sustained a complete transverse lesion below T6/7 due to a gunshot injury. While he was bedridden, because of the several pressure sores with which he had been admitted, and had to lie for many weeks in prone position, he started drawing and painting in oils. He continued this activity after discharge from the Centre and became a commercial artist in an advertising business, which kept him fully occupied for many years. However, through his drawings

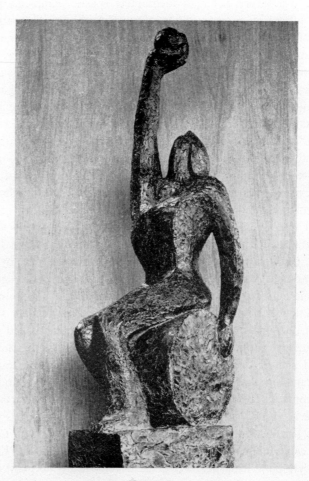

FIG. 273.

he became interested in architecture and in 1963 he took this up as a profession, passing all examinations, and now has his own business in Norwich, where he lives with his wife and adopted daughter. In his leisure hours he still continues painting.

G.S., an R.A.F. officer, at the age of 32, when instructing night fighter pilots to intercept enemy aircraft sustained in 1964 a complete paraplegia below T12. He became interested in teaching and, after passing a three-year course to enter teacher training college, he attempted to enter a training college but was refused by three colleges, which naturally dampened his spirits. Eventually, Culham College at Oxford accepted him. This college, built in 1853, was not designed to take paraplegics in wheelchairs, there being many steps and narrow staircases in the old building and even the new building had large steps to the entrance. However, the college carpenter made ramps to overcome these problems and all other setbacks were more than compensated for by the understanding attitude in which the college authorities viewed prospective candidates in wheelchairs. G.S. is now a fully established teacher of 9 year old pupils in a junior school in Berkshire, where the County Council has provided easy access. 'Children are wonderful,' he writes, 'completely natural and devoid of sophisticated sympathy. They are helpful and well behaved, for them life has no complications, everyone falls into some simple category and a teacher in a wheelchair is no exception. This makes teaching that

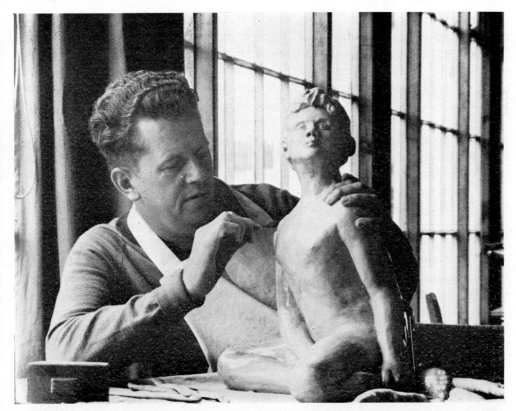

FIG. 274. Jim Laird of Glasgow, a skilled sculptor, paralysed below T3 in the Korean War.

much easier and consequently more enjoyable. I find myself happily established in the teaching profession. To anyone contemplating such a subject I would say "Go ahead" provided of course, he or she is prepared to work all hours in an under-rated, underpaid and overtaxed profession.'

I may add that several other paraplegics and even a tetraplegic had already taken that step many years before G.S. had done and are still employed as teachers, doing excellent work in educating the youth of our community.

Actually, the first person to become a teacher 'on wheels' was G.B., a female paraplegic, who at the age of 31 was admitted on 30 January 1950 with a complete transverse lesion below T11 following fracture-dislocation sustained in 1941. Following explorative laminectomy elsewhere, she was nursed on a plaster bed and remained for 3 months in hospital and was then sent home with her pressure sores unhealed, being provided with a spinal carriage, and since 1942 she had been nursed by her mother. It took us one year to control all her complications and return her to an active life in her wheelchair. Prior to her injury, she had taken up teaching and her most ardent desire was to return to this profession. In those days it was not easy to impress on the authorities concerned that a paralysed person in a wheelchair should not be prevented, because of this, from taking up teaching in an ordinary school. However, eventually in September 1951 she was accepted 'on probation' for 6 months. She has now been teaching for 23 years in classes of a complement of up to 40 children.

A further example of a paraplegic, who by sheer courage and endurance, has gained great achievement in his professional career, is an ex naval lieutenant of the Fleet Air Arm who, on 24 February 1960 had a crash and sustained a complete paraplegia below L2 in addition to a cerebral concussion and abducens paralysis on the left side. He made an excellent rehabilitation in spite of the severe injuries and was discharged on 29 September 1960 able to walk on crutches, which at home he continued to use as an exercise in spite of a great disincentive to continue walking involving putting on calipers, etc. He started a job as Education and Training Officer 5 weeks after leaving hospital and gradually regained self-confidence. He stayed in this job for 3 years but became frustrated and then joined the British Shoe Corporation as Personnel Officer at their headquarters. There he introduced new methods and, in due course, was appointed as Manpower Manager responsible for all personnel and training matters including industrial relations not only for the headquarters but also for the manufacturing division, retail division and 2,000 jobs throughout the British Isles, involving altogether 25,000 people. He travels some 23,000 miles per year in spite of his physical limitations. While carrying out his job he also studied for and obtained a professional qualification, and at present he is studying for a higher degree as an external university student. He has continued his sporting activities. He is secretary to the local Playing Field Trust Charity and has become one of the outstanding archers. He described his views on sport as follows: 'There are two major benefits to be gained from sports activities for paraplegics—the first is the obvious physical exercise and the second is the returning of the competitive spirit so necessary to succeed in both business and normal daily life. All in all it is a marvellous life and it has proved to me that a wheelchair invokes almost no limitations and one can enjoy a normal family and business life—*if you really want to*.'

These are only a few examples, to which many more could be added, to outstanding achievements of paraplegics.

Like able-bodied persons who are interested in the welfare of their fellow-men and are engaged in communal and social work, spinal paraplegics have also taken up social activities and are doing most valuable and essential work within the community, and have occupied important positions. Amongst them two have been elected mayors of their towns. One of our female patients is particularly interested in the education of Borstal boys and has been doing excellent work in a Borstal institution. She has also become president of the Red Cross Organization in her county and, on account of her social work, has become a Baroness and has taken her seat in the House of Lords. She and two other former patients of the Stoke Mandeville Centre have taken a leading part in the debate on the recent Chronically Sick and Disabled Persons Bill, which has now been accepted by the Houses of Parliament and become an Act. She received her paraplegia as a result of a riding accident. She became very soon interested in sport and became outstanding in swimming and table tennis and took part in many national and inter-national competitions with great success.

Our own results achieved in the social and industrial rehabilitation of paraplegics have been published since 1946 (Guttmann, 1946–68; Scruton, 1954). In recent years reports on the social aspects of paraplegics and tetraplegics, including domestic and industrial resettlement, have been published in increasing numbers, which just reveal the ever-increasing importance of spinal paraplegia and tetraplegia as a social problem. Hardy (1964) and Meinecke (1964) stressed the difficulties in the industrial resettlement of coalminers in Great Britain and Germany respectively, partly caused by high pensions and sickness benefit. Maury (1964) reported the results of a survey on the home condi-tions of his first 250 patients in France. Twenty-nine per cent of the patients were not able to get out of their homes by themselves because of architectural barriers and one-third had lavatories which they could not use. Tricot (1964) reported about a survey on the housing conditions in Belgium. As a result of this survey the Superior Council of the Institute du Lagement took immediate steps to adjust homes and houses for the special needs of neuro-motor disabled people. Damanski (1964) reporting on 300 patients showed a low percentage of cases being employed mainly owing to the high proportion of tetraplegics (107 out of 300). Thompson & Murray (1967) and Meine (1970) published surveys on paraplegics living at home and, in particular, that of Thompson and Murray is a comprehensive study of the conditions in Scotland. While in Great Britain for many years ex-service pensioners are surveyed regularly by medical and social workers, there is still a great lack of after-care for civilian paraplegics and tetraplegics in this respect. Unfortunately, spinal centres have not sufficient staff to carry out such surveys at the homes of paraplegics and tetraplegics themselves which would be, of course, the best guarantee for detailed assessment.

G · General Statistics and Legal Aspects

CHAPTER 39
GENERAL STATISTICS

Since the opening of the Stoke Mandeville Centre, over 5,000 paraplegics and tetraplegics have been admitted as in-patients by 1972. A previous statistic of the development of the Spinal Unit as a National Centre since 1951 when Stoke Mandeville Hospital was taken over by the National Health Service is shown in Table 36 which gives the turnover of the patients from 1952–64 (Guttmann, 1967). As mentioned before, the majority of patients are admitted by road, but in recent years transport by helicopter, especially of cervical injuries and those associated with other injuries, has steadily increased, and since January 1971–31 May 1972 36 patients were admitted by helicopter. Moreover, traumatic paraplegics and tetraplegics, in particular service personnel of the British Forces, have been transferred by plane within 48 hours of injury from as far afield as Germany, Aden and Singapore. The importance of immediate admission of acute spinal injuries to a Spinal Centre cannot be overstressed.

As shown in Table 36 the total turnover increased from 670 in 1952 to 2,780 in 1964. The yearly new admissions, due both to injuries and other causes, increased during the same period from 107 to 256, most of them being traumatic lesions. Readmissions increased from 198 in 1951–52 to 682 in 1963–64. In the following years until 1968–69 the new admissions varied between 228 and 269 but decreased between 1969 to 1971 varying between 168 and 203, as two of our wards had to be closed because of shortage of nursing staff. This closure of two wards inevitably resulted in delay of new admissions and, in particular, of early re-admission of former patients in need of specialized treatment. Accordingly the readmissions for routine check-ups and specialized treatment has fallen in this period, varying between 522 and 615. This shortage of nursing staff has, indeed, become a national and international problem for many hospitals in this country and abroad.

Of special interest is the development of the out-patient service from 63 in 1951–52 to 884 in 1963-64. This includes former in-patients for routine check-ups and patients sent for assessment from other hospitals and doctors. It may be noted that, while the number of new admissions and re-admissions decreased between 1968–69 and 1971–72, the number of out-patient attendances increased in that period from 1,092 to 1,408. The total turnover in that period varied between 2,817 and 2,865.

At the bottom of the columns of discharges in the statistic (Table 36), the number of deaths is given occurring every year, varying between 5 in 1952 and 21 in 1963–64. The number of deaths between the period of 1968–69 and 1971–72 varied between 13 and 21 (average 15).

TABLE 36

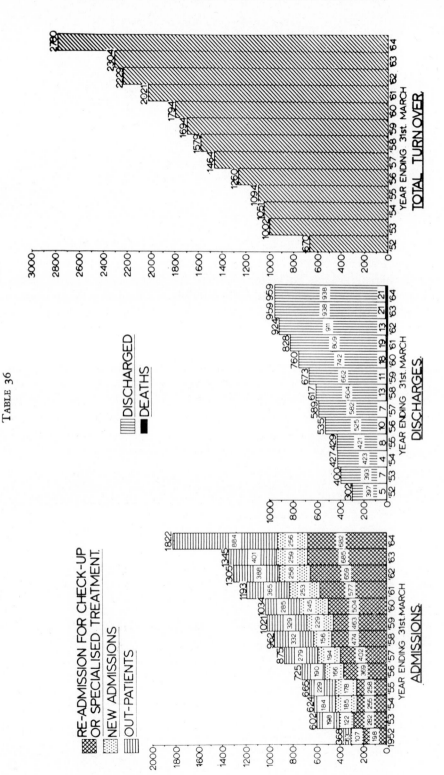

TOTAL TURNOVER

YEAR ENDING 31st. MARCH

2780 2304 2222 2021 1794 1694 1572 1464 1260 1194 1057 1002 670

DISCHARGES.

YEAR ENDING 31st. MARCH

DISCHARGED   DEATHS

959 959 924 828 760 673 617 589 535 429 427 400 302

938 938 911 809 742 662 604 582 525 421 423 393 397

21 21 13 19 18 11 13 7 10 8 4 7 5

ADMISSIONS.

YEAR ENDING 31st. MARCH

RE-ADMISSION FOR CHECK-UP OR SPECIALISED TREATMENT.
NEW ADMISSIONS
OUT-PATIENTS

1822 1345 1305 1193 1034 1021 962 875 725 665 624 602 368

884 401 388 365 329 285 332 279 190 229 184 198 53

256 259 258 253 245 229 156 194 166 178 185 122 107

682 685 659 577 504 463 474 402 369 258 256 282 198

22

TABLE 37. Analysis of 3,000 cases

	Servicemen and pensioners	Civilians	Total	Percentage
Traumatic lesions	753	1,210	1,963	65·4
Transverse myelitis	34	125	159	5·3
Poliomyelitis	89	63	152	5·1
Vascular processes	11	95	106	3·5
Spina bifida	—	62	62	2·1
Multiple sclerosis	41	80	121	4
Disc lesions	6	27	33	1·1
Miscellaneous	66	338	404	13·5
	1,000	2,000	3,000	100·00

Table 37 is an analysis of the first 3,000 patients admitted by May 1963 since 1944 divided into ex-service personnel and civilians (Guttmann, 1965). The majority (65·4 per cent), were traumatic lesions. The column headed 'Miscellaneous' consists of non-traumatic patients other than transverse myelitis, polio and spina bifida such as tuberculosis, syphilis, epidural abscesses, tumours, haemangioma, meningitis, syringomyelia, combined degeneration of the cord and congenital processes other than spina bifida and, last but not least, mishaps after surgical procedures. Table 37 shows an analysis of the 1963 traumatic lesions according to the level of the lesions and divided between complete and incomplete lesions.

A comparison between the statistic, shown in Table 37, and one of my previous statistics, published in 1953 on 458 traumatic cases out of a total of 570 admissions since 1944, demonstrates a considerable change in the ratio ex-servicemen/civilians. In the 1953 statistic there were 388 ex-servicemen and pensioners and only 70 civilians. Although

TABLE 38. Traumatic lesions

	Servicemen and pensioners	Civilians	Total	Percentage	
Cervical				23·6	
Complete	36	99	135		6·8
Incomplete	86	245	331		16·8
T1–5				9·8	
Complete	62	84	146		7·5
Incomplete	18	27	45		2·3
T6–12				43·1	
Complete	198	419	617		31·4
Incomplete	113	115	228		11·7
Cauda equina	240	221	461	23·5	23·5
	753	1,210	1,963	100	100

by 1963 the number of ex-servicemen and pensioners had almost doubled (753) there was a considerable increase of traumatic lesions amongst civilians (1,210) (Table 37).

Of particular interest is the increasing number of cervical injuries over the years. In the statistic of 1953 there were 41 cervicals amongst a total of 458 cord injuries (8·7 per cent). In a later statistic of our first 2,000 patients, published in 1962, the number of cervical lesions was 207 (15 per cent) out of 1,349 spinal cord injuries. The percentage of cervicals increased to 23·6 per cent amongst 1,963 traumatic lesions, as shown in Table 38. This experience is in accordance with the experience of other Spinal Injuries Centres in various countries.

The age of the patients at the time of injury varied from 6 to 80 years. However, the age groups mainly involved were those between 16 and 35 years—i.e. well over 50 per cent of the total.

TABLE 39. Aetiology of traumatic tetraplegia

	Complete lesions	Incomplete lesions	Total	Category totals
Road accidents				
Motor vehicle	42	92	134	
Motor cycle	20	21	41	209
Pedal cycle	3	20	23	
Hit by vehicle	2	9	11	
Industrial accidents				
Fall	9	13	22	
Hit by moving object	2	14	16	41
Caught in moving machinery or other object	1	2	3	
Knife wound	—	1	1	1
Bomb blast	1	6	7	7
Gunshot wound	4	19	23	23
Sport				
Diving	31	43	74	
Struck by diver	—	2	2	
Swimming other than diving	1	5	6	
Water skiing	1	—	1	
Football—Rugby	3	3	6	
Football—Association	—	3	3	111
Riding	1	2	3	
Climbing	1	—	1	
Wrestling	—	1	1	
Trampoline	1	—	1	
Other (vaulting horse, etc.)	5	8	13	
Aeroplane accidents	1	2	3	3
Fall	21	80	101	101
Miscellaneous	3	7	10	10
Totals	153	353	506	506

In analysing the various causes of traumatic tetraplegia, as shown in Table 39 of a statistic of 506 tetraplegics out of 2,078 traumatic spinal cord lesions (24·4 per cent) comprising a period of 20 years between 1 February 1944 to 31 January 1964, road accidents take, as one would expect, the first place, while sport injuries with 111 cases represent the second highest figure. Special attention must be drawn to the fact, that the majority of sport injuries, namely 83 out of 111, were due to water sport and of these no less than 74 occurred due to diving. If one realizes that diving accidents represent nearly three-quarters of all sports injuries, and that the victims are almost always in the prime of life, the youngest being only 13 years old, this is indeed a terrifying statistic. The most important measure in dealing with these dreadful injuries in young people is, of course, prevention, and it cannot be emphasized too strongly that this can only be achieved by systematic education of the public generally. In as much as schoolchildren and young adults are taught road safety measures to prevent accidents, the same should be applied in schools and public swimming pools with regard to the hazard of diving even from the lowest spring board and from the shallow end of a swimming pool. Moreover, when diving is practised in swimming pools, no swimmer must be in the water within the diving area because of the danger of being struck by the diver, as either the diver will break his neck or the swimmer in the water will sustain a thoracic injury. Parents, school teachers and swimming instructors should join in this educational problem of the public.

There is, moreover, another point in this connection where there is a great need for improvement: there are too few and too inconspicuous warning notices placed by local

TABLE 40

MORTALITY

TOTAL MATERIAL   3000 CASES

496 deaths   = 16.5%
343 corrected figure = 11.4%

TRAUMATIC PATIENTS
TOTAL 1963

331 deaths   = 16.9%
242 corrected figure = 12.3%

SERVICEMEN & PENSIONERS   CIVILIANS
TOTAL 753   TOTAL 1210
180 deaths   = 23.9%   151 deaths   = 12.5%
132 corrected figure = 17.5%   110 corrected figure = 9.0%

ANALYSIS OF SERVICEMEN & PENSIONERS
WORLD WAR I
TOTAL 67
39 deaths   = 58.2%
15 corrected figure = 22.4%

WORLD WAR II
TOTAL 468
125 deaths   = 26.7%
103 corrected figure = 22.0%

POST WAR PERIOD from 1946
TOTAL 218
16 deaths   = 7.3%
14 corrected figure = 6.4%

TABLE 41. Length of survival of deceased traumatics

	Under 7 days	+7-28 days	+1-6 mths	+6-24 mths	+2-5 yrs	+5-10 yrs	+10-15 yrs	+15-20 yrs	+20-25 yrs	+25-30 yrs	+30-35 yrs	+35-40 yrs	+40-45 yrs	+45-50 yrs	Total
Cervicals															
Complete	5	5	1	6	4	2	4	1							28
Incomplete	2	4	6	4	7	8	4	2			3	2	1		43
T1–5															
Complete	1			3	5	10	3	1					3		26
Incomplete	1				1	1	1						3		7
T6–12															
Complete	2	9	4	10	30	33	31	7		1			1		128
Incomplete		1			4	3	4	5	1		3	3	2	1	27
Cauda equina	1	2	2	4	7	19	7	9	4		3	7	6	1	72
Total	12	21	13	27	58	76	54	25	5	1	9	12	16	2	331

TABLE 42. Length of survival of living traumatics

	Under 2 yrs	+2-7 yrs	+7-12 yrs	+12-17 yrs	+17-22 yrs	+22-27 yrs	+27-32 yrs	+32-37 yrs	+37-42 yrs	+42-47 yrs	+47-52 yrs	Total
Cervicals												
Complete	31	53	17	3	2	1						107
Incomplete	81	127	31	17	25	4	2				1	288
T1–5												
Complete	20	36	31	8	23	2						120
Incomplete	2	11	8	6	8	1			1	1		38
T6–12												
Complete	48	150	111	77	94	5	2	1		1		489
Incomplete	34	45	37	11	52	9	1		7	5		201
Cauda equina	30	80	70	44	14	137			8	6		389
Total	246	502	305	166	218	159	5	1	16	13	1	1,632

authorities on river banks, lake sides and beaches to prevent children and, in particular, young adults from diving into shallow water. There is, indeed, a great need for the authorities concerned to ensure that the public are suitably warned of any danger of this kind. Only by these combined efforts will the number of victims of traumatic tetraplegia due to diving be diminished in future.

Mortality rate—survival rate

The death rate amongst the 3,000 patients is given in Table 40. It may be noted that these statistics include every patient who died either during treatment in the Centre or after discharge home or to other institutions. The uncorrected figures of 496 deaths (16·9 per cent) include causes of death quite independent of those as a direct result of paraplegia, such as tuberculosis of the lung, cancer, other diseases, cerebral haemorrhage and new accidents. Taking out these causes of death the corrected figure of death directly related to the spinal cord affliction is only 343 or 11·4 per cent. Table 40 also gives a more detailed mortality rate of the traumatic patients. It shows a very low mortality rate—i.e. 9 per cent of the 1,210 civilians and 6·4 per cent of the 218 ex-servicemen of the Second World War, many of whom had survived 18–20 years, was only 22·4 per cent.

Table 41 reveals the length of survival of the 331 deceased traumatic and Table 42 shows the length of survival of the 1,632 living traumatic paraplegics and tetraplegics at the time of the statistics in 1963.

Of special interest from both medical and social points of view is the increased life expectancy of tetraplegics. As shown in Table 42 of the statistics, out of 288 incomplete tetraplegics 49 (17 per cent) survived longer than 12 years and 32 longer than 17 years (11 per cent). However, the survival rate of complete tetraplegics, as one would expect, is much reduced. Nevertheless, 6 out of 107 survived longer than 12 years and of these 3 survived longer than 17 years. Since 1963, the number of survivors from incomplete as well as complete cervical injuries has increased, and so has the length of survival of those shown in Tables 41 and 42 up to 20 years and longer. Further statistics of survival rate of paraplegics and tetraplegics of the total material of over 5,000 patients treated at Stoke Mandeville Spinal Centre since its inception is being prepared, which will include the 3,000 patients reported in this book.

The increased number of tetraplegics has, naturally, created social problems, as many severe incomplete and complete tetraplegics need more or less constant attendance and special residential facilities for their care. Although the majority have succeeded in living with their families in houses adjusted to their severe disability, being provided with home nursing equipment, there will always be a group who cannot return home or whose families are unable to continue to look after them at home. For these, accommodation in residential hostels or other institutions had been established (see pages 12 and 645).

All these figures clearly demonstrate the dramatic change which has taken place since the introduction of the new concept of management in the prognosis of these men and women, who for thousands of years had no hope to live for any length of time. But, of course, as already pointed out, the aim was not just to prolong their life expectation but to make their lives worthwhile living as respected and contented citizens, to live with their families and become once again their breadwinners. It can be said today that this aim has been accomplished in a great number of paralysed people.

Domestic resettlement

Table 43 is an analysis of the domestic resettlement. Of the 2,504 survivors out of 3,000 patients (496 died as shown in Table 40) the very great majority, 2,059, had returned to their own homes—the ideal solution—once these were adjusted to their disability by the authorities concerned or privately, and only 240 who could not return home for one reason or another, were accommodated in paraplegic settlements, hostels or homes for the disabled (see chapter Domestic Resettlement).

TABLE 43

DOMESTIC RESETTLEMENT OF 3000 PATIENTS

LIVING AT HOME	2059	
LIVING IN PARAPLEGIC SETTLEMENTS, HOSTELS & HOMES FOR THE DISABLED	240	
		2299
PATIENTS UNDER TREATMENT AT STOKE MANDEVILLE	151	
PATIENTS UNDER TREATMENT IN OTHER HOSPITALS	54	
DEATHS	496	
		701
		3000

Employment statistics

Table 44 gives an analysis of the employment statistics of 2,012 paraplegics and tetraplegics available for employment at the time of the statistics of 1963. One thousand and ninety-seven were full-time employed (54·5 per cent) in a variety of jobs. Details of their occupations are given in the chapter Industrial and Professional Resettlement. Two hundred and ninety-four people were not employed at the time of the statistic. This does not mean that they were unemployable, but that in the majority of cases society had not yet been able to provide suitable employment. If one analyses the 1,718 actually employed people, the percentage of the full-time employed was 63·9 per cent.

Table 45 is a more detailed employment statistic according to level of the lesions of both traumatic and non-traumatic cases, polios and miscellaneous. Naturally, the statistics of employed paraplegics and tetraplegics must vary from year to year as it also does for the able-bodied. From the various statistics published since 1947 of our former patients the number of actually employed varied from 69 to 84 per cent of the total figures. As a rule paraplegics are able to carry out their work in many jobs and professions very satisfactorily and in many instances their absenteeism from work is less than that of able-bodied workers. Many have been in employment more than 20–25 years.

CHAPTER 39

TABLE 44

EMPLOYMENT STATISTICS ON 3000 PATIENTS

ANALYSIS

Deceased	496
Retired and Over Age	103
Physically Unfit (including 64 cervicals)	143
Under treatment at Stoke Mandeville	151
Under treatment at other hospitals	54
Not traced	41
	988
Available for employment	2012
Total	3000

AVAILABLE FOR EMPLOYMENT 2012

Full time	1097	54.5%
Part time	222	11.0%
Home occupations	399	19.9%
	1718	85.4%
Not working	294	14.6%
	2012	100.0%

ANALYSIS OF EMPLOYED

Full time	1097	63.9%
Part time	222	12.9%
Home occupations	399	23.2%
	1718	100.0%

TABLE 45. Statistics on 2,012 patients available for employment

	Full time	Part time	Home occupations	Not working	Total
Cervicals					
Complete	9	13	37	1	60
Incomplete	84	31	89	27	231
T1–5					
Complete	77	20	19	14	130
Incomplete	43	7	14	6	70
T6–12					
Complete	270	75	114	106	565
Incomplete	206	20	43	64	333
Cauda equina	277	35	52	61	425
Polio	99	6	16	4	125
Miscellaneous	32	15	15	11	73
Total	1,097	222	399	294	2,012
Percentage	54·5	11	19·9	14·6	100

CHAPTER 40

LEGAL ASPECTS

THE DISABLED PERSONS (EMPLOYMENT) ACT

There are two Parliament Acts in the United Kingdom, which have been fundamental in the social re-integration of paraplegics and other severely disabled persons. The first was the Disabled Persons (Employment) Act, which came into being during the Second World War in 1944. This charter of humanity really legalized the modern concept of rehabilitation of severely disabled, by promoting training and facilities for employment to enable the severely disabled to obtain employment or undertake work on their own account. Employers of not less than 20 persons are obliged by law to employ 3 per cent registered disabled persons of their total staff. Failure to employ this quota means that the employer concerned is not allowed to engage a person who is not a registered disabled person nor may he discharge a registered disabled person without reasonable cause, for this would leave him below his quota. Records showing compliance with the quota obligation may be produced for inspection by officers authorized by the Minister.

Sheltered employment

The Act empowers the Minister and local authorities to provide facilities for sheltered employment for those severely disabled persons who cannot obtain employment in ordinary competitive conditions but on the other hand are capable of carrying out remunerative work as distinct from diversionary occupation.

As early as 1945 Remploy Limited was set up for this purpose. This is a non-profit making company administered by a Board of Directors appointed by the Ministry. This company has over 80 factories set up since 1945 for sheltered employment for disabled people in which paraplegics take part. The company receives loans to cover capital expenditure and an annual grant to cover trading losses. The paraplegics and other severely disabled are employed in the production of articles for the ordinary commercial market and on contract work for industry and Government.

Local authorities also have the power to set up sheltered workshops for severely disabled persons and are supported financially by the Government. So, too, are voluntary organizations which run sheltered workshops and mention has already been made of the Residential Centres at Lyme Green, Cheshire; Chaseley, Eastbourne; and the Star and Garter Home in Richmond for paraplegic and tetraplegic ex-service pensioners.

Industrial rehabilitation units

These have been set up in various parts of the country in the main industrial centres to provide an opportunity for severely disabled people such as paraplegics to adjust themselves gradually to normal working conditions and occupational assessment for the type of work or training for which they are best suited. The average length of such assessment courses varies between 8 to 12 weeks, and the disabled people work under the supervision of selected craftsmen. During the course, the trainees receive maintenance allowances.

Vocational training courses

In nearly 40 different trades in special Training Centres the disabled are trained side by side with the able-bodied, and these centres are provided with special facilities for wheelchair cases. There are four Residential Centres run by voluntary organizations with financial support from the Ministry for those disabled people who are unable to travel daily to the Training Centres and need special care. These are:

1   Finchale Abbey Training Centre, Durham.
2   Portland Training College, Mansfield.
3   The Queen Elizabeth Training College, Leatherhead, which has also a Residential Rehabilitation Unit at Benstead and the Residential Sheltered Employment Centre, Dorincourt.
4   St Loyes College, Exeter.

Special aids to employment

There are special aids for blind and other severely disabled persons to take up employment. Paraplegics are entitled to a second wheelchair at the place of employment to facilitate their work, if this is certified by a consultant.

Allowances

The provision of social legislation includes various types of allowances for severely disabled persons:

National Insurance (Industrial Injuries Act 1946). The Industrial Injuries Scheme covers workers of all ages who work for an employer under a contract of service and are insured under the main National Insurance Scheme (so-called Class 1). It does not cover the self-employed persons (Class 2). This scheme provides:

(a) A Temporary Injury Benefit of a fixed weekly amount lasting 26 weeks following the accident, which is called the Injury Benefit Period.

(b) A Disablement Pension from the day after Injury Benefit ends, for the rest of the patient's life in the case of severe disablement such as paraplegia and tetraplegia. Paraplegics and tetraplegics who are unemployable may receive, in addition, a Supplementary Unemployment Benefit. This is given, if the disabled is unable to work and likely to remain so permanently.

Disabled people, whether employable or unemployable, are entitled to additional allowances:

Constant Attendance Allowance (C.A.A.). Paraplegics and tetraplegics are entitled to C.A.A. if they require constant attendance every day, although not necessarily the whole day, and that the attendance is likely to last for a prolonged period. This is not surrendered when the patient takes up employment.

In addition there is an allowance for the wife is she is not working. Furthermore, there are allowances for children and also a clothing allowance for paraplegics and tetraplegics who wear calipers and urinals, to cover the wear and tear of the clothing.

Persons with spinal cord injuries as a result of road accidents are entitled to compensation by insurances. The same applies to paraplegics and tetraplegics, who have suffered an industrial injury and who may claim damages from their employer, if there is evidence that safety precautions at work were at fault. The sum awarded in Court or settled out of Court is always high in complete lesions of the spinal cord or cauda equina, in particular for tetraplegics. In this connection, the assessment of life expectancy plays, of course, the most important part. When I had to give evidence in the Court in the early years of our work for paraplegics or tetraplegics the life expectancy was still considered very low by most of the medical experts on the opposite side, as a rule no longer than 2 to 5 years. There has been a dramatic change in this respect as the result of the high survival rate due to the advances made in the treatment and rehabilitation of spinal paraplegics and tetraplegics, and it has been proved that even tetraplegics with complete lesions below C5/6 may live 20 years and longer. Moreover, as most paraplegics are now employable, even for full-time work, in a job adjusted to their disability, the question often asked in the last 15 years by the defence counsel is why the paraplegic concerned is not employed. Here lies the fundamental change which has taken place in the whole outlook of these severely disabled people and which has to be taken into account by the legal profession when assessing damages.

Paraplegic and tetraplegic war pensioners are entitled to higher allowances. Although the basic pension of 100 per cent disablement is the same as the disabled pension for industrial injuries, additional allowances make the income of the war pensioner higher. The war pensioner, like the disabled civilian, is allowed to earn up to £104 a year without affecting his unemployability supplement. The dependants' allowances are higher and the wife's allowance stays as long as she earns less than £104 a year. There is also a Discretionary Educational Allowance for children. Moreover, to encourage service-pensioners to work they get an additional allowance of £2 when they are employed. The pension of a paraplegic ex-serviceman with a complete lesion who is entitled to the various additional allowances, is at present £24 and more per week. In spite of the high pension an ex-service paraparaplegic may receive from the State, a high percentage of war pensioners have been full-time employed for many years, because they have realized how important regular work is for their general well being. The pension of an unemployable married tetraplegic ex-serviceman with a complete lesion, with all special allowances (including children's allowance) amounts at present to £30–£35 per week. Having regard to the present inflationary trend in this and other countries adjustments of pensions are necessary. In recent years repeated adjustments of the allowances have been made, commensurate with the increase of inflation.

Non-industrial accidents

Insured persons who have become paraplegics through non-industrial accidents are treated in the same way as cases of any other disabling diseases, and are entitled to sickness benefit, which is free from income tax and given for an unlimited time up to the retirement pension age. The National Assistance Board will supplement their benefit, provided they pass the means test but their total income is just above subsistence level. Paraplegics, aged 16 or over, who are not in full-time employment can have their income supplemented by the National Assistance Board to the level at which their needs are assessed under the regulations. All persons in full-time work are disqualified from receiving help. Only if a person is self-employed and his earning power is reduced as compared with others similar occupied, because of his disability, he is not disqualified. The National Assistance Board also has the power to make additional grants over and above the normal scales to paraplegics in exceptional circumstances.

THE CHRONICALLY SICK AND DISABLED PERSONS ACT
(1970)

This Act of Parliament which came into being on 29 May 1970, makes further provision with respect to the welfare of the severely disabled. The provisions made by this new Act include information as to the need for and existence of welfare services, provision of welfare services and duties of local authorities. Of special importance is the provision of lectures, games, outings or other recreational facilities outside the disabled person's home as well as provision of educational facilities or assistance in travelling to and from his home and facilitating the taking of holidays. Furthermore, the Act stresses the need for access of the disabled to, and facilities at, premises open to the public. 'Any person undertaking the provision of any building or premises to which the public are to be admitted, whether on payment or otherwise, shall, in the means of access both to and within the building or premises, and in the parking facilities and sanitary conveniences to be available (if any), make provision, in so far as it is in the circumstances both practicable and reasonable, for the needs of members of the public visiting the building or premises who are disabled.' This regulation, if put into practice will be, indeed, a fundamental step forwards in breaking down the architectural barriers which today still confront all wheelchair-bound disabled people. This regulation also applies to university and school buildings. Special attention is also drawn by the new Act to the provision of public sanitary conveniences for the disabled, the use of which in most public premises, such as railway stations, airports, theatres, museums, restaurants, etc., is at present most difficult or impossible.

In the design of public buildings the following details should be considered:

Parking space
The parking space should be very near to the entrance of the building and adequate space should be reserved for disabled drivers.

Entrance
There should be at least one entrance at ground level, or if that is not possible, a ramp should be built, the gradient of which should not exceed 1 in 20. The kerb on the

pavement edge should be reduced to 30 or 50 cm in height and the pavement approaching the entrance should be of a firm and not loose material. The width of the entrance should be at least 80 cm. The entrance should be provided with automatically sliding doors with a contact mat, as is usually provided now in airports. If a public building is fitted with revolving doors, there should be an additional entrance for wheelchair bound disabled. Within the building, steps very often cannot be avoided; therefore, ramps should be used where variations in level are unavoidable, not exceeding a gradient of 1 in 12. Every building should be provided with lifts large enough to admit at least 4 wheelchair bound people (8–9 persons). Lifts should be provided with sliding doors.

Toilets

Should be at the same level as the entrance door or lift. The dimension of the toilet should be large enough to enable negotiation with a wheelchair, i.e. at least 2 m in depth and 1·5 m in width. The upper face of the WC should be between 48 to 50 cm above floor level. The WC should be provided with horizontal and vertical support rails to enable the paralysed to transfer from the wheelchair on to the toilet. Flushing handle should be suitably located to enable easy management. The same applies to the toilet paper. A small wash-basin should be fixed near the toilet so that the paralysed can reach it with his legs underneath the basin.

Urinals should be provided as slab urinals and a high step should be avoided.

Light switches should be arranged so that the wheelchair bound can reach them. The same applies to the telephone. The height of these appliances should be about 1·20 m above floor level.

MEDICAL AND LEGAL ASPECTS IN LITIGATION PROCEDURES

Spinal specialists are often called upon to provide medical reports to lawyers in legal compensation procedures and give evidence in Court either on behalf of the plaintiff or the defence if the case cannot be settled out of Court. One has to realize that the assessment of compensation in spinal cord injury cases is today a more complex problem than it was 25 to 30 years ago. In those days it was still the generally accepted view by both the medical and legal professions that life expectancy of paraplegics, let alone tetraplegics, was very limited, as a rule to 2 to 5 years, and the question of working capability and employability did not arise. Accordingly, the legal assessment of the compensation was relatively simple and the monetary award not high. This has changed dramatically as the result of the greatly improved early and long term management of traumatic paraplegics and tetraplegics, and consequently the greatly increased life expectancy of these patients is reflected in the much higher monetary awards. In England, a complete paraplegic may receive at present up to £70,000 and a tetraplegic up to £100,000; in the U.S.A. the compensation awards are 1,000,000 dollars and more.

Customarily, the plaintiff's lawyer tends to enhance the disability, while the defendant's lawyer's approach is to mitigate and minimize damages. Moreover, some patients themselves, being anxious for their economic security, aggravate their symptomatology due to neurotic overlay. This applies in particular to the problem of pain, which I have found often disappears or greatly diminishes after the case is settled. Furthermore, a Solicitor may dissuade his client, who otherwise would be capable of taking up employment, from doing so before the case is settled. Whenever I come across this attitude, I never hesitate to warn the patient that this may have just an adverse effect on the Court's decision.

As a rule, it takes a considerable time to settle litigation cases following injuries resulting in severe disability including spinal cord injuries. There are two reasons for this delay. The first concerns the medical adviser. The physician or surgeon in charge of the case has to wait with his final assessment until the optimum of the patient's readjustment to his permanent disability has been reached and the question of whether full-time or part-time attendance has to be considered. This applies in particular to complete lesions, while in incomplete paraplegics and tetraplegics who show functional recovery the optimum of recovery has also to be assessed. Moreover, the assessment of life expectancy in both complete and incomplete lesions depends on the risks of complications developing after discharge from hospital, in particular, ascending infection of the urinary tract, septic absorption from pressure sores and, in tetraplegics in particular, respiratory complications. Furthermore, the working capability of the paralysed to take up employment either full time or part-time in his former job or to be trained for another job adjusted to his disability has also to be considered in the assessment. It is not now unusual that Counsel for the Defence may ask the medical expert in Court about the reasons why the plaintiff is unemployable, in spite of his satisfactory physical condition—a question which would have never arisen 25 years ago.

The other reasons for the delay in settling the case concern the lawyers. There is a difference regarding the lawyer's fee in litigation cases between the English and American systems. In England, the lawyers on either side are paid for the amount of time they spend on the case, in the U.S.A. the Defence lawyers are paid per diem and the attorney (like the English Solicitor) must prove his fee. Therefore, the longer the case is delayed the larger the fee. On the other hand, the lawyer of the plaintiff in the U.S.A. receives what is called a contingency fee, which is the portion of the award the patient will receive if he is successful. If he is not successful, he will receive no award. Therefore, the plaintiff's attorney is anxious to bring the case to an end as soon as possible and is against procrastination (Golman, 1975). Finally, a further delay may be caused by the difficulty in fixing a date for the Hearing in Court, having regard to the great number of litigation cases.

H · The Ultimate Integration of the Spinal Man

CHAPTER 41

THE ESSENCE OF REHABILITATION

In the preceding chapters of this book, many details of the great complexity of the problem of spinal paraplegia and tetraplegia have been discussed. It now remains to weld the many facets of the mosaic into one entity: the spinal man.

Let us first summarize our findings on the physiological aspects of the integrative function of the central nervous system in the spinal man:

Physiological integration of the spinal man

In summarizing our findings on the physiological aspects, one cannot fail to become aware of the integrative action of the nervous system in the spinal man. The accomplishment of the spinal man's physiological integration lies in the restoration of a co-ordinated function between the isolated cord and the remaining components of the nervous system. A better understanding of the pathophysiology of the isolated cord and the effect of its undesirable reflex responses on the muscular and autonomic systems have led to the recognition and development of regulatory mechanisms, aimed at restoring and maintaining a suitable environment in the spinal man:

1 The part which the isolated cord plays in this process of integration lies in our realization, that the isolated cord is by no means as ineffectual as a regulatory reflex-organ as was previously accepted by clinicians and physiologists. In fact, it is capable of some re-adaptive metamorphosis which, by proper management, can be utilized in the rehabilitation of the spinal man (Guttmann, 1945–69). From all that has been said in the chapter on neurophysiological aspects, it can be concluded that the isolated cord under the influence of correct management in the initial stages following transection, in particular proper positioning and avoiding contractures, infection of the urinary tract and sepsis from pressure sores and by early and appropriate training, is adaptive to posture and can undergo such degree of functional adaptation that local reflex arcs become strong enough to be capable of producing useful static reflexes. Although the two-legged spinal man is, naturally, at some disadvantage in this respect, as compared with the quadruped spinal dog or cat, his static reflexes help in the restoration of standing and walking in parallel bars and, in thoracic lesions, walking on crutches. The intricate neural mechanism involved in this accomplishment within the spinal cord is still obscure, and more informa-

671

tion on the transmission of impulses to and from the isolated cord will be necessary. However, in the light of the work of cell physiologists, pre-eminently of Eccles and his school, our understanding of the excitatory and inhibitory function of synapses in the transmission of information from one neurone to another or from neuron to effector cell has greatly deepened, as has the recognition of the importance of the muscle spindle as a sensory organ and the elaboration of the detailed organization of its encapsulated structure in nuclear-chain and nuclear-bag fibres and their innervation.

2   The process of training and reconditioning of the isolated cord is enhanced and facilitated through the action of non-paralysed shoulder muscle groups, especially latissimus dorsi and trapezius and in lower lesions rectus abdominis, thanks to their segmental innervation in the cord above the level of transection and to their anatomical attachment on the pelvis and vertebral column in most patients with transection of the spinal cord. Thus, a re-connection between the paralysed parts of the organisms with the brain is established, which by training enables the paraplegic to restore his upright position.

3   In the process of reconditioning of the spinal man, the development of a new pattern of postural sensibility by re-orientation of the afferent system is a prerequisite for the compensatory action of the muscular system. This is accomplished, as pointed out, through proprioceptive impulses arising from any movement of the pelvis and transmitted centrally along the afferent pathways of the muscles mentioned above, which are innervated from segments of the cord above the transection. As described before, the new pattern of postural sensibility develops by training under visual control.

4   The analysis of the effects of postural changes on the cardio-vascular system in transection above T5, with a view to overcoming postural hypotension due to loss of the splanchnic control, has led to the mobilization and utilization of vasoconstrictor reflexes and other factors (exercises, sport and abdominal binder) to overcome the circulatory maladaptation in high cord lesions and secure sufficient cardiac output.

5   Another most striking evidence of the adjustment forces of the organism is the restoration of the vital capacity and ventilatory function of the lung in cervical lesions. This is achieved by the compensatory action of the remaining normal auxiliary respiratory muscles and, as described in detail also by adaptive reflex function of the paralysed intercostal muscles once a co-ordinating reflex function of the isolated cord has been established.

6   The loss of thermoregulation in cervical lesions, as a result of the interruption of autonomic mechanism subserving heat production and heat loss, which renders these patients poikilotherm in the acute and early stages following cord transection, by no means remains permanent. Our own studies and those of other workers in this field have clearly shown that homeothermia can be restored to a great extent by re-conditioning, even in these high lesions. In this connection, my observations during the Paraplegic Commonwealth Games in Jamaica, 1966, have been a great lesson on the adaptability of the spinal man to high temperature and humidity. Not only could men and women with complete lesions above T5 tolerate the high temperature and humidity, but they were able to indulge in strenuous sports activities. There could have been no better proof of applied physiological re-adaptation in the spinal man.

7   Last, but by no means least, the re-organization of bowel and bladder function has

been accomplished in one way or another, in the latter provided that infection of the urinary tract can be avoided and obstruction eliminated. Moreover, the generalization held dogmatically in the past, that the spinal man remains impotent and infertile has proved to be incorrect. One of the outstanding examples of readjustment in this respect is the ability of paraplegic and even tetraplegic women to become pregnant and bear children.

All those observations confirm Sherrington's dictum: 'Each and every part of the animal is integrative'. However, it must be remembered that the spinal man is not an animal like a cat or dog. He still remains a member of that species *Homo sapiens*, and is still endowed with all those intellectual faculties which distinguish him from all other types of mammal. He can use these faculties with sapientia—i.e. wisely—to modify the reflex functions of the isolated cord and thus re-connect them in one way or another with the control of the central nervous system, in order to re-integrate himself into the community. To achieve this, he has not only to utilize and develop his already known talents but to arouse and develop those hitherto dormant talents, which enable him to carve out a new and sometimes fuller life. This final achievement really represents the essence of rehabilitation in the spinal man. Thus the spinal man is a classical example of the integrative function of the central nervous system by transforming a chaotic multitude of components into a new functional unit and system activity.

THE MEANING OF TALENTS IN REHABILITATION

The word 'talent' can be interpreted either in general terms as an expression of high intelligence or more specifically as a gift of special aptitudes. In whatever sense it is used, talent even in our materialistic world is often looked upon as an emanation from Heaven. However, such unsophisticated simplification can hardly satisfy any scientific approach to define and analyse such a very complex spiritual quality. For, it disregards the intricate mechanism of neuronal activities of the brain, which conditions this extraordinary faculty as an outstanding feature in the formation of personality.

Throughout the years, theories based on anatomical, physiological and psychological studies have been put forward in an attempt to analyse the nature of talent. While no theory today denies the presence of some inherited or congenital feature in the pattern of talent nor disregards environmental forces, the differences lie mainly in the relative emphasis placed upon either of these two basic features.

In an attempt to analyse the nature of talent, three questions concerning the underlying neurophysiological mechanisms immediately arise:
1 Is talent the prerogative of man?
2 What role play experience and memory in the development of talents?
3 What is the significance of learning in relationship to experience and memory, and how does training contribute to promoting and retaining special memories over long periods in the development of special talents?

It is well known that certain specific aptitudes can be developed in various species of animals, which make them outstanding amongst their fellow creatures. Certain birds, especially the parrot group, develop the unique gift of imitating the human voice both for words and sounds including whistling. Certain species of dogs have the gift to act as guides for the blind, having been trained to develop visual, acoustic and olfactory associations. Certain species of monkeys can acquire more complex aptitudes, thanks to their more highly developed brain; for instance chimpanzees may be able to emulate human beings holding tea-parties. During a recent visit to Malaysia to advise on the setting up of a National Spinal Centre and National Paraplegia Service, I watched a monkey, tied to a very long lead, climb up a coconut tree and select carefully only ripe coconuts which it broke off and threw down to be picked up by its trainer—indeed an ingenious method of preventing spinal injuries in man!

While in all these animals the underlying anatomical and physiological processes of their talents is obscure, the importance of learning, resulting in the gaining of experience and the setting up as well as the retaining of memories over long periods, is beyond doubt. However, talents in animals remain fragmentary owing to their limited mental potentialities. It is only man, endowed with a highly differentiated brain, who distinguishes himself from all other mammals by manifold intellectual potentialities, which provide the basis of a great variety of talents. Hence, his designation as *Homo sapiens* within the philogenetic scale. Whether man always uses his talents fully and wisely is, of course, another matter. In this connection, one is reminded of the parable in the Gospel according to St Matthew, Chapter 25, 14–30, where the word talent is used in the terms of money. A man who was due to travel into a far land distributed five, two and one talents respectively to his three servants according to their individual abilities. The servant who received 5 talents, traded with them and doubled them and so did the servant who received 2, but the third, with his limited ability, was afraid to put his one talent into good use and buried it in the ground, thus gaining nothing. This allegoric story, applied to our interpretation of talent as a spiritual quality, indicates the diversity which exists in man's intellectual resources. These qualities, combined with an exceptional drive and imaginative creative power, may raise man's talent even to the height of genius. However, although genius cannot develop without creative thinking, yet through the lives of the geniuses of this world runs like a thread an infinite capacity for learning, training and concentrated effort to produce those highest degrees of performance which make their work and names immortal.

Music is indeed a good example for illustrating the complexity of talent, and in this respect Ludwig van Beethoven is a classical example.

In discussing the neuronal mechanism underlying the processes of learning and memory as essentials to talent, it must be remembered that the central nervous system is subjected to a continuous stream of multitudes of intrinsic and extrinsic impulses—that means stimuli emanating on the one hand from every part of the organism and on the other from the outside world. But only those impulses which arouse awareness and attention of the individual leave a lasting record, penetrating ganglion cells of the human brain by setting up structural impressions on them, generally called engrams. Although the definition of the word 'engram' is still a matter of discussion amongst physiologists and psychologists, it can be assumed that the perceptive neuronal elements affected by a stimulus and its emotional associations, be they visual, acoustic or olfactory, set into operation from early childhood inter-communications with other neurones through an intrinsic system of synapses, resulting in patterns of memories. The function of this complex neuronal network is to register and store the patterns of memories and consolidate them one with another and also to recall memories in the light of new experiences, either voluntarily or reflexly. Memories are only relatively static, as they are accessible to modifications and alterations, as a result of accumulation of new experiences by learning and training.

Where, in the human brain, the process of registration and storage of memories and their recall takes place is a matter of hypothesis and conjecture. No doubt, certain cortical areas with their communications with subcortical centres, especially thalamus, represent certain functions. The parietal lobe is connected with the motor and sensory functions, the temporal lobe with hearing, the occipital lobe with vision, the 2nd and 3rd convolutions of the frontal lobe with speech and the hippocampal zone with olfactory sensation. Destruction of one or several of these areas results in loss of the corresponding functional capacities. However, it is the frontal and temporal lobes, with their intercommunications with each other and with cortical as well as subcortical stations, in particular, the limbic system comprising the thalamus, hippocampus, amygdala, and mamillary bodies, which play an essential part in the perception and interpretation of experience and learning, as well as storage and recall of memories. There is abundant clinical evidence of the profound adverse effects which bilateral damage of the frontal and temporal lobes and their communications may have on learning and memory as a result of trauma and other pathological processes or surgical excisions. In this respect, the studies of Penfield and his associates on memories following excisions of parts of the temporal lobe area, are of particular interest and importance and have thrown some light on this complex process of memory and learning. For, they show conclusively that bilateral removal of the hippocampus and hippocampal gyrus in man results in loss of recent memory, while memory for the distant past is not lost, nor is the memory for words, speech, reasoning ability and previously acquired skill disturbed (Penfield & Milner, 1958; Penfield, 1958).

From all this, the importance of environmental forces on the creation and development of talent is undeniable. The reaction of the individual to environmental pressure, however, varies considerably. This is due to the personality construction of the individual, which is conditioned to a greater or lesser degree also by hereditary factors, whereby the alternating dominance from either of the parents may have an influence in making specified aptitudes apparent. There are well-known examples of outstanding talents of the same or different types in certain families, such as the mathematical talent amongst members of the Swiss family Bernouilli or the musical talents in the families of Bach, Mozart, Beethoven, Schumann, and our contemporary family of Yehudi Menuhin. Amongst these, Beethoven is of special interest.

He doubtless inherited his basic musical talent from his father and grandfather, both of whom were practising musicians. But, their artistic faculties remained limited, as neither of them possessed his unique power of creation and concentration, which remained indestructible throughout his whole life and even became intensified during the years of his severe disability.

Therefore, his case is a unique example to all concerned with rehabilitation of how either new talents can be discovered and developed or existing talents diverted into other channels when a person is stricken by a severe disability. At the age of 29 or 30, when Beethoven's prestige as a solo pianist was at its zenith, he became deaf. From his letters to his close friends, one gets an insight into his mental agony, especially during the early stage of his illness, when he rebelled, as is typical of so many disabled people and described in this book on paraplegia, against his fate, combined with the fear of being detected. In his letter of 1 January 1800, to Amenda, a theologian, he wrote: '. . . Your Beethoven is living an unhappy life, quarrelling with nature and its Creator, often cursing the latter because He surrenders His creatures to the merest accident that sometimes breaks and destroys the most beautiful blossoms. Know that my noblest faculty, my hearing, has gradually deteriorated.' In fact, in due course he became completely deaf.

It is a well-known fact that patients in the rebellious frame of mind against their disability curse not only God but also, naturally, their medical advisers, especially those who give false hopes to their patients, and, again, Beethoven is a classical example. In his famous 'Heiligenstadt Will', 1804, he recorded to his brothers his horror of his impending deafness: 'I was ever eager to accomplish great deeds but reflect now that for six years I have been a hopeless case, aggravated by senseless physicians, cheated year after year in the hope for improvement, finally compelled to face the prospect of a lasting malady. . . . For me there can be no recreation in the society of my fellows, refined intercourse and mutual exchange of thoughts, only just as little as the greatest needs demand do I mix with society, I must live like an exile.' Yet in the same document, one can already find the first signs of his determination to come to terms with his disability and to rise above it. He wrote—'I would have put an end to my life, only art it was that withheld me, it seemed impossible to leave the world until I produced all that I felt was called upon me to produce and so I endured this wretched existence. . . .' Actually, while his deafness made an end to his career as a solo pianist, his inner ear, fortunately for the community at large and for all times, remained unaffected by his illness, which, although forcing him to withdraw into loneliness, made him direct his indomitable creative energy to his compositions. Utilizing all his remaining spiritual potentialities, he rose through his disability to that brilliant genius which made his work and name immortal.

Everyone who has experience in the rehabilitation of the severely physically handicapped will agree, that all disabled are in some way like the servants described in the Gospel according to St Matthew. We have all been entrusted with talents in life, and when the challenge comes to some of us in the nature of some physical disaster we employ these talents according to our individual personalities, conditioned by environmental and hereditary factors. Some, like the servants entrusted with five or two talents, rise nobly to the occasion and with great courage and self-discipline use their talents to build up for themselves a new scheme of life. Some examples have been given in this book. They are rewarded for their endeavours by regaining their self-confidence and self-respect and, in spite of their remaining disability, become useful and respected members of society. But there are some who, like the third servant who buried his talent in the earth, make no effort to utilize their remaining spiritual potentialities but instead resign themselves hopelessly into their disability, regardless of whether they have been entrusted with one or many talents. For these, there is no reward of self-achievement and self-dignity, for, in addition to their physical handicap, their soul is crippled, which makes them outcasts of society.

From all these considerations, it is obvious that the essence of rehabilitation of the severely physically handicapped, such as spinal paraplegics and tetraplegics, must lie in restoring activity of mind and promoting their determination to utilize those talents which are already apparent and manifest, in addition to encouraging new talents by awakening and mobilizing those intellectual potentialities which are still dormant. In this process, early education and training of the disabled child and teenager and retraining of the adult with mature brain are the indispensable essentials. Education and training should be the guiding principles in our work in rehabilitating the disabled of any age, to counteract from the start those adverse psychological effects which follow almost inevitably in the wake of severe disability—namely, frustration, apathy and resignation. Only then can new and dormant talents of the disabled be mobilized to enable him to become once again a respected and useful member of the community.

In the previous chapter I have given only a few outstanding examples of paraplegics and tetraplegics, who have developed old talents and mobilized new talents, but they could be amplified by hundreds and thousands, all over the world.

One could only wish that the community at large would also recognize the new talents exhibited by paraplegics and other severely disabled in the field of training and employment. The old prejudice towards a person in a wheelchair dies hard. Indeed, there is still a great need for educating the public as a whole to give their disabled fellow men, women and children fair chances for their social re-integration by providing more and better facilities both in places of employment and in particular in ordinary schools and universities, to give wheelchair users the opportunity to be educated in company with their able-bodied fellows. Although some progress has been made since we started our work on spinal cord sufferers 32 years ago there is still much to be desired.

In conclusion, there is a wealth of talent lying dormant in human beings, and paradoxically and ironically enough, it often takes a disaster in life resulting in severe disability to bring it out! But, when the disabled, with determination and concentrated effort, develops his dormant talents, with what pride and satisfaction is he rewarded and with what priceless treasures the community enriched!

REFERENCES

A. INTRODUCTION

Chapters 1–6

ADAMS F. (1891) *The Genuine Works of Hippocrates*, Vol. II, pp. 114–123. New York.

ALLEN D. (1967) Spinal unit at the Star and Garter Home. *The Cord*, **17**, 14.

AMAKO T. (1967) Workshops for paraplegics in Japan. *Paraplegia*, **5**, 131–132.

AVICENNA (980–1037) *Avicennae Operum de Rex Medica*, Vol. II, pp. 100, 284–285. Venice, 1544.

BEARSTED J.H. (1930) *The Edwin Smith Surgica Papyrus*, Vol. 1, pp. 316–342, 425–428. Chicago.

BEDBROOK G. (1967) *Organisation of a Spinal Injuries Unit at Royal Perth Hospital, Perth, Western Australia*.

BELL, SIR CHARLES (1824) *Observations on Injuries of the Spine and the Thigh Bone*, pp. 3–31.

BORS E. (1967) The Spinal Cord Injury Center of the Veteran Administration Hospital, Long Beach, California, U.S.A. Facts and Thought. *Paraplegia*, **5**, 126–130.

BOTTERELL, E.H., JOUSSE A.T., KRAUS A.S., THOMPSON M.G., WYNNE-JONES M. & GEISLER W.O. (1975) A model for the future care of acute spinal cord injuries. *Ann. Roy. Coll. Phys. & Surg. of Canada*, **00**, 193.

CALOT T.P. (1896) Des Moyens de guérir la boss du mal de Pott. *France méd.*, **52**.

CELSUS A.C. (100 BC) *Of Medicine*, Transl. by James Greive, pp. 494, 509–510. London, 1756.

COOPER, SIR ASTLEY (1824) *Principles and Practice of Surgery*, London.

CUSHING H. (1927) *The Med. Dept. United States Army in World War Surgery II*, Part 1, 757.

DICK T.B.S. (1949) Rehabilitation in chronic paraplegia, M.D. Thesis, University Manchester.

DICK T.B.S. (1969) Traumatic paraplegia pre-Guttmann, *Paraplegia*, **7**, 173–178.

EVERTS W.H. & WOODHALL B. (1944) *J. Amer. Med. Ass.*, **126**, 145.

GALEN (AD 131) *Omnie Opera*, Carolus Kühn edition, pp. 237–250. Leipzig 1821.

GOLDING J. (1964) *First Symposium on Rehabilitation*, Kampala, Uganda. Nat. Fund for Crippling Dis., London.

GOWLAND E.L. (1934) *Med. Press*, **188**, 81.

GOWLAND E.L. (1941) *Brit. Med. J.*, i, 814.

GREGG T. (1967) Organisation of a spinal injury unit within a rehabilitation centre. *Paraplegia*, **5**, 163–166.

GUTTMANN L. (1966) Establishing spinal injuries units in Africa. *2nd Symposium on Rehabilitation*, pp. 178–179. Nat. Fund for Crippling Dis., London.

GUTTMANN L. (1967) History of the National Spinal Injuries Centre, Stoke Mandeville Hospital, Aylesbury, *Paraplegia*, **5**, 115–126.

JACOBSON S.A. & BORS E. (1970) Spinal cord injury in Vietnamese combat. *Paraplegia*, **7**, 263–281.

LOUIS A. (1762) quoted by KUHN R.A. (1947) *J. Neurosurg.*, **4**, 40.

MAGLIO A. (1967) Organisation of an autonomous spinal unit as part of a national accident insurance organisation (Italy). *Paraplegia*, **5**, 176–178.

MALING R.G. & CLARKSON D.C. (1963) Electronic control for the tetraplegic. *Paraplegia*, **1**, 161–174.

MEINECKE F.W. (1967) The situation of a spinal unit in an accident hospital. *Paraplegia*, **5**, 147–150.

ORIBASIUS (324–400) *Oeuvres d'Oribase*, Darenberg edition, Vol. IV, pp. 242–243, 449–451. Paris 1862.

PAESLACK V. (1967) Organisation of a spinal injuries unit within a university hospital. *Paraplegia*, **5**, 140–142.

PARÉ A. (1564) *Dix-Livres de Chirurgie*. Paris.

PAULUS OF AEGINA (625–690) *Adams F.*, Vol. II, pp. 493–497. London, 1846.

ROLAND OF PARMA (1210) *Chirurgia*.

ROPER A. (1964) *First Symposium on Rehabilitation*, Kampala, Uganda. Nat. Fund for Crippling Dis., London.

ROSSIER A. (1967) Organisation and function of the French Swiss Paraplegic Centre. *Paraplegia*, **5**, 166–170.

SARRIAS, DOMINGO M. (1967) Organisation of an autonomous spinal injuries unit (Spain). *Paraplegia*, **5**, 170–176.

SÖMMERING J. (1793) *Bemerkungen über Verrenkung und Bruch des Rückgraths*, pp. 3–40. Berlin.

THOMSON-WALKER, SIR J. (1917) *Lancet*, i, 173.

THOMSON-WALKER, SIR J. (1937) *Proc. Royal Soc. Med.*, **30**, 1233.

VELLACOTT P.N. & WEBB-JOHNSON A.E. (1919) *Lancet*, i, 173.

VIDUS VIDIUS (1544) *Chirurgia è Graeco in Latinum connersa*, Paris.

WILSON D.H. (1966) Paraplegia in tropical Africa. *Proc. 2nd Symposium on Rehabilitation in Africa*, pp. 171–177. Nat. Fund for Crippling Dis., London, Vincent Square.

B. ANATOMY, NEUROPATHOLOGY AND REGENERATION

Chapter 7 Anatomical Data on Vertebral Column and Spinal Cord

ADACHI B. (1928) *Das Arteriensystem der Japaner*. Maruzen, Kyoto.

ADAMKIEWICZ A.S.B. (1881) *Akad. Wiss. Wien. Math.-Nat.Kl.*, **84**, 496.

ADAMKIEWICZ A.S.B. (1882) *Akad. Wiss. Wien. Math.-Nat.Kl. Abt.*, **85**, 101–130.

BALTHASAR K. (1952) Morphologie der spinalen tibialis — und peroneus — Kerne bei der Katze. *Arch. Psychiat. Z. Neurol.*, **199**, 345.

BIKELES G. & FRANKE M. (1905) Die Localization im Rückenmark für motorische Nerven der vorderen und hinteren Extremtät. *Dtsch. Z. Nervenhk*, **29**, 171.

BOLTON R. (1939) The blood supply of the human spinal cord. *J. Neurol. & Psychiat*, **2**, 137.

BRADFORD F. & SPURLING R. (1945) *The Intervertebral Disc*. Enke, Stuttgart.

BROCHER J.E.W. (1955) *Die Occipital-Cervical-Gegend*. G. Thieme, Stuttgart.

CAJAL, S. RAMON (1935) Die Neuronenlehre. In *Handbuch der Neurologie*, Vol. I, pp. 887–899. Bumke und Foerster (eds.).

CLARKE J.A.L. (1851) *Philos. Tr. Soc., London*, **141**, 607–621.

DOMISSE G.E. (1975) *The arteries and veins of the human spinal cord from birth*. Churchill Livingstone, Edinburgh.

ECCLES J. (1963) *The Physiology of Synapses*. Springer, Berlin.

FOREL A. (1887) Einige hirnanatomische Betrachtungen und Ergebnisse. *Arch. Psychiat. Nervenkr.*, **18**, 162–198.

FRETTS L. (1911) Über die Variabilität der Wirbelsäule. *Gegenbaur morph. Jb.*, **43**, 449.

FRYKHOLM R. (1970) Die cervicalen Bandscheibenschäden. In *Handbuch der Neurochirurgie*, pp. 62–163. Springer, Berlin.

GALLAND U. (1930) Le nucleus pulposus. *Press méd.*, 16th April.

GARCIA R., ZÜLCH K., LAZORTHES G. & GRUNNER J. (1962) *Pathologie Vasculaire de la Moelle*. Masson, Paris.

GEHUCHTEN A. VON & NEEF C. DE (1900) Les noyaux noteurs de la moelle lombo-sacree chez l'homme. *Le Névraxe*, **1**, 1.

GERLACH J. (1871) Von dem Rückenmarke. In *Handbuch der Lehre von den Geweben*, Vol. 2, Stricker (ed).

GLEES P. (1961) *Experimental Neurology*, p. 163. Clarendon Press, Oxford.

GOLGI C. (1886) *Sulla Fina Anatomia Degli Organi Centralis Del Sistema Nervoso*. Hoepli, Milan.

GUTTMANN L. (1936) Physiologie und Pathologie der Liquormechanik und Liquordynamik. In *Handbuch der Neurologie*, Vol. VII/2, pp. 1–114, Foerster und Bumke (eds). Springer, Berlin.

HAYMAKER, WEBB (1956) *Bing's Local Diagnosis in Neurological Diseases*. C. V. Mosby, St Louis.

HELD H. (1905) Zur Kenntnis einer neurofibrillären Continuität des Zentralnervensystems der Wirbel. *Arch. Anat. Physiol.*, 55–78.

HELD H. (1929) Die Lehre von den Neuronen und vom Nervencytium. *Fortschr. naturw. Forsch.* N.F., H.8.

HIS W. (1886) *Zur Geschichte des menschlichen Rückenmarks und der Nervenwurzeln*. Leipzig.

JELLINGER K. (1966) *Zur Orthologie und Pathologie der Rückenmarksdurchblutung*. Springer, Wien.

KADYI H. (1889) *Über die Blutgefässe des menschlichen Rückenmarks*. Gubrinowicz und Schmidt, Lemberg.

LAZORTHES G., POULHES J., BASTIDE G., ROULLEAU J. & CHANCHOLLE A. (1958) La vascularisation artérielle de la moelle. *Neuro-Chirurgie*, **4**, 3–19.

LOB A. (1954) *Die Wirbelsaulenverletzungen und ihre Ausheilung*. Georg Thieme, Stuttgart.

MAIR W.S.P. & DRUCKMAN R. (1953) The pathology of spinal cord lesions and their relation to the clinical feature in protrusion of cervical intervertebral discs. *Brain*, **76**, 70–91.

MEHLER F.A. (1848) *Neuroanatomy*, pp. 33–35. Mosby, St Louis.

MIXTER W.J. & BARR J.S. (1934) Rupture of the intervertebral disc with involvement of the spinal cord. *New Engl. J. Med.*, **211**, 210.

NISSL F. (1903) *Die Neuronenlehre und ihre Anhänger*. Fischer, Jena.

PISCOL K. (1972) Blood supply of the Spinal Cord. Springer, Berlin.

POLLACK E. (1935) Anatomie des Rückenmarks. In *Handbuch der Neurologie*, Vol. 1, p. 265. Bumke und Foerster (eds), Springer, Berlin.

PÜSCHEL J. (1930) *Beitr. path. Anat.*, **84**.

RIO-HORTEGA, DEL. P. (1921) La glia de escasus radiacones (oligodendro glia). *Bol. Soc. Hist. Nat.*, **21**, 63–92.

RIO-HORTEGA, DEL. P. (1932) In *Cytology and Cellular Pathology of the Nervous System*, Vol. 2, p. 485. Penfield W. (ed.), Hoeber, New York.

ROMANES G.J. (1951) *The Motor Cell Columns of the Lumbo-sacral Spinal Cord of the Cat*.

ROMANES G.J. (1965) The arterial blood supply of the human spinal cord. *Paraplegia*, **2**, 199.

SCHLÜTER K. (1964) Spannungsoptische Modelversuche zu den Rissformen im Bereich der Zwischenwirbelscheibe. *Fortschr. Med.*, **82**, 135.

SCHMORL G. (1927–32) In *Die gesunde und die kranke Wirbelsaule in Röntgenbild und Klinik*, 5th Ed. G. Thieme, Stuttgart.

SCHMORL G. & JUNGHANNS H. (1927–32) In *Die gesunde und die kranke Wirbelsäule in Röntgenbild und Klinik*. 5th Ed. Georg Thieme, Stuttgart.

SHARRARD W.J. (1956) *British Surgical Progress*, p. 83.

SHERRINGTON C. (1897) The central nervous system. In *Textbook of Physiology*, Vol. 3. Macmillan, London.

SPIELMAYER W. (1922) *Histopathologie des Nervensystems I*. Springer, Berlin.

SUH T.H. & ALEXANDER L. (1939) Vascular system of the human spinal cord. *Archs Neurol. Psychiat. Chicago* **41**, 659–677.

TANON L. (1908) *Thèse de Paris*, p. 98. Vigot Frères.

TONDURG G. (1958) *Entwicklungsgeschichte und Fehlbildungen der Wirbelsäule*. Stuttgart.

TÖNNIS D. (1963) Rückenmarkstrauma und Mangeldurchblutung. *Beitr. zur Neurochirurgie*.

TUREEN L. (1938) Circulation of the spinal cord and the effect of vascular occlusion. *A. Res. Nerve. Ment. Dis. Proc.*, **18**, 394–437.

TURNBULL I., BRIEG A. & HASSLER O. (1966) *J. Neurosurg.*, **24**, 951–965.

WALMSLEY R. (1950) *Edinb. Med. J.* **60**.

ZÜLCH K.J. (1954) Mangeldurchblutung an der Grenzzone zweier Gefässgebiete etc. *Deutche Ztschr. Nervenheilk.*, **172**, 81–101.

Chapter 8 Neuropathology of Spinal Cord and Spinal Roots

BECKER J. & HESS F. (1954) Zur Frage der Spätlähmungen bei Wirbelsäulendeformitäten. *Dtsch. Z. Nervenhk.*, **171**, 228.

BECKER J. (1958) Zur Klinik der spinalen Durchblutungsstörungen. *Nervenarzt.*, **29**, 16.

DAVISON C. (1945) Trauma of the central nervous system. *Proc. Ass. Res. nerve, ment. Dis.* 24. Publ. Williams and Wilkins.

FOERSTER O. (1929) Die traumatischen Läsionen des Rückenmarks auf Grund der Kriegserfahrungen. In *Handbuch der Neurologie*, pp. 1722–1933, Bumke und Foerster (eds). Springer, Berlin.

GREENFIELD J.G. (1958) Traumatic lesions of the spinal cord. In *Neuropathology*, pp. 426–431. Arnold, London.

GUILLAIN G. & BARRÉ J.A. (1917) Etude anatome-clinique de 15 cas de section totale de la moelle. *Ann. Méd.*, 1917.

HARANDI A., ABAZARI M. & ZAHIR, A. (1975) Vertebral haemangiomatosis causing paraplegia. *Paraplegia*, **13**, 89.

HARTMANN F. (1900) Klinische und pathologisch-anatomische Untersuchungen über die unkomplizierten Rückenmarkserkrankungen. *Jb. Psychiatr.*, **19**, 380.

HASSIN S.B. (1923) *Archs Neurol. Psychiat., Chicago*, **10**, 194.

L'HERMITTE J. (1932) Étude de la commotion de la moelle. *Rev. neurol.*, **39**, I, 210.

HUGHES J.T. (1964) *Pathology of the Spinal Cord*, pp. 1–196. Lloyd-Luke, London.

JACOB A. (1919) Zur Pathologie der Rückenmarkserschüttreung. *Z. Neur.*, **51**, 244.

JELLINGER K. (1966) *Zur Orthologie und Pathologie der Rückenmarksdurchblutung*. Springer, Wien and New York.

KIENBÖCK A. (1902) Kritik der sogenannten 'traumatischen Syringomyelie'. *Jb. Psychiat.*, **21**, 50.

KLAUE R. (1969) Die traumatischen Schädigungen des Rückenmarks und seiner Hüllen. In *Handbuch der Neurochirurgie*, Vol. VII, 1, pp. 375–400, Olivecrone O. & Tönnis W. (eds). Springer, Berlin.

MARBURG O. (1936) Die traumatischen Erkrankungen des Gehirns und Rückenmarks. In *Handbuch der Neurologie*, Vol. XI, pp. 1–177, Bumke und Foerster (eds). Springer, Berlin.

MAYER E.T. & PETERS G. (1971) Pathologische Anatomie der Rückenmarkverletzungen. In *Neuro-Traumatologie*, Vol. II. *Rückenmark*, Sir Ludwig Guttmann (ed.). Urban und Schwarzenberg, München.

OBERSTEINER L. (1879) Über Erschütterung des Rückenmarks. *Wien. med. Jb.*, 531.

ROUSSY J. & L'HERMITTE J. (1918) *Blessures de la Moelle et de la Queue de Cheval*. Masson, Paris.

SCARFF J.E. & POOL J.L. (1946) Factors causing massive spasm following transection of the cord in man. *J. Neurosurg.*, **3**, 4, 285.

SCHNEIDER R.C. (1955) The syndrom of acute anterior spinal cord injury. *J. Neurosurg.*, **12**, 95.

TÖNNIS D. (1963) Rückenmarkstrauma und Mangeldurchblutung. In *Beiträge zur Neurochirurgie*, W. Tönnis (ed.). J. Ambr. Barth, Leipzig.

WOLMAN L. (1965) The neuropathology of traumatic paraplegia. *Paraplegia*, **1**, 233–251.

ZÜLCH (1954) *Dtsch. Z. Nervenheilk*, **172**, 81.

ZÜLCH (1967) Die spinale Mangeldurchblutung und ihre Folgen. *Verh. dtsch. Ges. inn. Med.*, **72**, 1007–1059.

Chapter 9 Spinal Cord Ischaemia

ADAMS H.D. & VAN GEERTRUYDEN H.H. (1956) Neurologic complications of aortic surgery. *Ann. Surg.*, **144**, 574.

ALLEN A.R. (1911) Surgery of experimental lesion of spinal cord equivalent to crush injury of fracture dislocation of spinal column: A preliminary report. *J. Am. med. Ass.*, **57**, 878–880.

ALLEN A.R. (1914) Remarks on the histopathological changes in the spinal cord due to impact. An experimental study. *J. nerv. ment. Dis.*, **41**, 141–147.

BLACK P. & MARKOWITZ R.S. (1971) Experimental spinal cord injury in monkeys; Comparison of steroids and local hypothermia. *Surg. Forum.*, **22**, 409–411.

CAMPBELL J.B., DECRESCITO V., TOMASULA J.J. *et al.* (1971) *Biolectric prediction of permanent post-traumatic paraplegia.* Read before the 1971 meeting of the American Association of Neurological Surgeons, Houston, 20 April 1971.

DANIELL H.B., FRANCIS W.W., LEE W.A. & DUCKER T.B. (1975) A method of quantitating injury inflicted in acute spinal cord studies. *Paraplegia*, **13**, 137.

DOHRMANN G.D., WAGNER F.C. JR., WICK K.M. & BUCY P.C. (1971) Fine structural alterations in transitory traumatic paraplegia. *Proc. XVIII Vet. Admin. Spinal Cord Inj. Conf.*, 5–7 October 1971. 6–8.

FERGUSON L.R.J., BERGAN M.D., CONN, J. JR. & YAO J.S.T. (1975) Spinal ischemia following abdominal aortic surgery. *Ann. Surg.*, **181**, 267–272.

GUMP F.E. (1969) Paraplegia after resection of aneurysm. *New Engl. J. Med.*, **281**, 798.

HARA M. & LIPIN, R.J. (1960) Spinal cord injury following resection of abdominal aortic aneurysm. *Archs Surg.*, **80**, 419.

JELLINGER K. (1967) Spinal cord arteriosclerosis and progressive vascular myelopathy. *J. Neurol. Neurosurg. Psychiat.*, **30**, 195.

KIRCHGASSER G. (1897) Experimentalle Untersuchungen uber Ruckenmarkserschutterung. *Deutsche Z. Nervneh*, **11**, 408–419.

PASTERNAK B.M., BOYD D.P. & ELLIS F.H. JR. (1972) Spinal cord injury after procedures on the aorta. *Surgery Gynec. Obstet.*, **135**, 29.

RICHARDSON H.A. & NAKAMURA S. (1971) An electron microscopic study of spinal cord edema and the effect of treatment with steroids, manniton, and hypothermia. *Proc. XVIII Vet. Admin. Spinal Cord Inj. Conf.*, 5–7 October, 1971, 0–16.

SCHMAUS H. (1890) Beitrage zur pathologischen anatomie der ruckenmarkserschutterung. *Virchows Arch.*, **122**, 470–495.

SHER M.H. & HEALY E.H. (1971) Paraplegia following infrarenal aneurysmorrhaphy. *Vasc. Surg.*, **5**, 171.

SPILLER W.G. (1899) A critical summary of recent literature on concussion of the spinal cord with some original observations. *Am. J. med. Sci.*, **118**, 190–198.

TARLOV I.M., KLINGER H. & VITALE S. (1953) Spinal cord compression studies: 1. Experimental techniques to produce acture and gradual compression. *Archs Neurol. Psychiat.*, **70**, 813–819.

TARLOV I.M. & KLINGER H. (1954) Spinal cord compression studies: II. Time limits for recovery after acute compression in dogs. *Archs Neurol. Psychiat.*, **71**, 271–290.

TATOR C.H. (1971) Experimental circumferential compression injury of primate spinal cord. *Proc. XVIII Vet. Admin. Spinal Cord Inj. Conf.*, 5–7 October 1971, 2–5.

TATOR C.H. (1971) Experimental circumferential compression injury of primate spinal cord. *Proc. Annu. Clin. Spinal Cord Inj. Conf.*

TATOR C.H. & DEECKE L. (1973) Value of normothermic perfusion and durotomy in the treatment of experimental acute spinal cord trauma. *J. Neurosurg.*, **39**, 52–64.

WAGNER F.C., GREEN B.A. & BUCY P.C. (1971) Spinal cord edema associated with paraplegia. *Proc. XVIII Vet. Admin. Spinal Cord Injury Conf.*, 5–7 October 1971, 9.

YEO J., PAYNE W. & HINWOOD B. (1975) The experimental contusion injury of the spinal cord in sheep. *Paraplegia*, **12**, 275.

Chapter 10   Regeneration of the Spinal Cord

BABBINI R. (1956) Suture medullaire. *Neuro-Chirurgie*, T2, N2.

CAJAL, RAMON Y. (1928) *Degeneration and Regeneration of the Nervous System.* Oxford, Univ. Press.

CAMPBELL (1967) *16th Clin. Spinal Cord. Conf.* Long Beach, U.S.A., p. 102.

CAPOROSO L. (1889) Sulla rigenerazione del midollo spinale della coda dei tritoni. *Beitr. path. Anat.*, **5**, 67–98.

FOERSTER O. (1936) *Handbuch der Neurologie*, Vol. V. Springer, Berlin.

FOWLER G.R. (1905) A case of suture of the spinal cord, following a gunshot injury involving complete severance of the structure. *Ann. Surg.*, **42**, 507–513.

FREEMAN L.W. (1952) Return of function after complete transection of the spinal cord of the rat, cat and dog. *Ann. Surg.*, **136**, 193–205.

FREEMAN L.W. (1954) Return of spinal cord function in mammals after transecting lesions. *Ann. N.Y. Acad. Sc.*, **58**, 564–569.

GUTTMANN L. (1936) Röntgendiagnostik des Gehirns und Rückenmarks durch Kontrastverfahren. In *Handbuch der Neurologie*, Vol. VII/2, 187–491, pp. 481–483. Foerster und Bumke (eds) Springer, Berlin.

HAMBURGER V. (1948) The mitotic pattern in the spinal cord of the chick embryo and their relation to histogenic processes. *J. Comp. Neur.*, **88**, 221–284.

HARTE R.H. & STEWART E.T. (1902) A case of severed spinal cord in which myeloraphy was followed by partial return of function. *Tr. Am. Surg. Ass.*, **20**, 28–38.

MARINESCO G. & MINEA J. (1906a) Recherches sur la régéneréscence de la moelle. *N. iconog. Salpétrière*, Par. **19**, 417–440.

MARINESCO G. & MINEA J. (1906b) Note sur la régéneréscence de la moelle chez l'homme. *C. rend. Sco. biol.*, **60**, 1027–1028.

MARINESCO G. & MINEA J. (1910/11) Nouvelles contribution à l'étude de la régéneréscence de la moelle et du cervelet. *J. Psychol. Neur.*, **1**, 2, 17, 116–143.

MINEA I. (1928) Sur quelques réactions des axones dans la sclérose en plaques. *C. rend. Soc. biol.*, **98**, 1474–1479.

MÜLLER H. (1864–65) Über Regeneration der Wirbelsäule und des Rückenmarks bei Tritonen und Eidechsen. *Abb. Senken. naturf. Ges., Frankfurt*, **5**, 113–136.

STREET D.M. (1967) Traumatic paraplegia treated by vertebral resection, excision of the spinal cord, suture and interbody fusion. In *Proc. 16th Clin. Spinal Cord Conf., Amer. Adm. Hosp.*, Long Beach, pp 92–99.

TARLOW I.M. (1957) *Spinal Cord Compression*. Ch. Thomas, Springfield, Ill.

THOMERET G. (1960) Suture de la moelle épinière (a propos deux cas). *Memoires de l'Academie de Chirurgie*, No. 1 et 5.

WINDLE W.F. (1955) *Regeneration in the Central Nervous System*. Ch. Thomas, Springfield, Ill.

WOLMAN L. (1966) Axon regeneration after spinal cord injury. *Paraplegia*, **4**, 175–183.

C. FRACTURES AND DISLOCATIONS OF THE VERTEBRAL COLUMN

Chapters 11–12   Mechanism—Classification

BARNES R. (1948) Paraplegia in cervical spine injuries. *J. Bone & Joint Surg.*, **30B**, 239.

BARNES R. (1951) Mechanism of cord injury without vertebral dislocation. *J. Bone & Joint Surg.*, **33B**, 494.

BARWOOD A.J. (1975) Sources of ejection injury. *Proc. roy. Soc. Med.*, **68**, 721.

BEDBROOK G. (1969) Intrinsic factors in the development of spinal deformities with paralysis. *Paraplegia*, **6**, 222–232

BEDBROOK G. (1969) Are cervical fractures ever unstable? *Western Pacific Orthop. Ass.*, **6**, 7.

BEDBROOK G. (1971) Stability of spinal fractures and fracture dislocations. *Paraplegia*, **9**, 23–32.

BERGMANN E.W. (1949) Fractures of the ankylosed spine. *J. Bone & Joint Surg.*, **31A**, 669.

BRAAKMAN R. & PENNING L. (1971) Injuries of the cervical spine. *Excerpta Medica, Amsterdam*.

BÖHLER L. (1937) Behandlung von Wirbelbrüchen mit und ohne Lähmung. *Zbl. Chir.*, 2210.

BÖHLER L. (1963) *Technik der Knochenbruchbehandlung (Erganzungsband)*. W. Mandrich, Wien.

BURKE D.C. (1971) Spinal cord trauma in children. *Paraplegia*, **9**, 1–12.

BURKE D.C. & BERRYMAN D. (1971) The place of closed manipulation in the management of flexion-rotation dislocation of the cervical spine. *J. Bone & Joint Surg.*, **53B**, 165–182.

BURTON L.G. (1938) Reduction of fracture-dislocations of cervical vertebrae by skeletal traction. *Surg. Gyne. & Obst.*, **67**, 94.

CHESHIRE D.J.E. (1969) Stability of the cervical spine following conservative treatment of fractures and fracture-dislocations. *Paraplegia*, **7**, 192–203.

CLOWARD R.B. (1958) The anterior approach for removal of ruptured cervical discs. *J. Neurosurg.*, **15**, 602.

CLOWARD R.B. (1961) Treatment of acute fracture and fracture dislocation of the cervical spine by vertebral-body fusion. *J. Neurosurg.*, **18**, 2, 201–209.

COMARR A.E. (1959) Laminectomy in patients with injuries of the spinal cord. *J. Intern. Coll. Surgeons*, **31**, 437.

CONE W. & TURNER W. (1939) The treatment of fracture-dislocations of the cervical vertebrae by skeletal traction and fusion. *J. Bone & Joint Surg.*, **19**, 584.

DURBIN F.C. (1957) Fracture dislocation of cervical spine. *J. Bone & Joint Surg.*, **39B**, 23.

EVANS D.K. (1961) Reduction of cervical dislocation. *J. Bone & Joint Surg.*, **43B**, 552.

FORSYTH H.F. & WINSTON-SALEM A. (1958) Extension injuries of the cervical spine. *J. Bone & Joint Surg.*, **46A**, 1792–1795.

FRANKEL, H., HANCOCK D., HYSLOP G., MELZAK J., MICHAELIS L., UNGAR G., VERNON J. & WALSH J. (1969) The value of postural reduction in the initial management of closed injuries of the spine with paraplegia and tetraplegia. *Paraplegia*, **7**, 179–192.

GALLIE W.E. (1937) Skeletal traction in treatment of fractures and dislocations of the cervical spine. *Ann. Surg.*, **106**, 770.

GALLIE W.E. (1939) Fractures and dislocations of the cervical spine. *Ann. J. Surg.*, **46**, 495.

GRIFFIN C.R. (1975) Spinal ejection injuries. *Proc. Roy. Soc. Med.*, **68**, 722.

GUTTMANN L. (1931) Trauma und Wirbelsäule (Trauma and Spine). *Hefte z. Unfallheilk.*, **8**, 37.

GUTTMANN L. (1949) Surgical aspects of the treatment of traumatic paraplegia. *J. Bone & Joint Surg.*, **31B**, 322.

GUTTMANN L. (1961) Errors and hazards of the treatment of traumatic paraplegia. *Langenbecks Arch. Kln. Chir.*, **298**, 184.

GUTTMANN L. (1963) Initial treatment of traumatic paraplegia and tetraplegia. *Proc. Symp. Spinal Injuries*, Harris P. (ed.). Roy. Coll. Surg., Edinburgh.

GUTTMANN L. (1966) Traumatic paraplegia and tetraplegia in ankylosing spondylitis. *Paraplegia*, **4**, 188–203.

GUTTMANN L. (1971) Principien und Methoden in der Behandlung und Rehabilitation von Rückenmarksverletzten. In *Neuro-Traumatologie*, Vol. II, Guttmann L. (ed.). Urban und Schwarzenberg, München.

GUTTMANN L. & FRANKEL H. (1966) The value of intermittent catheterisation. *Paraplegia*, **4**, 63–84.

HALL, McK. (1940) Clay shoveller's fracture. *J. Bone & Joint Surg.*, **22**, 63.

HARALSON R.H. & BOYD H.B. (1969) *J. Bone & Joint Surg.*, **51A**, 561.

HARRIS P. (1963) Some neurosurgical aspects of traumatic paraplegia. *Proc. Symp. Spinal Injuries*, Roy. Coll. Surg., Edinburgh, pp. 101–112.

HARDY A.G. (1965) *Paraplegia*, **3**, 112.

HOEN T.A. (1936) A method of skeletal traction for treatment of fracture dislocations of cervical vertebrae. *Archs Neurol. Psychiat.*, **36**, 158.

HOLDSWORTH F.W. & HARDY A.C. (1953) Early treatment of paraplegia from fractures of the thoracic and lumbar spine. *J. Bone & Joint Surg.*, **35B**, 540.

HOLDSWORTH F.W. (1963) *Proc. Symp. on Spinal Injuries*, Harris, P. (ed.). Roy. Coll. Surg., Edinburgh, pp 43–101 and 160–61.

HOWORTH B.M. & PETRIE G. (1964) *Injuries of the Spine*. Williams and Wilkins, Baltimore.

JEFFERSON, SIR G. (1920) Fracture of the atlas vertebrae. *Brit. J. Surg.*, **7**, 407.

JEFFERSON, SIR G. (1940) Discussion on fractures and dislocations of cervical vertebrae. *Proc. Roy. Soc.*, **33**, 657.

KAHN E.A. (1959) Paraplegia in cervical spinal injuries. *J. Bone & Joint Surg.*, **41A**, 6.

KUHLENDAHL H. (1966) Schleudertrauma der Halswirbelsäule. *Arch. Klin. Chir.*, **316**, 470–475.

LONERBLAD L. (1934) Disruption fracture of spinous processes as a trade injury. *Arch. chir scandinav.*, **74**, 434.

MADERSBACHER H. (1975) Urinary flow and flow pattern in paraplegics. *Paraplegia*, **13**, 95.

MATHES H.G. (1935) Dornfortsatzabrisse, eine typische Verletzung bei schweren Erdarbeitern. *Chirurg*, **7**, 665.

MAYER E.T. & PETERS G. (1971) Pathologische Anatomie der Rückenmarksverletzungen. In *Neuro-Traumatologie*, Vol. II pp. 44–45. Guttmann L. (ed.). Urban und Schwarzenberg, München.

MORGAN T.H., WHARTON G.W. & AUSTIN G.N. (1971) The results of laminectomy in patients with incomplete spinal cord injuries. *Paraplegia*, **1971**, 14–23.

MUNRO D. (1966) The factors that govern the stability of the spine. *Paraplegia*, **3**, 219–228.

PETRIE G. (1964) Flexion injuries of the cervical spine. *J. Bone & Joint Surg.*, **1964**, 1800–1806.

ROAF R. (1960) A study of the mechanics of spinal injuries. *J. Bone & Joint Surg.*, **42B**, 810.

ROAF R. (1972) International classification of spinal injuries. *Paraplegia*, **10**, 78.

ROWLAND L.P., SHAPIRO J.H. & JACOBSON H.S. (1958) *Archs Neurol. Psychiat.*, **80**, 286.

STIASMY H. (1933) Fractur der Halswirbelsäule bei spondylarthritis ankylopoetica. *Zentralbl. Chir.*, **60**, 998.

TAYLOR A.R. & BLACKWOOD W. (1948) Paraplegia in hyperextension. *J. Bone & Joint Surg.*, **30B**, 245–248.

VINKE T.H. (1948) A skull traction apparatus. *J. Bone & Joint Surg.*, **30A**, 527.

WADIA N.H. (1967) *Brain*, **90**, 449.

WAGNER W. & STOLPER P. (1898) *Die Verletzungen der Wirbelsäule und des Rückenmarks*. Enke, Stuttgart.

WATSON-JONES R. (1931) *J. Bone & Joint Surg.*, **13**, 383.

WATSON-JONES R. (1955) *Fractures and Joint Injuries* (4th Ed.). Livingstone, Edinburgh.

WITLEY J.E. & FORSYTH H.F. (1960) The classification of cervical injuries. *Am. J. Roentgenol.*, **83**, 633–644.

Chapter 13 Management of Spinal Fractures

ABRAMSON A.S. (1966) Early management of patients with trauma to the spinal cord. *Med. Serv. J. Canada*, **22**, 522. Discussion to Geister *et al.*

ALBIN M.S., WHITE R.J., ACOSTA RUA G., YASHON D. (1968) Cooling after Spinal Cord Injuries in Primates. *J. Neurosurg.*, **29**, 113.

ASCOLI R. (1970) In defence of the Foster-Stryker turning bed. *Paraplegia*, **8**, 117–118.

AUDIC B. & MAURY M. (1969) *Secondary Vertebral Deformities in Childhood and Adolescence.*

BAND D. (1963) *Proc. Symp. Spinal Injuries*, p. 47, Roy. Coll. Surg., Edinburgh.

BARTON L.G. (1938) *Surg. Gynec.-Obstet.*, **67**, 94.

BATCHELOR (1964) In *Injuries of the Spine*. p. 1964 Howorth M. & Petrie J. (eds.). Baltimore.

BEATSON T.R. (1963) *J. Bone & Joint Surg.*, **45B**, 21.

BEDBROOK G. (1963) Some pertinent observations on the pathology of traumatic paralysis. *Paraplegia*, **1**, 215–227.

BEDBROOK G. (1966) Pathological principles in the management of spinal trauma. *Paraplegia*, **4**, 43–56.

BEDBROOK G. (1971) Stability of spinal fractures and fracture dislocations. *Paraplegia*, **9**, 23–32.

BEDBROOK G.M. & EDIBAM R.C. (1973) The study of spinal deformity in traumatic spinal paralysis. *Paraplegia*, **10**, 321.

BELL, SIR CHARLES (1824) *Observations on Injuries of the spine and of the Thigh Bone*, pp. 3–31. London.

BENASSY J., BLANCHARD J. & LECOQ A. (1967) Neurological recovery rate in Para- and Tetraplegia. *Paraplegia*, **4**, 259–261.

BENĖS V. (1968) *Spinal Cord Injury*. Baillière, Tindall, Cassel, London.

BÖHLER L. (1935) *The Treatment of Fractures*. Wright & Son, Bristol.

BUCKLEY R.E. (1964) *Proc. 13th Clin. Spinal Cord Inj. Conf.*, p. foll. 6. Am. Vet. Admin., Richmond.

BUERGI H. (1963) Medizinische Forderungen bei der Versorgung von Notfallpatienten. *Schweiz. Aerztezeitung*, **44**, 219.

BURKE D. (1971) Hyperextension injuries of the spine. *J. Bone & Joint Surg.*, **53B**, 3–12.

BURKE D. & BERRYMAN D. (1971) *J. Bone & Joint Surg.*, **53B**, 165–182.

BURKE D.C. & TIONG T.S. (1975) Stability of the cervical spine after conservative treatment. *Paraplegia*, **13**, 191.

BURKLE-DE-LA CAMP (1940) Funktionelle Wirbelbruchbehandlung oder Bohlersohe Wirbelauf-richtung. *Langenbecks. Arch. Clin. Med.*, **200**, 321.

CHAHAL A.S. (1975) Results of continuous lumbar traction in acute dorso-lumbar spinal injuries with paraplegia. *Paraplegia*, **13**, 1.

CALOT T.F. (1896) Des moyens de guérir la boss du mal de Pott. *France méd.*, **52**.

CAREY P.C. (1965) Neurosurgery and Paraplegia. *The Cord*, **17**, 3, 14.

CLOWARD R.B. (1961) Treatment of acute fractures and fracture-dislocations of the cervical spine by vertebral body fusion. *J. Neurosurg.*, **18**, 2, 201–209.

CLOWARD R.B. (1962) Treatment of dislocations and fracture-dislocations of the cervical spine. *Neurosurgical News*, **2**, 1, 3–6.

COMARR A.E. (1959) Laminectomy in patients with injuries of the spinal cord. *J. Intern. Coll. Surgeons*, **31**, 47.

CONE W. & TURNER W.G. (1937) Treatment of fracture-dislocations of the cervical spine by skeletal traction and spinal fusion. *J. Bone & Joint Surg.*, **19**, 584.

COOPER, SIR ASTLEY (1824–27) *Principles and Practice of Surgery*. London.

COVALT D., COOPER I., HOEN T. & RUSK H. (1953) *Am. med. J.*, **151**, 89.

CRUTCHFIELD W.G. (1933) Skeletal traction for dislocation of the cervical spine. *Southern Surgeon*, **2**, 156.

CUTLER C.W. (1945) *J. Am. Med. Ass.*, **129**, 153.

DAVIS A.G. (1929) *Bone, Joint Surg.*, **11**, 1929.

DEL SEL J.M., CIBERIA J.B., ESPAGNOL R.O., DELSEL G.M. & DEL SEL H.J. (1975) Stability following fracture-dislocations of the cervical spine. *Paraplegia*, **13**, 208.

DICK I.L. (1953) *Edinburgh Med. J.*, **60**, 249.

DICK T.B. (1949) Rehabilitation in chronic paraplegia. M.D. Thesis, Manchester University.

DUCKER T.B. & HAMIT H.F. (1969) Experimental treatments of acute spinal cord injury. *J. Neurosurg.* **30**, 693–697.

DUNLOP J. & PARKER C.H. (1930) Correction of compressed fractures of vertebrae. *J. Am. Med. Ass.*, **94**, 89.

DUNLOP J. & PARKER C.H. (1933) *J. Bone & Joint Surg.*, **15**, 153.

DURBIN F.C. (1957) Fracture-dislocations of the cervical spine. *J. Bone & Joint Surg.*, **39B**, 23.

EHNI G. (1965) *Tex. St. J. Med.*, **61**, 746.

EVANS D.K. (1961) *J. Bone & Joint Surg.*, **43B**, 552.

FOERSTER O. (1929) Symptomatologie der Erkrankungen bei Rückenmarks. In *Handbuch der Neurologie*, Vol. 5, Springer, Berlin.

FRANKEL H. (1929) Ascending cord lesions in the early stages. *Paraplegia*, **7**, 111–116.

FRANKEL H., HANCOCK D.O., HYSLOP G., MELZAK J., MICHAELIS L., UNGAR G., VERNON J. & Walsh J. (1969) *The Value of Postural Reduction in the Initial Management of Closed Injuries of the Spine with Paraplegia and Tetraplegia. Paraplegia*, **7**, 179–192.

GEISLER W.O., WYNNE-JONES M. & JOUSSE A.T. (1966) *Med. Serv. J. Canada*, **22**, 512–523.

GREGG T. & WILMOT C. (1964) Flying squad. *Paraplegia*, **2**, 15.

GUTTMANN L. (1946) Postural reduction. *Nursing Times*, **42**, 798.

GUTTMANN L. (1949) Treatment and rehabilitation of spinal cord injuries. *Proc. Roy. Soc. Med.*, **40**, 219.

GUTTMANN L. (1954a) Statistical survey on 1000 paraplegics and initial treatment of traumatic paraplegia. *Proc. Roy. Soc. Med.*, **47**, 12.

GUTTMANN L. (1954b) Statistics on 1000 traumatic paraplegics and initial treatment of traumatic paraplegia. *Proc. Roy. Soc. Med.*, **47**, 5.

GUTTMANN L. (1954c) Statistical survey on 1000 paraplegics and initial treatment of traumatic paraplegia. *Proc. Roy. Soc. Med.*, **47**, 12.

GUTTMANN L. (1956) Initial treatment of traumatic paraplegia. *The Practitioner*, **176**, 157.

GUTTMANN L. (1965) A new turning-tilting bed. *Paraplegia*, **3**, 193–196.

GUTTMANN L. (1967) New turning-tilting bed and head-traction unit. *Br. med. J.*, **1**, 288.

GUTTMANN L. (1968) Principles of initial treatment of traumatic paraplegics and tetraplegics, *Festschrift for Sir Harry Platt* pp 18–28. Nat. Fund for Research into Crippling Diseases, London.

GUTTMANN L. (1969) Spinal deformities in traumatic paraplegics and tetraplegics following surgical procedures. *Paraplegia*, **7**, 38–49.

GUTTMANN L. (1971) Principien und Methoden in der Behandlung und Rehabilitation von Ruckenmarksverletzten. In *Neuro-Traumatologie* Vol. II, pp. 77–163. (ed.). Guttmann L. Urban & Schwarzenberg, Munich.

HACHEN H.J. (1974) Emergency transportation in the event of acute spinal cord lesion. *Paraplegia*, **12**, 33.

HANCOCK D.O. (1967) Congenital narrowing of the spinal canal. *Paraplegia*, **5**, 89–96.

HARDY A.G. (1965) Treatment of paraplegia due to fracture-dislocation of the dorso-lumbar spine. *Paraplegia*, **3**, 112.

HARDY A.G. (1969) *Paraplegia*, **7**, 51–52.

HARGEST T.S. (1975) The air fluidised bed as a solution. *Proceed. Congress Univ. Strathclyde*, p. 101.

HARRINGTON R. (1962) Treatment of scoliosis. **44A**, 591–610.

HARRIS P. (1963) *Proc. Symp. Spinal Injuries*, p. 105. Roy. Coll. Surg., Edinburgh.

HARRIS P. & WHATMORE W.J. (1969) Spinal deformity after spinal cord injury. *Paraplegia*, **6**, 232–238.

HAYNES W.G. (1946) *Am. J. Surg.*, **72**, 42.

HINCK V.L. & SACHDEV N.S. (1966) *Brain*, **89**, 27.

HOEN T.A. (1936) A method of skeletal traction for treatment of fracture-dislocations of cervical vertebrae. *Archs Neurol. Psychiat.*, **36**, 158.

HOLT E.P. (1964) Fallacy of cervical discography. Report of 50 cases in normal subjects. *J. Am. med. Ass.*, **188**, 799–801.

HOLT E.P. (1975) Further reflections on cervical discography. *J. Am. med. Ass.*, **231**, 613–614.

HOLDSWORTH F.W. & HARDY A.G. (1953) *J. Bone & Joint Surg.*, **35B**, 540.

HOLDSWORTH F.W. (1954) Personal Communication.

HOLDWORTH F. (1963) Early orthopaedic treatment of patients with spinal injuries. In *Proc. Symp, Spinal Injuries*, pp. 93–101, 160 and 162. Harris P. (ed.). Roy. Coll. Surg, Edinburgh.

JACKSON R.W. (1975) Surgical Stabilisation of the spine. *Paraplegia*, **13**, 71.

KAPLAN L., POWELL B., GRYNBAUM B. & RUSK H. (1966) *Comprehensive Follow-up Study on Spinal Cord Dysfunction*, p 13. New York.

KATZNELSON A.M. (1969) Stabilisation of the spine in traumatic paraplegia. *Paraplegia*, **7**, 33–37.

KEANE F. (1966) Roto-Rest. *Paraplegia*, **7**, 254–258.

KEMPE L. (1964) *Proc. 13th Clin. Spinal Cord Injury Confer*, p. 64. Am. Vet. Admin., Richmond.

KERR SUTCLIFFE A. (1956) Meeting Ass. Brit. Neurologists and Neurosurgeons, London.

KEY A. (1975) Cervical spine dislocations with unilateral facet interlocking. *Paraplegia*, **13**, 208.

LEIDHOLT J.D., YOUNG J., HAHN R.E., JACKSON R., GAMBLE W.E. & MILES T.S. (1969) Evaluation of late spinal deformities with fracture dislocation of the dorsal and lumbar spine in paraplegia. *Paraplegia*, **7**, 16–23.

LEIMBACH G. (1962) *Unfallchirurgische Operationen an Knochen und Gelenken*, pp. 251. Hippocrates Verlag, Stuttgart.

LOUGHEED W.M. & KAHN D.S. (1955) Circumvention of anoxia during arrest of cerebral circulation for intracarnial surgery. *J. Neurosurg.*, **12**, 226–239.

MACCRAVEY A. (1945) *J. Amer. Ass.*, **129**, 152.

MAGNUS G. (1931) Die Behandlung der Wirbelbrüchel. *Orthop. und Unfall Chir.*, **29**, 277–283.

MCSWEENEY T. (1969) Spinal deformity after spinal cord injury. *Paraplegia*, **6**, 212.

MCSWEENEY T. (1975) Discussion on treatment of spinal injuries. *Paraplegia*, **13**, 217.

MEINECKE F.W. (1964) Early treatment of traumatic paraplegia. *Paraplegia*, **3**, 262–270.

MERLE D'AUBIGNE, BENASSY J. & RAMADIER (1956) *Chirurgie Orthopédique des Paralysies*. Masson, Paris.

MORGAN T.H., WARTON G.W. & AUSTIN G.W. (1971) The results of laminectomy in patients with incomplete spinal cord lesions. *Paraplegia*, **9**, 14–23.

MUNRO D. (1945) *New Engl. J. Med.*, **233**, 453.

MUNRO D. (1965) The role of fusion or wiring in the treatment of acute traumatic instability. *Paraplegia*, **3**, 97–109.

MYERS P.W. (1967) Management of the complications of anterior cervical fusion. In *Proc. 16th Clin. Spinal Cord Conf.* pp. 33–38. Amer. Vet. Admin., Long Beach.

NEGRIN J. JR. & KLAUBER, L. (1960) Local hypothermia of the central nervous system. *N.Y. Neur. Soc., Sec. Neur. N.Y. Acad. Med. 1959; Proc. Arch. Neur.*, **3**, 122.

NEGRIN J. Jr. (1973) Spinal cord hypothermia in the neurosurgical management of the acute and chronic post-traumatic paraplegic patient. *Paraplegia*, **10**, 336.

NEUHEISER (1937) *Surg. Gynec. Obstet. Internat. Abstracts*, **104**, 521.

NISSEN C. (1941) *Proc. Roy. Soc. Med.*, **34**, 457.

PENNYBACKER J. (1953) *J. Bone & Joint Surg.*, **35B**. Editorial.

RIDDOCH G. (1941) *Brain*, **64**, 197.

ROGER L. (1941) *Surgery of Modern Warfare*. Hamilton Bailey, Edinburgh.

ROGERS W.A. (1930) An extension frame for reduction of fracture of vertebral body. *Surg. & Gynec. Obstet.*, **50**, 101.

ROGERS W.A. (1942) Treatment of fracture-dislocation of cervical spine. *J. Bone & Joint Surg.*, **24**, 245.

ROSOMOFF H.L. (1955) Protective effects of hypothermia against pathological processes of the nervous system. *Ann. N.Y. Acad. Sci.*, **80**, 775.

RUGE D. (1969) *Spinal Cord Injuries*, p. 29. Ch. Thomas, Springfield, Ill.

SCARFF J.E. & POOL J.L. (1946) *J. Neurosurg.*, **3**, 285.

SCHMIEDEN V. (1927–32) In: JUNGHANNS H. *Die gesunde und kranke Wirbelsäule in Röntgenbild und Klinik*, p. 331. Thieme, Stuttgart.

SMITH G.W. (1959) The normal cervical discogram. *Am. J. Roentgenol. Radium Ther. Neul. Med.*, **81**, 1006–1010.

SELMO A. (1939) In *Injuries of the Spine*, p. 103. Howorth M. & Petrie J., Baltimore, 1964.

SOUSTELLE (1951) In *Injuries of the Spine*, p. 103. Howorth M. & Petrie J., Baltimore, 1964.

ST. CLAIRE STRANGE F.G. (1973) An area accident service. *R.S.H.*, **1**, 31.

STREET D.M. (1967) *Proc. 16th Clin. Spinal Cord Inj. Conf.* pp. 92 Amer. Vet. Admin., Long Beach.

TALBOT H. (1966) Early management of patients with trauma to the spinal cord. *Med. Serv. J. Canada*, **22**, 523.

TATOR C.H. & DEECKE L. (1973) Studies of the treatment and pathophysiology of acute spinal cord injury in primates. *Paraplegia*, **10**, 344.

TAYLOR A.S. (1929) *Am. Surg.*, **90**, 321.

VERBIEST, H. (1962) *J. Neurosurg.*, **19**, 389.

VERBIEST H. (1963) Surgery of the cervical vertebral body in cases of traumatic deformity in dislocation. In *Proc. Symp. Spinal Injuries*, pp. 110–120. Harris P. (ed.). Roy. Coll. Surg., Edinburgh,

VIDUS VIDIUS (1544) De Machinamentis (Oribasius). In *Chirurgia, è Graeco in Latinum connersa*, Paris.

VINKE T.H. (1948) A skull traction apparatus. *J. Bone & Joint Surg.*, **30A**, 522.

WALTON G.L. (1889) *Boston, M. & S. J.*, **120**, 277.

WALTON G.L. (1893) A new method of reducing dislocation of cervical vertebrae. *J. Nerv. & Ment. Dis.*, **20**, 609.

WATSON-JONES R. (1931) Manipulative reduction of crush fracture spin. *Br. med. J.*, **1**, 300.

WATSON-JONES, R. (1955) *Fractures and Joint Injuries*, Vol. II, pp. 1004–1005. Livingstone, Edinburgh.

WEISS M. (1975) Dynamic spine alloplasty (spring-loading devices) after fracture and spinal cord inury. In *Clinical Orthopaedics and Related Research*, pp. 150–158. Urist M. (ed.). Lippincott, Philadelphia.

WHITE R.J. see Albin *et al* (1968).

YAMADA K. & IKATA T. (1969) Early treatment of traumatic paraplegia and tetraplegia by a new method, using a 'rolling plaster jacket' or a 'rocking plaster shell'. *Paraplegia*, **6**, 238.

D. GUNSHOT INJURIES AND STAB WOUNDS

Chapter 14 Gunshot Injuries

BERGMANN E. (1922) *Z. Neurol.*, **12**, 270.

COLLIER (1917) *Proc. Roy. Soc. Med.*, **10**, 38.

CUSHING H. (1927) Part 1, Surgery *The medical department, United States Army in World War I.* 57.

DIETLEN A. (1920) *Bruns. Beitr. Klin.-Chir.*, **101**, 320.

EISELSBERG Q. (1916) *Arch. Chir.*, **108**.

FOERSTER O. (1929) Läsionen des Rückenmarks auf Grund der Kriegserfahrungen. In *Handbuch der Neurologie*. Bumke und Foerster (eds). Springer, Berlin.

FRANGENHEIM B. (1916) *Munch. Med. Wschr.*, **43**.

GREENFIELD J. & RUSSELL D. (1958) *Neuropathology*, p. 461. E. Arnold, London.

GUILLAIN G. (1920) *Travaux Neurologiques de Guerre*. Masson, Paris.

GUTTMANN L. (1945) *New Hope for Spinal Cord Sufferers*. M.Times New York,.

GUTTMANN L. (1953) Treatment and rehabilitation of patients with injuries to the spinal cord and cauda equina. *Vol. Surgery, Br. Med. History of World War II*, pp. 422–516. H.M. Stationery Office, London.

HAYNES W.G. (1946) *Amer. J. Surg.*, **72**, 424.

HEAD H. & RIDDOCH G. (1917) *Brain*, **40**, 188.

HEINEKE B. (1917) Lehrbuch der Kriegschirurgie. *Verletzungen der Wirbelsäule und des Rüchenmarks*. J.A.Barth, Leipzig.

HOLMES G. (1915) *Brit. Med. J.*, **11**, 769.

JOURDAN P. (1915) Reunion Med. IV armee 12th Decembre.

KRAHN P., WHITTERIDGE D. & ZUCKERMAN S. (1942) *Lancet*, **1**, 252.

LERI A. (1918) *Rev. gén Path. guerre.*

LEVA M. (1915) *Dtsch. med. Wschr.*, 844.

MARBURG O. (1918) *Kriegsverletzungen des Zentralnervensystems*. Wiesbaden.

MARBURG O. & RANZI E. (1917) Über Rückenmarksschüsse. *Wien, Klin. Wschr.*, **1**, 652.

MARINESCO G. (1918) *Rev. neurol.*, **25**, 329.

MATSON D.M. (1948) *The Treatment of Acute Compound Injuries of the Spinal Cord due to Missiles*, pp. 1–64. Ch.Thomas, Springfield, Ill.

MAIRET A. & DURANTE G. (1919) *Revue neurol.*, **26**, 97.

MINGAZZINI (1917) *Policlinico, Sez. prat.*, 329.

MOTT F.W. (1916) *Lancet*, i, 441, 545.

OSTERHOLM J.L. & MATHEWS G.J. (1971) A proposed biochemical mechanism for traumatic spinal cord haemorrhagic necrosis; successful therapy for severe injuries by metabolic blockade. *Trans. Am. Neurol. Assoc.*, **96**, 187–191.

OSTERHOLM J.L. & MATHEWS G.J. (1972) Altered norepinephrine metabolism following experimental spinal cord injury. 1. Relationship to haemorrhagic necrosis and post-wounding neurological deficits. *J. Neurosurg.*, **36**, 386–394.

POOL (1945) Gunshot wounds of the spine. *Surg. Gynec. Obstet.*, **81**, 617.

REINHARDT F. (1915) *Dtsch. med. Wschr.*

RIDDOCH G. (1918) *Lancet*, ii, 838.

ROTHMANN I. (1915) *Dtsch. med. Wschr.*, 237.

ROUSSY & L'HERMITTE (1918) *Blessures de la Moelle*. Masson, Paris.

SCALES J.T., LUNN H. F., JENEID P.A., GILLINGHAM M.E. & REDFERN S. J. (1974) The prevention and treatment of pressure sores using air-support systems. *Paraplegia*, **12**, 118.

SCHLAGWITZ F. (1920) *Med. Klinik*, 927.

SELBERG H. (1917) *Z. Chir.*, 18.

SIMMONDS A. (1915) *Dtsch. med. Wschr.*, 1053.

SOLLIER A. (1918) *Press méd.*, 70.

SOUQUES F. & MÉGEVANT E. (1916) *Revue neurol.*, 280.

THOMPSON-WALKER J. (1937) *Proc. Roy. Soc. Med.*, **30**, 1233.

THORBURN W. (1922) *Br. official history of the Great War*. Ser. v., **2** 118.

VELLACOTT P. & WEBB JOHNSON A. (1919) *Lancet*, i, 733.

WOLMAN L. (1967) Blast injuries. *Paraplegia*, **5**, 89.

ZUCKERMAN S. (1941) *Proc. Roy. Soc. Med.*, **34**, 171.

Chapter 15   Stab Wounds

FOERSTER O. (1929) Symtomatologie der Erkrankungen des Rückenmarks. In *Handbuch der Neurologie*, Vol. 5. Springer, Berlin.

GUTTMANN L. (1949) *Brit. Surg. Pract.*, **6**, 455.

KEY A. & RETIEF P.J.H. (1970) Spinal cord injuries. *Paraplegia*, 243–249.

KEY A. (1971) Personal Communication.

LIPSCHITZ R. (1967) Stabwounds of the spinal cord. *Paraplegia*, **5**, 75–82.

LIPSCHITZ R. (1971) Stichverletzungen der Wirbelsäule. In: *Neurotraumatologie*. Guttmann L. (ed.) Urban und Schwarzenberg, München.

LIPSCHITZ R. & BLOCK J. (1962) *Lancet*, i, 169–172.

PETREN K. (1910) *Arch. Physiol.*, **47**, 495–557.

RAND C.W. & PATTERSON G.H. (1929) *Surg. Gynec. Obstet.*, **48**, 652.

ROSENBERG A.W. (1957) *Bull. Los Angeles Neurol. Soc.*, **22**, 79.

ST JOHN T.R. & RAND C.W. (1953) *Bull. Los. Angeles Neur. Soc.*, **18**, 1.

E. COMPLICATIONS

Chapter 16   Associated Injuries

BÉNASSY J. (1968) Associated fractures of the limbs in traumatic paraplegia and tetraplegia. *Paraplegia*, **5**, 209–211.

FRANKEL H. (1968) Associated chest injuries. *Paraplegia*, **5**, 221–225.

GUTTMANN L. (1963) Initial treatment of traumatic paraplegics and tetraplegics. In *Proc. Symp. Spinal Injuries*, p. 81. Roy. Coll. Surg., Edinburgh.

HARRIS P. (1968) Associated injuries in traumatic paraplegia and tetraplegia. *Paraplegia*, **5**, 215–220.

MC.SWEENEY (1968) The early management of associated injuries in the presence of co-incidental damage to the spinal cord. *Paraplegia*, **5**, 189–196.

MEINECKE F.W., REHN J. & LEITZ G. (1967) *Spinal Cord Injury Conf.*, p. 77, Long Beach, U.S.A.

MEINECKE F.W. (1968) Frequency and distribution of associated injuries in traumatic paraplegia and tetraplegia. *Paraplegia*, **5**, 196–211.

SILVER J. (1968) Chest injuries and complications in the early stages of spinal cord injury. *Paraplegia*, 226–243.

TRICOT A. & HALBOT R. (1968) Traumatic paraplegia and associated fractures. *Paraplegia*, **5**, 211–215.

Chapter 17   Venous Thrombosis and Pulmonary Embolism

BENASSY J. (1965) *Paraplegia*, **3**, 211.

BERGQUIST D., DAHLGREN S., EFSING O. & HALLBÖÖK (1975) Thermographic diagnosis of deep vein thrombosis. *Brit. med. J.*, **4**, 684.

COOKE E.D. & PILCHER M.D. (1974) *Brit. J. Surg.*, **61**, 971.

DOTT H. & LYONS H.A. (1956) *The Pathology and Surgery of the Veins of the Lower Limbs.* Livingstone, Edinburgh.

GUTTMANN L. (1963) *Proc. Symp. Spinal Injuries*, p. 83. Harris P. (ed.). Livingstone, Edinburgh.

HACHEN H.J. (1974) Anticoagulant therapy in patients with spinal cord injury. *Paraplegia*, **12**, 176.

HARRIS P. (1965) *Paraplegia*, **3**, 210.

MURLEY R.S. (1950) *Ann. Roy. Coll. Surgeons, Engl.*, **6**, 283.

PHILIPPS R.S. (1963) The incidence of deep venous thrombosis in paraplegia. *Paraplegia*, **1**, 116–130.

PROVAN T.L. (1965) *Brit. med. J.*, **2**, 538.

SILVER J.R. (1974) The prophylactic use of anticoagulant therapy in the prevention of pulmonary emboli in one hundred consecutive spinal injury patients. *Paraplegia*, **12**, 188.

WAKIN K., TERRIER J., ELKINS E. & KRUSEN F. (1948) *Amer. J. Physiol.*, **153**, 183.

WALSH J. J. & TRIBE C. (1965) Phlebo-thrombosis and pulmonary embolism in paraplegia. *Paraplegia*, **3**, 209.

WATSON N. (1974) Anticoagulant therapy in the treatment of venous thrombosis and pulmonary embolism in acute spinal injury. *Paraplegia*, **12**, 197.

Chapter 18   Respiratory Disturbances

BALDWIN E. DE F., COURNAND A. & RICHARDS D.W. (1948) Medicine. *Baltimore*, **27**, 243.

BERGSTRÖM O. & DIAMANT H. (1960) *Archives of Otolaryngology*, **71**, 628–634.

BREMNER C.G. (1962) *Brit. J. Chest.*, **56**, 39.

BÜRGI H. (1964) *Lancet*, ii, 64.

CAMERON G.S., SCOTT J.W., JOUSSE A.J. & BOTTERELL E.H. (1955) *Ann. Chir.*, **141**, 451.

CAMPBELL E.J.M. (1958) *The Respiratory Muscles.* Lloyd Luke, London.

CHOO-KANG (1970) *Brit. med. J.*, **4**, 465.

CHESHIRE D. & COATS D. (1966) Respiratory and metabolic management in acute tetraplegia. *Paraplegia*, **4**, 1–23.

COOPER J.D. & GRILLO H.C. (1969) The evolution of tracheal injury due to ventilatory assistance through cuffed tubes. *Ann. Surg.*, **169**, 334.

COURNAND A., RICHARDS D. & DARLING R. (1939) *Amer. Rev. Tuberc.*, **40**, 487.

DAVIS P.R. & MOORE R.E. (1962) *Proc. Phys. Soc. J. Physiol.*, **162**, 8.

DAVIS H., KRETSCHMER E. & BRYCE SMITH R. (1953) *J. Am. Med. Ass.*, **153**, 1156.

DOLLFUS P. & FRANKEL H. (1965) Cardiovascular reflexes in tracheostomised tetraplegics. *Paraplegia*, **2**, 227–231.

DUCHENNE G.B. (1866) *Physiologie der Bewegungen* (German Transl. by C.Wernicke, 1885). T.Fischer, Berlin.

FEARON B. (1966) *Clinical Trends, July.*

FLEXER S.Y. (1970) *Pediatriya*, **11**, 39–43.

FRANKEL H. (1968) Associated chest injuries. *Paraplegia*, **5**, 221–225.

FRANKEL H. (1970) Tracheal stenosis following tracheostomy. *Paraplegia*, **8**, 172–174.

GIBSON P. (1967) *Thorax*, **22**, 1.

GILLIATT R., GUTTMANN L. & WHITTERIDGE D. (1948) Inspiratory vasoconstriction after spinal injuries. *J. Physiol.*, **107**, 67.

GREEN N.M. (1959) *New Engl. J. Med.*, **261**, 846.

GROSSIORD A., BUZACOUX J., MAURY M. & BARTHES G. (1963) Studies on motor metamerisation of upper and lower limbs. *Paraplegia*, **1**, 81–97.

GUTTMANN L. (1970) *Paraplegia*, **8**, 175–176.

GUTTMANN L. & BELL D. (1958) In *Suspension Therapy*, pp. 107–108. Hollis M. & Roper M. (ed.). Baillière, Tindall & Cox, London.

GUTTMANN L. & SILVER J. (1965) Electromyographic studies on reflex activity of the intercostals and abdominals in cervical cord lesions. *Paraplegia*, **3**, 1.

HARDCASTLE B. (1966) Prolonged intubation and subglottis stenosis. *Brit. Med. J.*, **2**, 826.

HAMILTON W.F., PALMER K.N. & GENT M. (1970) *Brit. med. J.*, **3**, 260.

HARLEY H.R. (1971) Laryngotracheal obstruction complicating tracheostomy or endotracheal intubation with assisted respiration. *Thorax*, **26**, 493–533.

HEMINGWAY A., BORS E. & HOBBY R.P. (1958) *J. clin. Invest.*, **37**, 775.

HERMANNSEN J. (1933) *Z. ges. exper. Med.*, **90**, 130.

HUTCHINSON J. (1846) *Med.-chir. Trans.*, **29**, 137.

JACKSON C.L. (2921) High tracheostomy and other errors the chief causes of chronic laryngeal stenosis. *Surg. Gyn. Obstet.*, **32**, 392.

JACKSON C.L. (1954) Tracheostomy. In *Lewis', Practice of Surgery*. pp. 24–44. Walters, W. (ed.). Vol. 4, 7, Prior, Hagerstown, Maryland.

JOHNSON J.B., WRIGHT J.S. & HERCUS V. (1967) Tracheal stenosis following tracheostomy. *J. thoracic. cardiovasc. Surg.*, **53**, 206.

LUSTMAN F. (1970) *Practitioner*, **205**, 213.

MATHOG R.H., KENAN P.D. & HUDSON W.R. (1971) *Laryngoscope*, **81**, 107–119.

NEFFSON A.H. (1949) *Acute Laryngotracheobronchitis.* Grune & Stratton, New York.

NELSON T.G. (1957) *Amer. Surg.*, 660, 750, 841.

RABUZZI D.D. & REED G.F. (1971) *Laryngoscope*, **81**, 939–946.

READING P. (1958) *J. Lar. Otol.*, **72**, 785–798.

REID C.L. & BRACE D.E. (1940) *Surg. Gynec. Obstet.*, **70**, 157.

SALMON L.F.W. (1975) Tracheostomy. *Proc. Roy. Soc. Med.*, **68**, 447.

SARA C. (1965) *Med. J. Aust.*, **1**, 99.

SILVER J. & MOULTON A. (1969) The physiological and pathological sequelae of paralysis of the intercostal and abdominal muscles in tetraplegic patients. *Paraplegia*, **7**, 131–139.

STEPHENSON H.E. (1958) *Cardiac Arrest and Resuscitation*, p. 73. Mosley, St Louis.

STURGIS C., PEABODY F., HALL F. & FREEMONT-SMITH F. (1922) *Arch. Intern. Med.*, **29**, 236.

TALBOT H.S., ROCCO A.G., CONROY M.E. (1957) *Proc. 6th Conf. Spinal Cord Injury*, p. 20. Amer. Vet. Admin.

TAYLOR A.B. (1960) *Br. J. Dis. Chest*, **54**, 157.

WATTS J.McK. (1963) Tracheostomy in modern practice. *Br. J. Surg.*, **50**, 954.

WHITE R.J. (1973) Current status of spinal cord cooling. *Clinical Neurosurgery*, Williams & Wilkins Company, Baltimore. pp. 400–407.

WILKS S. (1860) *Guy's Hospital Reports*, **6**, 97.

WINGO G.F. (1957) *Proc. 6th Conf. Spinal Cord Injury* p. 23. Amer. Vet. Admin.

WOLFF, G., KELLERHALS B., SCHUMANN L., GRÄDEL E. (1973) Eine nene methode der cuffblähung. *Anaesthesist*, **22**, 317.

Chapter 19 Metabolic Disturbances of the Skeletal System

BARTELHEIMER H. (1956) Osteopathien, die den Internisten angehen. *Internist*, **3**, 233.

BARTELHEIMER H. & SCHMIDT-RHODE J.M. (1962) Osteoporosen als Krankheitsgeschehen Ergeb. inn. *Med. Kinderheilk*, **7**, 454.

COMARR E., HUTCHINSON R. & BORS E. (1962) Extremity fractures of patients with spinal cord injuries. *Am.J. Surg.*, **103**, 732.

DULL T.A. & HENNEMAN P.H. (1963) *New Engl. J. Med.*, **268**, 132.

EDWARDS K., GUTTMANN L. & MEHRA N.C. (1973) Studies on mineral metabolism following spinal cord injuries. *Paraplegia* (in press).

EICHENHOLTZ S.N. (1962) Management of long-bone fractures in paraplegic patients. *J. Bone & Joint Surg.*, **45A**, 299–300.

EGER W. (1962) Allgemeine morphologische Physiologie und Pathologie der Knochengewebe unter Berücksightigung calcipenischer Osteopathien. *Internist*, **3**, 267.

FOURMAN P. (1960) *Calcium Metabolism and the Bone*. Blackwell, Oxford.

FREEHAFER A. & LOWRY R. (1963) *Proc. Spinal Cord Injury Conf.* pp. 23–29. Amer. Vet. Admin. Hines Hosp.

GUTTMANN L. (1953) *Brit. Med. History of World War II*, Vol. Surgery, p. 447. H.M. Stationery Office, London.

GUTTMANN L. (1953) *Brit. Med. History of World War II*, Vol. Surgery, p. 447. H.M. Stationery Office, London.

KLEIN LE ROY, NOORT, ST.V.DEN & DE JAK J.J. (1966) Sequential studies of urinary hydroxyproline and serum alkaline phosphatase in acute paraplegia. *Med. Services Journ. Canada*, **22**, 524–533.

NORRDIN B.E. (1962) L'osteoporose. *Schweiz. med. Wschr.*, **92**, 892.

PAESLACK V. (1965) *Internistische Störungen beim Paraplegiker*, pp. 53–54. G.Thieme, Stuttgart.

ZIFF M., KIBRICK A., DRESSNER, GRIBETZ H. (1956) Excretion of hydroxyproline in patients with rheumatic and nonrheumatic diseases. *J. Clin. Invest.*, **35**, 579.

Chapter 20 Soft Tissue Calcifications and Ossifications

ABRAMSON A. (1948) Bone disturbances in injuries of the spinal cord and cauda equina. *J. Bone & Joint Surg.*, **30A**, 982.

ABRAMSON A & KAMBERG G. (1949) *J. Bone & Joint Surg.*, **31A**, 982.

BÉNASSY J., MEZABRAUD A., DIVERRES J.C. (1963) *Rozhl. Chir.*, **34**, 239.

BÉNASSY J., BOISSIER J., PATTE D. & DIVERRES J.C. (1960) *Presse med.*, 811.

BRAILSFORD J.F. (1941) *Br. med. J.*, **1**, 320.

COUVÉE L.M. (1971) *Paraplegia*, **9**, 89.

DAMANSKI M. (1961) *J. Bone & Joint Surg.*, **43B**, 286.

EBEL A. (1966) *Medical Services J., Canada*, **22**, 477.

EICHHORST H. (1895) *Arch. path. Anatomie*, **139**, 193.

FINKFFMAN I. (1965) *Proc. 5th Conf. Spinal Cord Injury, Amer. Vet. Admin. Hines Hosp.*, p. 74.

FINKLE J.R. (1956) *Proc. 5th Conf. Spinal Cord Injury, Amer. Vet. Admin. Hines Hosp.*, p. 72.

FREEHAFER A., YURICK R. & MAST A. (1966) Para-articular ossification in spinal cord injury. *Med. Services J., Canada*, **22**, 471–477.

GREGONO M.C. (1966) *Medical Services J., Canada*, **22**, 478.

GUTTMANN L. (1953) *Brit. Med. History of World War II*, Vol. Surgery. H.M. Stationery Office London.

GUTTMANN L. & MEDAWAR P.B. (1942) Chemical inhibition of fibre regeneration and neuroma formation in peripheral nerves. *J. Neur. Psychiat., London*, **5**, 130.

HARDY A. & DICKSON J.W. (1963) Pathologic ossification in traumatic paraplegia. *J. Bone & Joint Surg.*, **45B**, 76.

HEILBORN N. & KUHN W. (1947) *Radiology*, **48**, 579.

KLUMPKE-DÉJÉRINE C. (1918) *Rev. neurol.*, **25**, 159, 207, 348.

KLUMPKE-DÉJÉRINE C. & CEILLIER A. (1919) Para-osteo-arthropathies des paraplegiques par lésions médullaires. *Ann. Med.*, **34**, 399.

LIBERSON M. (1953) *J. Am. Med. Ass.*, **152**, 1010.

MICHAELIS L.S. (1964) *Orthopaedic Surgery of the Limbs in Paraplegia*, pp. 30–33. Springer, Berlin.

MILLER L. & O'NEILL P. (1949) *J. Bone & Joint Surg.*, **A31**, 283.

PAESLACK V. (1965) *Internistische Störungen bein Paraplegiker*, pp. 59–60.

POPPE E. & MYERS J. (1953) *T. norske Laegeforen*, **73**, 774.

RIEDEL B. (1883) *Verh. dtsch. Ges. Chir.*, **12**, 93.

ROSAK K. (1961) *Z. Orthop.*, **94**, 576.

ROSSIER A.B., BUSSAT PH., INFANTE F., ZENDER R., COURVOISIER B., MUHEIM G., DONATH A., VASEY H., TAILLARD W., LAGIER R., GABBIANI G., BAUD C.A., POUEZAT J.A., VERY J.M. & HACHEN H.J. (1973) Current facts on para-osteo-arthropathy (POA). *Paraplegia*, **11**, 36.

SKOTNIKOV V.J. (1958) *Vop. Nejrchir.*, **22**, 32.

SOULE A.B. (1945) Neurogenic ossifying fibromyopathies. *J. Neurosurg.*, **2**, 485.

STOREY D. & TEGNER W. (1955) *Ann. Rheum. Dis.*, **14**, 176.

WHARTON G.W. & MORGAN T.H. (1970) *J. Bone & Joint Surg.*, **52A**, 105.

WORMS R. & GOUGEON (1947) *Rev. neurol.*, **79**, 346.

F. NEUROPHYSIOLOGICAL AND CLINICAL ASPECTS OF SPINAL CORD INJURIES

Chapter 23   Patterns of Reflex Disturbances

ARCANGEL L.S., JOHNSTON B. & BISHOP B. (1971) The H reflex in normal, spastic and rigid subjects. *Archs Neurol. Psychiat., Chicago*, **8**, 591.

ASHBY P., VERRIER M. & LIGHTFOOT E. (1974) Segmental reflex pathways in spinal shock and spinal spasticity in man. *J. Neurol. Neurosurg. Psychiat.*, **37**, 1352.

BABINSKI J. (1896) Sur le réflexe cutané plantaire dans certain affections organique de systeme nerveux central. *Soc. biol.*, **3**, 207–208.

BARNES D.C., JOYNT R.J. & SCHOTTELINS B.A. (1962) Motoneuron resting potentials in spinal shock. *Amer. J. Physiol.*, **203**, 1113.

BARRÉ L. (1915) *Revue neurol.*, 768.

BOYD I.A., EYZAGUIRRE C., MATTHEWS P.B. & RUCHWORTH G. (1964) The role of the gamma system in movement and posture. New York Assoc. for the aid of crippled children.

BROWN M.C., ENGBERG L. & MATTHEWS P.B. (1967) The relative sensitivity to vibration of muscle receptors of the cat. *J. Physiol.*, **192**, 773.

BURKE D., ANDREWS C. & LANCO J.W. (1972) Tonic vibration in spasticity. *Neurological Sciences*, **15**, 321.

COLLIER (1916) Gunshot wounds and injuries of the spinal cord. *Lancet*, iv, 711–716.

COLLIER (1917) *Proc. Roy. Soc. Med.*, **10**, 4; *Sect. neur.*, **38**.

COOPER S. & DANIEL P.M. (1956) *J. Physiol.*, **133**, 1.

DELWAIDE P.J. (1973) Human monosynaptic reflexes and presynaptic inhibition. In *New Development in Electromyography and Clinical Neurophysiology*, Vol. 3, p. 508. Karger, Basel.

DENNY-BROWN D. & LIDDELL E.G.T. (1927a) The stretch reflex as a spinal process. *J. Physiol.*, **63**, 144–150.

DENNY-BROWN D. & LIDDELL E.G.T. (1928) Extensor reflexes in the fore-limb. *J. Physiol.*, **65**, 305–326.

DESMEDT J.E., Ed. (1973) In *New Development in Electromyography and Clinical Neurophysiology*, Vol. 3. *Human reflexes. Pathophysiology of motor system*. Karger, Basel.

DIAMANTOPOULOS E. & OLSON P.Z. (1967) Excitability of motoneurones in spinal shock in man. *J. Neurol. Neurosurg. Psychiat.*, **30**, 427.

DICK T.S. (1949) Rehabilitation in chronic paraplegia. M.D. Thesis, Manchester University.

DIETRICHSEN G. (1973) The role of the fusomotor system in spasticity and Parkinsonian rigidity: In *New Development in Electromyography and Clinical neurophysiology*, Vol. 3, p. 496. Karger, Basel.

ECCLES J.C. (1964) *The Physiology of Synapses*. Springer, Berlin.

ECCLES & LUNDBERG A. (1957a) Synaptic actions of motoneurons in relation to the two components of the Group I muscle afferent volley. *J. Physiol.*, **136**, 527–546.

ECCLES & LUNDBERG A. (1957b) The convergence of monosynaptic afferents on the many different species of alpha motor neurones. *J. Physiol.*, **137**, 22–50.

ECCLES & LUNDBERG A. (1957c) Synaptic actions on motoneurones caused by impulses in Golgi tendon organ afferents. *J. Physiol.*, **138**, 227–252.

ECCLES J.C. & LUNDBERG A. (1958) The action potentials of the alpha motoneurones supplying fast and slow muscles. *J. Physiol.*, **142**, 275–291.

ECCLES & SCHADÉ T.P. (1964) *Physiology of spinal neurones*. Amsterdam, Elsevier.

EKLUND G. (1971) On muscle vibration in man; an amplitude dependent inhibition, inversely related to muscle strength. *Acta physiol. scand.*, **83**, 425.

ELKINS C.W. & WEGNER W.R. (1946) *Ann. Surg.*, **123**, 516.

FOERSTER O. (1908) Über eine neue Methode zur Behandlung spastischer Lähmungen mittels Resektion hinterer Rückenmarks Wurzeln. *Z. orthop. Chir.*, **22**, 203–223.

FOERSTER O. (1911) Resection of posterior spinal nerve-roots in the treatment of gastric crises and spastic paralysis. *Proc. Roy. Soc. Med.*, **4**, 226–246.

FOERSTER O. (1936) Symtomotologie der Erkrankungen des Rückenmarks. In *Handbuch der Neurologie*, Vol. 5, p. 94. Springer, Berlin.

FULTON J.F., LIDDELL E.G.T. & RIOCH D. McK. (1930a) The influence of experimental lesions of the spinal cord upon the knee-jerk. *Brain*, **53**, 311–326.

FULTON J.F., LIDDELL E.G.T. & RIOCH D. McK. (1930b) The influence of unilateral destruction of the vestibular nuclei upon posture and the knee-jerk. *Brain*, **53**, 327–343.

FULTON J. & McCOUCH G.P. (1937) The relation of the motor area of primates to the hyporeflexia (spinal shock) of spinal transection. *J. Nerve and Ment. Dis.*, **86**, 125–196.

GILLIES J.D., LANCE J.W., NEILSON P.D. & TASSNARI C.A. (1969) Presynaptic inhibition of the monosynaptic reflex by vibration. *J. Physiol.*, **205**, 329.

GOLTZ F.L. (1869) *Beitrage zur Lehre von den Funktionen der Nervenzentren des Frosches*. Hirschwald, Berlin.

GRANIT R. (1966) *Muscular Afferent and Motor Control*. Almquist & Wisksell, Stockholm.

GUTTMANN L. (1946) Rehabilitation after injuries to the spinal cord and cauda equina. *Brit. J. Physical Med.*, **9**, 130–162.

GUTTMANN L. (1952) Studies on reflex activity of the isolated cord in the spinal man. *J. Nerv. & Ment. Dis.*, (Festschrift to R.Wartenberg.) Haymaker (ed.) 957–972.

GUTTMANN L. (1953) The treatment and rehabilitation of patients with injuries of the spinal cord. In *Brit. Med. History of World War II*, Vol. Surgery, pp. 431–516.

GUTTMANN L. (1967) The re-orientation of posture and locomotion in spinal man. *Kovacs-Mem. Lecture, Proc. Roy. Soc. Med.*, **1**, 47.

GUTTMANN L. (1970) Spinal shock and reflex behaviour in man. *Paraplegia*, **8**, 100–110, 112–116.

HALL, MARSHALL (1841) *On the Diseases and Derangements of the Nervous System*, p. 256. Baillière, London.

HUNTER J. & ROYLE N. (1924) The symptomatology of complete transverse lesions of the spinal cord. *Austral. J. Exper. Biol.*, **1**, 57–72.

KUHN R.A. (1950) Functional capacity of the isolated human spinal cord. *Brain*, **73**, 1–50.

LUNDBERG A. (1964) Supraspinal control in reflex paths to motoneurones and primary afferents. *Progr. Brain Res.*, **12**, 197–219.

McCOUCH G. (1964) Physiology of the spinal cord. In *The Spinal Cord*. Austin G. (ed). C. Thomas, Springfield, Ill.

MONAKOW C. VON (1914) *Die Lokalisation im Grosshirn und der Abbau der Funktionen durch Kortikale Herde bei einigen Saugetieren und beim Menschen*, p. 257. Bergmann, Wiesbaden.

PHILIPP C.G. (1970) An outline of recent work on the spinal cord of the cat. *Paraplegia*, **8**, 86–100.

REMARK E. (1893) Zur Lokalisation der spinalen Hautreflexe der Unterextremitäten. *Neurol. Centralbt*, **12**, 506–512.

RESWICK J.B. & ROGERS J. (1975) Experience at Rancho Los Amigos Hospital with devices and techniques to prevent pressure sores. *Proc. Congress Univ. Strathclyde*, p. 113.

RIDDOCH G. (1917b) The reflex function of the completely divided spinal cord in man, compared with those associated with less severe lesions. *Brain*, **40**, 264–402.

RUCH T.C. & WATTS J.W. (1934) Reciprocal changes in reflex activity of the fore limbs induced by postbrachial 'cold-block' of the spinal cord. *Amer. J. Physiol.*, **110**, 362–375.

RUSHWORTH G. (1960) Spasticity and rigidity. *J. Neurol. Neuro-surg. & Psychiat.*, **23**, 90.

RUSHWORTH G. (1966) Some studies on the pathophysiology of spasticity. *Paraplegia*, **4**, 130–141.

SCARFF J.E. & POOL J.L. (1946) Factors causing massive spasms following transection of cord in man. *J. Neurosurg.*, **3**, 285.

SCARFF J.E. (1952) Injuries of the vertebral column and spinal cord. In *Injuries of the Brain, Spinal Cord and Covering*, pp. 510–586, Brock S. (ed.).

SHERRINGTON, SIR CHARLES (1897) The central nervous system, In *A Textbook of Physiology*, Foster, (ed.). Macmillan, London.

SHERRINGTON, SIR CHARLES (1947) *The Integrative Action of the Nervous System*. Yale University Press, New Haven.

STEWART I.M. (1970) The sand bed. *J. Bone Jt. Surg.*, 52-B, **4**, 799.

WEAVER R.A., LANDAU W.M. & HIGGINS J.F. (1963) Evidence of fusomotor depression in human spinal shock. *Archs Neurol.*, **9**, 127.

WHITTERIDGE D. (1966) The spinal cord and spasticity. *Paraplegia*, **4**, 127–130.

Chapter 24 Symptomatology

BENNETT A.E. & FORTES A. (1945) Meningeoma obstructing the foramen magnum. *Archs Neurol. Psychiat., Chicago*, **53**, 131.

BROWN S. (1892) On hereditary ataxy with a series of 21 cases. *Brain*, **15**, 250.

BROWN-SÉQUARD C.E. (1850) De la transmission croisée des impressions sensitives par la moelle epinière. *C.R. Soc. biol.*, **2**, 70.

BRUNS, LAZARUS, FLATAN, EDINGER, BING, VILLIGER (see Foerster O.) (1927) Specielle Anatomy und Physiologie der peripheren Nerven *Handbuch der Neurologie*, Ergänzungsband, p. 966.

ELSBERG C.A. (1929) Tumors of the spinal cord. *Archs Neurol. Psychiat.*, **22**, 949.

FOERSTER O. (1927) Spezielle Anatomie und Physiologie der peripheren Nerven. *Handbuch der Neurologie*, Ergänzungsband, p. 966. Springer, Berlin.

FOERSTER O. (1936) *Handbuch der Neurologie*, Vol. 5, p 106. Springer, Berlin.

GROSSIORD A., BUZACOUX M., MAURY M. & BARTHES (1963) Studies on motor metamerisation of the upper and lower limbs. *Paraplegia*, **1**, 81–97.

GUTTMANN L. (1964) Problems in the initial treatment of traumatic tetraplegia. *Proc. IV. Intern. Congress of Physical Med., Paris. Excerpta Medica*, 593–596.

GUTTMANN L. (1969) *Handbook of Clinical Neurology*, Vol. 2, pp. 1, 103. Vinken & Bruyn (eds)., North-Holland Publ. Co., Amsterdam.

MARIE, PIERRE (1892) *Leçons sur les Maladies de la Moelle*. Masson, Paris.

NAFFZIGER H.C. & BROWN H.A. (1933) Hour-glass tumors of the spine. *Archs Neurol. Psychiat., Chicago*, **29**, 561.

SCHNEIDER R., CHERRY G. & PANTEK H. (1954) The syndrome of acute central cervical cord injury with special reference of mechanism involved in hyperextension injuries of the cervical spine. *J. Neurosurg.*, **11**, 546.

SYMONDS P. & MEADOWS S.P. (1937) Compression of the spinal cord in the neigbhourhood of the foramen magnum. *Brain*, **60**, 52–84.

Chapter 25 Disturbances of Sensibility

BAYLISS (1901) *J. Physiol*, **26**, 728–748.

BECK K. (1949) Zur Physiologie des Rückenmarks. *Dtsch. Z. Nervenheilk*, **160**, 55.

BECKER H. (1949) Über Storüngen des Körperbildes und über Phantomerlebnisse bei Rückenmarksverletzten. *Arch. Psychiat. Nervenkr.*, **182**, 97.

BISHOP (1946) *Physiol. Rev.*, **26**, 77.

VAN BOGAERT (1930) *Revue Neur.* **2**, 149.

BORS E. (1951) Phantom limbs of patients with spinal cord injuries. *Archs Neurol. Psychiat.*, **66**, 610.

BOWLEY A.A. (1890) *Med. chir. Trans.*, **73**, 317.

BRAIN, RUSSELL W. (1951) *Diseases of the Nervous System*, p. 114. Oxford Univ. Press, London.

CRAWFORD J.P. & FRANKEL H.L. (1971) Abdominal 'visceral' sensation in human tetraplegia. *Paraplegia*, **9**, 153–158.

CRITCHLEY (1949) *Brain*, **72**, 538–561; *Brain*, **106**, 1.

DUSSER DE BARENNE J.S. (1935) Central levels of sensory integration. *Res. Publ. nerv. ment. Dis.* **15**, 279–288.

FOERSTER O. (1933) *The Dermatomes in Man.*

FOERSTER O. (1936) Rückenmark. In *Handbuch der Neurologie*, Vol. 5, pp. 308–399. Springer, Berlin.

GERSTMANN (1924) Fingeragnosie. *Wien. Klin. Wschr.*, **37**, 1010.

GROSSMAN M. & STEIN I. (1948) *J. Applied Physiol.*, **1**, 263.

GUTTMANN L. (1946) *Brit. J. Physical Med.*, 130 and 162.

GUTTMANN L. (1953) *Brit. Medical History of World War II*, Vol. Surgery, pp. 422–516. H.M. Stationery Office, London.

GUTTMANN L. (1957) The problem of pain and paraesthesia. *Proc. Int. World Congr. I.S.W.C.*, p. 443.

GUTTMANN L. (1962) Sport and the disabled. In *Sport Medicine*, pp. 367–391. Arnold, London.

GUTTMANN L. (1967) The re-orientation of posture and locomotion. Kovacs Me-Lecture, *Proc. Roy. Soc.* **1**, 47.

GUTTMANN L. (1969) Phantom sensation. In *Handbook Clinical Neurology*, Vol. 3, p. 187. Vinken & Bruyn, (eds). North-Holland Publ. Co., Amsterdam.

GUTTMANN L. & WITTERIDGE D. (1947) Effects of bladder distension on autonomic mechanisms after spinal cord injuries. *Brain*, **70**, 36.

HAGBARTH E.E. (1973) The effect of muscle vibration in normal man and patients with motor disorders. In *New Development in Electromyography and Clinical Neurophysiology*. Vol. 3, Karger, Basel.

HEAD H. (1893) *Brain*, **16**, Part I.

HEAD H. & HOLMES G. (1920) Sensation and the cerebral cortex. *Brain*, **41**, 57–253.

HEAD H. & RIDDOCH G. (1917) The automatic bladder, excessive sweating and some other reflex conditions in gross injuries of the spinal cord. *Brain*, **40**, 188–263.

HEILPORN A. & NOEL G. (1968) *Paraplegia*, **6**, 122–127.

L'HERMITTE (1939) *L'image de Notre Corps*. Paris.

HEYE H.L. (1956) *J. Neurosurg.*, **13**, 184.

HOPKINS A. & RUDGE P. (1973) Hyperpathia in the central cervical cord syndrome. *J. Neurol. Neurosurg. Psychiatr.*, **36**, 637–642.

JAMES, A. H. (1957) *The Physiology of Gastric Digestion*. London.

JONES M.H. (1956) *Science*, **124**, 442.

KEEGAN (1943) *Archs. Neurol. Psychiat., Chicago*, **50**, 47–83.

KEELE C.A. (1957) *Proc. Roy. Soc. Med.*, **50**, 477.

KEELE C.A. (1957) *Anatomy of Pain*. Oxford.

KELLGREN (1939) *Clin. Sc.*, **4**, 35, 303.

LANCE J.W., BURKE D. & ANDREWS C.J. (1973) The reflex effects of muscle vibration. In *New Development in Electromyography and Clinical Neurophysiology*, Vol. 3, p. 444. Karger, Basel.

LANDAU W. & BISHOP G.H. (1958) *Arch. Neurol. & Psychiat.*, **69**, 490.

LENNANDER R. (1902) *Mitt. a.d. Grenzgeb. d. Med. und Chir.*, **10**, 38.

LENNANDER R. (1906) *Mitt. a.d. Grenzgeb. d. Med. und Chir.*, **15**, 465.

LEWIS, SIR T. (1927) *The Blood Vessels of the Human Skin and their Responses*. Shaw & Son, London.

LEWIS, SIR T. (1941) *Pain*. The Macmillan Co., New York.

MACKENZIE M. (1909) *Symptoms and their Interpretation*. Shaw & Sons, London.

MONEY J. (1960) Phantom orgasm in the dreams of paraplegic men and women. *Am. J. Gener. Psych.*, **3**, 373–382.

PICHLER E. (1954) Störungen des Körpererlebens bei Rückenmarksquerschnittsläsionen. *Wien, Z. Nervenheilk*, **10**, 43.

POLLOCK L., BOSHES B., ARIEFT A., FINKELMAN I., BROWN M., DOBIN N., KESERT B., PYZIK J., FINKLE E., TIGAG E. & ZIVIN I. (1957) Phantom limb in patients with injuries to the spinal cord and cauda equina. *Surg. Gynec. Obstet.*, **104**, 409.

RIDDOCH G. (1917) The reflex function of the completely disabled spinal cord in man compared with those associated with less severe lesions. *Brain*, **40**, 264–402.

RIDDOCH G. (1941) Phantom limbs and body shape. *Brain*, **64**, 197.

ROSS C. (1888) *Brain*, **10**, 333.

SCHILDER (1935) *The Image and Appearance of the Human Body*. London.

SCHULTE W. (1947) Die Psyche von Rückenmarksquerschnittsverletzten. *Nervenarzt*, **18**, 28.

SHERRINGTON, SIR C. (1898) *Philos. Trans.*, **190B**, 45–186.

STURGE A. (1883) *Brain*, **5**, 492.

WENGER M.A. (1950) In: *Feelings and emotions*. Morehead Symp. Regmith M. (ed.). McGraw-Hill.

WRIGHT S. (1965) *Applied Physiol.*, 11th Ed., revised by C.A.Keele. Neil & Jepson, London.

Chapter 26   Disturbances of Vasomotor Control

ALDERSON J.D. & THOMAS D.G. (1975) The use of halothane anaesthesia to control autonomic hyperreflexia during trans-urethral surgery in spinal cord injury patients. *Paraplegia*, **13**, 183–188.

BARRON D.H. & MATTHEWS B.H. (1935) 'Recurrent Fibres' of dorsal roots. *J. Neurophys.*, **3**, 403–406.

BENEDICT F. & LEE R. (1938) New York, Carnegie Instit. Publ. No. 497.

BENZINGER (1959) *Proc. nat. Acad. Sci. U.S.*, **45**, 645.

BENZINGER (1960) *Federation Proc.* **19**, Suppl. 5, 32.

BICKFORD (1939) *Clin. Sci.*, **4**, 159.

BIGELOW W., LINDSAY W., HARRISON R., GORDON R. & GREENWOOD F. (1950) Oxygen transport and utilization in dogs at low body temperatrues. *Am. J. Physiol.*, **160**, 125.

BRADBURY S. & EGGLETON C. (1927) Postural hypotension: autopsy on case. *Amer. Heart*, **3**, 105–106.

BRESLAUER F. (1921) *Beitr. z. Klin. Chir.*, **121**, 301.

BRIDGEN W., HOWARTH S. & SHARPEY-SCHAFER E. (1950) Postural changes in the peripheral blood flow of normal subjects with observations on vaso-vagal fainting reactions as a result of tilting, Lordotis position pregnancy and spinal anaesthesia. *Clin. Sci.*, **9**, 79–91.

BUCY C.P. & PRIBRAM K.H. (1943) Localized sweating as part of a localized convulsive seizure. *Archs Neurol. Psychiat.*, **50**, 456–461.

BURGI S. (1953) *Les Regulations Neuro-végéatives*, pp. 89–113. Doin, Paris.

CHESHIRE D. & COATS A. (1966) Respiratory and metabolic management in acute tetraplegia. *Paraplegia*, **4**, 1–23.

CLARK G. (1940) *The Hypothalamus*. Williams & Wilkins, Washington.

COOPER K., FERRES, H. & GUTTMANN L. (1963) Vasomotor responses in the foot to raising temperature in the paraplegic. *J. Physiol.*, **136**, 547.

CORBETT J.L., FRANKEL H.L. & HARRIS P.J. (1971) Cardiovascular reflexes in tetraplegia. *Paraplegia*, **9**, 113.

DIEDEN F. (1915) Über die Innervation der Schweissdrüsen. *Dtsch. Arch. Klin. Med.*, **117**, 180.

ERICKSON T.C. (1938) Neurogenic hyperthermia. *Brain*, **62**, 172–190.

FOERSTER O. (1936) *Handbuch der Neurologie*, Vol. 5. Springer, Berlin (see his references of 1924 and 1927).

FREUND & STRASSMANN (1912) Zur Kenntuis des nervösen Mechanismus der Wärmeregulation. *Arch. exp. Pharm.*, **69**, 12.

FREWIN D.B., LEVITT M., MYERS S.J. & DOWNEY J.A. (1973) Catecholamine responses in paraplegia. *Paraplegia*, **11**, 238.

GAGEL O. (1930) Zur Frage der Existenz efferenter Fasern in den hinteren Wurzeln des Menschen. *Z. Neur.*, **126**, 405.

GILLIAT L.R., GUTTMANN L. & WHITTERIDGE W. (1948) Inspiratory vasoconstriction after spinal injuries. *J. Physiol.*, **107**, 67.

GUTTMANN L. (1931) Die Schweissekretion des Menschen in ihren Beziehungen zum Nervensystem. *Z. ges. Neurol. & Psychiat.*, **135**, 1–48.

GUTTMANN L. (1933) Epidemiologische, Klinische und histologische Erfahrungen während der Polyomyelitis Epidemie 1932 in Schlesien. *Med. Klin.*, 1–12.

GUTTMANN L. (1933) Motorische und autonome Grenzzonenreflexe *Z. ges Neurol. & Psychiat.*, **147**, 292–307.

GUTTMANN L. (1936) *Handbuch der Neurologie*, Vol. VII/2, p. 326. Bumke & Foerster (eds). Springer, Berlin.

GUTTMANN L. (1937) Ein neues einfaches colorimetrisches Verfahren zur Untersuchung der Schweissdrüsenfunktion. *Klin. Wsche.*, **35**, 212–214.

GUTTMANN L. (1938a) Über reflecktorische Beziehungen zwischen Viszera und Schweissdrüsen und ihre Bedentung bei der Erkrankung innerer Organe (der viscero-sudorale Reflex). *Confinia Neurologica*, **1**, 296–310.

GUTTMANN L. (1938b) Zur Wiederherstellung der Schweiss-Sekretion in Hauttransplantaten. *Dermatol. Zeitschr.*, 73–76.

GUTTMANN L. (1946) *Brit. J. Phys. Med.* **9**, 130, 162.

GUTTMANN L. (1947) Management of the Quinizarin-Test. *Postgrad. med. J.*, **23**, 353–366.

GUTTMANN L. (1953) *Brit. Med. History of World War II*, Vol. Surgery, p. 422–516. H.M. Stationery Office.

GUTTMANN L. (1954) *Visceral Activity and Peripheral Circulation* Ciba Found. Sympos. T. & A. Churchill, London.

GUTTMANN L. (1969) Clinical symptomatology of spinal cord lesions. Sweating. In *Handbook of Clinical Neurology*, Vol. 2, Chapter 9, pp. 200–201, 209. Vinken & Bruyn, (eds). North-Holland Publ. Co., Amsterdam.

GUTTMANN L. & LIST C.F. (1928) Zur Topik and Pathophysiologie der Schweiss sekretion. *Z. ges. Neurol. & Psychiat.*, **116**, 504–535.

GUTTMANN L., MUNRO A., ROBINSON R. & WALSH J. (1963) Effects of tilting on the cardio-vascular responses on plasma catecholamine levels in spinal man. *Paraplegia*, **1**, 1.

GUTTMANN L., SILVER J. & WYNDHAM C. (1958) Thermoregulation in the spinal man. *J. Physiol.*, **142**, 406–418.

GUTTMANN L. & WHITTERIDGE (1944) *Brain*, **70**, 361.

HARA Y. (1932) *Jap. J. Med. Sci. Biophys.*, **2**, 215.

HARDY A. & SODERSTRON (1938) Heat loss from the nude body and peripheral blood-flow at temperatures of 22°C–35°C. *J. Nutr.*, **15**, 477–497.

HASAMA B. (1940) Pharmakologische und physiologische Studien über die Schweisszentren. *Arch. exper. Path. Pharmakol.*, **146**, 129–161.

HAYMAKER W. & ANDERSON E. (1955) Disorders of the hypothalamus and pituitary gland. In *Clinical Neurology*, Vol. 2, pp. 1160–1215. Baker (ed.). Hoeber, New York.

HEAD H. & RIDDOCH G. (1917) The autonomic bladder, excessive sweating and some other reflex conditions in gross injuries of the spinal cord. *Brain*, **40**, 188–263.

HENSEL H. & ZOTTERMAN Y. (1951) The response to mechanoreceptors to thermal stimulation. *J. Physiol.*, **115**, 16.

HILL L. (1895) The influence of the force of gravity on the circulation of the blood. *J. Physiol.*, **18**, 15.

HINSEY J.C. (1934) Are there efferent fibres in the dorsal roots? *J. comp. Neurol.*, **59**, 117–137.

HOLMES G. (1915) *Brit. med. J.*, **2**, 815.

HORVATH S., HUTT G., SPURR G. & STEVENS G. (1953) Some metabolic responses of dogs having low body temperature. *Science*, **118**, 100.

INGRAM W.R. (1940) Nuclear connection and chief connections of the primate hypothalamus. *Res. Publ. Ass. nerv. ment. Dis.*, **20**, 195–244.

JOHNSON R.H., LEE DE J., OPPENHEIMER D.R. & SPALDING J.K. (1966) Autonomic failure with orthostatic hypotension due to intermediolateral column degeneration. *Quart. J. Med.*, **35**, 276–292.

JOHNSON R.H., PARK D.M. & FRANKEL H.L. (1971) Orthostatic hypotension and the renin-angio-tensin system in paraplegia. *Paraplegia*, **9**, 146–152.

JOHNSON R.H. & SPALDING J.M. (1964) The effect of surface and central temperature on hand blood-flow in subjects with complete transection of the spinal cord. *J. Physiol.*, **171**, 14P–15P.

JONASSON P. (1947) *Proc. Roy. Soc. Med.*, **40**, 222.

KARPLUS J.P. (1937) Die Physiologie der vegetativen Zentren. In *Handbuch der Neurologie*, **2** 402–475, Bumke & Foerster (eds.).

KARPLUS J.P. & KREIDL A. (1909) Gehirn und Sympathicus. *Pflug. Arch. ges. Physiologie*, **129**, 138–144.

KARPLUS J.P. & KREIDL A. (1910) *Ein Sympathienszentrum im Zwischenhirn*, **135**, 401–416.

KELLER A.D. (1938) Separation in the brain stem of the mechanisms of heat loss from those of heat production. *J. Neurophysiol.*, **1**, 543–557.

KELLER A.D. & HARE W.K. (1932) The hypothalamus and heat regulation. *Proc. Soc. exp. Biol. N.Y.*, **29**, 1060–1070.

KEN KURE (1930) *Pflügers Arch.*, 129, 135 and 153.

KENDRICK W., SCOTT J., JOUSSE A. & BOTTERELL H. (1953) *Reflex Sweating and Hyptertension in Traumatic Transverse Myelitis.*

LANGWORTHY O.R. & RICHTER C.P. (1930) The influence of efferent cerebral pathways upon sympathetic nervous system. *Brain*, **53**, 178–193.

LEWIS, SIR T. (1927) *The Blood Vessels of the Human Skin and Their Responses*. Shaw & Sons, London.

LEWIS T. & GRANT R. (1925) Observations upon reactive hyperaemia in man. *Heart*, **12**, 73–120

LEWIS T. & MARVIN A. (1927) *J. Physiol.*, **64**, 27.

LIST C.F. & PEET M.M. (1938–1939) Sweat secretion in man. *Archs Neurol. Psychiat, Chicago*, **99**, 1228–1237; **40**, 27–43; **40**, 269–290; **40**, 443–470; **40**, 1098–1127.

LIST C.F. & PIMENTA A.D. (1944) Spinal reflex sweating. *Archs Neurol. Psychiat.*, **51**, 501–507.

MILLER L.R. (1931) *Lebensnerven und Lebenstriebe*. Springer, Berlin.

MINOR V. (1927) *Z. ges. Neur. Psychiat.*, **47**, 800.

MUNRO A. & ROBINSON R. (1960) *J. Physiol.*, **154**, 244.

OKELBERRY A.M. (1935) Efferent nerve fibres in the lumbar roots of the dog. *J. comp. Neurol.*, **62**, 1–15.

OPPENHEIMER D., PALMER E., WEDDELL G. (1962) Nerve endings in the conjunctiva. *J. Anat.*, **92**, 321.

PEMBREY (1897) The temperature in man and animals after section of the spinal cord. *Brit. Med. J.*, **2**, 883–884.

PEMBREY (1897) Animal heat. In *Textbook of Physiology*, Vol. 1, p. 61, Schäfer E.A. (ed.). Pentland, Edinburgh.

PENFIELD W.G. & BOLDREY E. (1937) Somatic motor and sensory representation in the autonomic system. *Brain*, **60**, 389–443.

PFLÜGER F. (1878) *Pflügers Arch. ges. Physiol.*, **18**, 321.

RANDALL W.C. (1946) Quantitation and regional distribution of sweat glands in man. *J. clin. Invest.*, **25**, 761.

RANDALL W., COX W., ALEXANDER K., COLDWATER K. & HERTZMAN A. (1953) Direct examination of the sympathetic outflow in man. *J. Appl. Physiol.*, **7**, 688–698.

RANDALL W.C. & SECKENENDORF S. (1961) *J. appl. Physiol.*, **16**, 761.

RANSON S.W., FISCHER C. & INGRAM W. (1937) Hypothalamic regulation of temperature in the monkey. *Archs Neurol. Psychiat.*, *Chicago*, **38**, 445–466.

RANSON S. & MAGOUN H.W. (1939) The hypothalamus. *Ergeb. Physiol.*, **41**, 56–163.

RANSON S. (1940) Regulation of body temperature. *Res. Publ. Ass. nerv. ment. Dis.*, **20**, 342–399.

RIDDOCH G. (1917) *Brain*, **40**, 264–402.

SCHWARTZ H.G. (1937) Effect of experimental lesions of the cortex on the 'Psychogalvanic Reflex' in the cat. *Neurol. Psychiat.*, **38**, 308–320.

SHEEHAN D. (1935) Some problems relating to the dorsal spinal nerve roots. *Yale J. Biol. Med.*, 7 425–440.

SHEEHAN D. (1941) Spinal autonomic outflow in man and monkey. *J. comp. Neurol.*, **75**, 341–370.

SHERRINGTON CH.S. (1924) Notes on temperature after spinal transection with some observation on shivering. *J. Physiol.*, **58**, 405.

SILVER J. (1970) Vascular reflexes in spinal shock. *Paraplegia*, **8**, 231–241.

SMITH L. & FAY T. (1940) Observations on human beings with cancer, maintained at reduced temperatures of 75°–90°. *Amer. J. clin. Path.*, **10**, 1.

SOMOGY R. (1913) Das vagotonische Pupillenphänomen. *Wien. Klin. Wschr.*, **26**, 1331.

SPALDING J.M.K. (1969) Autonomic nervous system. In *Handbook of Neurology*, Vol. 2 1P pp. 107–127, Vinken & Bruyn (eds.). North-Holland Publ. Co., Amsterdam.

STEAD E.A. & EBERT R.V. (1941) Postural hypotension: disease of sympathetic system. *Arch. intern. Med.*, **67**, 546–562.

STORY M., CORBIN K. & HINSEY J. (1936) Further observations on dorsal roots components. *Proc. Soc. exp. Biol. N.Y.*, 309–311.

STRICKER S. (1876) Untersuchungen über die Gefässnervenwurzeln des Ischiaticus. *Arch. Wiss. Wien* (Math. Nat. Kl. Abt), **74**, 173–185.

TEAGUE R.S. & RANSON S.W. (1936) The role of the anterior hypothalamus in temperature regulation. *Am. J. Physiol.*, **117**, 562–570.

THAUER S. (1931) Der Mechanismus der Wärmeregulation. *Ergebn. Physiol.*, **41**, 607–805.

THOMAS A. (1921) *Le Reflêxe Pilomoteur*. Masson, Paris.

TOENNIES J.F. (1938) Reflex discharges from the spinal cord over dorsal roots. *J. Neurophysiol.* **1**, 378–390.

TOPORKOFF N. (1925) Die lokale Schweiss secretion bei Epilepsie. *Z. Neur*, **98**, 277–283.

TROLL G.F. & DOHRMANN G.J. (1975) Anaesthesia of the spinal cord injured patient: cardio-vascular problems and their management. *Paraplegia*, **13**, 162–171.

VEREL D. (1951) Postural hypertension: the localisation af the lesion. *Brit. Heart J.*, **13**, 61–67.

WANG G.H. & LU T.W. (1930) Galvanic skin reflex induced in cat by stimulation of the motor area of the cortex. *Clin. J. Physiol.*, **4**, 303–326.

WEDDELL G. (1941) The pattern of cutaneous innervation in relation to cutaneous sensibility. *J. Anat.*, **75**, 346.

WEDDELL G., PALMER E., PALLIE W. (1955) Nerve endings in mammalian skin. *Biol. Rev.*, **30**, 159.

WELPLY N.C., MATHIAS C.J. & FRANKEL H.L. (1975) Circulatory reflexes in tetraplegics during artificial ventilation and general anaesthesia. *Paraplegia*, **13**, 172–182.

WERZILOFT (1896) Zur Frage der vasomotorischen Funktion der hinteren Wurzeln. *Zbl. Physiol.*, **10**, 194–198.

Chapter 27 Disturbances of Bladder and Upper Urinary Tract

ABEL B.J., COSBIE-ROSS J., GIBBON N.O.K. & JAMESON R.M. (1975) Urethral pressure measurement after division of the external sphincter. *Paraplegia*, **13**, 37.

ABRAMSON A.S., BOYARSKY S., ROUSSAN M.S. & FREEDMAN H. (1962) Simultaneous cystometry and electromyography. A method for studying the dynamics of voiding. *Proc. 11th Ann. clin. spinal inj. conf.*, pp. 107–117. Am. Vet. Admin. Hosp., Bronx, N.Y.

ADLER A. (1920) 6 ber organisch (kirtikale) und funktionell-nervöse Blasenstörungen. *Dtsch. Z. Nervenheilk.*, **5**, 72–152.

ALEXANDER S. & ROWAN D. (1968) *Lancet*, i, 728.

ANDREW J. & NATHAN P.W. (1964) Lesions of the anterior frontal lobes and disturbances of micturition and defecation. *Brain*, **87**, 233–262.

ARDRAN G.M., HAMILL J. & SIMMONS C.A. (1956) Further observations of the female urethra and bladder. *Proc. Roy. Soc. Med.*, **49**, 647–652.

ARDUINO L.J. & MILLER E.V. (1960) *J. Urol.*, **84**, 609.

ASCOLI R. (1968) Le tratement des vessies neurogenes. *Acta urol. belg.*, **33**, 76–83.

AUERBACH S., MAINWARING R. & SCHWARZ F. (1963) Renal and ureteral damage following clinical use of ranacidin. *J. Amer. med. Ass.*, **183**, 61–63.

BAKER W.J., CARNEY J.F. & DE ROSA F.P. (1950) Transurethral resection for relief of urinary retention in patients with neurologic lesions. *J. Urol.*, **63**, 309–318.

BARKER N.W. & WALTER W. (1940) *Proc. Staff Meet. Mayo Clinic*, **15**, 475.

BARRINGTON F.J.F. (1915) The nervous mechanism of micturition. *Quart. J. exp. Physiol*, **8**, 33–71.

BARRINGTON F.J.F. (1921) The relation of the hind brain to micturition. *Brain*, **44**, 25–53.

BARRINGTON F.J.F. (1925) The effect of lesion of the hind and midbrain on micturition in the cat. *Quart. J. exp. Physiol.*, **15**, 181–202.

BARRINGTON F.J.F. (1928) The central nervous control of micturition. *Brain*, **51**, 209–220.

BARRINGTON F.J.F. (1931) The component reflexes of micturition in the cat. Part I and II. *Brain*, **54**, 177–188.

BARRINGTON F.J.F. (1933) The localization of the paths subserving micturition in the spinal cord of the cat. *Brain*, **56**, 126–148.

BARRINGTON F.J.F. (1941) The component reflexes of micturition in the cat. Part III. *Brain*, **64**, 239–243.

BARRY K.G., BROOKS M. & HANO J.E. (1967) The prevention of acute renal failure. In *Renal Failure*. Chapter 32, pp. 259–271. Brest A.N. & Moyer J.H. (eds.). Pitman, London.

BERNSTEIN-HAHN L., CIBEIRA J.B. & ZONZINI J. (1965) The urinary tract in myelomeningocele. *Paraplegia*, **3**, 203–206.

BISCHOFF P. (1962) Symptomatologie et traitement chirurgical du mégaurètere congénital. *Acta urol. belg.*, **30**, 257–285.

BITKER M.P. & PAGNOT J. (1964) L'exploration radio-manométrique de la vessie dans l'etude du reflux vésico-urétéral classification des reflux et indications thérapeutiques. *J. d'Urol. et Néph.*, **70**, 485–503.

BLOCKSOM B.H. (1957) *J. Urol.*, **78**, 398.

BLOCK A. (1923) *Z. of Urol. Chir.*, **12**, 239.

BORS E. (1951) Urologic aspects of rehabilitation in spinal cord injuries. *J. amer. med. Ass.*, **146**, 225–229, 19 May.

BORS E. (1952) Segmental and peripheral innervation of the urinary bladder. *J. nerv. ment. dis.*, **116**, 572–578.

BORS E. (1952) Effect of electric stimulation of the pudendal nerves on the vesical neck, its significance for the function of cord bladders: a preliminary report. *J. Urol.*, **67**, 925–935.

BORS E. (1955) Therapeutic procedures of the pudendal nerve for the treatment of cord bladder. Postgrad. meeting North Central Sect. A.U.A. at Rochester, Minn. Postgraduate Sem., pp. 177–187.

BORS E. (1957) Neurogenic bladder. *Urolog. Survey*, **7**, 177–250.

BORS E. (1963) Some anatomical and physiological aspects of the urinary bladder. In *Proc. of Symp. at Royal College of Surgeons*, (ed.) P. Harris, Edinburgh.

BORS E. (1967) Intermittent catheterization in paraplegic patients. *Urologia internationalis*, **22**, 236–249.

BORS E. & BLINN K.A. (1957) Spinal reflex activity from the vesical mucosa in paraplegic patients. *Archs Neurol. Psychiat.*, **78**, 339–354.

BORS E. & COMARR A.E. (1952) Vesico-ureteral reflux in paraplegic patients. *J. Urol.*, **68**, 691–698.

BORS E. & COMARR A.E. (1954) Effect of pudendal nerve operations on the neurogenic bladder. *J. Urol.*, **72**, 666–670.

BORS E. & COMARR A.E. (1971) *Neurological Urology. Physiology of Micturition. Its Neurological Disorders and Sequelae.* S.Karger, Basel, Munchen, Paris, New York.

BORS E., COMARR A.E. & REINGOLD I.M. (1954) Striated muscle fibers of the vesical neck. *J. Urol.*, **72**, 191–196.

BORS E., COMARR A.E. & MOULTON S.H. (1950) The role of nerve blocks in management of traumatic cord bladders: spinal anesthesia, subarachnoid alcohol injections, pudendal nerve anaesthesia and vesical neck anaesthesis. *J. Urol.*, **63**, 653–666.

BORS E., COMARR A.E., EBAL A., HABIB H.N., SUSSET A. & TALBOT H. (1963) *Proc. Clin. Spinal Cord Conf.* p. 97. Amer. Vet. Admin. Hosp., Hines, U.S.A.

BOSHAMER K. (1951) Splanchnicotomy for prevention and treatment of urologic disturbances in diseases of the spinal cord. *J. int. Coll. Surg.*, **15**, 424–426.

BOSHAMER K. (1960) Die Behandlung der Querschnittsverletzten nach Durchführung der Erstversorgung. *Zbl. Neurochir.*, **20**, 193–215.

BOWLEY A.A. (1890) *Med. chir. Trans.*, **73**, 317.

BOYARSKY S., LABAY P., KRUGMAN A., GLENN J.F. & NEWMARK T. (1966) Clinical evaluation of bladder pressure studies in urological patients by combined cystometry and uroflowmetry. *J. Urol.*, **95**, 778–790.

BOYARSKY S. (1967) Neurogenic Bladder. Symposium Duke University, 306 pages. William & Wilkins, Baltimore.

BOURA A.L. & GREEN A.F. (1963) *Brit. Pharmacol. J.*, **20**, 30.

BRADLEY W.E. (1967) Ontogeny of central regulation of visceral reflex activity in the rabbit. *Amer. J. Physiol.*, **212**, 335–340.

BRADLEY W.E., CHOU S.N. & FRENCH L.A. (1963) Further experience with radio transmitter receiver unit for the neurogenic bladder. *J. Neurosurg.*, **20**, 953–960.

BRENDLER H., KRUEGER E.G., LERMAN P., HARPER J.G.M., BRADLEY D., BERMAN M.H., HERTZBERG A.D., LERMAN F. & DEAN A.L. (1953) Spinal root section in treatment of advanced paraplegic bladder. *J. Urol.*, **70**, 223–229.

BREST A.N., ONESTI G., SELLER R., RAMIREZ O., HEIDER C. & MOYER J.H. (1965) Pharmacodynamic effects of a new diuretic drug: ethacrynic acid. *Amer. J. Cardiol.*, **16**, 99.

BRICKER E.M. (1950) Bladder substitution after pelvic evisceration. *Surg. Clin. N. Amer.*, 1511.

BUDGE J. (1884) Über den Einfluss des Nervensystems auf die Bewegungen der Blase. *Z. rationelle Med.*, **21**, 1.

BROWN C.B., GLANCY J.J., FRY I.K. & CATTELL W.R. (1970) A high-dose excretion urography in oliguric renal failure. *Lancet*. ii, 952.

BULL G.M., JOÉKES A. & LOWE K. (1949) *Lancet*, ii, 229.

BULL M.B., HILLMAN R.S., CANNON P.J. & LARAGH J.H. (1966) The control of renin and aldosterone secretion: Influence of sodium and potassium balance and changes in blood volume. *J. Clin. Invest.*, **45**, 992.

BUNTS R.C. (1958) Management of urological complications in 1,000 paraplegics. *J. Urol.*, **79**, 733–741.

BUNTS R.C. (1959) Preservation of renal function in the paraplegic. *J. Urol.*, 720–727.

BUNTS R.C. (1964) Electrical stimulation of the neurogenic bladder. *V.A. Urologists News Letter* 16 Nov.

BUMPUS H.C., NOURSE M.H. & THOMPSON G.J. (1947) Urologic complications in injury of the spinal cord. *J. amer. med. Ass.*, **133**, 366–368.

BURGHELE T.H., ICHIM V. (1969) Erfahrungen über die Electrostimulation der neurogenen Harnblase. In *Neurogene Blasenstörungen*, pp. 39–44. Thieme, Stuttgart.

BURGHELE T.H. & ICHIM V. (1972) Research on anatomy and physiology of the neurogenic bladder. *Second Neurol-Urolog. Conference*, Mulhouse, France. In *Neurogene Blasenstörungen*, pp. 1–10. Thieme, Stuttgart.

BURNS E. & KITTREDGE W.G. (1958) Surgical procedures on the vesical neck. *J. Urol.*, **79**, 751–754.

BUTLER A.M. (1937) Chronic pyelonephritis and hypertension. *J. Clin. Invest.*, **16**, 889.

CAESAR R., EDWARDS G.A. & RUSKA H. (1957) Architecture and nerve supply of mammalian smooth muscle tissue. *J. biophys. biochem. Cytol.*, **3**, 867–878.

CALDWELL K.P.S. (1967) *Annals of Royal College of Surgeons, England*, **41**, 447.

CALDWELL K.P.S. (1969) Behandlung der Blaseninkontinenz durch Electro-stimulation, In *Neurogene Blasenstörungen*, pp. 56–58. Thieme, Stuttgart.

CANNON P.J. & LARAGH J.H. (1963) Treatment of hypertension with alpha-methyldopa. *Pharmakotherap.*, **1**, 171.

CANTEROVICH F., GALLI C., BENEDETTI L., CHENA C., CASTRO L., CORREA C., PEREZ LOREDO J., FERNANDEZ J.S., LOCATELLI A. & TIZADO J. (1973) High dose frusemide in established acute renal failure. *Brit. med. J.*, **4**, 449.

CARTER R.E. & JACKSON G.G. (1972) *Paraplegia*, **10**, 11.

CASHION E.L. & MOELLER B.A. (1975) Long-term results of sacral rhizotomy for ureteral reflux in the spinal cord injured. *Paraplegia*, **13**, 153.

CIBEIRA J.B. (1970) *Paraplegia*, **7**, 249.

CIBEIRA J.B. (1970) Some conclusions on a study of 365 patients with spinal cord lesions. *Paraplegia*, **7**, 4, 249–254.

CIBET J., REVOL M. & RIGONDET G. (1958) Troubles vésicaus d'origine nervaise tratés par iléocystoplastie de substitution. *J. Urol.*, **64**, 256–257.

COLLEY E.W. & FRANKEL H.L. (1964) Pencillin G. treatment of urinary infection in paraplegia. *Paraplegia*, **2**, 132–140.

COMARR A.E. (1955) A long term survey of the incidence of renal calculosis in paraplegia. *J. Urol.*, **74**, 447–452.

COMARR A.E. & BORS E. (1951) Pathological changes in urethra of paraplegic patients. *J. Urol.*, **66**, 355–361.

COMARR A.E. & BORS E. (1955) An unusual urethral fistula site. *Amer. J. Surg.*, **90**, 151–152.

COMARR A.E. & BORS E. (1955) Further observations on vesico-ureteral reflux. *J. Urol.*, **74**, 59–66.

COMARR A.E. & BORS E. (1958) Perineal urethral diverticulum; complication of removal of ischium. *J. Amer. med. Ass.*, **168**, 13 Dec, 2000–2003.

COMARR A.E. (1959) The practical urological management of the patient with spinal cord injury. *Brit. J. Urol.*, **31**, 1–46.

COMARR A.E., KAWAICHI G. & BORS E. (1962) Renal calculosis of patients with traumatic cord lesions. *J. Urol.*, **87**, 647–657.

CORREY & VEST (1954) Electropotential changes in the isolated mammalian bladder. *Surg. Gynec. Obstet.*, **98**, 91–95.

COOK J.B. & SMITH P.H. (1970) Second Neurol-Urolog. Conference, Mulhouse, France, pp. 95–98. Thieme, Stuttgart.

COOPER A. & CRANSTON G. (1957) *Lancet*, i, 396.

CRUIKSHANK W. (1790) *The Anatomy of the Absorbing Vessels of the Human Body*. London.

CUNNINGHAM D., GUTTMANN L., WHITTERIDGE D. & WYNDHAM C.H. (1953) Cardiovascular responses to bladder distension in paraplegic patients. *J. Physiol.*, **121**, 581–592.

DAMANSKI M. & GIBBON N. (1956) The upper urinary tract in the paraplegic: a long term survey. *Brit. J. Urol.*, **28**, 24–38.

DAMANSKI (1961) *Br. J. Urol.*, **33**, 67.

DAVIS L. & MARTIN J. (1948) *Surg. Gynec. Obstet.*, **86**, 535.

DENNING H. (1924) Untersuchungen über die Innervation der Harnblase und des Mastdarmes. *Zeitschrift für Biologie*, **80**, 239–254.

DENNY-BROWN D. & ROBERTSON E.G. (1933) The state of the bladder and its sphincters in complete transverse lesions of the spinal cord and cauda equina. *Brain*, **56**, 397–462.

DENNY-BROWN D. & ROBERTSON E. (1933) On the physiology of micturition. *Brain*, **56**, 149–199.

DE WARDENER H.E. & MILES B.E. (1952) The effect of haemorrhage on the circulatory autoregulation of the dog's kidney perfused *in situ*. *Clin. Sc.*, **11**, 267.

DOGGART J.R., GUTTMANN L. & SILVER J.R. (1966) Comparative studies on endogenous creatinine and urea clearance in paraplegics and tetraplegics. *Paraplegia*, **3**, 229–242.

DOLLFUS P. & MOLE L. (1969) *Paraplegia*, **7**, 204–206.

DOLLFUS P., JURASCHECK F., ALBI F. & CHATUIS A. (1976) Impairment of erection after external sphincter resection. *Paraplegia*, **14**, 290.

DONOVAN H. (1947) *Lancet*, i, 515.

DUZEN, VAN R.G. (1935) *Sth. Med. J.*, **28**, 785–791.

EHALT W. (1965) *Experiences on recent traumatic paraplegics in 25 years. Paraplegia* **3**, 66.

ELLIOTT T.R. (1907) The innervation of bladder and urethra. *J. Physiol.*, **35**, 367–445.

EMMETT J.L. (1945) Transurethral resection in treatment of true and pseudo-cord bladder. *J. Urol.*, **53**, 4.

EMMETT J.L. (1954) Neurogenic vesical dysfunction (cord bladder) and neuro-muscular ureteral dysfunction. In *Urology*, Vol. 2, Sec. XI, Chapter I, pp. 1285–1383. Meredith Campbell (ed.). W.B.Saunders, Philadelphia, London.

ERSLEV A.J. (1960) Control of red cell production. *Ann. Rev. Med.*, **11**, 315.

ERSLEV A.J. (1967) Anaemia in renal failure. In *Renal Failure*, Chapter 16. Brest A.N. & J.H. Moyer (eds.).

EVANS J.P. (1936) Observations on the nerve supply to the bladder and urethra of the cat with a study of their action potentials. *J. Physiol.*, **86**, 396–414.

FELTON L.M. & READ P.M. (1960) *J. Urol.*, **84**, 619.

FISHBERG A.M. (1954) *Hypertension and Nephritis*. Baillière, Tindall & Co, London.

FOERSTER O. (1936) *Handbuch der Neurologie*, Vol. **5**, p. 193. Springer, Berlin.

FOERSTER O. & GAGEL O. (1933) Über afferente Nervenfasern in den vorderen Wurzeln. *Z. ges. Neurol. Psychiat.*, **144**, 313–324.

FOSTVEDT G.A. & BARNES R.W. (1963) Complications during lavage therapy for renal calculi. *J. Urol.*, **89**, 329–331.

FREEMAN L.W. (1949) *J. Amer. med. Ass.*, **140**, 949, 1015.

FRY B. & QUENU L. (1965) *Physiologie Normale et Pathologique des Voies Urinaire Superieurs*, pp. 480–583. Springer, Berlin.

GARNIER B., GERTSCH B., STEINMANN B. (1964) *Cardiologie*, **44**, 167.

GARNIER B., IMHOF P., HEDIGER F. & STEINMANN B. (1963) Über das Verhalten des Blutdrucks beim Paraplegiker. *Cardiologie*, **42**, 103–110.

GARNIER B. & GERTSCH R. (1964) *Schweiz. med. Wschr.*, **94**, 124.

GENEST J. (1961) Angiotensin aldosterone and human arterial hypertension. *Canad. Med. Ass. J.*, **84**, 403.

GIBBON N.O.K. (1956) A case of herpes zoster with involvement of the urinary bladder. *Brit. J. Urol.*, **28**, 417–421.

GIBBON N.O.K., ROSS J.C. & DAMANSKI M. (1965) Bladder neck resection in the paraplegic. Report on over 100 cases. *Paraplegia*, **2**, 264–276.

GIBBON N.O.K., ROSS J.C. & SILVER J.R. (1969) Changes in the upper urinary tract following various types of initial treatment. *Paraplegia*, **7**, 2, 63–77.

GJONE R. & SETEKLEIV J. (1963) Excitatory and inhibitory bladder responses to stimulation of the cerebral cortex in the cat. *Acta physiol. scand.*, **59**, 337–348.

GLAHN B.E. (1970) Manual provocation of micturition contraction in neurogenic bladder. *Scand. J. Urol. Nephrol.*, **4**, 25.

GLAHN, B.E. (1974) Neurogenic bladder in spinal cord injury. *Urologic Clinics of North America*, **Vol. 1, N1**, 163.

GOLDBLATT H., LYNCH J., HANZAL R.F. & SUMMERVILLE W.W. (1934) Studies on experimental hypertension: production of persistent elevation of systolic blood pressure by means of renal ischemia. *J. Exp. Med.*, **59**, 847.

GOLDING (1958) Third African Rehabilitation Conference, Lusaka, Zambia.

GRIFFITH J. (1895) *J. Anat. Physiol.*, **29**, 61.

GRIFFITHS I.H. & WALSH J.J. (1961) Diverticula and fistulae of the urethra in paraplegics. *Brit. J. Urol.*, **33**, 374–380.

GUTTMAN D. & NAYLOR S.R. (1967) Dip-slide, an aid to quantitative urine culture in general practice. *Brit. med. J.*, **3**, 343.

GUTTMANN L. (1943) Studies on suture material. *Brit. J. Surg.*, **30**, 370.

GUTTMANN L. (1946) *Brit. J. Physical Med.*, **9**, 130, 162.

GUTTMANN L. (1947) Discussion on the treatment and prognosis of traumatic paraplegia. *Proc. Roy. Soc. Med.*, **40**, 219–225.

GUTTMANN L. (1949) Management of paralysis. In: Intermittent catheterization. *Brit. Surg. Pract.*, **6**, 445. Butterworth, London.

GUTTMANN L. (1949) Pituitrin therapy in hydronephrosis. *Roy. Soc. Med.*, **42**, 545–546.

GUTTMANN L. (1953) *Official Medical History of the Second World War*, Vol. Surgery, pp. 422–516, Sir Zachary Cope(ed.). Autonomic hyperreflexia, pp. 440–474, Intermittent catheterization, p. 465. H.M. Stationery Office, London.

GUTTMANN L. (1954) Statistical survey on one thousand paraplegics and initial treatment of traumatic paraplegia. *Proc. Roy. Soc. Med.*, **47**, 1099–1109.

GUTTMANN L. (1958) *Modern Trends in Diseases of the Spinal Column*, p. 258, Butterworth, London

GUTTMANN L. (1961) *The Medical Annual*, p 25. Wright, Bristol.

GUTTMANN L. (1963) In *Proc. Symp. Spinal Injuries*, p. 80. Harris P. (ed.). Roy. Coll. Surg., Edinburgh,

GUTTMANN L. (1963) Observations on the aetiology of vesico-ureteric reflux. *Paraplegia*, **1**, 184.

GUTTMANN L. (1968) Erfahrungen mit der konservativen Behandlung der neurogenen Blase. pp 1–10. *Conference on Neurogenic Bladder, Homburg*. Thieme, Stuttgart.

GUTTMANN L. (1969) Disturbances of bladder function. In *Handbook of Clinical Neurology*, Vinken & Bruyn (eds). Vol. 2, 9, pp. 188–193. North-Holland Publishing Co., Amsterdam.

GUTTMANN L. & FRANKEL H. (1966) The value of intermittent catheterization in the early management of traumatic paraplegia and tetraplegia. *Paraplegia*, **4**, 63–84.

GUTTMANN L. & WHITTERIDGE D. (1947) Effects of bladder distension on autonomic mechanisms after spinal cord injuries. *Brain*, **70**, 361–405.

HACHEN H. (1976) Late results of bilateral endoscopic sphincterotomy in patients with upper motor neuron lesions. *Paraplegia*, **14**, 268–274.

HAMILTON M. & KOPELMAN H. (1963) Treatment of severe hypertension with methyldopa. *Brit. med. J.*, **1**, 151.

HAGMAN J., FLANIGAN S. HARVARD B.M. & GLENN W.W. (1966) Electromicturition by radio frequency stimulation. *Surg. Gynec Obstet.*, **123**, 808–811.

HAGNER F. (1912) *Surg. Gynec. Obstet.*, **15**, 510.

HALL M. (1941) *On the Diseases and Derangements of the Nervous System*. Baillière, London.

HARDY A.G. (1966) Experience with intermittent catheterisation in acute paraplegia. *Med. Services J. Canada*, 438–544.

HARDY A.G. (1968) *Paraplegia*, **6**, 5–10.

HARTCROFT P.M., NEWMARK L.N. & PITCOCK J.A. (1959) Relationship of renal juxtaglomerular cells to sodium intake, adrenal cortex and hypertension. In *Hypertension*. Moyer. J. (ed.). W.B.Saunders, Philadelphia.

HARTCROFT P.M. (1966) The renal juxtaglomerular complex. *Ann. Rev. Med.*, **17**, 113.

HEAD H. (1893) *Brain*, **16**, Part I.

HEAD H. & RIDDOCH G. (1917) The automatic bladder, excessive sweating and some other reflex conditions in gross injuries of the spinal cord. *Brain*, **40**, 188–263.

HEPINSTALL R.H. (1966) *Pathology of the Kidney*. Little Brown, Boston.

HINMAN F., MILLER G., NICKEL E. & MILLER E. (1954) Vesical physiology demonstrated by cine-radiography and serial roentgenography. *Radiology*, **62**, 713–719.

HODGSON N.B. & WOOD J.A. (1958) Studies of the nature of paroxysmal hypertension in paraplegics. *J. Urol.*, **79**, 719–721.

HOPKINS B.R. (1972) *Annals of Royal Coll. of Surgeons, England*, **50**, 92.

HOVELACQUE A. (1927) *Anatomie*. Paris: Doin et Cie.

HUNSICKER W.C. & SPIEGEL E.A. (1934) Conduction of cortical impulses to the autonomic system. *Proc. Soc. exp. Biol. and Med.*, **31**, 974–976.

HUTCH J.A. (1957) *J. Urol.*, **123**.

HUTCH J.A. (1962) The role of the ureterovesical junction in the natural history of pyelonephritis. *J. Urol.*, **88**, 354–362.

HUTCH J.A. (1963) Ureteric advancement operation: anatomy, technique and early results. *J. Urol.*, **89**, 180–184.

IGGO A. (1955) Tension receptors in the stomach and the urinary bladder. *J. Physiol.*, **128**, 593–607.

INGELMAN-SUNDBERG A. (1957) An operation for the relief of urinary retention caused by paralysis of the detrusor muscle. *Urol. int.*, **4**, 247–253.

INGERSOLL E.H., JONES L.L. & HEGRE E.S. (1954) Urinary bladder response to unilateral stimulation of hypogastric nerves. *J. Urol.*, **72**, 178–190.

INGERSOLL E.H., JONES L.L. & HEGRE E.S. (1955) Urinary bladder responses to unilateral stimulation of pelvic nerves. *Soc. Exper. Biol. and Med.*, **88**, 46–49.

JACOBSON L.O., GOLDWASSER E., FRIED W. & PIZAK L. (1957) Role of the kidney in erythropoiesis. *Nature*, **179**, 633.

JACOBSON S.A. & BORS E. (1970) Spinal Cord Injury in Vietnamese Combat. *Paraplegia*, **7**, 4, 263–281.

JOHNSON D., KITCHIN A., LOWTHER C. & TURNER R. (1966) Treatment of hypertension with methyldopa. *Brit. med. J.*, **1**, 133.

JOHNSTON A., PRICHARD B. & ROSENHEIM M. (1962) *Lancet*, ii, 996.

JÖNSSON & ZEDERFELDT B. (1957) A study of cetiprin as a urologic drug. *Urol. int.*, **4**, 293–305.

JOUSSE A., MACDONALD M. & WYNNE-JONES (1964) Bladder control in the female paraplegic patient. *Paraplegia*, **2**, 146–152.

KABAT H., MAGOUN H.W. & RANSON S.W. (1939) Electrical stimulation of the hypothalamus. *Proc. Soc. exp. Biol.*, **31**, 541.

KARAFIN L. & KENDALL A.R. (1966) Vesicostomy in the management of neurogenic bladder disease secondary to meningomyelocele in children. *J. Urol.*, **96**, 723–728.

KASS E.H. & SOSSEN H.S. (1959) Prevention of infection of urinary tract in presence of indwelling catheter. Description of electromechanical valve to provide intermittent drainage of the bladder. *J. Amer. med. Ass.*, **169**, 1181–1183.

KAWAICHI S. (1960) *Pro. 9th Ann. Clin. Cord Injury Conf.*, pp. 104–105.

KINTER W.B. & PAPPENHEIMER J.R. (1956) Role of red blood corpuscles in regulation of renal blood flow and glomerular filtration rate. *Amer. J. Physiol.*, **185**, 399.

KIRKENDALL W.M. & FITZ A.E. (1967) The functional role of the juxtaglomerular apparatus. In, *Renal Failure*, Chapter 3. Brest A.N. & Moyer. J.H. (eds). Pitman Medical.

KJELLBERG S.R., ERICSSON N.O. & RUDHE U. (1957) *The Lower Urinary Tract in Childhood; Some Correlated Clinical and Roentgenologic Observations*. Yearbook publishers.

KLEIST (1934) *Gehirupathologie*, Leipzig.

KRAHN H., MORALES P. & HOTCHKISS R. (1964) Experience with tubeless cystostomy. *J. Urol.*, **91**, 246–252.

KRETSCHMER H. & GREER J. (1915) *Surg. Gynec. Obstet.*, **21**, 228.

KUNTZ A. & SACCOMANO G. (1944) *J. Neurophysiol.*, **7**, 163–170.

KURU M. & HUKAVAI G. (1954) *Jap. J. Physiol.*, **4**, 175.

KURU M., MAKNYA A. & KOYAMA (1961) *J. Comp. Neurol.*, **117**, 161.

KURNICK N.B. (1956) Autonomic hyperreflexia and its control in patients with spinal cord lesions. *Ann. Intern. Med.*, **44**, 678–686.

KYLE E. (1968) The complications of indwelling catheter. *Paraplegia*, **6**, 1–6.

LANGWORTHY O.R. & KOLB L.C. (1933) The encephalic control of tone in the musculature of the urinary bladder. *Brain*, **56**, 371–382.

LANGWORTHY O.R., REEVES, D.L. & TAUBER E.S. (1934) Autonomic control of urinary bladder. *Brain*, **57**, 266–290.

LANGWORTHY O.R. & MURPHY E.L. (1939) Nerve endings in the urinary bladder. *J. comp. Neurol.*, **71**, 487–504.

LANGWORTHY O.R., DREW J.E. & VEST S.A. (1940) Urethral resistance in relation to vesical activity. *J. Urol.*, **43**, 123–141.

LANGWORTHY OR., KOLB L.C. & LEWIS L.G. (1950) *Physiology of Micturition*. Williams & Wilkins, Baltimore.

LAPIDES J. (1948) The physiology of the intact human ureter. *J. Urol.*, **59**, 501–533.

LAPIDES J. (1964) Urecholine regimen for rehabilitating the atonic bladder. *J. Urol.*, **91**, 658–659.

LAPIDES J., SWEET R.B. & LEWIS L.W. (1955) Function of striated muscle in control of urination. II. Effect of complete muscle paralysis. *Clin. congr. amer. Coll. Surg.*, 31 Oct.–4 Nov., Chicago.

710 REFERENCES

LAPIDES J., AJEMIAN E.P., STEWART B.H., BREAKEY B.A. & LICHTWARDT J.R. (1960) Further observations on the kinetics of the urethrovesical sphincter. *J. Urol.*, **84**, 86–94.

LAPIDES J., AJEMIAN E. & LICHTWARDT J. (1960) *J. Urol.*, **84**, 609.

LAPIDES J., AJEMIAN E. & LICHWARDT J. (1962) *J. Urol.*, **88**, 735.

LAPIDES J., BOURNE R. & LANNING R. (1964) *Trans. Amer. Ass. Gen-urin. Surg.*, **56**, 78.

LASZKOWSKI T. & BRANTLEY-SCOTT F.B. (1965) Cutaneous vesicostomy as means of urinary diversion: 3 years experience. *J. Urol.*, **94**, 549–555.

LAVER C.H. (1917) An automatic bladder irrigator. *Guy's Hosp. Gaz.*, **31**, 71–74.

LEAL J.F. (1963) *Proc. Clin. Spinal Cord Conf.*, p. 95. Amer. Vet. Admin. Hosp. Hines, U.S.A.

LEARMONTH J.R. (1931) A contribution to the neurophysiology of the urinary bladder in man. *Brain*, **54**, 147–176.

LEGNER F. (1970) *Symposium on neurogenic bladder*, Mulhouse.

LE GROS-CLARK F. (1883) Some remarks on the anatomy and physiology of the urinary bladder and of the sphincters of the rectum. *J. Anat. and Physiol.* **17**, 442–459.

LEE L.W. (1950) The clinical use of urecholine in dysfunctions of the bladder. *J. Urol.*, **62**, 300–307.

LERICHE A.V., ARCHIMBAUD J.P., BERARD E., MINAIRE T. & BOURRET J. (1976a) Pathology of the striated urethral sphincter in spinal cord injury patients: indications and results of external sphinterotomy. *Paraplegia*, **14**, 275–279.

LERICHE A.V., ARCHIMBAUD J.P., BERARD E., MINAIRE T. & BOURRET J. (1976b) Differential diagnosis and limitations of external sphincterotomy. *Paraplegia*, **14**, 280–285.

LEWIS C.T., HOLLAND E.A., MARSHALL V.R., TRESIDDLER G.L. & BLANDY J.P. (1975) Analgesic abuse, ureteric obstruction and retroperitoneal fibrosis. *Brit. med. J.* **1**, 76.

LEWIS L.G. (1945) Treatment of bladder dysfunction after neurologic trauma. *J. Urol.*, **54**, 284–295.

LINDAN, R. & BELLOMY V. (1975) Effect of delayed intermittent catheterization on kidney function in spinal cord injury patients. *Paraplegia*, **13**, 49.

LLOYD F.A. (1963) *Proc. Clin. Spinal Cord Conf.*, p. 97. Amer. Vet. Admin. Hosp. Hines, U.S.A.

LUTZEIER W. (1963) Harnleiterdruckmessung. Eine zusätzliche diagnostische Methode zur Erfassung der Harnleiterfunktion. *Urol. int.*, **16**, 1–15.

MACALPINE J.B. (1948) *Textbook of Genito-urinary Surgery*, p. 356, Winsbury-White H.P. (ed.). Livingstone, Edinburgh.

MCCREA D. (1926) The musculature of the bladder. *Proc. roy. Soc. Med.*, **19**, 35–43.

MCINTOSH J.F. & WORLEY G. (1955) *J. Urol.*, **73**, 820.

MCLELLAN F.C. (1939) *The Neurogenic Bladder*. Ch. Thomas, Springfield, Ill.

MCMAHON S. (1937–1938) An anatomical study by injection technique of the ejaculatory ducts and their relations. *J. Anat.*, **72**, 556–574.

MARKLAND C., CHOU S., BRADLEY W., WESTGATE H. & WOLFSON J. (1966) Some problems in the use of intermittent vesical electronic stimulation. *Invest. Urol.*, **4**, 168–173.

MASGAGNI P. (1787) *Vasorum Lymphaticorum Corpus Humani*, Siena.

MAURY M. & AUDIC B. (1963) Les injections sous-arachnoidiennes d'alcool absolu dans les paraplegiques. *Soc. Med. d'Hopitaux de Paris*, **114**, 387–396.

MEIROWSKY A.M., SCHEIBERT C.D. & HINCHEY T.A. (1950) Studies on the sacral reflex arc in paraplegia; response of the bladder to surgical elimination of sacral nerve impulses by rhizotomy. *J. Neurosurg.*, **7**, 33–38.

MELZAK J. (1966) The incidence of bladder cancer in paraplegia. *Paraplegia*, **4**, 85–96.

MERTENS H.G., HARMS H.S. & JUNGMANN H. (1960) The regulation of the circulation in patients with cervical cord transection. *German Medical Monthly*, **5**, 189–193.

MILNER P.R. (1963) *J. Clin. Path.*, **16**, 39.

MITCHELL G.A.G. (1935–1936) The innervation of the kidney, ureter, testicle and epididymis. *J. Anat.*, **70**, 10–32.

MITCHELL G.A.G. (1950) The nerve supply of the kidney. *J. Anat.*, **84**, 70–71.

MITCHELL G. (1965) The use of haemodialysis in renal failure complicating paraplegia. A report of 5 cases. *Paraplegia*, **2**, 254–263.

MOORE C. (1957) The concept of relative bone marrow failure. *Amer. J. Med.*, **23**, 1.

MOSSO, A. & PELLACANI, P. (1882) Sur les fonctions de la véssie. *Arch. ital. biol.*, **1**, 97–128, 291–324.

MÜLLER L.R. (1924) *Lebensnerven und Lebenstriebe*, pp. 641–657.

MÜLLNER S.R. & FLEISCHNER F.G. (1949) Normal and abnormal micturition: a study of bladder behaviour by means of the fluorscope. *J. Urol*, **61**, 233–241.

MÜLLNER S.R. (1951) The physiology of micturition. *J. Urol.*, **65**, 805–810.

MÜLLNER S.R. (1958) The voluntary control of micturition in man. *J. Urol.*, **80**, 473–478.

MULVANEY W.P. (1959) A new solvent for certain urinary calculi: a preliminary report. *J. Urol.*, **82**, 546–548.

MULVANEY W.P. (1960) The clinical use of renacidin in urinary calcifications. *J. Urol.*, **84**, 206–212.

MULVANEY W.P. (1963) Hydrodynamics of renal irrigations; with reference to calculus solvents. *J. Urol.*, **89**, 765–768.

MULVANEY W.P. (1964) Prevention of calcification of indwelling catheter. *Arch. Phys. Med. Rehab.*, **45**, 610–613.

MUNRO D. (1936) Activity of the urinary bladder as measured by a new and inexpensive cystometer. *New Eng. J. Med.*, **214**, 617–624.

MUNRO D. (1943) Tidal drainage and cystometry in the treatment of sepsis associated with spinal cord injuries; a study of 165 cases. *New Eng. J. Med.*, **229**, 6–14.

MUNRO D. (1945) The treatment of patients with injuries of the spinal cord and cauda equina preliminary to making them ambulatory. *Clinics*, **4**, 448–474.

MUNRO D. (1947) The rehabilitation of patients totally paralysed below the waist with special reference to making them ambulatory and capable of earning their living. III. Tidal drainage, cystometry and bladder training. *New Eng. J. Med.*, **236**, 223–235.

MUNRO D. (1950) Two year end results in the total rehabilitation of veterans with spinal cord and cauda equina injuries. *New Eng. J. Med.*, **242**, 1–16.

MUNRO D. (1952) Anterior rootlet rhizotomy. A method of controlling spasm with retention of voluntary motion. *New Eng. J. Med.*, **246**, 161–166.

MUNRO D. & HAHN J. (1935) *New Engl. J. Med.*, **212**, 229.

MURPHY J.J. & SCHOENBERG H.W. (1960) Observations on intravesical pressure changes during micturition. *J. Urol.* **84**, 106–110.

NAETS J.P. (1960) The role of the kidney in erythropoiesis. *J. Clin. Invest.*, **39**, 102.

NARATH P.W. (1951) *Renal Pelvis and Ureter*. Grune & Stratton, New York.

NASH D.F.E. (1967) Urinary diversion in congenital paraplegia. *Paraplegia*, **4**, 216–225.

NATHAN P.W. (1952) Thermal sensations in the bladder. *J. Neurol. Neurosurg. Psychiat.*, **15**, 150–151.

NATHAN P.W. & SMITH M.C. (1958) The centrifugal pathway for micturition within the spinal cord. *J. Neurol. Neurosurg. Psychiat.*, **21**, 177–189.

NESBIT R.M., LAPIDES J., VALK W.W., SUTLER M., BERRY R.L., LYONS R.H., CAMPBELL K.N. & MOL G.H. (1947) The effects of blockade of the autonomic ganglia on the urinary bladder in man. *J. Urol.*, **57**, 242–250.

NOIX M. (1960) La motricité cysto-urétrale au cours de la miction son étude radiocinématographique. *Acta urol. belg.*, **28**, 532–538.

NOLAN B. (1972) Transplantation of the kidney. In *Renal Disease*, page 521. Sir Douglas Black (ed.). Blackwell Scientific Publications, Oxford.

O'FLYNN J.D. (1972) External sphincterotomy for the relief of outlet obstruction in neurogenic bladder. *Paraplegia*, **10**, 29.

OLIVECRONA (1935) *Parasagital Meningeomas*. Thieme.

OWATSU A. (1961) A study of the urinary reflux in paraplegic patients. *Abstr. jap. Med*, **1**, 1047.

PAESLACK V. (1965) *Internistische Störungen beim Paraplegiker*, pp. 6, 30, 43, 44, 93.

PAESLACK V. (1969) Asepsis und Chemotherapie in der Behandlung der neurogenen Blase. In *Neurogene Blasenstörungen*. pp. 22–27. Thieme, Stuttgart.

PATE V.A. & BUNTS C.R. (1948) Faulty healing of suprapubic sinus resulting in fatal peritonitis. *J. Urol.*, **60**, 915–921.

PEART W.S. (1965) The renin-angiotensin system. *Pharmacol. Rev.*, **17**, 143.

PÉLOT G. & VOEGTLIN R. (1961) Colocystoplastie chez les traumatisés medullaires. *J. Urol. Néphrol.*, **67**, 180–188.

PÉLOT M.G. (1963) Enterocystoplasty in contracted bladder complicated by hydronephrosis. *Paraplegia*, **1**, 55–61.

PERKASH I. (1976) Modified approach to sphincterotomy in spinal cord injury patients. *Paraplegia*, **14**, 247–260.

PETERSEN I., STENER I., SELLDEN U. & KOLLBERG S. (1962) Investigation of urethral sphincter in women with simultaneous electro-myography and micturition urethrocystography. *Acta neurol.*, Suppl. 3, **38**, 145–151.

PETROFF R. & LUCAS F. (1946) *Ann. Surg.*, **123**, 808.

PICKERING G. & HEPINSTALL R.H. (1953) *Quart. J. Med. N.S.*, **22**, 1.

PICKERING G. (1955) *High Blood Pressure*. Churchill, London.

PIEPER A. (1951) Beitrag zur Nervenversorgung des Ureters. *Z. Urol.*, **44**, 17–23.

POLITANO V.A. & LEADBETTER W.F. (1958) An operative technique for the correction of vesicoureteral reflux. *J. Urol.*, **79**, 932–941.

PRATHER G.C. (1944) Suprapubic Cystotomy. *Bull, U.S. Army Med. Dept.*, **81**, 96.

PRATHER G.C. (1947) Spinal cord injuries: calculi of the urinary tract. *J. Urol.*, **57**, 1097–1104.

PRATHER G.C. (1959) *Surgery in World War II*, Vol. 22, pp. 90, 99. Washington, D.C.

PULASKI E.J. (1946) *Ann. Surg.*, **124**, 392.

REINGOLD I.M. (1960) The pathology of selected cases of spinal cord injuries. In *Proc. 9th Spinal Cord Injury Conf.* Amer. Vet. Admin. Hospital, Long Beach, U.S.A.

REISSMANN K.R., NOMURA T., GUNN R.W. & BROSIUS F. (1960) Erythropoietic response to anaemia or erythropoietin injection in uremic rats with or without functioning renal tissues. *Blood*, **16**, 1411.

REITE A.E. & COMARR A.E. (1954) Complications of neurogenic bladder. A case report. *J. Urol.*, **72**, 41–44.

RENYI-VAMOS F. (1960) Anatomische Probleme der Lymphforschung, Fol. *Angiol.*, **6**, 13.

RETIEF P.J.M. & KEY A.G. (1967) Urinary diversion in paraplegia. *Paraplegia*, **4**, 225–231.

RICHES E.W. (1943) *Brit. J. Surg.*, **31**, 135.

RIDDOCH G. (1917) *Brain*, **40**, 264.

ROSENHEIM (1963) Vesico-ureteric reflux in general medicine. *Paraplegia*, **1**, 180.

ROSENTHAL A.M., ROLNICK D. & BLUM J.A. (1967) Experience with cutaneous vesicostomy for paraplegics and quadriplegics. *Arch. Physic. Med. & Rehab.*, **48**, 85–88.

ROSS J.C. (1960) *Handbuch der Urologie*, pp. 12, 80. Springer, Berlin.

ROSS J.C. & DAMANSKI M. (1953) Pudendal neurectomy in treatment of the bladder in spinal injury. *Brit. J. Urol.*, **25**, 45–50.

ROSS J.C., GIBBON N.O.K. & DAMANSKI M. (1958) Division of the external urethral sphincter in the treatment of the paraplegic bladder. *Brit. J. Urol.*, **30**, 204–212.

ROSS J.C., GIBBON N.O.K. & DAMANSKI M. (1963) Further experiences with division of the external urethral sphincter in the paraplegic. *J. Urol.*, **89**, 692–695.

ROSS J.C. (1966) Neuromuscular Dysfunction and Paraplegia, In *Handbuch der Urologie*, Vol. 12. pp. 58–111. Springer, Berlin.

ROSS J.C. (1967) Diversion of the urine in the neurogenic bladder. *Brit. J. Urol.*, **39**, 708–711.

ROSS J.A., J.A., EDMOND P. & GRIFFITHS J.M.T. (1967) The action of drugs on the intact human ureter. *Brit. J. Urol.*, **29**, 26–30.

ROSSIER A. & BORS E. (1962) Urological and neurological observations following anesthetic procedures for bladder rehabilitation of patients with spinal cord injuries. I. Topical anesthesias. *J. Urol.*, **87**. 876–882.

ROSSIER A. & BRUMER V. (1964) Zur initialen Behandlung der frischen Querschnittsläsion. *Schweiz. med. Wschr.*, **94**, 362–370.

ROSSIER A. & BORS E. (1965) Problems of the aged with spinal cord injuries. *Paraplegia*, **3**, 34–45.

ROTHFIELD S.H. & RABINER A.H. (1954) Vesical sphincter and nervous system. *N.Y. J. Med.*, **54**, 368–371.

ROUSSAU M., FREEDMAN H., BOYARSKI S., & ABRAMSON A.S. (1962) *Proc. 11th Clinical Spinal Injury Conf.* p. 122. Amer. Vet. Admin., Bronx.

RUCH T.C. & TANG P.C. (1967) The higher control of the bladder, In *Neurogenic Bladder* pp. 34–35. Boyarsky S. (ed.). Williams & Wilkins, Baltimore.

RUTISHAUSER G. (1962) Zur Pathogenese der Ureterkolik. *Helv. chir. Acta*, **29**, 461–465.

SCHEIBERT C.D. (1954) Sacral nerve interruption in paraplegia. *Proc. Third Ann. Clin. Paraplegia Conf.*, V.A. Hosp., Roxbury, 24–29.

SCHELLHAMMER P.F., HACKLER R.H. & BUNTS R.C. (1974) External sphincterotomy: rationale for the procedure and experiences with 150 patients. *Paraplegia*, **12**, 5.

SCOTT F.B., QUESEDA E.M., CARDUS D. & LASKOWSKI T. (1965) Electronic bladder stimulation: dog and human experiments. *Invest. Urol.*, **3**, 231–243.

SCRIBUTIS (1963) *Proc. Clin. Spinal Cord Conf.*, p. 96. V.A. Hosp., Hines, U.S.A.

SCRIBUTIS B., VALADKA, LLOYD F., POWERS L. & ROGERS W. (1962) *Proc. 11th Clinical Spinal Injury Conf.*, pp. 80–88. Amer. Vet. Admin., Bronx.

SELLER R.H. (1967) Pathogenesis of renal edema. In *Renal Failure*, Brest A.N. & Moyer J.H. (eds.). Pitman, London.

SEMANS J.H. (1949) Neurogenic disease of the bladder: the surgical management of its complications. *J. Urol.*, **62**, 820–832.

SEMANS J.H. (1961) Membranous urethroplasty: Indications and postoperative results 15 years later. *J. Urology*, **85**, 45–54.

SILVER J., MARTINDALE, J.H. & MOULTON A. (1970) The forgotten complication of paraplegia. *Paraplegia*, **8**, 128–141.

SILVER J.F. (1971) Vascular reflexes in spinal shock. *Paraplegia*, **8**, 231–242.

SKALOL S. & MORALES P. (1966) Ureteral activity in paraplegia. *J. Urol.*, **96**, 875–884.

SMITH R.D. (1966) Further observation on uretero-neocystostomy. *Brit. J. Urol.*, **38**, 432–434.

SMITH P.H., COOK J.B. & ROBERTSON R.G. (1969) Stone Formation in Paraplegia. *Paraplegia*, **7**, 2, 77–85.

STICKLER D.J., WILMOT C.B. & O'FLYNN J.D. (1971) The mode of development of urinary infection in intermittently catheterised male paraplegics. *Paraplegia*, **8**, 4, 243–252.

STÖHR JR (1926) Uber die Innervation der Harnblase und der Samenblase beim Menschen. Zugleich ein Beitrag über die Beziehung zwischen Nerv und glatter Muskulatur. *Z. Anat. Entw. Gesch.*, **78**, 556–584.

STOTT R.B., OGG C.S., CAMERON J.S. & BEWICK M. (1972) Management of acute renal failure. *Lancet*, ii, 75.

STRAUB L.R., RIPLEY H.S. & WOLFE S. (1949) Disturbances of bladder function associated with emotional states. *J. Amer. med Ass.*, **141**, 1139–1143.

SUBY H., SUBY R. & ALBRIGHT F. (1942) *J. Urol.*, **48**, 549.

SUSSET J.G., TAGUCHI Y., DEDOMENICO I. & MACKINNON K.J. (1966) Hydronephrosis and hydroureter in ileal conduit urinary diversion. *Canad. J. Surg.*, **9**, 141–145.

SUSSET J.G. (1966) *Med. Services J.*, Canada, **22**, 564–568.

SUSSET J.G., BOCTOR Z.N., ROSARIO F., RABINOVITCH H. & MACKINNON K.J. (1966) Implantable electrical vesical stimulator: review of the literature and report of a successful case. *Canada, ed. Ass. J.*, **95**, 1128–1131.

TALAAT M. (1937) Afferent impulses in the nerves supplying the urinary bladder. *J. Physiol.*, **89**, 1–13.

TALBOT H.S. & BUNTS R.C. (1949) Late renal changes in paraplegia: hydronephrosis due to vesicoureteral reflux. *J. Urol.*, **61**, 870–880.

TALBOT H.S. & BUNTS R.C. (1966) Renal disease and hypertension in paraplegics and tetraplegics. *Med. Services J., Canada*, **22**, 570–576.

TALBOT H.S. (1949) Renal disease and hypertension in paraplegics and tetraplegics. *Med. Services J. Canada*, **61**, 265.

TALBOT H.S. (1946) *Virginia. Med. Mon.*, **52**, 449.

TALBOT H.S. (1963) Management of neurogenic vesical dysfunction. *Bull. N.Y. Acad. Med.*, **39**, 71–89.

TALBOT H., EDWARD A., MAHONEY M., JARRETT J. & COBB O. (1967) *Paraplegia*, **5**, 97–103.

TANAGHO E.A. & PUGH R.C.B. (1963) The anatomy and function of the ureterovesical junction. *Brit. J. Urol.*, **35**, 151–165.

TANG P.C. & RUCH T.C. (1955) Non-neurogenic basis of bladder tone. *Amer. J. Physiol.*, **181**, 249–257.

TANG P.C. & RUCH T.C. (1956) Localization of brainstem and diencephalic areas controlling the micturition reflex. *J. comp. Neurol.*, **106**, 213–246.

TARABULCY E., MORALES P.A. & SULLIVAN F.A. (1967) Vesicoureteral reflux in paraplegia: Results of various forms of management. In *Proc. 16th clinical Spinal Cord. Injuries Conf.* V.A. Hosp., Long Beach, Calif.

THOMAS D.J. (1976) The effect of transurethral surgery on penile erections in spinal cord injured patients. *Paraplegia*, **14**, 286–289.

THOMPSON C.E. & WITHAM A.C. (1948) Paroxysmal hypertension in spinal cord injuries. *New Engl. J. Med.*, **239**, 291–294.

THOMPSON-WALKER J. (1937) *Proc. Roy. Soc. Med.*, **30**, 1233.

TOBIAN L. (1966) Physiological and clinical aspects of the juxtaglomerular apparatus and its role in hypertension. In: *Hormones and Hypertension.* Manger W.M. (ed.). Ch. Thomas, Springfield, Ill.

TRIBE C.R. (1963) Causes of death in early and late stages of paraplegia. *J. Paraplegia*, **1**, 19–47.

TRIBE C.R. & SILVER J.R. (1969) *Renal Failure in Paraplegia.* Pitman Medical, London.

TRUC E., LEVALLOIS, M., GRASSET D. & BADOSA J. (1962) Colo-cystoplastie pour véssie neurogène chex un paraplegique. A propos d'un nouveau cas. *J. Urol. Nephrol.*, **68**, 797–798.

TUCKER J.L., HANNA H., KAISER C.J. & DARROW D.C. (1963) Cardiac necrosis accompanying potassium deficiency and administration of corticosteroids. *Cir. Res.*, **13**, 420.

TULLOCH A.G.S. & ROSSIER A.B. (1975) The autonomic nervous system and the bladder during spinal shock—an experimental study. *Paraplegia*, **13**, 42.

UHLENHUTH E., HUNTER, DE WITT T. & LOECHEL W.E. (1953) *Problems in the anatomy of the pelvis. An atlas.* J.B.Lippincott, Philadelphia/London/Montreal.

URSILLO R.C. (1961) Electrical activity of the isolated nerve—urinary bladder strip preparation of the rabbit. *Amer. J. Physiol.*, **201**, 408–412.

VELLACOTT P. & WEBB JOHNSON A. (1919) *Lancet*, i, 733.

VERMET A., DUCKERT A. & MULLER A.F. (1956) Hypokalimie et oedème par dèperdition intestinale de potassium. *Helv. med. Acta*, **23**, 490.

VINCENT S.A. (1968) Electrical and mechanical means of achieving bladder control. *Proc. Roy. Soc. Med.*, **61**, 906.

VIVIAN J.M. & BORS E. (1974) Experience with intermittent catheterisation in the southwest regional system for treatment of spinal injury. *Paraplegia*, **12**, 158.

WALDEYER W. (1892) Über die sogenannte Ureterscheide. *Anat. Anz.*, **7**, 259–260.

WALSH J.J. (1967) Discussion. Proc. 1966 Scientific Meeting, Intern. Med. Soc. Paraplegia. *Paraplegia*, **4**, 232–234.

WALSH J.J. (1968) Results on intermittent catheterization. Paraplegia,**6**, 74.

WALSH J.J. (1970) Pyonephrosis in paraplegia. *Paraplegia*, **8**, 2, 121–127.

WALTZ W. (1922) Über die Blasensensibilität. *Dtsch. Z. Nervenheilk.*, **74**, 278–284.

WARD O. & RICHES E.W. (1944) *Surgery of Modern Warfare*, Hamilton Bailey (ed.). E. & S. Livingstone, Edinburgh.

WERTHEIMER P. & MICHON L. (1928) La névrotomy du nerf honteux interne Indication, technique, résultats. *J. Chir.*, **31**, 497–509.

WESSON M.B. (1920) Anatomical, embryological and physiological studies of the trigone and neck of the bladder. *J. Urol.*, **4**, 279–307.

WINTER C.C. (1966) Clinical application of an operation to correct vesico-ureteral reflux. *Amer.J Surg.*, **112**, 20–22.

WOODBURNE R.T. (1960) Structure and function of the urinary bladder. *J. Urol.*, **84**, 79–85.

WOODBURNE R.T. (1965) The ureter, ureterovesical junction and vesical trigone. *Anat. Rec.*, **151**, 243–249.

YATES-BELL J.G. (1949) Pituitrin therapy in hydronephrosis. *Proc. Roy. Soc. Med.*, **42**, 541–546.

YOUNG B.W. (1953) The retropubic approach to vesical neck obstruction in children. *Surg. Gyn. Obstet.*, **96**, 150–154.

YOUNG H.H. & WESSON M.B. (1921) The anatomy and surgery of the trigone. *Arch. Surg.*, **3**, 1–37.

YOUNG H.H. & DAVIS D.M. (1926) *Young's Practice of Urology*. Saunders, London.

Chapter 28   Disturbances of Intestinal Function

ATKINSON M., EDWARDS D.A., HONOUR A.J. & ROWLANDS D.N. (1957) *Lancet*, ii, 918.

BAYLISS W.M. & STARLING E.H. (1900) *J. Physiol.*, **26**, 107.

BEATTIE J. (1938) *Functional Aspects of the Hypothalamus*. Henderson Trust Lectures, Edinburgh.

BEATTIE J. & SHEEHAN D. (1934) The effect of hypothalamic stimulation on gastric motility. *J. Physiol.*, **81**, 218–227.

BORS E. & BLINN (1958) *Arch. Neurol. & Psychiat.*, **78**, 339–354.

CONNELL A.M. (1962) *Gut*, **3**, 342.

CONNELL A.M., FRANKEL H., GUTTMANN L. (1963) The motility of the pelvic colon following complete lesions of the spinal cord. *Paraplegia*, **1**, 98.

CONNELL A.M., HILTON C., IRVINE G., JONES J. & MISIEWICZ J. (1965) *Brit. Med. J.*, **2**, 1095.

CONNELL A.M. & ROWLANDS E.N. (1960) *Gut*, **1**, 266.

DAGRADI A.E. (1953) *Proc. Ann. Clin. Paraplegic Conf.*, p. 6. Amer. Vet. Admin. Hospital, Long Beach, Calif.

DENNY-BROWN D. & ROBERTSON E.G. (1935) *Brain*, **58**, 256.

FRANKEL H. (1967) Bowel training. *Paraplegia*, **4**, 254–256.

FULTON J. (1945) *Physiology of the nervous system*, p. 437. Oxford Med. Publications.

GARRY R.C. (1933) *J. Physiol.*, **78**, 208.

GOWERS W.R. (1899) *Manual of Diseases of the Nervous System I*, p. 246. London.

GUTTMANN L. (1954) *Peripheral Circulation in Man*, p. 192. Churchill, London.

GUTTMANN L. (1959) *The Regulation of Rectal Function in Spinal Paraplegia*. Proc. Royal Soc. Med. **52**, 86.

GUTTMANN L. & WHITTERIDGE (1947) *Brain*, **70**, 36.

HEAD H. & RIDDOCH G. (1917) *Brain*, **40**, 188.

HURST A.F. (1921) *Constipation and Allied Intestinal Disorders*. London.

LEARMONTH T.R. & RANKIN F.W. (1930) *Amer. Surg.*, **52**, 75.

LISTER J. (1858) see RUDOLF L.R. (1932) *Brit. J. Surg.*, **20**, 195.

MASIUS P. (1868) *Bull. Acad. R. Sci., Belge*, **1**, 491.

MELZAK J. & PORTER N.B. (1964) Studies on the reflex activity of the external sphincter ani in man. *Paraplegia*, **3**, 77–296.

MUNRO D. (1953) Control of bowel emptying. *New Engl. J. Med.*, **248**, 43.

NATHAN P.W. & SMITH M.C. (1953) Spinal pathways subserving defaecation and sensation from the lower bowel. *J. Neur.*, **16**, 245.

PAESLACK V. (1965) *Intermistische Störungen beim Paraplegiker*, p. 25. Thieme, Stuttgart.

PAESLACK V. (1967) Disorders of bowel functions in spinal lesions. *Paraplegia*, **4**, 254–256.

ROWLANDS E.N., HONOUR A.J., EDWARDS D.A. & CORBETT B.D. (1953) *Clin. Sc.*, **12**, 299.

Chapter 29   The Sexual Problem

ADAMS J. & ALEXANDER A. (1958) *Obstet. Gynec.*, **12**, 542.

ANDRES P. (1972) Sexual and genital prognosis in adult paraplegics. *Paraplegia*, **10**, 218.

BORS E. (1963) Sexual function in patients with spinal cord injuries. *Proc. Symp. Spinal Injuries*, pp. 62–70. Harris. P. (ed.). R. Coll., Surg., Edinburgh.

BORS E., ENGLE E., ROSENQUIST R. & HOLLIGER V. (1950) *J. Clin. Endocrinol.*, **10**, 381.

BORS E. & COMARR E. (1960) *Urol. Survey*, **10**, 191.

BURGES A., WATERMANE G. & CUTTS F. (1936) *Arch. int. Med.*, **58**, 433.

COMARR E. (1962) *Proc. 11th Spinal Cord Injury Conf.*, pp. 209, 211. Amer. Vet. Admin. Bronx Hosp.

COMARR E. (1966) Observations on menstruation and pregnancy among female spinal cord injury patients. *Paraplegia*, **3**, 263–272.

COOPER S. & HOEN T. (1949) *J. Neurosurg.*, **6**, 187.

DEYOE F.S. (1972) Marriage and family patterns with long-term spinal cord injury. *Paraplegia*, **10**, 219.

ESPERSEN T. & JORGENSEN J. (1947) *Acta med. scand.*, **127**, 494.

FOERSTER O. (1936) *Handbuch der Neurologie*, Vol. 5, p. 290. Springer, Berlin.

FRANKEL H.L., MATHIAS C.J. & WALSH J.J. (1974) Blood pressure, plasma catecholamines and prostaglandins during artificial erection in a male tetraplegic. *Paraplegia*, **12**, 205.

GERSTMANN J. (1926) *Mschr. Geburtsh. Gynäk.*, **83**, 253.

GÖLLER H. & PAESLACK V. (1970) Our experience about pregnancy and delivery of paraplegic woman. *Paraplegia*, **8**, 161–170.

GÖLLER H. & PAESLACK V. (1972) Pregnancy damage and birth-complications in the children of paraplegic women. *Paraplegia*, **10**, 213.

GOLMAN S.J. (1975) Medicine and the law. *Paraplegia*, **12**, 237.

GOLTZ F. & EWALD J. (1896) Der Hund mit verkürztem Rückenmarks. *Pflüg. Arch. ges. Physiol.*, **63**, 362–400.

GUTTMANN L. (1937) *Klin. Wschr.*, **25**, 1212–1214.

GUTTMANN L. (1947) *Postgrad. med.*, **23**, 353.

GUTTMANN L. (1953) Sexual disturbances. In *Brit. Med. History of World War II*, Vol. Surgery, pp. 482–486. H.M. Stationery Office, London.

GUTTMANN L. (1954) *Ciba Foundation Symp. on Peripheral Circulation in Man*, pp. 192–203. Churchill, London.

GUTTMANN L. (1956) Victory over paraplegia. In *Conquest of Disability*. pp. 56, 383. Sir Ian Fraser, (ed.). Odhams, London.

GUTTMANN L. (1961) The sexual problem in spinal paraplegia. *Proc. Scient. Meeting, Inter. Stoke Mandeville Games*, Rome, pp. 63–60.

GUTTMANN L. (1963) The paraplegic patient in pregnancy and labour. *Proc. Roy. Soc. Med.* **56**, 383.

GUTTMANN L. (1964) The married life of paraplegics and tetraplegics. *Paraplegia*, **2**, 182–188.

GUTTMANN L. (1969) *Handbook of Clin. Neurology*, Vol. 2, Part 1, pp. 196–198, Vinken & Bruyn (eds.). North-Holland Publ. Co., Amsterdam.

GUTTMANN L. & WHITTERIDGE D. (1947) *Brain*, **70**, 361.

GUTTMANN L., FRANKEL H., & PAESLACK, V. (1965) Cardiac irregularities during labour in paraplegic women. *Paraplegia*, **3**, 144–151.

GUTTMANN L. & WALSH J.J. (1971) Prostigmin assessment test of fertility in spinal man. *Paraplegia*, **9**, 40–51.

HARDY A. & WARRELL (1965) Pregnancy and labour in complete tetraplegia. *Paraplegia*, **3**, 182–186.

HARVEY C. & JACKSON M.H. (1945) Assessment of male fertility by semen analysis. *Lancet*, 28 July and 5 Aug., 1–11.

HEAD H. (1898) *Die Sensibilitätsstörungen der Haut bei Visceralarkrankungen* (German Transl. by W.Seiffer). Hirschwald, Berlin.

HEGLIN R. & HOLZMANN M. (1937) *Dtsch. Arch. of Klin. Med.*, **180**, 681.

HORNE H.W., PAUL D.A. & MUNRO D. (1948) *New Engl. J. Med.*, **239**, 959.

HUTCHINSON H.T. & VASICKA A. (1962) *Obstet. Gynec.*, **20**, 675.

JACKSON R.W. (1972) Sexual Rehabilitation after Cord Injury. *Paraplegia*, **10**, 50.

JUNG H. & SCHMIDT K. (1962) *Zentralbl. f. Gynäkol.*, **84**, 1105.

KREMER M. (1942) Action of intrathecally injected prostigmine, acetylcholine and esarine on the central nervous system in man. *Quart. J. exp. Physiol.*, **31**, 337.

KUHN B.H. (1950) *Brain*, **73**, 1.

MORTELL E. & WHITTLE J. (1945) *J. clin. Endocrin.*, **5**, 396.

RAAB W. (1953) *Wien. Zschr. f. inn. Med.*, **31**, 241.

REUBEN (Quoted by Jackson, 1972)

ROBERTSON STR. (1963) The paraplegic patient in pregnancy and labour. *Proc. Roy. Soc. Med.*, **56**, 380.

ROBERTSON D.N.S. (1972) Pregnancy and labour in the paraplegic. *Paraplegia*, **10**, 209.

ROSSIER A., RUFFREUX M. & ZIEGLER W. (1969) Pregnancy and labour in high traumatic spinal cord lesions. *Paraplegia*, **7**, 210–215.

ROSSIER A., ZIEGLER W., DUCHOSAL A. & MAYLAN J. (1971) Sexual function and dysreflexia. *Paraplegia*, **9**, 51–58.

SPIRA R. (1956) Artificial insemination after intrathecal injection of neostigmine in a paraplegic. *Lancet*, i, 670.

TALBOT H.S. (1949) A report on sexual function in paraplegics. *J. Urol.*, **61**, 265.

TALBOT H.S. (1955) The sexual function in paraplegics. *J. Urol.*, **3**, 91.

TALBOT H.S. (1971) Psycho-social aspects of sexuality in spinal cord injury patients. *Paraplegia*, **9**, 37.

TARABULCY E. (1972) Sexual function in the normal and in paraplegia. *Paraplegia*, **10**, 201.

THOMPSON C. & WITHAM A. (1948) *New Engl. Med. J.*, **239**, 291.

WARE H.H. (1934) *J. Amer. med. Ass.*, **102**, 133.

ZEITLIN A.B., COTTRELL T. & LLOYD F. (1957) *Fertility and Sterility*, **8**, 337.

Chapter 30 Psychological Aspects

BOSHES B. (1963) Traumatic paralysis: diagnosis and non-surgical treatment. *Med. Clin. N. Amer.*, **47**, 1629–1645.

FORDYCE W.E. (1965) Personality characteristics in men with spinal cord injury as related to manner of disability. *Arch. Phys. Med.*, **45**, 321.

GUNTHER M.S. (1969) Emotional aspects. In *Spinal Cord Injuries*. Ruge R. (ed.). Ch.Thomas, Springfield, Ill.

GUTTMANN L. (1945) New hope for spinal cord sufferers. *N.Y. Med. Times*, **73**, 318.

GUTTMANN L. (1953) *Brit. Med. History of World War II*, Vol. Surgery, pp. 496–499.

KENNEDY R.H. (1946) *Am. Surg.*, **124**, 1057.

LABHARDT F. (1962) Psychosomatic problems in paraplegics. *Psychiat. Univ. Lin. Basel Ther. Umsch.*, **19**, 259.

MICHAELIS J.J. (1950) *J. Amer. med. Ass.*, **7**, 33, 39.

MUELLER A.D. (1962) Psychologic factors in rehabilitation of paraplegic patients. *Arch. Phys. Med.*, **43**, 151.

NAGLER B. (1950) *Amer. J. Psychiat.*, **107**, 49.

POER D.H. (1945) *J. Amer. med. Ass.*, **129**, 162.

WEISS F. & BORS E. (1948) *J. Social Case Work*, **29**, 60.

Chapter 31   Care of the Skin—Pressure Sores

ARREGUI J., CANNON B., MURRAY J. & O'LEARY J. (1965) *Plast. reconstr. Surg.*, **36**, 583.

BAILEY B.N. (1967) *Bedsores*. E.Arnold, London.

BARKER D.E. (1945) *J. Amer. med. Ass.*, **129**, 160.

BARKER D.E. (1946) *Ann. Surg.*, **123**, 523.

BLOCKSMA R., KOSTRUBALA J. & GREELEY P. (1947) *Plast. reconstr. Surg.*, **4**, 123.

BORS E. & COMARR E. (1948) *Surg. Gynec. Obstet.*, **87**, 68.

BROWN-SÉQUARD E. (1953) *Experimental Researches Applied to Physiology and Pathology*. Bailliére, New York.

CARREL A., HARTMANN R. & LECOMTE DU NONY (1918) *J. exp. Med.*, **27**.

CHARCOT J.M. (1879) *Lectures on the Diseases of the Nervous System*. H.C.Lea, Philadelphia.

CHASE R. & WHITE W. (1959) *Plast. reconstr. Surg.*, **24**, 445.

COMARR E. (1951) Radical ischialectomy in decubitus ischial ulcers complicating paraplegia. *Ann. West. Med. & Surg.*, **5**, 210.

COMARR E. (1964) An interesting decubitus ulcer closure. *Paraplegia*, **3**, 271–276.

CONWAY H., KRAISSL C., CLIFFORD R., GELB J., JOSEPH J. & LEVERIDGE L. (1947) *Surg. Gyn. Obstet.*, 321–332.

CONWAY H. & GRIFFITH B.H. (1956) *Amer. J. Surg.*, **91**, 946–975.

DAVENPORT L.F. (1962) The use of enzymes in the treatment of chronic ulcers. *Proc. 11th Clin. Spinal Cord Injury Conf.*, pp. 220–222. Am. Veter. Admin.,

DICK T. (1949) M.D. Thesis, Univ. Manchester.

EXTON-SMITH A.N. & SHERWIN R.W. (1961) *Lancet*, ii, 1124–1126.

FANTUS B. (1935) Therapy of bedsores. *J. Amer. Med. Ass.*, **104**, 46.

GALLAGHER J.P. & GESCHICHTER C.P. (1964) *J. Amer. Med. Ass.*, **189**, 928–933.

GIBBON J.H. & FREEMAN L.W. (1946) The primary closure of decubitus ulcers. *Ann. Surg.*, **124**, 1148.

GILLIS L. & LEE S.T. (1951) Cancer as a sequel to war wounds. *J. Bone & Joint Surg.*, **33B**, 167–179.

GRIFFITH B.H. (1969) Pressure sores. In *Spinal Cord Injuries*, pp. 125–143. Ruge D. (ed.). Ch. Thomas, Springfield, Ill.

GUTTMANN L. (1945) *Med. Times, N.Y.*, **73**, 318.

GUTTMANN L. (1946) *Brit. J. Phys. Med.*, **9**, 130 and 160.

GUTTMANN L. (1949) Management of paralysis. In *Brit. Surg. Practice*, Vol. 6, p. 445. Butterworth, London.

GUTTMANN L. (1953) *Brit. History of World War II*, Vol. Surgery, pp. 486–496. H.M. Stationery Office, London,

GUTTMANN L. (1955) The problem of treatment of pressure sores in spinal paraplegia. *Brit. J. Plast. Surg.*, **7**, 196–213.

GUTTMANN L. (1957) The problems of Spina Bifida Cystica. *Roy. Soc. Med.*, **50**, 742.

GUTTMANN L. (1961) *Langenbeck's Arch. Klin. Surg.*, **298**, 187.

GUTTMANN L. (1970) *Paraplegia*, **8**, 185.

KERMANI R., SIDDIQUI M., LAIN S. & KAZI Z. (1970) Biochemical studies on pressure sore-healing in paraplegia. *Paraplegia*, **8**, 36–41.

LATIMER E.O. (1934) Treatment of decubitus with tannic acid. *J. Amer. Med. Ass.*, **102**, 751.

LINDENBERG W. (1953) *Nervenarzt*, **24**, 127.

MUNRO D. (1945) *New Engl. J. Med.*, **233**, 453.

MUNRO D. (1952) *The Treatment of Injuries to the Nervous System*, p. 72. Saunders, Philadelphia.

NISSEN C. (1941) *Proc. Roy. Soc. Med.*, **34**, 457.

NUSEIBEH I.M. (1974) Split skin graft and the treatment of pressure sores. *Paraplegia*, **12**, 1.

ODEN P.H. (1967) *Gold Leaf Occlusive Therapy on the Management of Decubitus Ulcers*, pp. 72–74.

OSBORNE R. (1955) *Brit. J. Plast. Surg.*, **8**, 214.

PAGET J. (1873) Clinical lecture on bed sores. *Students J. Hosp. Gazette, London*, **1**, 144–146.

POER (1946) *Amer. Surg.*, **123**, 510.

RIDDOCH G. (1917) *Brain*, **40**, 264.

STOOP J.W. (1970) Treatment of pressure sores in paraplegic patients with animal collagen. *Paraplegia*, **8**, 177–181.

STREET D.M. (1958) *Proc. 7th Clin. Parapl. Conf.*, Am. Vet. Admin. p. 9.

TRUMBLE H.C. (1930) The skin tolerance for pressure and pressure sores. *Austr. med. J.*, **2**, 724.

URSU G. (1970) Bed sores treated with negative air-ions. *Paraplegia*, **8**, 182–185.

WANKE M. & GRÖZINGER K.H. (1965) *Klin. Wschr.*, **43**, 975.

Chapter 32   Clinical Management of Spasticity

AIRD R. & SEIFERT J. (1952) *J. nerv. ment. dis.*, **116**, 912.

APOLINARIO E., DOMINELLI J.C., FERNANDEX M. & SOTELANO F. (1966) Follow-up of a series of phenol spinal blocks. *Paraplegia*, **4**, 162.

BERGER F.M. & BRADLEY W. (1946) Mode of action of Myanasin. *Brit. J. Pharmacol.*, **1**, 265.

CAIN H.D. (1965) Subarachnoid block in the treatment of pain and spasticity. *Paraplegia*, **3**, 152–160.

CARTER C.H. (1959) Trancopal. *I. Florida M.A. XLVI*, 709–712.

CORBETT M., FRANKEL H.L. & MICHAELIS L. (1972) *Paraplegia*, **10**, 19.

DEJAK J.I. & LOWRY R. (1956) *Proc. 13th Ann. Clin. Conf. Spinal Cord Injury Conf.*, p. 78. Amer. Vet. Admin.

DICK T.S. (1949) Rehabilitation in chronic paraplegia. M.D. Thesis, Manchester University.

EGGLETON G. (1942) *J. Physiol.*, **101**, 72.

ELKINS C.W. & WEGNER W.R. (1946) *Am. Surg.*, **123**, 516.

FOERSTER O. (1911) Resection of posterior spinal nerve-roots in the treatment of gastric crises and spastic paralysis. *Proc. Roy. Soc. Med.*, **4**, 226–246.

FREEMAN L.W. & HEIMBURGER R.F. (1947) The surgical relief of spasticity in paraplegic patients. I. Anterior rhyzotomy. *J. Neurosurg.*, **4**, 435–443.

FREEMAN L.W. & HEIMBURGER R.F. (1948) The surgical relief of spasticity in paraplegic patients. II. Peripheral nerve section, posterior rhyzotomy and other procedures. *J. Neurosurg.*, **5**, 556–561.

GANZ S.E. (1959) Clinical evaluation of a new muscle relaxant (Chlormethazonone). *J. Indiana State Med. Ass.*, **52**, 1134.

GINGRAS G. (1948) Intrathecal alcohol block. *Treat. Serv. Bull. Dept. Vet. Canada*, **3**, 56.

GLASS A. & HANNAH A. (1974) A comparison of dantrolene sodium and diazepam in the treatment of spasticity. *Paraplegia*, **12**, 170.

GRIFFITH B.H. (1969) Spasticity. In *Spinal Cord Injuries*, p. 150. Ruge D. (ed.). Springfield, Ill., Ch. Thomas.

GUTTMANN L. (1929) Störungen der Liquorzirkulation and Liquorresorption bei Psychosen. *Deutsche Zeitschr. Nervenhlk*, **111**, 159.

GUTTMANN L. (1931) Posterior rhyzotomy in spasticity and cordotomy (in discussion to Foerster on cordotomy). *Med. Klinik*, **37**, 1–2.

GUTTMANN L. (1946) Intrathecal alcohol block in intractable spasticity. *Proc. Roy. Soc. Med.*, **42**, 546.

GUTTMANN L. (1949) The principles of physiotherapy in the treatment of spinal paraplegia. *Physiotherapy*, October 1949, 1–8.

GUTTMANN L. (1953) The treatment and rehabilitation of patients with injuries to the spinal cord and cauda equina. *Brit. med. History of World War II*, Vol. Surgery, pp. 452–458.

GUTTMANN L. & ROBINSON R. (1956) The absorption of ethyl alcohol following intrathecal injection in spinal paraplegia. *Proc. 2nd intern. cong. neuropathology*, London, pp. 579–583. Excerpta Med. Found., Amsterdam.

KATZENELBOGEN S. (1935) The cerebrospinal fluid and its relation to the blood. p. 73. John Hopkins Press, Baltimore, U.S.A.

KELLY R.E. & GAUTIER-SMITH P.C. (1959) Intrathecal phenol in the treatment of reflex spasm and spasticity. *Lancet*, ii, 1102–1105.

KERR W.G. (1966) The use of Diazopem (Valium) in the relief of spasticity. *Paraplegia*, 4, 149–152. Discussion by Maglio, Ungar, Pool, Weiss, Michaelis, Cibeira, Jousse, Frankel, Guttmann, Walsh & McSweeney, pp. 152–154.

KERR SUTCLIFFE, A. (1966) Anterior rhyzotomy for the relief of spasticity. *Paraplegia*, 4, 154–160.

KENNEDY R.H. (1946) *Ann. Surg.*, **124**, 1057.

KREMER M. (1942) Action of intrathecally injected prostigmine, acetylcholine and eserine on the central nervous system in man. *Quart. J. Exper. Physiol.*, **31**, 33.

KHALILI A.A. & BETTS H.B. (1967) Peripheral nerve block with phenol in the management of spasticity. In *Spinal Cord Injuries*. Ruge D. (ed.). Ch.Thomas. Springfield, Ill.

LACOMBE M., AUDIC B. & MAURY M. (1966) Motor point injections with diluted alcohol and intrathecal injections through the vertebral foramine with absolute alcohol. *Paraplegia*, 4, 165.

LEE W.J., McGOVERN J.P. & DUVALL E.N. (1950) *Arch. Physical Med.*, **31**, 366–771.

LEVINE I.M. (1961) Muscle relaxants in neurospastic diseases. *Med. Clin. North America*, **45**, 1017–1026.

LIVERSIDGE L.A. & MAHER R.M. (1960) Use of phenol in relief of spasticity. *Brit. med. J.*, **2**, 31–33.

MACDONALD J.B., McKENZIE K.G. & BOTTERELL E.H. (1946) *J. Neurosurg.*, **3**, 421.

MacCARTHY C.S. (1954) The treatment of spastic paraplegia by selective spinal cordectomy. *J. Neurosurg.*, **11**, 539–545.

MAHER R.M. (1955) *J. Amer. med. Ass.*, **129**, 153.

MALTBY G. (1945) *J. Amer. med. Ass.*, **129**, 153.

MARTIN J. & DAVIS L. (1948) Studies upon spinal cord injuries. Altered reflex activity. *Surg. Gynec. Obstet.*, **86**, 535–542.

MAYFIELD F. (1945) *J. Amer. med. Ass.*, **129**, 153.

MEIROWSKI M., SCHEIBERT C. & HINCHLEY T. (1948) *J. Neurosurg.*, **5**, 154.

MICHAELIS L. (1965) *Orthopaedic Surgery of the Limbs in Paraplegia*, pp. 8–12. Springer, Berlin.

NATHAN P.W. (1959) Intrathecal phenol to relieve spasticity in paraplegia. *Lancet*, ii, 1099–1102.

NATHAN P.W. & SEARS T.A. (1962) Effect of phenol in nervous conduction. *J. Physiol.*, **150**, 565–580.

NATHAN P.W. (1970) *J. Neurol. Ser.*, **10**, 33.

NEILL R.W. (1965) *Proc. 13th Ann Clin.. Conf. Spinal Cord Injury Conf.* p. 30. Amer. Vet. Admin.

O'HARE J.M. (1962) The use of phenol blocks for spasm. *Proc. 11th Clin. Spinal Cord Injury Conf.* Amer. Vet. Admin. pp. 215–216.

O'ROURKE F.I., GERSHON S., TRANTNER E.M. & SHAW F.H. (1960) The use of Tigloidine in the treatment of spastic paraplegia. *Med. J. Aust.*, **1**, 73.

RIDDOCH G. (1917b) The reflex function of the completely divided spinal cord in man, compared with those associated with less severe lesions. *Brain*, **40**, 264–402.

SAVITZ, M.H. & MALIS L.I. (1973) Intractable pain treated with intrathecal isotonic iced saline. *J. Neurol., Neurosurg., Psychiatr.*, **36**, 417.

SCHLESINGER E.B. (1946) Curare: Review of its therapeutic effects and their physiological basis. *Am. J. Med.*, **1**, 518–530.

SELIG R.C. (1914) *Arch. Clin. Chir.*, **103**, 994.

SHELDON C.H. & BORS E. (1948) Subarachnoid alcohol block in paraplegia. *J. Neurosurg.*, **5**, 389–391.

VOGEL M., WEINSTEIN L. & ABRAMSON A.S. (1955) Use of tetanizing current for Spasticity. *Physical Ther. Review*, **35**, 435–437.

WEISS A.A., D'OROUZIO G., EBEL A. & LINDENAUER (1956) *Proc. Clin. Conf. Paraplegia*, pp. 53–64. Vet. Admin. Hosp. Hines, Ill.

WEISS M., RUDNICKI S., HAFTEK J. & WIRSKI J. (1966) Phenolisation of spinal roots and peripheral nerves in spastic paralysis. *Paraplegia*, **4**, 165.

WILSON L.A. & McKECHNIE A.A. (1966) *Scot. med. J.*, **11**, 46.

Chapter 33 Surgical Reconstruction of the Tetraplegic Hand

BEDBROOK G. (1969) Discussion to Freehafer. *Paraplegia*, **7**, 130.

FOWLER B. (1959) Surgery of the paralytic hand. *Am. Acad. of Orth. Surg.*, St Louis, Mosby, **16**, 85–87.

FREEHAFER A.A. & MAST W.A. (1967) Transfer of the brachiaradialis to improve wrist extension in high spinal cord injury. *J. Bone & Joint Surg.*, **49A**, 648.

FREEHAFER A.A. (1969) Care of the hand in cervical spinal cord injuries. *Paraplegia*, **7**, 118–129.

GARRETT A.L., PERRY J. & NICKEL V.L. (1964) Traumatic paraplegia. *J. Amer. med. Ass.*, **187**, 7.

GUTTMANN SIR L. (1969) Discussion to Freehafer. *Paraplegia*, **7**, 130.

LAMB D.W. (1963) The management of the upper limbs in cervical cord injuries. *Proc. Symp. on Spinol Injuries*, pp. 120–127. Harris E.D. (ed.). Roy. Coll. Surg., Edinburgh.

LAMB D.W. & LANDRY R.M. (1972) The hand in quadriplegia. *Paraplegia*, **9**, 204–212.

LIPSCOMB P.R., ELKINS E.C. & HENDERSON E.D. (1958) Tendon transfers to restore function of hands in tetraplegia, especially after fracture dislocation of the 6th cervical vertebra on the 7th. *J. Bone & Joint Surg.*, **40A**, 1071.

McSWEENEY T. (1969) Discussion to Freehafer. *Paraplegia*, **7**, 129.

NAPIER J.R. (1956) The prehensile movements of the human hand. *J. Bone & Joint Surg.*, **38B**, 902–913.

RIORDAN D. (1959) Surgery of the paralytic hand. *Am. Acad. of Orth. Surg.*, St Louis, Mosby, **16**, 79–90.

SARRAFIAN S.K. (1959) Surgical reconstruction of the hand in spinal cord injuries, pp. 189–201, Ruge D. (ed.).

STREET D. (1958) *Proc. of 7th Ann. Clinical Paraplegia Conf.* Amer. Vet. Admin., p. 81.

THOMPSON T.C. (1942) Modified operation of opponents' paralysis. *J. Bone & Joint Surg.*, **24**, 632.

WILSON J.N. (1956) Providing automatic grasp by flexor tenosesis. *J. Bone & Joint Surg.*, **38A**, 1019.

ZANCOLLI E.A. (1942) Claw-hand caused by paralysis of the intrinsic muscles. A simple surgical procedure for this correction. *J. Bone & Joint Surg.*, **24**, 632.

Chapters 34–35 Principles and Techniques of Physiotherapy

ALTENBURGER H. & GUTTMANN L. (1928) Chronaxie und Aktionsstrombild bei Ermüdung durch Willkürkontraktion. *Z. Neur.*, **115**, 1–12.

BELL D. (1954a) Some aspects in the physical rehabilitation and training of paraplegic children. *Proc. 6th World Compr. Itern. Soc. for the Welfare of Cripples,* pp. 186–190.

BELL D. (1954b) Principles and technique in the treatment of spinal paraplegia. *Physiotherapy,* **40,** 84.

CHOR H., CLEVELAND D., DAVENPART H., DOLCART R. & BEARD G. (1939) *J. Amer. med. Ass.,* **113,** 1029.

DAID C.W. (1951) *Calif. Med.,* **35,** 217–218.

DENLY O. (1964) The user's viewpoint. *Paraplegia,* **2,** 42–48.

DOUPE J., BARNES R. & KERR A.S. (1943) *J. Neurol., Psychiat.,* **6,** 136.

FISCHER E. (1939) *Amer. J. Physiol.,* **127,** 605.

FLOYD W., GUTTMANN L., PARKER K. & WARD J. (1966) A study on the space requirement of wheelchair users. *Paraplegia,* **3,** 24.

FRENKEL-HEYDEN S. (1900) *Die Behandlung der tabischen Ataxie mit Holf der Übung.* Leipzig.

GUTHRIE-SMITH O.F. (1943) *Rehabilitation Exercises.* Baillière, Tindall & Cox, London.

GUTMANN E. & GUTTMANN L. (1942) The effect of electrotherapy on denervated muscles in rabbits. *Lancet,* i, 169.

GUTMANN E. & GUTTMANN L. (1944) The effect of galvanic exercise on denervated and re-innervated muscles. *J. Neurol. Neurosurg.,* **7,** 7.

GUTTMANN L. (1946) Rehabilitation after injury to the spinal cord and cauda equina. *Brit. J. Physical Med.,* **9,** 130–160.

GUTTMANN L. (1948) Readjustment to a new life (II—Physical aspects). *The Cord,* II, **1,** 55.

GUTTMANN L. (1949a) Principles of Physiotherapy in the treatment of spinal paraplegia. *Physiotherapy,* **35,** 157.

GUTTMANN L. (1949b) Readjustment to a new life (II—Physical aspects). *The Cord* II, **2,** 21.

GUTTMANN L. (1950) Rehabilitation after injuries to the spinal cord and cauda equina. In *Rehabilitation,* Guthrie-Smith (ed.). Tindell, Cox & Baillière, London.

GUTTMANN L. (1951) Problems of physiotherapy in poliomyelitis (Editoria). *Brit. J. Physical Med.,* **14,** 73.

GUTTMANN L. (1952) Principles of rehabilitation in disseminated sclerosis. *Brit. J. Physical Med.,* **189,** 15, 8.

GUTTMANN L. (1953) Physiotherapy. In: *Brit. History of World War II,* Vol. Surgery. H.M. Stationery Office, London,

GUTTMANN L. (1954) A symposium on the wheelchair. *Paraplegia,* **2,** 64–67, 68 and 69.

GUTTMANN L. (1960) The management of the spinal paraplegic child. *J. Mother and Child,* Vol. August, 3–7.

GUTTMANN L.A. Symposium on the wheelchair (1964) *Paraplegia* **2,** 64–69.

GUTTMANN L. (1967) Water therapy and water sport for the physically handicapped with special reference to the paralysed. *J. Institute of Bath Management.* Proc. 37th Ann. Conf., Blackpool, 128–140.

GUTTMANN L. & MALING R.C. (1965) Demonstration of a special electric control for a power-driven wheelchair for high spinal cord lesions. *Paraplegia,* **3,** 197.

HINES H.M. (1942) *J. Am. med. Ass.,* **120,** 527.

HINES H., THOMSON J. & LAZERE B. (1942) *Amer. J. Physiol.,* **100,** 407.

HOBSON E.P.G. (1956) *Physiotherapy in paraplegia,* pp. 1–110. Churchill, London.

HUCKSTEP R.L. (1968) Bracing the paraplegic. *Proc. 4th Pan-Pacific Rehab. Conf., Hong Kong,* pp. 276–277. Int. Soc. for Rehabilitation of the Disabled.

HUNT S.S.M. & HUCKSTEP R.L. (1967) Wheelchairs for developing countries. *E. Afr. med. J.,* **44,** 377.

JACKSON SH. (1945) The role of galvanism in the treatment of denervated voluntary muscles in man. *Brain,* **68,** 300–330.

JOLLY D.W. (1964) Ministry practice. *Paraplegia,* **2,** 20–24.

LANGLEY J.N. & KATO T. (1915) *J. Physiol.,* **49,** 432.

LANGLEY J.N. & KATO T. (1915) *J. Physiol.*, **50**, 335.

MOLANDER C., STEINITZ F., & ASHER R. (1941) *Arch. phys. Ther.*, **21**, 154.

POOL G.M. & WEERDEN G.J.v. (1973) Experiences with frog breathing tetraplegic polio victims as telephone operators. *Paraplegia*, **11**, 253.

REID J. (1841) Edinburgh Month. *J. Med. Science*, May.

SOLANDT D.Y. & MAGLADERY J.W. (1940) *Brain*, **63**, 255.

TOWER S. (1939) The reaction of muscle to denervation. *Physiol. Rev.*, **19**, 1–48.

WALKER J. (1964) Factors influencing the specification of wheelchairs supplied by the Ministry of Health for the Domestic use of invalids. *Paraplegia*, **2**, 25–30.

WALSH J.J. (1964) Wheelchairs for paraplegics. *Paraplegia*, **2**, 30–34.

Chapter 36   Sport

BLEASDALE N. (1975) Swimming and the paraplegic. *Paraplegia*, **13**, 124.

FRANKEL H. (1975) Aqualung diving for the paralysed. *Paraplegia*, **13**, 128.

GUTTMANN L. (1945) New hope for spinal cord sufferers. *New York Med. Times*, **73**, 318.

GUTTMANN L. (1949a) Readjustment to a new life. *The Cord*, **2**, 21.

GUTTMANN L. (1949b) *The Cord*, **3**, 24.

GUTTMANN L. (1952) On the way to an international sports movement for the paralysed. *The Cord*, **5**.

GUTTMANN L. (1953) *Br. Medical History of World War II*, Vol. Surgery, pp. 505–506. H.M. Stationery Office.

GUTTMANN L. (1954) De paralyserades olympaid. *Varlshorisont, Goteburg*, **2**, 3–6.

GUTTMANN L. (1957) The significance of sport in the rehabilitation of the disabled. *Proc. 7th World Conf. I.S.W.C., London*, pp. 295–299.

GUTTMANN L. (1960) The international Stoke Mandeville games in Rome. *The Cord*.

GUTTMANN L. (1962a) Sport and the disabled. In *Sports Medicine*, pp. 367–391. Arnold, London.

GUTTMANN L. (1962b) The first 10 years of the international Stoke Mandeville games for the paralysed. *The Cord*, **14**, 30–39.

GUTTMANN L. (1964) The international Stoke Mandeville games for the paralysed in Tokyo. *Physiotherapy*.

GUTTMANN L. (1965) Reflections in sport for the physically handicapped. *Physiotherapy*.

GUTTMANN L. (1967a) The Stoke Mandeville games *Abbotempo Univ. Ltc.*, **3**, 2.

GUTTMANN L. (1967b) Sport for the disabled as a world problem. Proc. Intern. Seminar, Brit. Council for Rehabilitation, Brighton. *Rehabilitation*.

GUTTMANN L. (1973) Sport and Recreation for the Mentally and Physically Handicapped. pp. 1–6. Conference on Sport for All. *Royal Soc. of Health*, London.

HÜLLEMANN K.D., LIST M., MATTHES D., WIESE G. & ZIKA D. (1975) Spiroergometric and telemetric investigations during the XXI International Stoke Mandeville Games 1972 in Heidelberg. *Paraplegia*, **13**, 109.

Chapters 37–38   Recreational Activities—Occupational Therapy—Rehabilitation by Work

DAMANSKI M. (1964) The paraplegic patient as a social problem. *Paraplegia*, **2**, 169–177.

GUTTMANN L. (1946) Rehabilitation after injury to the spinal cord and cauda equina. *Brit. J. Phys. Med.*, **9**, 130 and 162.

GUTTMANN L. (1949a) Annual Stoke Mandeville games. *The Cord*, **3**, 24.

GUTTMAN L. (1949b) Readjustment to a new life. (Resettlement aspects.) *The Cord* II, **4**, 18–23.

GUTTMANN L. (1953) *Brit. Med. History of World War II*, Vol. Surgery, pp 506–513. H.M. Stationery Office, London.

GUTTMANN L. (1959) The place of our spinal-paraplegic fellowmen in society. Second Dame Georgina Buller Memorial Lecture. *Rehabilitation J.*, **30**, 15–27.

GUTTMANN L. (1963) The rehabilitation of the traumatic paraplegic by work and sport. *Proc. 14th Internat. Congr. of Occupational Health, Madrid*, pp. 1–15. Excerpta Medica Foundat.

GUTTMANN L. (1965) Services for the treatment and rehabilitation of spinal paraplegics in Great Britain. In *Trends in Social Welfare*, pp. 319–336. Pergamon Press.

GUTTMANN L. (1968) New talents for the community. *Proc. 4th Pan-Pacific Conf., Hong Kong*, pp. 7–12. Int. Soc. for Rehabilitation of the Disabled.

HARDY A. (1964) Resettlement problems of paraplegic coal-miners. *Paraplegia*, **2**, 157–163.

MAURY M. (1964) The future of paraplegics. *Paraplegia*, **2**, 156–157.

MEINE E. (1970) On after-care of paraplegic patients in their home. *Paraplegia*, **8**, 154–157.

MEINECKE F.W. (1964) Social aspects of paraplegic coalminers in Germany. *Paraplegia*, **2**, 163–169.

SCRUTON J. (1954) Resettlement problems in the rehabilitation of spinal paraplegics. *Proc. 6th World Congr. Intern. Soc. for the care of cripples*, pp. 194–199, The Hague.

THOMPSON M. & MURRAY W. (1967) *Paraplegia at Home*, pp. 1–43. E. Livingstone, Edinburgh.

TRICOT A. (1964) Special housing for paraplegics. *Paraplegia*, **2**, 178–182.

G. GENERAL STATISTICS AND LEGAL ASPECTS

Chapters 39–41

COLMAN S.J. (1975) Medicine and the law. *Paraplegia*, **12**, 237.

GUTTMANN L. (1953) The treatment and rehabilitation of patients with injuries of the spinal cord. Monograph in *Brit. Medical History of World War II*, Vol. Surgery, pp 425–427.

GUTTMANN L. (1962) The National Spinal Injuries Centre, Stoke Mandeville Hospital. *Monthly Bull. of Min. of Health and Publ. Health Labor. Service* **21**, 60–71.

GUTTMANN L. (1965) Services for the treatment and rehabilitation of spinal paraplegics and tetraplegics in Great Britain. In *Trends in Social Services*, pp. 319–336, Farndale W. (ed.). Pergamon Press, London.

GUTTMANN L. (1967) History of the national spinal injuries centre, Stoke Mandeville Hospital, Aylesbury. *Paraplegia*, **5**, 115–125.

INDEX